The Practice of
Cardiac Anesthesia

The Practice of Cardiac Anesthesia

Edited by

Frederick A. Hensley, Jr., M.D.
Associate Professor of Anesthesia, The Pennsylvania State University
College of Medicine; Director of Cardiac Anesthesia, University
Hospital, The Milton S. Hershey Medical Center, Hershey

Donald E. Martin, M.D.
Associate Professor of Anesthesia, The Pennsylvania State University
College of Medicine; Director of Clinical Anesthesia, University
Hospital, The Milton S. Hershey Medical Center, Hershey

Foreword by

Joel A. Kaplan, M.D.
Horace W. Goldsmith Professor and Chairman, Department of
Anesthesiology, Mount Sinai School of Medicine, New York

Little, Brown and Company
Boston/Toronto/London

To our families

Contents

Contributing Authors

William R. Camann, M.D.
Instructor in Anesthesia, Harvard Medical School; Attending
Anesthesiologist, Brigham and Women's Hospital, Boston

David B. Campbell, M.D.
Associate Professor of Surgery, The Pennsylvania State University
College of Medicine; Attending Surgeon, University Hospital, The
Milton S. Hershey Medical Center, Hershey

Frederick W. Campbell, M.D.
Assistant Professor of Anesthesia, University of Pennsylvania School of
Medicine; Attending Anesthesiologist, Hospital of the University of
Pennsylvania and The Children's Hospital of Philadelphia, Philadelphia

Scott K. Clark, M.D.
Assistant Professor of Anesthesia, The Pennsylvania State University
College of Medicine; Attending Anesthesiologist, University Hospital,
The Milton S. Hershey Medical Center, Hershey

Thomas J. Conahan III, M.D.
Associate Professor of Anesthesia, University of Pennsylvania School of
Medicine; Attending Anesthesiologist, Hospital of the University of
Pennsylvania, Philadelphia

John R. Cooper, Jr., M.D.
Clinical Assistant Professor of Anesthesia, University of Texas Medical
School at Houston; Attending Anesthesiologist, Texas Heart Institute,
Houston

Norig Ellison, M.D.
Professor of Anesthesia, University of Pennsylvania School of Medicine;
Attending Anesthesiologist, Hospital of the University of Pennsylvania
and The Children's Hospital of Philadelphia, Philadelphia

Frederick A. Hensley, Jr., M.D.
Associate Professor of Anesthesia, The Pennsylvania State University
College of Medicine; Director of Cardiac Anesthesia, University
Hospital, The Milton S. Hershey Medical Center, Hershey

Paul R. Hickey, M.D.
Associate Professor of Anesthesia, Harvard Medical School; Senior
Associate in Anesthesiology, The Children's Hospital, Boston

Kane M. High, M.D.
Assistant Professor of Anesthesia, The Pennsylvania State University
College of Medicine; Attending Anesthesiologist, University Hospital,
The Milton S. Hershey Medical Center, Hershey

Peter G. Hild, M.D.
Assistant Professor of Anesthesia, University of Alabama School of
Medicine; Attending Anesthesiologist, Cardiovascular Anesthesia
Division, University of Alabama Medical Center, Birmingham

Jan C. Horrow, M.D.
Associate Professor of Anesthesiology, Hahnemann University School of
Medicine; Director, Cardiothoracic Anesthesia, Hahnemann University
Hospital, Philadelphia

David R. Jobes, M.D.
Associate Professor of Anesthesia, University of Pennsylvania School of Medicine; Attending Anesthesiologist, Hospital of the University of Pennsylvania and The Children's Hospital of Philadelphia, Philadelphia

W. Andrew Kofke, M.D.
Assistant Professor of Anesthesiology/CCM and Neurosurgery, University of Pittsburgh School of Medicine; Attending Anesthesiologist, Presbyterian University Hospital, Pittsburgh

Mark Kurusz, B.A., C.C.P.
Clinical Instructor of Cardiothoracic Surgery, University of Texas Medical Branch; Chief Perfusionist, John Sealy Hospital, Galveston

David R. Larach, M.D., Ph.D.
Associate Professor of Anesthesia, The Pennsylvania State University College of Medicine; Attending Anesthesiologist, University Hospital, The Milton S. Hershey Medical Center, Hershey

Jerrold H. Levy, M.D.
Assistant Professor of Anesthesiology, Emory University School of Medicine; Associate Director, Cardiothoracic Intensive Care Unit, The Emory Clinic, Atlanta

Jerry C. Luck, M.D.
Associate Professor of Medicine, Division of Cardiology, The Pennsylvania State University College of Medicine; Attending Cardiologist, University Hospital, The Milton S. Hershey Medical Center, Hershey

Wayne K. Marshall, M.D.
Associate Professor of Anesthesia, The Pennsylvania State University College of Medicine; Attending Anesthesiologist, University Hospital, The Milton S. Hershey Medical Center, Hershey

Donald E. Martin, M.D.
Associate Professor of Anesthesia, The Pennsylvania State University College of Medicine; Director of Clinical Anesthesia, University Hospital, The Milton S. Hershey Medical Center, Hershey

Robert G. Merin, M.D.
Professor of Anesthesiology, University of Texas Medical School at Houston, Houston

Roger A. Moore, M.D.
Associate Professor of Anesthesia, The University of Pennsylvania School of Medicine; Co-Chairman, Department of Anesthesia, The Deborah Heart and Lung Center, Browns Mills, New Jersey

John L. Myers, M.D.
Assistant Professor of Surgery and Pediatrics, The Pennsylvania State University College of Medicine; Attending Surgeon, University Hospital, The Milton S. Hershey Medical Center, Hershey

Christopher J. Peterson, M.D.
Research Fellow in Anesthesia, The Pennsylvania State University College of Medicine; Resident in Anesthesia, University Hospital, The Milton S. Hershey Medical Center, Hershey

William S. Pierce, M.D.
Evan Pugh Professor of Surgery and Jane A. Fetter Professor of Surgery, The Pennsylvania State University College of Medicine; Staff Cardiothoracic Surgeon and Chief, Division of Artificial Organs, University Hospital, The Milton S. Hershey Medical Center, Hershey

Mark E. Romanoff, M.D.
Staff Anesthesiologist, Wilford Hall U.S.A.F. Medical Center, Lackland AFB, San Antonio

George W. Rung, M.D.
Assistant Professor of Anesthesia, The Pennsylvania State University College of Medicine; Attending Anesthesiologist, University Hospital, The Milton S. Hershey Medical Center, Hershey

Garfield B. Russell, M.D., FRCP(C)
Assistant Professor of Anesthesia, The Pennsylvania State University College of Medicine; Attending Anesthesiologist, University Hospital, The Milton S. Hershey Medical Center, Hershey

Paul N. Samuelson, M.D.
Professor of Anesthesiology, The University of Alabama School of Medicine; Attending Anesthesiologist, Cardiovascular Anesthesia Division, University of Alabama Medical Center, Birmingham

Thomas M. Skeehan, M.D.
Assistant Professor of Anesthesia, The Pennsylvania State University College of Medicine; Attending Anesthesiologist, University Hospital, The Milton S. Hershey Medical Center, Hershey

Michael T. Snider, M.D., Ph.D.
Professor of Anesthesia and Associate Professor of Physiology, The Pennsylvania State University College of Medicine; Chief, Division of Respiratory and Intensive Care, University Hospital, The Milton S. Hershey Medical Center, Hershey

Mark W. Stull, M.D.
Instructor in Anesthesia, The Pennsylvania State University College of Medicine; Cardiac Anesthesia Fellow, University Hospital, The Milton S. Hershey Medical Center, Hershey

Daniel M. Thys, M.D.
Associate Professor of Medicine and Director, Division of Cardiothoracic Anesthesia, Mount Sinai School of Medicine, New York

John A. Waldhausen, M.D.
John W. Oswald Professor and Chairman, Department of Surgery, The Pennsylvania State University College of Medicine; Chief of Cardiothoracic Surgery, University Hospital, The Milton S. Hershey Medical Center, Hershey

G. Scott Wickey, M.D.
Assistant Professor of Anesthesia, The Pennsylvania State University College of Medicine; Attending Anesthesiologist, University Hospital, The Milton S. Hershey Medical Center, Hershey

Dennis R. Williams, C.C.P.
Director, Perfusion Technology, Department of Surgery, The Pennsylvania State University College of Medicine; Chief Clinical Perfusionist, University Hospital, The Milton S. Hershey Medical Center, Hershey

Craig B. Wisman, M.D.
Assistant Professor of Surgery, The Pennsylvania State University College of Medicine; Attending Surgeon, University Hospital, The Milton S. Hershey Medical Center, Hershey

Foreword

Anesthesiology continues to expand its base of clinical knowledge at a rapid rate, which has led to the lengthening of our training programs and the formation of more subspecialties. Cardiac anesthesia is the largest and most attractive of the subspecialties due to the challenges presented by the pathophysiology, pharmacology, monitoring, and acute nature of the problems encountered. This field requires an in-depth understanding of cardiology, cardiac surgery, cardiovascular pharmacology, internal medicine, and critical care medicine in addition to the basic principles of anesthesiology. In order to keep up with rapidly evolving concepts and practices, this subspecialty has generated numerous textbooks, a journal, multiple societies and associations, refresher courses, and now a true pocket-size manual of cardiac anesthesia.

Cardiac anesthesia and surgery have come a long way since 1954 when Gibbon performed the first open heart operation using cardiopulmonary bypass in a girl with an atrial septal defect. Anesthetic agents have progressed from Morton and Long's use of ether in 1846 to new drugs such as sufentanil and etomidate that have minimal cardiovascular effects. The use of cardiovascular monitoring has increased dramatically since a finger on the pulse and a precordial stethoscope were considered state of the art. Today, the pulmonary artery catheter is routine and transesophageal echocardiography is being widely used during cardiac surgical procedures. New vasoactive substances, such as intravenous nitroglycerin and esmolol, have been developed and tested by cardiac anesthesiologists for use during both cardiac and noncardiac surgery. This book highlights all of these developments and makes the information available at a glance. It will be useful in the management of patients undergoing cardiac surgery, for which it was primarily intended, as well as for the cardiac patient undergoing noncardiac surgery.

Cardiac anesthesia is a full time specialty. Those who do it well spend many hours reviewing the current literature in the field. For those anesthesiologists who have only occasional or brief exposure to this area (e.g., residents on cardiac anesthesia rotations), the amount of available information can be overwhelming. This concise manual initiated by the Cardiac Anesthesiology Group from The Pennsylvania State University College of Medicine at Hershey will provide information regarding doses of drugs rarely used outside of cardiac surgery, protocols and algorithms for various techniques in the initiation and termination of cardiopulmonary bypass, and the use of new instruments such as the intra-aortic balloon pump and left heart assist device. The book will also serve as a good introduction to the achievements of cardiac anesthesiologists who have (1) led the recent major advances in the field of anesthesiology, (2) helped cardiac surgery develop to its present level, and (3) whose innovative ideas will lead the future expansion of both specialties.

Joel A. Kaplan, M.D.

Preface

Since the first clinical use of cardiopulmonary bypass in the 1950s, the techniques used to monitor, anesthetize, and support patients during cardiac surgery have become increasingly specialized and complex. Likewise, the literature in the field of cardiac anesthesia has become more sophisticated and more voluminous. Therefore, the practitioner beginning training in cardiac anesthesia may easily be overwhelmed. This handbook provides an easily accessible, practical reference designed to help the practitioner prepare for and manage cardiac anesthetics. It has been designed for ease of use in the operating room and the intensive care unit by residents and fellows as well as accomplished practitioners reentering the arena of cardiac anesthesia.

The book is organized into three main areas. The first ten chapters address the perioperative management of a routine adult cardiac case, including patient evaluation, cardiac operating room design and organization, cardiovascular pharmacology, and intraoperative/postoperative care. This section is primarily designed for the cardiac anesthesia resident's first exposure to the cardiac patient.

The second eight chapters address in a more detailed fashion anesthetic management of specific cardiovascular disorders. More theoretical information is presented in these eight chapters in addition to practical tips regarding patient management. The chapter on congenital heart disease is particularly detailed since the management of pediatric patients is very often specific for a particular cardiac lesion.

The last six chapters provide a comprehensive, unique description of mechanical support of the circulation. Four of these deal with support of the patient undergoing routine open heart surgery. Included are three chapters dealing with bypass circuits, pathophysiology of cardiopulmonary bypass, and myocardial preservation during cardiopulmonary bypass. A chapter discussing brain protection during cardiac surgery is included. Many recent advances in monitoring as well as therapy are unfolding. Many aspects of brain protection are related to pharmacological intervention but also include the mechanical aspects of cardiopulmonary bypass. The remaining two chapters in this section deal with longer term circulatory support. Included is a chapter devoted to circulatory assist devices, ranging from the intra-aortic balloon pump to the total artificial heart, and another describing extracorporeal membrane oxygenation. The intricacy and physiology of veno-veno bypass and veno-arterial extracorporeal membrane oxygenation and their comparison to conventional bypass circuitry are of educational value for the resident in training. In addition, many cardiac anesthesiologists manage this technology at an increasing number of centers.

The experience of thirteen other institutions in addition to The Pennsylvania State University College of Medicine have been blended to provide the reader with a broad-based feel for the way cardiac surgical patients are managed across the country.

We appreciate Betsy Dressler's extensive assistance in the preparation and typing of this handbook.

F.A.H.
D.E.M.

Anesthetic Management for Cardiac Surgery

The Cardiac Patient

Donald E. Martin, Frederick A. Hensley, Jr., and Jerry C. Luck

I. Patient presentation
   A. Age and sex
   B. Primary surgical problems and procedures
II. Clinical assessment of cardiac disease
   A. Angina pectoris
   B. Prior myocardial infarction
   C. Congestive heart failure
   D. Dysrhythmias
   E. Cyanosis
III. Noninvasive cardiac diagnostic studies
   A. Electrocardiogram
   B. Chest roentgenogram
   C. Exercise tolerance testing
   D. Echocardiography and nuclear imaging technique
IV. Cardiac catheterization
   A. Assessment of coronary anatomy
   B. Assessment of left ventricular function
   C. Assessment of valvular function
   D. Assessment of pulmonary vascular compliance
V. Systemic disease
   A. Atherosclerotic vascular disease
   B. Hypertension
   C. Pulmonary disease
   D. Hepatic dysfunction
   E. Renal disease
   F. Diabetes mellitus
   G. Coagulation
VI. Management of preoperative cardiac medications
   A. Calcium channel blockers
   B. Beta-adrenergic blockers
   C. Digitalis
   D. Vasodilators
   E. Antidysrhythmics
VII. Informed consent
   A. Risks of invasive monitoring
   B. Awareness
   C. Myocardial infarction
   D. Blood transfusions
VIII. Premedication

Cardiovascular disease is classified by many as our society's number one health problem. It is estimated that 15 million Americans have some form of cardiac disease, 10 million suffering from coronary artery disease, 4 million from valvular heart disease, and 1 million from congenital heart disease. More than 1 million of these patients undergo surgery of some type each year; approximately one-quarter of these procedures are performed on the heart itself.

By the time the anesthesiologist is consulted, a definitive cardiac diagnosis has usually been established, supported by invasive and noninvasive diagnostic studies, and the decision to undergo surgery has been made. The prime goal of preoperative evaluation is to prepare the cardiac patient for surgery (Fig. 1-1).

How, then, can we best prepare these 250,000 patients for cardiac surgery each year? What characteristics do they share? How can we identify and interpret the factors that increase morbidity during anesthesia and surgery, and how can we plan our anesthetic course to avoid known pitfalls? Key findings, as outlined below, that are important in determining perioperative morbidity and anesthetic management must be assessed carefully for each patient.

I. **Patient presentation**
   A. **Age and sex**
      1. **Advanced age,** especially age over 70, is associated with high cardiovascular morbidity. In patients undergoing noncardiac surgery, Goldman found that age greater than 70 was one of nine independent predictors of morbidity and death[6]. In patients undergoing cardiac revascularization, the Collaborative Study in Coronary Artery Surgery (CASS) found an increased operative mortality in men over age 50–60 years[7] (Fig. 1-2).

         However, it may be difficult to separate the risk of advanced age from that of aging-related diseases, and controversy still exists about the value of age alone as a predictor of perioperative cardiac morbidity.
      2. **Sex.** When patients of all ages are considered, operative mortality is more than twice as great among women as among men during coronary artery surgery (Fig. 1-2).
   B. **Primary surgical problem and procedure.** Even though a single patient may have multiple cardiac lesions, such as aortic stenosis and coronary artery disease, it is important to predict the relative impact of each lesion on the patient's hemodynamic status during surgery and anesthesia.

      The complexity of the surgical procedure itself may be the most important predictor of perioperative morbidity for many patients. Valvular and other intracardiac procedures present the risk of systemic and coronary air emboli. Procedures requiring ventriculotomy imply damage to ventricular muscle. Procedures on multiple heart valves, or on both the aortic valve and coronary arteries, carry a statistical morbidity much higher than that for procedures involving only a single valve or coronary artery bypass grafting alone. Finally, any procedure requiring more than 40 minutes on cardiopulmonary bypass is associated with greater morbidity, which increases with the duration of bypass.
II. **Clinical assessment of cardiac disease.** Four basic disease processes— coronary artery disease, myocardiopathy, structural heart disease (congenital and valvular), and disease of the conducting system—may require surgical intervention. Of these basic diseases, cardiac surgery is performed mainly for coronary artery disease and structural heart disease, each

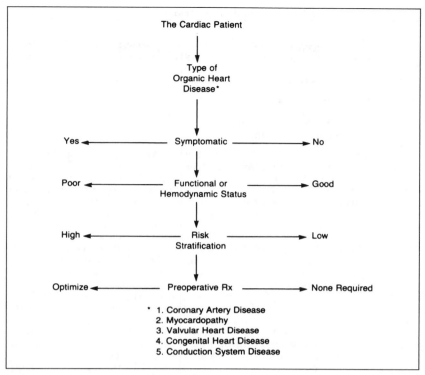

Fig. 1-1. Preoperative evaluation of the cardiac patient.

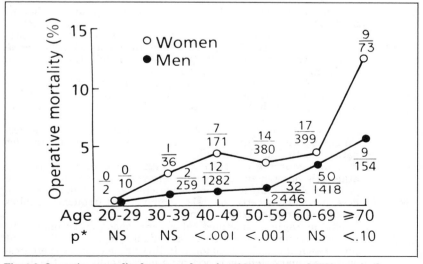

Fig. 1-2. Operative mortality by age and sex for 1061 women and 5569 men in the CASS study. (From J.W. Kennedy, G.C. Kaiser, L.D. Fisher, et al. Clinical and angiographic predictors of operative mortality from the Collaborative Study in Coronary Artery Surgery [CASS]. *Circulation* 63:796, 1981. With permission.)

manifest by some combination of five symptom complexes: angina pectoris, myocardial infarction, heart failure, cyanosis, and dysrhythmias (Fig. 1-3).

A. Angina pectoris

Key clinical findings
Exercise tolerance
Unstable "crescendo" angina
Ischemia without angina

1. **Definition and causes of ischemia.** Angina pectoris is classically described as an aching, heavy, or squeezing sensation in the chest, chest tightness, or chest pressure. Most often it affects an area about the size of a clenched fist and may radiate to the neck, jaw, either arm, back, or abdomen. It occurs most notably with exertion, after eating, or with emotion. This symptom complex signifies ischemia of the cardiac muscle that occurs whenever the energy demands of the myocardium exceed the supply. Usually, however, ischemia can be presumed to result from obstruction to coronary artery blood flow. Fixed atherosclerotic coronary disease is the most common cause. In the absence of specific coronary lesions, the myocardium may be rendered ischemic by other mechanisms (Table 1-1).

    Because the location, type, and severity of angina often do not indicate the extent of myocardium at risk, the clinician must depend for this information on other characteristics of the anginal syndrome, such as its relationship to exercise and the progression of symptoms.

2. **Exercise-induced angina pectoris** is related primarily to an increase in myocardial oxygen demand when supply is fixed. The working myocardium requires more oxygen than resting muscle. Thus, as an atherosclerotic lesion gradually obstructs blood flow, its effect will be noticed first during exercise. Angina of this type usually persists from 1–5 minutes following cessation of exercise, and myocardium is not permanently damaged. Myocardial dysfunction almost always does occur during the ischemic event. With exercise, the patient's heart rate and blood pressure rise to a level that precipitates angina. This "angina threshold" (heart rate and blood pressure known to cause angina pectoris) is an important guide to perioperative hemodynamic management.

    The level of exercise producing angina, described by the New York Heart Association or Canadian Cardiovascular Society Classification, will help to predict the risk of ischemic damage and operative mortality (Table 1-2).

    During coronary revascularization procedures, operative mortality for patients with Class IV symptoms is almost double that for patients with Class I angina[7].

3. **Angina occurring at rest** implies either subtotal obstruction by atherosclerotic plaque, coronary artery spasm, or spasm around a partially obstructing lesion. In the patients with valvular heart disease, particularly aortic stenosis, angina at rest frequently implies coexisting coronary artery disease.

4. **Unstable angina,** sometimes called "crescendo" or "preinfarction" angina, describes the new onset of anginal symptoms or the recent progression of existing symptoms. In this circumstance the progression of coronary stenosis is occurring more rapidly than the development of collateral circulation. Progressive coronary stenosis may be caused by growth of an atheromatous plaque, repeated episodes of coronary spasm, embolus, or hemorrhage into plaque. Patients in

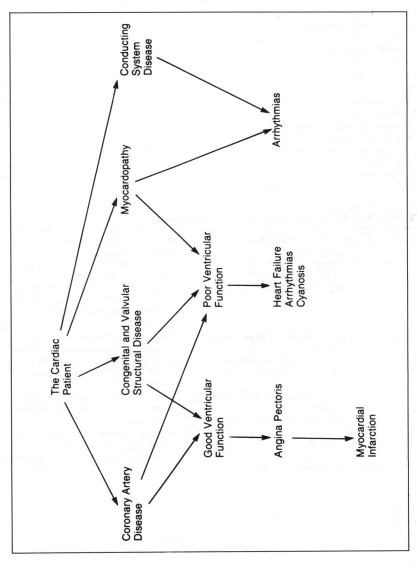

Fig. 1-3. Manifestations of cardiac disease.

Table 1-1. Cardiovascular diseases causing angina pectoris

Coronary artery disease
  Atherosclerotic
  Spasm
  Vasculitis
  Trauma
Valvular heart disease
  Aortic stenosis or insufficiency
  Mitral stenosis or insufficiency
  Pulmonic stenosis
Myocardiopathy
Myocardial hypertrophy
  Hypertension
Dysrhythmias
  Supraventricular tachycardia
Congenital anomaly
  Anomalous coronary artery
  Cyanotic lesion
  Aortic coarctation

Table 1-2. Functional classification of anginal syndrome

Functional class	New York Heart Association classification	Canadian Cardiovascular Society classification
I	Cardiac disease without limitation of physical activity	No angina with ordinary physical activity (walking or climbing stairs). Angina with strenuous or prolonged exertion
II	Slight limitation of physical activity Ordinary physical activity results in fatigue or angina	Slight limitation of ordinary activity. Limitation of walking or climbing stairs rapidly, walking uphill, after meals, in cold wind
III	Marked limitation of physical activity Comfortable at rest	Marked limitation of physical activity. Walking 1–2 blocks on level
IV	Angina at rest, increased with activity	Unable to carry on any physical activity without discomfort; angina may be present at rest

this category have a higher incidence of myocardial infarction and sudden death, increased incidence of left main occlusive disease, and an operative mortality 3.5 times the average of that for all myocardial revascularization procedures[7].

5. **Myocardial ischemia without angina** may occur and may be manifest by fatigue, rapid onset of pulmonary edema, cardiac arrhythmias, syncope, or an "anginal equivalent," most often characterized as indigestion or jaw pain. Some patients show ischemic changes on the electrocardiogram, either resting or with exercise, with no other symptoms. More than half of all patients with chronic stable angina have daily episodes of silent ischemia, and these episodes are most common during the morning hours. Such silent ischemia is particularly common in elderly and diabetic patients and is responsible for at least 15–35% of all myocardial infarctions. Perhaps because of coexisting disease or because patients with silent ischemia undergo treatment only when their disease is far advanced, silent ischemia has been associated with an unfavorable prognosis. **Over half of perioperative infarctions associated with all types of surgery are thought to be "silent."**

B. **Prior myocardial infarction**

Key clinical findings
Interval between infarction and surgery
Location and extent of infarction
Complications of infarction—heart failure or dysrhythmias
Residual dysfunction

1. **Recurrent myocardial infarction during *noncardiac surgery.***
One of the significant dangers in a patient with a history of prior myocardial infarction is a new infarct in the perioperative period. In patients undergoing noncardiac surgery, the risk of another infarct in the perioperative period is closely related to the time interval between the last prior infarct and the date of surgery. If the prior infarct has occurred within 3 months of surgery, the risk of reinfarction at surgery was found in the 1970s to be from 27–37%[11]. This risk has been recently shown in one study to be reduced to 5.7% with the use of aggressive invasive monitoring and intensive care unit support[8]. If the prior infarction occurred from 3-6 months before surgery, the risk of perioperative infarction is less—16–26% for conventional management and 2.3% with use of aggressive management. For patients who have had a prior infarction more than 6 months before surgery, the risk of reinfarction is still lower—4–6%—and can be reduced still further by the aggressive monitoring used in Rao's series to 1.9%. For patients without a history of a prior infarction, the risk of perioperative infarction is only approximately 0.1–0.7%. Perioperative infarction occurs most often in the first 2–3 postoperative days and has a very high (50–70%) mortality, much higher than that for myocardial infarctions not occurring in the setting of surgery, perhaps because perioperative infarctions are commonly "silent" and therefore untreated.

2. **Recurrent myocardial infarction during *cardiac surgery.*** In patients undergoing coronary revascularization procedures, the risk of death after perioperative infarction is lower, perhaps because the surgical procedure itself alters the course of the disease. In the CASS, 63% of all patients undergoing myocardial revascularization had had a myocardial infarction at unspecified times prior to surgery, but only 6% of patients suffered a perioperative infarction[7]. Further, mortality from a perioperative infarction in these patients was approximately 25% compared to 50–70% in patients undergoing non-

cardiac surgery. In the CASS patients, operative mortality was not increased by a history of prior infarction[7].

3. **Perioperative myocardial infarction in patients with *prior coronary bypass.*** In patients who have undergone coronary artery bypass surgery and have returned to the operating room for noncardiac procedures, the risk of perioperative infarct and perioperative cardiac death is low (0.1–0.6%) and is similar to that in patients with no prior infarction. It is not clear whether this improved perioperative infarction rate is a result of the beneficial effect of coronary artery bypass surgery or the fact that surviving the prior cardiac procedure was a type of natural "selection" process. Most studies from which this infarction rate has been calculated were published between 1978 and 1981 and may not apply to subgroups of patients with advanced disease seen today.

4. **Location and extent of infarction.** An anterior infarct is more likely to be associated with left ventricular failure whereas an inferior infarction is likely to be associated with bradycardia and heart block. A history of complications, such as heart failure or dysrhythmias, in the early postinfarction period may further help to predict perioperative problems. The location of a prior infarction may influence the risk of reinfarction[5] associated with anesthesia and surgery.

C. **Congestive heart failure**

Key clinical findings
Dyspnea on exertion, orthopnea, nocturnal dyspnea
History of congestive heart failure
Digitalis use
Diuretic use
Rales on physical examination

1. **Clinical assessment of ventricular function.** Questions such as "What is the most strenuous thing you can do?", "Do you find yourself getting tired more easily?", "Do you do housework or yard work?", as well as the more standard "Can you climb a flight of stairs?", give a very good index of the patient's ventricular reserve. It is sometimes difficult, however, to assess ventricular function by history. Valvular and congenital heart diseases are usually characterized by a gradual progression of the symptoms characteristic of congestive heart failure. Frequently, patients with coronary artery disease lack any symptoms of heart failure until the occurrence of an ischemic "event," which may cause sudden worsening of cardiac failure. Ventricular dysfunction occurs almost immediately in association with the ischemic event and may persist chronically as a result of myocardial infarction.

2. **Perioperative morbidity.** Any evidence of congestive heart failure or ventricular dysfunction preoperatively is associated with an increased operative mortality. In fact, diminished ventricular function may be the **single greatest risk factor** for patients undergoing cardiac surgery. The "congestive heart failure score" used in the CASS[7] is helpful in grading the severity of heart failure:

Congestive Heart Failure Score

Symptom or Sign	Points
History of congestive heart failure	1
Digitalis therapy	1
Diuretic therapy	1
Rales on physical examination	1
Total	0–4

Patients with a congestive heart failure score of 4 have an operative mortality of approximately 8 times that of patients without heart failure undergoing cardiac procedures[7].

D. Dysrhythmias

Key clinical findings

Palpitations—chronic or acute
Dizziness
Syncope or near-syncope
Association with angina or dyspnea
Drug therapy
Predisposing factors

1. **Incidence.** Cardiac dysrhythmias are common in patients presenting for cardiac surgery. In the perioperative period, abnormal rhythms occur in more than 75% of patients, whereas serious, life-threatening dysrhythmias occur in less than 1%.
2. **Supraventricular tachycardia (SVT).** Supraventricular tachycardias appear most often in the preoperative history as palpitations or near-syncope. Atrial fibrillation and flutter, the most common SVTs, increase in frequency with age and in association with organic heart disease. Atrial fibrillation and flutter are nonspecific signs of generalized cardiac disease. Paroxysmal SVT is frequently seen in young individuals without apparent heart disease. These dysrhythmias usually cause no direct hemodynamic deterioration. However, in patients with ventricular dysfunction, mitral valve or aortic valve disease, a hypertrophied left or right ventricle, or pulmonary disease, the loss of the atrial contribution to ventricular filling caused by an SVT may reduce cardiac output severely. In patients with an intraaortic balloon pump in place, the presence of SVT may make it difficult for the device to inflate at the appropriate time.
3. **Ventricular tachycardia (VT).** Ventricular dysrhythmias may lead directly to ventricular fibrillation, especially if they occur in the setting of acute or recent infarction. Ventricular dysrhythmias that have been present for many years, especially in elderly patients, and dysrhythmias that improve with exercise are more likely to be benign. Multifactorial indices of cardiac risk in patients undergoing noncardiac surgery established by Goldman and modified recently by Detsky include both atrial and ventricular dysrhythmias (more than five premature ventricular contractions/min) as factors that increase perioperative cardiovascular risk[4,6]. The frequency of ventricular dysrhythmias is increased by metabolic derangement (hypokalemia), digitalis intoxication, and progressive heart failure. All are common causes of ventricular tachydysrhythmias perioperatively.
4. **Bradycardia.** Two syndromes are associated with most clinically relevant bradycardias—sick sinus syndrome and atrioventricular block (heart block). Anesthetics frequently affect sinus node automaticity (both directly and indirectly) but rarely cause complete heart block. Asymptomatic patients with electrocardiogram (ECG)-documented atrioventricular conduction disease (PR prolongation, bundle branch block, and so on) rarely require temporary pacing perioperatively. Symptomatic patients, however, probably require preoperative evaluation for permanent pacing.

Patients with left bundle branch block in whom a Swan-Ganz catheter is being placed may need a transcutaneous pacemaker because of the risk of inducing right bundle branch block, and thus complete heart block, during passage of the pulmonary artery catheter. Patients with a left bundle branch block and right coronary artery disease may be at particular risk during the passage of a Swan-Ganz catheter.

E. Cyanosis. Cyanosis is a bluish discoloration of the skin caused by the presence of deoxygenated hemoglobin in the blood. It is important to note that it is not the ratio of oxygenated to deoxygenated hemoglobin that determines cyanosis but rather the absolute amount of deoxygenated hemoglobin. More than 5 volumes % of deoxygenated hemoglobin is required to produce visible cyanosis. Thus cyanosis is a common finding in some forms of congenital heart disease and in secondary polycythemic states. However, in anemic states, tissue hypoxemia may exist in the absence of cyanosis because the required amount (5 volumes %) of deoxygenated hemoglobin may not exist owing to the low total amount of hemoglobin.

Both blood flow and skin thickness in various regions of the body affect the degree of cyanosis that is present clinically. Thus, cyanosis is most apparent in the fingers and nail beds (poorly perfused tissue), lips, and mucous membranes (thin skin).

Cyanosis may be secondary to a number of cardiorespiratory dysfunctional states. Low output states (e.g., cardiogenic shock), pneumonia, adult respiratory distress syndrome, and physiologic intracardiac right-to-left shunts (e.g., atrial or ventricular defects, thebesian veins) may all cause varying degrees of cyanosis.

III. Noninvasive cardiac diagnostic studies
A. Electrocardiogram

Key clinical findings
Rate
Rhythm
Axis
Ischemia
Infarction
Hypertrophy

All patients undergoing open heart procedures should have a preoperative ECG performed. Rate, rhythm, axis, QRS complexes, and ST segments should be examined in turn, looking for signs of malignant arrhythmias, ischemia, infarction, and hypertrophy. Depending on the cardiac lesion involved, one or more of these key features may be abnormal.

In patients with ischemic heart disease the preoperative ECG should be performed no more than 24–48 hours before the procedure to rule out any silent preoperative ischemic changes or infarction. Obviously, if the patient has a prolonged episode of chest pain prior to the surgical procedure, regardless of the time interval, this patient should undergo an electrocardiogram immediately. The ECG performed within 24 hours of surgery also provides a baseline for comparison in the operating room before induction. In one series a high incidence (18%) of new ischemic changes occurred on arrival in the operating room in patients with ischemic heart disease[9]. Often there is no good correlation between severity of coronary disease and ischemic changes on the resting ECG. It is not uncommon to find that a patient with severe occlusive left main disease manifests a normal-appearing **resting** ECG.

B. Chest roentgenogram

Key clinical findings
Heart size
Pulmonary vascular flow

1. A chest roentgenogram is also necessary prior to all cardiac surgical procedures. An increase in heart size or prominent pulmonary vascularity usually represents cardiac failure, specifically left-sided failure. In the absence of congenital or valvular heart disease an increase in heart size of greater than 50% of the width of the thorax is usually indicative of ventricular dysfunction. Increased pulmonary vascular markings may be due to elevated pulmonary venous pressures caused in turn by left ventricular dysfunction. If a congenital lesion such as a large atrial septal defect is present, prominence of the pulmonary vasculature may result from increased anterograde pulmonary blood flow.

Important surgical landmarks visible on a chest roentgenogram can be referred to by the surgeon during the operation. Inspection of a lateral chest roentgenogram before a cardiac reoperation will show the relationship of the right ventricular free wall to the sternum and may change the technique for opening the chest surgically.

C. **Exercise tolerance testing (ETT)**

Key clinical findings
Ischemic threshold
Cardiac location of ischemia
Ventricular dysfunction
Dysrhythmias

1. Unlike the chest roentgenogram and ECG, the exercise tolerance test may not be performed in all patients preoperatively. It is often the initial diagnostic test performed in a patient with stable or questionable symptoms of ischemic disease with a borderline or normal resting ECG. It is performed to determine functional capacity and prognostic stratification in patients with evidence of ischemic disease prior to therapeutic interventions such as coronary bypass surgery. In addition, ETT is utilized to risk-stratify patients after myocardial infarction and to monitor the effect of antianginal medications.

Many protocols exist for ETT. The primary goal behind the test is to increase the workload of the heart and elicit maximal myocardial oxygen consumption.

a. The level of exercise used is dependent on expected patient performance. The Naughton protocol utilizes a low initial workload and small increments and is used for patients who have had a recent infarction, for debilitated patients, and for those with reduced functional capacity due to moderate angina pectoris.

b. The Bruce protocol has a higher initial workload and greater increments and is excellent for patients with mild symptoms without physical disability. Symptom-limited testing is preferred to submaximal exercise testing.

c. The amount of work can be given in metabolic equivalents (METs), which are multiples of resting oxygen consumption in ml/kg/min.

d. Patients who, on preoperative exercise testing, can exercise at a level of at least 5 MET appear less likely to die or suffer perioperative infarction than patients who cannot achieve this exercise level[2].

e. Exercise tolerance testing can provide information in three areas: (1) ischemia, (2) ventricular dysfunction, and (3) cardiac dysrhythmias. Ischemia may be manifest by angina pectoris, ST-segment depressions, or ventricular ectopic complexes. Ventricular dysfunction may be manifest by an inability to perform at average workloads. A 12-lead ECG test is preferred to single or three-channel ECG recordings for evaluation of ischemia. The most widely accepted exercise ECG criterion for ischemia is ST-segment depression of at least 0.1 mV (1 mm) at 0.08 seconds after the end of the QRS complex. If the exercise test elicits ischemia (angina pectoris, dysrhythmias, or ST-segment depression) at a certain heart rate, an **"anginal threshold"** has been established. One then has a rough idea that ischemic changes or dysrhythmias can be expected at a similar heart rate in the operating room. When ischemia or dysrhythmias occur at rest following exercise, the prognosis is more ominous. The blood pressure and wall tension changes, however, may be different during awake exercise stress testing than during anesthesia and surgery.

D. **Echocardiography and nuclear imaging techniques**

Key clinical findings
Segmental wall motion
Ejection fraction
Valvular function
Anatomic defects

1. In some cases these noninvasive studies are utilized as the sole diagnostic tool prior to cardiac operation, particularly in the pediatric population, in whom concern about the presence or extent of coronary disease is not usually an issue. Most commonly, these studies complement cardiac catheterization or are part of the diagnostic workup leading to cardiac catheterization. Segmental wall motion and ejection fraction can be assessed fairly accurately noninvasively. In addition, the extent of valvular dysfunction (stenosis and regurgitation) can be assessed by echocardiographic and Doppler flow studies. By knowing the peak velocity of blood flow distal to an obstruction, one can calculate a pressure drop (gradient) across a stenotic valve (Fig. 1-4). Color Doppler flow mapping has become a valuable modality in assessment of valvular regurgitation and shunt flow and in localization of septal defects and other structural abnormalities.

In some patients, such as those with critical aortic stenosis, severe left ventricular failure, or allergy to radiographic contrast material, left ventriculography may not be possible, and neither an ejection fraction calculation nor regional wall motion may be assessed at cardiac catheterization. Both echocardiography and nuclear ventriculography can be helpful in assessing ventricular function.

In patients who cannot undergo exercise tolerance testing because of systemic disease, nuclear imaging after coronary vasodilation with dipyridamole—the so-called dipyridamole-thallium scan—can be used to evaluate the ability of coronary blood flow to increase in response to stress.

IV. **Cardiac catheterization**

Key clinical findings
Coronary anatomy
Ventricular function
Valvular function
Pulmonary vascular compliance

A. **Introduction.** Cardiac catheterization is still considered the gold standard for diagnosis of cardiac pathology prior to most open heart operations and is essential for definition of lesions of the coronary vessels. More than 95% of all patients undergoing open heart operations have had catheterization prior to the procedure. The remainder (5%) are assessed only by noninvasive techniques (echocardiography, Doppler flow studies, and so on) prior to their procedure. They have path-

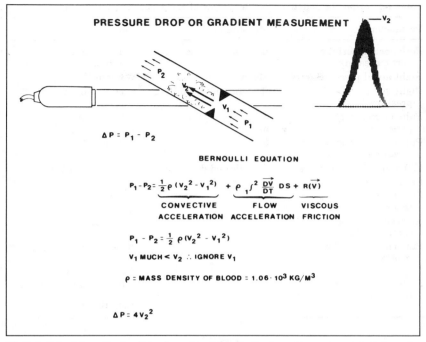

Fig. 1-4. Principles of using Doppler echocardiography to measure a pressure drop or gradient across an obstruction. P_2 = pressure distal to an obstruction; V_2 = blood velocity distal to an obstruction; V_1 = velocity proximal to an obstruction; P_1 = pressure proximal to an obstruction. (From H. Feigenbaum. *Echocardiography* [4th ed.]. Philadelphia: Lea & Febiger, 1986. P. 211. With permission.)

ologies such as an atrial septal defect (ASD) or ventricular spetal defect (VSD) that are adequately defined by noninvasive means.

The following general description of catheterization data and their interpretation is an introduction to the general concepts of catheterization reporting and the types of information available from cardiac catheterization. Specific hemodynamic patterns will be discussed in sec. II of this book along with each specific cardiac lesion. In addition, intracardiac shunt detection and diagnostic "saturation runs" will be discussed in Chap. 13.

Most formal catheterization reports contain:

1. A brief summary of indications for the catheterization procedure
2. A description of the catheterization procedure itself
3. Hemodynamic data, including chamber pressures and cardiac output
4. Qualitative descriptive information on coronary anatomy, ventricular function, and valvular regurgitation
5. Calculation of derived parameters including valve areas, ejection fraction, and pulmonary and systemic vascular resistances

If only coronary anatomy is to be delineated, often only a systemic-arterial or left-sided catheterization will be performed. However, if any degree of left ventricular dysfunction, valvular abnormality, severe pulmonary disease, or impaired right ventricular function exists clinically, a right-sided (Swan-Ganz) catheterization will also be per-

Table 1-3. Normal hemodynamic values obtained at cardiac catheterization

Parameter	Measurement	Value
Peripheral arterial or aortic pressure	Systolic/diastolic Mean	$\leq$ 140/90 mm Hg $\leq$ 105 mm Hg
Right atrial pressure	Mean	$\leq$ 6 mm Hg
Right ventricular pressure	Systolic/end-diastolic	$\leq$ 30/6 mm Hg
Pulmonary artery pressure	Systolic/diastolic Mean	$\leq$ 30/15 mm Hg $\leq$ 22 mm Hg
Pulmonary artery wedge pressure	Mean	$\leq$ 12 mm Hg
Left ventricular pressure	Systolic/end-diastolic	$\leq$ 140/12 mm Hg
Cardiac index		2.5–4.2 liters·min^{-1}·m^{-2}
End-diastolic volume index		< 100 ml/m^{-2}
Arteriovenous O_2 content difference		$\leq$ 5.0 volumes %
Pulmonary vascular resistance		20–130 dynes·sec·cm^{-5} or 0.25–1.6 Woods units
Systemic vascular resistance		700–1600 dynes·sec·cm^{-5} or 9–20 Woods units

formed. A range of normal hemodynamic values obtained from right- and left-sided catheterization is included in Table 1-3.

Interpretation of catheterization data emphasizes the following areas.

B. Assessment of coronary anatomy
  1. Procedure. Radiopaque dye is injected through a catheter placed at the coronary ostia. The coronary anatomy of both the right and left coronary arteries is then delineated. Multiple views are important to rule out artifacts (e.g., points at which coronary vessels cross) and to determine more clearly the extent of stenosis. Two common projections of the coronary arteries are the right anterior oblique (RAO) and the left anterior oblique (LAO) views (Fig. 1-5).
  2. Interpretation. The degree of vessel stenosis is generally assessed by the percent reduction in diameter of the vessel, which in turn correlates with the reduction in cross-sectional area of the vessel at the point of narrowing. Lesions that reduce vessel diameter by more than 50% are considered significant. Lesions are also characterized as either focal or segmental. There is a great deal of interobserver variability in interpretation of the degree of stenosis in the range of 40–80%.

A detailed discussion of coronary anatomy and blood flow is included in Chap. 11.
C. Assessment of left ventricular function. Both global and regional measures of ventricular function can be obtained from catheterization data.
  1. Global ventricular measurements
    a. Left ventricular end-diastolic pressure (LVEDP) measurement. An elevated value above 15 mm Hg **usually** indicates some

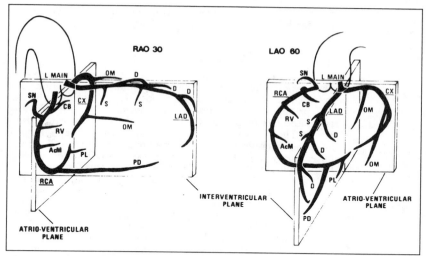

Fig. 1-5. Representation of coronary anatomy relative to the interventricular and atrioventricular valve planes. Coronary branches are L Main (left main), LAD (left anterior descending), D (diagonal), S (septal), CX (circumflex), OM (obtuse marginal), RCA (right coronary), CB (conus branch), SN (sinus node), AcM (acute marginal), PD (posterior descending), PL (posterolateral left ventricular). (From D.S. Baim, and W. Grossman. Coronary Angiography. In W. Grossman [ed.], *Cardiac Catheterization and Angiography* [3rd ed.]. Philadelphia: Lea & Febiger, 1986. P. 185. With permission.)

degree of ventricular dysfunction. LVEDP is an index that may reflect either systolic or diastolic dysfunction and is acutely affected by preload and afterload. Without examining other indices of function, an isolated measurement of elevated LVEDP simply indicates that something is abnormal. Associated with a normal left ventricular contractile pattern and cardiac output, an elevated LVEDP measurement may indicate a decrease in left ventricular compliance. Many patients with left ventricular hypertrophy (hypertension, aortic stenosis) and ischemia have good systolic function, but an elevated LVEDP value points instead to decreased diastolic compliance. Aortic and mitral regurgitation tend to cause volume overload of the ventricle, causing dilatation and a more compliant left ventricle (LV). The LVEDP measurement remains normal until LV dysfunction is far advanced in these lesions.

b. **Forward cardiac output–cardiac index.** Forward cardiac output is the total amount of blood pumped past the aortic valve into the systemic circulation. It is generally determined today by the thermodilution method. The green dye dilution method (see Chap. 4) is more accurate but is rarely used because it is difficult to perform. Cardiac output determined by angiography may exaggerate the true forward cardiac output in the presence of aortic or mitral regurgitation.

c. **Left ventricular ejection fraction**

(1) **Calculation.** The ejection fraction (EF) is defined as the volume of blood ejected (stroke volume) per beat divided by the volume in the left ventricle before ejection (end-diastolic volume). The stroke volume (SV) is equal to the end-diastolic

volume (EDV) minus the end-systolic volume (ESV). The equation for EF determination is therefore:

$$EF = \frac{[EDV - ESV]}{EDV} = \frac{SV}{EDV}$$

End-systolic and end-diastolic volume determinations are extrapolated from data gained from left ventriculography. In this procedure, radiopaque dye is used to define the left ventricle and motion pictures (cines) are taken for several cardiac cycles. The cines are then analyzed by tracing the two-dimensional **areas** highlighted by the radiopaque dye either by computer analysis or by hand. The areas are calculated during both systole and diastole. These areas are then converted to **volumes** based on a formula for an ellipse that most closely represents the ventricular chamber dimension. These volume measurements are most accurate when two views are used, (i.e., RAO and LAO) for the calculations. An ejection fraction calculation using the volume measurements calculated from just one projection (RAO) is frequently misleading.

(2) **Angiographic versus forward cardiac output.** The ejected volume of blood (EF) can either pass forward out the aorta or, in the presence of valvular lesions, proceed in a direction through the mitral valve or the aortic valve. Hence, the **angiographic** or **total cardiac output** calculated as stroke volume times heart rate takes into account both **forward** and **backward** flow. With valvular regurgitation, the **angiographic** cardiac output will be greater than the forward cardiac output.

(3) **Normal valves.** We generally consider an EF of greater than 50% to be normal. However, in the presence of significant mitral regurgitation, an EF of only 50–55% suggests moderate LV dysfunction, since part of the volume is ejected backward into a low-resistance pathway (i.e., into the left atrium). Furthermore, the EF, like any other indirect measurement of contractility, is reflective of only one point in time and can be influenced by the heart rate, preload, and afterload.

d. **Diastolic volume index.** The end-diastolic volume indexed to the patient's body surface area is another global measure of ventricular performance. It can, however, be elevated in patients with regurgitant or volume overload lesions with preserved left ventricular function (similar to the LVEDP measurement). A normal index is considered less than 100 ml/m^2.

e. **Arterial-venous O$_2$ content difference.** The Fick equation relates cardiac output to oxygen extraction by the body as follows:

$$\text{Cardiac output} = \frac{O_2 \text{ consumption}}{O_2 \text{ content difference}}$$

Thus, cardiac output is inversely related to arteriovenous O$_2$ content difference, assuming that oxygen consumption is constant. A normal value of arteriovenous O$_2$ difference is less than 5 volumes %. A low cardiac output state would be represented by an increased extraction of oxygen resulting in a widened arteriovenous O$_2$ content difference (> 5 volumes %).

2. **Regional assessment of ventricular function.** Uniform rapid inward contraction of the entire left ventricle (observed during left ventriculography) is representative of a normal contractile pattern.

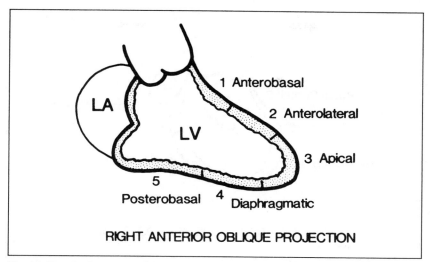

Fig. 1-6. Terminology for left ventricular segments 1–5 analyzed from right anterior oblique ventriculogram. LV = left ventricle; LA = left atrium. (From Principal investigators of CASS and their associates. National Heart, Lung, and Blood Institute Coronary Artery Surgery Study. *Circulation* [Suppl.] Part II. 63:1-14, 1981. With permission.)

This sign provides a qualitative assessment of overall ventricular function but is not as specific as the calculated ejection fraction.

Qualitative regional differences in contraction may be evident. For examination, the heart is divided into a number of segments, and the motion of these segments is studied. The anterior, posterior, apical, basal, inferior (diaphragmatic), and septal regions of the left ventricle are examined (Figs. 1-6 and 1-7). Motion of each one of these particular regions is defined as normal, hypokinetic (decreased inward motion), akinetic (no motion), or dyskinetic (outward paradoxical motion) in relation to the other normally moving inward segments.

One wall (e.g., the anterior wall) may appear hypokinetic and the rest of the ventricle may contract normally. Despite this one area of abnormal motion, however, global ventricular function may still be preserved. Obviously, if half of the left ventricle is mildly hypokinetic, global measurements of ventricular function should reflect this by also being depressed.

Regional wall motion abnormalities are usually secondary to prior infarction or acute ischemia. However, very infrequently myocarditis as well as rare infiltrative processes by myocardial tumors may lead to wall motion abnormalities.

D. Assessment of valvular function. This section will be limited to a brief discussion of the methods utilized to study lesions of the aortic and mitral valves. The specific hemodynamic patterns of acute and chronic valvular disease will be discussed in Chap. 12.

  1. Regurgitant lesions

  a. Qualitative assessment. A relative scale of 1 + to 4 + (4 + being the most severe) is used to quantitate the severity of valvular incompetence during the injection of dye at ventriculography (for mitral regurgitation) and during an aortic root injection (for aortic

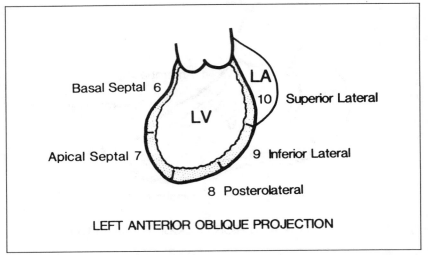

Fig. 1-7. Terminology for left ventricular segments 6–10 analyzed from left anterior oblique ventriculogram. LV = left ventricle; LA = left atrium. (From Principal Investigators of CASS and their Associates. National Heart, Lung, and Blood Institute Coronary Artery Surgery Study. *Circulation* [Suppl.] Part II. 63:1-14, 1981. With permission.)

regurgitation). For both valves, visual inspection is utilized to determine the intensity and rapidity of washout of dye from the ventricle (aortic regurgitation) or left atrium (mitral regurgitation) after dye injection. The intensity and rapidity of washout is related to the severity of valvular regurgitation.

b. Calculation of regurgitant fraction. The percentage of regurgitant blood flow can be calculated by the following equation:

$$\text{Regurgitant fraction} = \frac{\text{SV angiographic} - \text{SV forward}}{\text{SV angiographic}}$$

where forward stroke volume refers to the volume calculated from a forward cardiac output method (thermodilution or green dye) divided by simultaneous heart rate. The angiographic stroke volume is determined during left ventriculography. If there is a large difference in heart rate when the two different output measurements are obtained, this calculation would be erroneous. If both aortic and mitral regurgitation occur in combination, the amount contributed by each valve to the total amount of regurgitation can be detected only by viewing the cineangiograms qualitatively.

c. Pathologic V waves. In patients with mitral regurgitation the pulmonary capillary wedge trace may manifest giant V waves. Normal or physiologic V waves are seen in the left atrium at the end of systole and are secondary to filling from the pulmonary veins against a closed mitral valve. With valvular incompetence the regurgitant wave into the left atrium is superimposed on a physiologic V wave, producing a giant V wave (Fig. 1-8). One would expect that this giant V wave would occur earlier in the cardiac cycle. However, transmission of the wave to the pulmonary

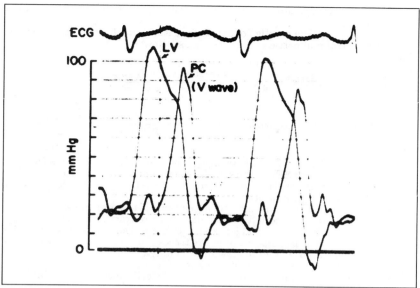

Fig. 1-8. Left ventricular (LV) and pulmonary capillary wedge (PC) pressure tracings taken in a patient with ruptured chordae tendineae and acute mitral insufficiency. The giant V wave results from regurgitation of blood into a relatively small and non-compliant left atrium. Electrocardiogram (ECG) illustrates the timing of the PC V wave, whose peak follows ventricular repolarization, as manifested by the T wave of the ECG. (From W. Grossman. Profiles in Valvular Heart Disease. In W. Grossman [ed.], *Cardiac Catheterization and Angiography* [3rd ed.]. Philadelphia: Lea & Febiger, 1986. P. 365. With permission.)

capillary wedge catheter is dependent on a number of factors including compliance of the left atrium and the pulmonary venous circuit. A giant V wave need not be present even with severe regurgitation if there is a huge compliant left atrium. With chronic regurgitation the left atrium dilates owing to the volume overload; it thus becomes highly compliant and absorbs the back pressure wave. In this situation a giant V wave may not exist.

2. Stenotic lesions

    a. The severity of valvular stenosis can be determined only by knowing the size of the pressure drop across the stenotic valve **and** the amount of flow across the stenosis. One cannot uniformly assess the severity of stenosis solely by examining the pressure gradient (either peak to peak or mean) across the valve.

        Gorlin developed an equation for determining valve area based on these two factors. A simplified version of this equation is:

$$\text{Valve area} = \frac{\text{cardiac output (l/min)}}{\sqrt{\text{pressure gradient} \times \text{constant}}}$$

It can be seen that in the situation of a low cardiac output, even a small pressure gradient may indicate a significant reduction in valve area. Conversely, a large pressure gradient in the face of a hyperdynamic output may reveal only a small decrease in valve area.

The detailed equation for actual calculation of both the mitral and aortic valve areas is as follows:

$$\text{Valve area} = \frac{\text{flow through valve}}{44.3*\sqrt{\text{mean pressure gradient}}}$$

$$\text{where flow through valve (ml/sec)} = \frac{\text{cardiac output (ml/min)}}{\text{DFP or SEP (sec/beat)} \times \text{heart rate (beat/min)}}$$

DFP is the diastolic filling period, used for mitral valve calculations, and SEP is the systolic ejection period, used for aortic valve calculations. These periods represent the time period of flow through the valve of interest.

The **mean pressure gradient** is the area of common overlap (aortic and left ventricular pressure traces for aortic stenosis; left ventricular and left atrial pressure traces for mitral stenosis) on the superimposed pressure traces (Fig. 1-9). The area of overlap is traced by planimetry and then divided by the time interval of the overlap area to give the mean pressure.

A simplistic or "poor man's" Gorlin formula is as follows:

$$\text{Valve area} = \frac{\text{cardiac output (liters/min)}}{\sqrt{\text{mean pressure gradient}}}$$

This equation is simplified because heart rate, DFP or SEP, and the constant approximately and usually cancel to unity. Hence, if the mean pressure gradient is given on the catheterization report a quick estimate of either aortic or mitral valve area can be made.

In examining combined regurgitant and stenotic lesions of the same valve, the total or angiographic cardiac output must be used in the calculation; otherwise the severity of stenosis will be overestimated. Values for normal and abnormal valve areas are discussed in Chap. 12.

E. **Assessment of pulmonary vascular compliance.** Pulmonary artery hypertension can be a result of increased anterograde pulmonary flow or elevated pulmonary venous pressures. Increased anterograde pulmonary flow is characteristic of atrial or ventricular septal defects. An increase in pulmonary venous pressure occurs with left ventricular failure, mitral valve disease, and, less commonly, aortic valve disease. Either situation (i.e., an increased anterograde flow or elevated pulmonary venous pressure) may induce pulmonary vascular changes and result in elevated pulmonary vascular resistance. Normal values for pulmonary artery pressure and resistance are included in Table 1-3.

Remember that catheterization data represent only *one* point in time, and medical management may have changed the hemodynamic pattern and catheterization results at the time of cardiac operation.

V. **Systemic disease**

A. **Atherosclerotic vascular disease**

Key clinical findings
Carotid bruits

*For mitral valve calculations 37.7 is used as the constant.

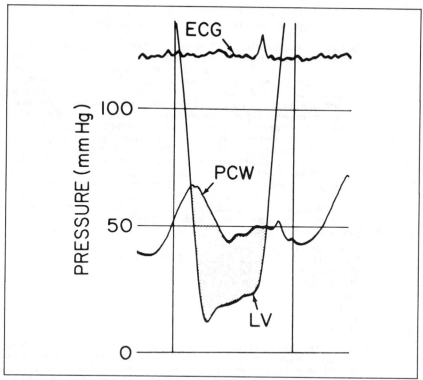

Fig. 1-9. Superimposed left ventricular (LV) and pulmonary capillary wedge pressure trace (PCW) in a patient with mitral stenosis. The area of common overlap is calculated by planimetry and is divided by the diastolic time period to give the mean pressure gradient. A similar calculation would be performed for patients with aortic stenosis. (Modified from B.A. Carabello, and W. Grossman. Calculation of Stenotic Valve Orifice Area. In W. Grossman [ed.], *Cardiac Catheterization and Angiography* [3rd ed.]. Philadelphia: Lea & Febiger, 1986, P. 147. With permission.)

Transient ischemic attack
Cerebrovascular accident
Hypertension
Azotemia
Claudication

1. **Coronary and major vascular disease.** Aortic, carotid, and peripheral vascular disease are frequently associated with coronary artery disease. Further, the presence of major vascular disease certainly affects anesthetic management, blood pressure control, and use of diuretics in patients scheduled to undergo cardiopulmonary bypass procedures.

   a. **Carotid disease.** Symptoms of transient ischemic attack or visual disturbance should be sought in all preoperative cardiac patients. The presence of these symptoms or of an asymptomatic carotid bruit should warrant at least noninvasive Doppler carotid flow studies before cardiac surgery. Even in the absence of symptoms, it is wise to assume that every patient over age 70 with coronary

artery disease also has some cerebrovascular disease and intraoperative blood pressure management should be planned accordingly.
  b. **Renovascular disease.** Severe recent-onset or recently progressive hypertension, abdominal bruits, or renal insufficiency should prompt a thorough investigation of the renal vasculature, including renin measurement. Renal vascular disease, if present, requires increased concern in patients with hypotension on cardiopulmonary bypass and in those with radiopaque dye loads in the immediate preoperative period as well as use of mannitol and other diuretics to preserve renal function intraoperatively.
  c. **Peripheral vascular disease.** Symptoms of claudication should be sought, and peripheral pulses should be examined in both arms and legs in patients with generalized vascular disease. Preoperative assessment of pulse strength is necessary to form a baseline for postoperative evaluation, to determine the most appropriate sites for arterial cannulation, and to locate the best peripheral insertion site for an intraaortic balloon pump or arterial cardiopulmonary bypass cannula should the need arise.
B. **Hypertension**
  Key clinical findings
  Range of resting and admission blood pressures
  Duration of hypertension
  Drug history
  Azotemia
  Hypokalemia
  Palpitations
  Headache

  1. **Etiology.** The contribution of hypertension to perioperative morbidity and the implications for anesthetic management depend on (1) the etiology of hypertension, (2) blood pressure level, both with stress and at rest, (3) preexisting complications of hypertension, and (4) physiologic changes due to drug therapy. Most hypertension is so-called primary or essential hypertension, probably related to an alteration of membrane handling of sodium, potassium, or calcium. It is important preoperatively, however, to exclude several treatable causes of secondary hypertension (Table 1-4).
  2. **Severity.** Evaluation of all cardiac patients, and hypertensive patients in particular, should include a determination of the *range* of blood pressures within which the patient usually functions. Intraoperative cardiac morbidity in the form of dysrhythmias and ischemic ECG changes has been observed in association with intraoperative blood pressure lability in untreated hypertensive patients with awake diastolic blood pressures of greater than 110 mm Hg. Increased perioperative risk in patients with diastolic blood pressures of between 90 and 110 mm Hg are more controversial.
  3. **"Pseudo" normotension.** It is very rare for essential hypertension to actually resolve without treatment. The hypertensive patient who becomes normotensive for no apparent reason presents a special dilemma. A myocardial ischemic event or progression of stenotic valvular disease may cause this apparent resolution of hypertension in which the patient may indeed become normotensive only because his heart cannot generate sufficient cardiac output to produce hypertension any longer. His response to any surgical or anesthetic stress may well be immediate cardiac failure.
  4. **Sequelae of hypertension.** The hypertensive state can lead to sequelae most evident in the heart, central nervous system, and kidney.

Table 1-4. Causes of hypertension

Cause	Incidence (percent)	Distinctive signs and symptoms
Essential hypertension	85–95	Duration greater than 1 year Family history Racial origin
Chronic renal disease	2–5	Elevated BUN or creatinine levels Volume expansion Polyuria or oliguria Hyperkalemia Metabolic acidosis
Renovascular disease	1–3	Accelerated course Abdominal bruits Elevated renin levels
Aortic coarctation	2–5	Diminished lower extremity pulses Rib notching Heart murmur
Oral contraceptives	4	History
Primary hyperaldosteronism	0.1–0.5	Hypokalemia Alkalosis Muscle weakness Fatigue
Cushing's syndrome	0.2	Muscle weakness Osteoporosis "Moon" facies "Buffalo" hump Hirsutism
Pheochromocytoma	0.2	Episodic hypertension Palpitations Headache Diaphoresis

Findings that should be sought in patients with established hypertension include (1) left ventricular hypertrophy leading to decreased ventricular compliance, (2) neurologic symptoms such as headache, dizziness, tinnitus, and blurred vision that may progress to cerebral infarction, and (3) renal vascular lesions leading to proteinuria, hematuria, and decreased glomerular filtration progressing to renal failure.

5. **Sequelae of antihypertensive therapy.** Most antihypertensive agents have beneficial effects in the perioperative period, reducing vascular reactivity and myocardial workload, and they should be continued until the morning of the operation. Beta-blockers and clonidine, in particular, must be continued throughout the perioperative period to avoid a "rebound" phenomenon. Antihypertensive therapy, however, often leads to hypovolemia and hypokalemia, which must be recognized and treated preoperatively. Most current antihypertensives have other hemodynamic effects that may be important to intraoperative management (Table 1-5).

C. **Pulmonary disease**

Key clinical findings
Cigarette smoking

Table 1-5. Common antihypertensives

Classification	Agents	Effects
Diuretics		
Saluretic	Indapamide (Lozol) Metolazone (Diulo, Zaroxolyn) Guanethazone (Hydromox)	Mild hypokalemia Orthostasis Decreased response to norepinephrine Sensitivity to tubocurarine barbiturates, narcotics Some authors recommend discontinuation prior to anesthesia
Loop	Bumetanide (Bumex) Ethacrynic acid (Edecrin) Furosemide (Lasix) Chlorthalidone (Hygroton, Thalitone)	Hypovolemia Hypokalemia Ototoxicity
Potassium-sparing	Amiloride (Midamor, Moduretic) Spironolactone (Aldactone) Triamterene (Dyrenium, Maxzide)	Hyperkalemia Azotemia Sensitivity to muscle relaxants
Thiazides	Bendroflumethiazide (Naturetin) Benzthiazide (Exna) Chlorothiazide (Diuril) Hydrochlorothiazide (Hydroduril, Esidrix, Oretic) Hydroflumethiazide (Diucardin, Saluron) Methyclothiazide (Aquatensen, Enduron) Polythiazide (Renese) Trichlormethiazide (Metahydrin, Naqua)	Hypovolemia Hypokalemia Azotemia
Catecholamine-depleting	Quanadrel (Hylorel) Guanethidine (Ismelin) Rescinnamine (Moderil) Reserpine (Serpasil, Raudixin)	Orthostatic hypotension Sensitivity to direct-acting pressors Sensitivity to anesthetics (some authors recommend stopping 48–72 h preoperatively)
Central-acting Alpha-2 agonists	Clonidine (Catapres) Guanabenz (Wytensin) Guanfacine (Tenex)	Hepatic dysfunction Withdrawal hypertension

Drug Class	Drugs	Adverse Effects
Central-acting alpha-1 inhibitors	Methyldopa (Aldomet)	
	Prazosin (Minipress)	Resistance to indirect-acting pressors
Direct vasodilators	Hydralazine (Apresoline)	Hypotension
	Minoxidil (Loniten)	Reflex tachycardia
Angiotensin-converting enzyme inhibitors	Captopril (Capoten)	Hypotension
	Enalapril (Vasotec)	Pancytopenia
		Hyperkalemia
Alpha-1 adrenergic blocker	Terazosin (Hytrin)	Orthostasis
Beta-adrenergic blockers	Acebutolol (Sectral)	Bradycardia
	Atenolol (Tenormin)	Orthostasis
	Metoprolol (Lopressor)	Hypoglycemia
	Nadolol (Corgard)	Bronchospasm
	Pindolol (Viskin)	Congestive failure
	Propranolol (Inderal)	
	Timolol (Blocadren)	
Alpha and beta blockers	Labetalol (Normodyne, Trandate)	Orthostasis
		Hepatic failure
Ganglionic blocker	Mecamylamine (Inversine)	Orthostasis
		Choreiform movement
		Sensitivity to pressor amines

Sputum production
Dyspnea
Wheezing
Recent respiratory infection
Age
Weight
Type of cardiac disease

Cardiac surgery requires exposure of the thorax, leading to increased risk of postoperative ventilatory complications. Risk factors for postoperative pulmonary insufficiency and the need for prolonged mechanical ventilation should be sought on preoperative evaluation. They include:

1. **Smoking history.** A smoking history is common in adults with heart disease and raises several questions. Does smoking in the absence of other risk factors increase surgical risk? Is recent smoking a more important risk factor than chronic smoking? If so, how long a smoke-free interval is necessary to reduce risk?

   A smoking history in the absence of any signs or symptoms of respiratory disease does little to increase anesthetic risk. However, a history of prolonged smoking is almost invariably associated with signs and symptoms of bronchitis or obstructive pulmonary disease, and it increases the significance of these symptoms. Abstinence from smoking for as little as 8 weeks before surgery reverses some of the changes in the tracheobronchial tree and decreases pulmonary complications in patients undergoing cardiac surgery[12]. However, discontinuing smoking 1–3 days preoperatively confers little beneficial effect except that it does allow carbon monoxide levels in the blood to decrease.

2. Patients with chronic lung disease manifest by dyspnea on exertion or at rest, sputum production, or audible wheezes on physical examination have 2–6 times the rate of pulmonary complications found in normal patients after thoracic surgery.

3. **Recent respiratory infection.** Controversy exists about the need to postpone surgery in a patient with an upper respiratory infection who is undergoing a peripheral surgical procedure. In a cardiac or major thoracic procedure, however, the difficulty encountered in clearing an increased volume of tenacious bronchial secretions can easily lead to postoperative atelectasis or pneumonia. Especially in infants and young children, purulent secretions can lead to mucous plugging of the bronchi and, in our experience, recurrent occlusion of a small endotracheal tube, requiring emergency reintubation in the early postoperative period. For all these reasons, we recommend postponement of elective cardiac surgery in patients, especially children, with evidence of an upper or lower respiratory infection manifest by cough, hoarseness, or purulent nasal discharge within 2 weeks of surgery. In patients undergoing emergent surgery, special efforts to clear secretions by suctioning or bronchoscopy will be needed in the early postoperative period.

5. **Age.** Resting PO_2 decreases almost linearly with age. However, the risk of pulmonary complications increases significantly only after age 70-80 years in patients with no other pulmonary risk factors.

6. **Weight.** Obesity, or weight in excess of 10% of ideal body weight, is sufficient to increase the chances of atelectasis. With further increases in body weight, severe chronic atelectasis can occur, in the extreme case of the morbidly obese patient with Pickwickian syndrome, such atelectasis can lead to pulmonary hypertension and right heart failure.

Table 1-6. Spirometry—risk indices

Low risk
  Forced vital capacity (% predicted) + FEV_1 (% FVC) > 150
Moderate risk
  150 > forced vital capacity (% predicted) + FEV_1 (% FVC) > 100
High risk
  Forced vital capacity (% predicted) + FEV_1 (% FVC) < 100
  Forced vital capacity < 20 ml/kg
  Postbronchodilator FEV_1/FVC < 50%

Source: From B.A. Shapiro. *Evaluation of Respiratory Function in the Perioperative Period.* ASA Refresher Course Lecture No. 222. Park Ridge, Ill.: American Society of Anesthesiologists, Inc., 1979. With permission.

7. **Cardiac disease.** Valvular heart disease, particularly mitral valve disease, as well as chronic congestive heart failure is associated with postoperative respiratory failure and the need for prolonged ventilation. Pulmonary hypertension from these or other causes is one mechanism by which cardiac disease contributes directly to perioperative pulmonary insufficiency.

8. **Pulmonary function testing.** In patients judged to be at increased perioperative risk based on clinical criteria, and especially in all patients with aortic or mitral valve disease, spirometry is indicated to further evaluate perioperative lung function. Shapiro divided patients into groups with low, moderate, or high risk of acute respiratory failure in the first postoperative 24 hours based on preoperative spirometry (Table 1-6).

D. **Hepatic dysfunction**

Key clinical findings
  History of hepatitis
  Ascites
  Serum bilirubin greater than 3
  Serum albumin less than 3
  Elevated prothrombin time

1. **Acute hepatitis.** Acute viral, alcoholic, or toxic hepatitis is associated with high perioperative morbidity for approximately 1 month after the onset of the disease or until AST returns to normal. Therefore, no elective surgery should be performed during this period. If patients with acute hepatitis must undergo emergency surgery, high morbidity and mortality must be expected.

1. **Chronic hepatic disease.** The severity of liver function impairment and its impact on operative outcome can be gauged from criteria such as those developed by Child (see Table 1-7).

    The laboratory abnormalities listed in the table may be simplified into the "rule of three's."

    Bilirubin greater than 3   High risk of liver failure
    Albumin less than 3

3. **Clotting abnormalities.** Patients with severe liver dysfunction often have an elevated prothrombin time due to deficits of clotting factors II, VII, IX, and X, which are manufactured in the liver. In these patients vitamin K therapy should be used first, but, if the liver still cannot produce sufficient clotting factors, transfusions of fresh frozen plasma are indicated before and during surgery, keeping in mind the danger of fluid overload in patients with congestive heart failure or poor left ventricular function. Also, use of intravenous vitamin K

Table 1-7. Child's criteria—classification of hepatic function

	Low risk	Moderate risk	High risk
Functional impairment	Minimal	Moderate	Severe
Serum bilirubin (mg/dl)	< 2	2–3	> 3
Serum albumin (g/dl)	> 3.5	3.0–3.5	< 3
Ascites	None	Easily controlled	Poorly controlled
Neurologic disorder	None	Minimal	Moderate to severe
Nutrition	Good	Adequate	Poor, wasted

Source: From C. G. Child, III. *The Liver and Portal Hypertension.* Philadelphia: Saunders, 1964. P. 50. With permission.

in an attempt to correct coagulopathy quickly can cause severe hypotension and a life-threatening anaphylactic response. In any patient with liver function that is limited enough to prolong the prothrombin time, a slowed drug metabolism with prolonged drug action should be expected. Infusion of vasoactive drugs (lidocaine and aminophylline in particular) must be done at a reduced rate in these patients.

4. **Abnormal electrolyte measurements.** Hyponatremia, hypokalemia, and metabolic acidosis occur with liver dysfunction and are often secondary to hyperaldosteronism or diuretic use.

E. Renal disease

Key clinical findings
Daily urine output
Serum creatinine
Body weight
Serum electrolytes
Hematocrit

1. **Renal failure and cardiopulmonary bypass.** Renal disease impairs the ability to maintain body fluid, electrolyte and acid base balance in the face of operative stress and to excrete waste products and drug metabolites. For patients undergoing cardiopulmonary bypass, however, particular concern exists because of (1) the large fluid load typically administered with a crystalloid cardiopulmonary bypass prime and (2) the potassium usually administered as part of the cardioplegic solution. Oliguric patients are usually in more danger than polyuric patients from both fluid and potassium administration.

2. **Metabolic acidosis.** Most patients with established renal failure have some degree of metabolic acidosis. When preoperative acidosis becomes severe, however (plasma bicarbonate less than 18 mEq/liter), the extra acid load that may be generated during surgery may lead to acidemia and a subsequent decrease in myocardial function.

3. **Anemia.** Patients with chronic renal failure are anemic, with hemoglobin ranging between 7 and 8 gm/dl. Therefore, use of a crystalloid cardiopulmonary bypass prime could reduce hemoglobin to levels that would seriously reduce oxygen-carrying capacity in these patients.

4. **Pericarditis.** Patients with chronic renal failure have a high incidence of pericarditis, which may lead to adhesions, making the surgical procedure more difficult, longer, and more bloody.

F. Diabetes mellitus

Table 1-8. Perioperative insulin administration

Management plan	Technique	Reference
Subcutaneous insulin	One-third to one-half usual daily dose of NPH insulin 5% dextrose infusion	Alberti, K.G.M.M. *Br. J. Anaesth.* 51:693, 1979
No glucose, no insulin	Administer no glucose, no insulin	Fletcher, J., et al. *Lancet* 2:52, 1965
Continuous IV glucose and insulin infusion	Give 500 ml of 5% dextrose in first hour, then 125 ml/h 5% dextrose; give a 2-unit priming dose followed by with 2 units/h regular insulin; give a 1-unit priming dose followed by 1 unit/h regular insulin for patients taking < 20 units of insulin/day	Taitelman, U. *J.A.M.A.* 237:658, 1977
	Prepare 500 ml of 10% dextrose containing 7.4 mEq KC1 and 5 units of regular insulin if blood glucose is < 108 mg/dl and 10 units if blood glucose is > 108 mg/dl; administer at 100 ml/h	Alberti, K.G.M.M. *Br. J. Anaesth.* 51:693, 1979

Key clinical findings
Duration
Insulin requirement
Fasting blood glucose
Autonomic instability
Renal insufficiency

1. **Silent ischemia.** Diabetic patients are at increased risk of ischemic heart disease even at a young age. Diabetics are more likely to suffer myocardial infarction. If infarction does occur it is more likely to be fatal than in nondiabetics. Further, because of autonomic neuropathy, an infarct, if it occurs, is more likely to be **silent.**
2. **Glucose management.** Difficulties likely to be encountered with intraoperative glucose management, especially the risk of intra-operative hypoglycemia, can be predicted from the duration of the disease, the usual blood glucose level, and the preoperative insulin requirement. If insulin is not required for preoperative management, none is likely to be required with the decreased glucose load intra-operatively, and oral agents should simply be held 24 hours before surgery. Long-acting oral hypoglycemics like chlorpropamide should be held for 2 days preoperatively. Regimens used for perioperative management of insulin-dependent diabetes fall into one of three cat-egories (Table 1-8).
3. **Autonomic instability.** Patients with autonomic instability man-ifested by either orthostatic hypotension or lack of heart rate vari-ation with deep breathing are at increased risk for sudden death and will need continuous cardiac monitoring throughout the perioperative period.
4. **NPH** stands for neutral protamine hagedorn. Therefore, patients taking NPH insulin are at increased risk of allergic reaction to pro-tamine received after cardiopulmonary bypass.

Table 1-9 Drugs inducing hemostatic defects

Platelet inhibitors
Aspirin
Indomethacin
Nonsteroidal antiinflammatory agents
Phenylbutazone
Tricyclic antidepressants
Coumadin potentiators
Alcohol
Amiodarone
Cimetidine
Clofibrate
Mefenamic acid
Nalidixic acid
Phenformine
Phenylbutazone
Sulfonamide
Tolbutamide

G. **Coagulation**

Key clinical findings
Patient or family history of abnormal bleeding
Drugs inhibiting coagulation
Liver dysfunction
Abnormal coagulation studies
(1) Prothrombin time
(2) Partial thromboplastin time
(3) Platelet count
(4) Fibrinogen studies

1. **Bleeding history.** A history of abnormal bleeding is perhaps the best indicator of an underlying hemostatic defect. A history of small bruises, petechiae, epistaxis, and gastrointestinal bleeding is common in patients with platelet disorders. Large bruises and hematomas, hemarthrosis, and hematuria are common in patients with defects of the intrinsic or extrinsic coagulation pathway.

2. **Screening studies.** In patients planning to undergo cardiopulmonary bypass, three screening tests are indicated: (1) platelet count, (2) prothrombin time (PT), and (3) partial thromboplastin time (PTT). These tests will detect virtually all significant coagulopathies and will ensure that any bleeding after cardiopulmonary bypass is not due to a preexisting condition. Only if one of these tests is abnormal is it necessary to pursue further laboratory studies.

3. **Anticoagulants.** Most perioperative bleeding disorders in our current patient population are drug induced. Preparations containing aspirin and nonsteroidal anti-inflammatory agents are common in patients requiring cardiac surgery. It is not sufficient to inquire about aspirin. Each patient should also be asked about Bufferin, Ecotrin, or any other pain or arthritis medication (Table 1-9). A more complete discussion of the factors surrounding perioperative coagulation defects is found is Chap. 18. In patients taking coumadin, particularly those with prosthetic valves in place, the drug should be stopped 4-5 days before surgery and heparin substituted until the night before the operation. Coagulation status should be monitored by PT and PTT throughout this period.

VI. Management of preoperative cardiac medications

A. Calcium channel blockers.
Calcium channel blockers are used to treat ischemic heart disease, supraventricular dysrhythmias, and occasionally systemic hypertension. They improve the myocardial oxygen supply-demand ratio by both increasing the supply and reducing the demand. Calcium channel blockers reduce coronary vascular resistance and are especially useful in relieving coronary vasospasm. Simultaneously, they reduce inotropy, dilate the systemic vasculature, and possibly provide direct protection to the ischemic myocardium from calcium-related injury. Diltiazem and verapamil reduce inotropy in the intact heart, although nifedipine and nicardipine do not. All these effects are theoretically beneficial in the perioperative period. We have found in a randomized prospective study that the preoperative administration of diltiazem, in moderate doses, has no adverse hemodynamic effects. Similarly, others have found no detrimental effects from chronic oral calcium channel blockers given in the preoperative period. Therefore, the administration of calcium channel blockers—diltiazem, nifedipine, and verapamil—should be continued preoperatively, giving the last dose the morning of surgery.

Although the preoperative administration of calcium entry blockers is safe and of theoretical benefit, Slogoff and Keats found that patients treated with these medications had no lower incidence of perioperative ischemic events than did untreated patients[10].

B. Beta-adrenergic blockers.
Beta-adrenergic blockers are used primarily for the treatment of stable exercise-induced angina without coronary vasospasm in patients with good ventricular function. These drugs can also be used to treat supraventricular tachycardia including that due to preexcitation syndromes, hypertension, and the manifestations of systemic disease ranging from hyperthyroidism to migraine headaches. Beta blockers decrease the rate and force of myocardial contraction and decrease renin production by blocking beta-1 receptors. They cause bronchial and vascular smooth muscle constriction, reduction of glucose and insulin production, and extracellular movement of potassium by blocking the beta-2 receptors. Beta-blocker therapy is generally beneficial in the perioperative period, and abrupt withdrawal of β blockers can lead to a "rebound" phenomenon, manifest by nervousness, tachycardia, palpitations, hypertension, and even myocardial infarction, ventricular arrhythmias, and sudden death. Both Chung et al.[3] and Slogoff and Keats[10] found that preoperative treatment with beta blocking agents, in contrast to calcium entry blockers, reduces perioperative tachycardia and lowers the incidence of ischemic events. Therefore, administration of beta-blockers should continue until the morning of surgery. However, it may be wise to substitute a shorter acting β blocker for a long-acting drug such as nadolol on the day of surgery.

C. Digitalis.
Digitalis is used preoperatively both as an inotropic agent in patients with chronic symptoms of congestive heart failure and to control the ventricular rate in patients with atrial flutter or fibrillation.

1. The risks of digitalis toxicity are increased in the perioperative period by fluid shifts, hypokalemia, and hyperventilation. Further, the benefit of digitalis in treating heart failure is often marginal, and more effective intravenous inotropes with a wider margin of safety are available. Therefore, digitalis used preoperatively as an inotrope should not be given on the day of surgery; other inotropes can be substituted if needed.

2. Digitalis used to treat a rapid ventricular response to atrial fibrillation or flutter, on the other hand, is very effective and is easy to titrate using the heart rate as a guide. Preoperatively, the adequacy

of digitalization may be assessed by observing the changes in heart rate that result with exercise, such as walking in the hall. Stability of the heart rate indicates adequate digitalization. Digitalis should be continued in these patients until the morning of the operation and should be supplemented intraoperatively with small intravenous doses if needed to keep the ventricular rate under 100. Serum potassium must be carefully monitored in patients maintained on digitalis.

D. **Vasodilators.** Oral or sublingual nitrates (nitroglycerin, isosorbide dinitrate, or pentaerythritol tetranitrate) are used to prevent coronary artery constriction and to maintain dilation of venous capacitance vessels (to decrease myocardial ischemia) in patients with coronary artery disease. Because sudden withdrawal of nitrates in these patients may precipitate ischemia, sublingual and oral preparations should be replaced by nitroglycerin ointment applied to the skin preoperatively and by intravenous nitroglycerin given intraoperatively. Because nitroglycerin ointment has a long duration of action, however, it is essential to remove it from the skin before surgery or before the use of intravenous nitroglycerin begins.

Arteriolar vasodilators such as hydralazine or prazosin as well as nitroglycerin may be used to control systemic vascular resistance in patients with aortic or mitral insufficiency or severe ventricular failure. These vasodilators should be continued until approximately 6 hours prior to the operation. If additional vasodilation is needed, rapidly titratable intravenous agents such as sodium nitroprusside should be substituted.

E. **Anti-dysrhythmics.** Preoperative dysrhythmias are usually treated with quinidine, disopyramide, or procainamide but may also require any of a large number of oral antidysrhythmic agents, including those shown in Table 1-10. Therapy for ventricular dysrhythmias should be continued perioperatively. Disopyramide, in particular, has been associated with difficulty in terminating cardiopulmonary bypass in our patients. Therefore, we recommend that another agent be substituted, if at all possible, even on the day before the operation. Similarly, encoinide and flecainide should be used only for life-threatening dysrhythmias, since recent data indicate an increased mortality in post myocardial infarction patients treated with these drugs.

VII. **Informed consent.** Cardiac surgery by definition is major surgery involving risks that are rare in other operating rooms. It is important to convey by manner, tone, and particular phrases chosen, **a realistic** assessment of the risks for each particular patient. The following information should be included in the discussion with the patient.

A. **Risks of invasive monitoring.** Thrombosis of an arterial catheter could lead to digital ischemia, and placement of a pulmonary artery catheter could cause pulmonary hemorrhage, thrombosis, or infarction. Placement of a transesophageal echocardiographic probe could cause bleeding, sore throat, or the potential for an esophageal tear, though none have been reported to date.

B. **Awareness.** Awareness during cardiac surgery, though not common, is very possible, especially during termination of cardiopulmonary bypass. It has been our experience in using modern narcotic-based anesthesia that awareness, when it occurs, has not been associated with pain. Therefore, the properly prepared patient has not, and should not, be disturbed by the experience.

C. **Myocardial infarction.** The risk of myocardial infarction ("heart damage"), cerebral infarction ("stroke"), or even death should at least be mentioned in discussing all cardiac surgery. In pediatric cardiac pa-

Table 1-10 Antidysrhythmics

Drug	Anti-dysrhythmic class	Dosage forms	Duration of action	Myocardial contractility	Vascular resistance
Quinidine	IA	Oral, IM, IV	6 h	↓	↓ ↓
Procainamide	IA	Oral, IM, IV	4 h	↓	↓ ↓
Disopyramide	IA	Oral	6 h	↓ ↓	↑
Lidocaine	IB	IV	15 min		
Mexilitine	IB	Oral	12 h	↓	↓
Tocainide	IB	Oral	12 h		
Flecainide	IC	Oral	20 h		
Encainide	IC	Oral	8 h		
Beta-adrenergic blockers	II	Oral, IV	10 min–20 h	↓	↑
Amiodarone	III	Oral	20–50 days	↓	↓
Bretylium	III	IV	6–12 h		
Calcium channel blockers	IV	Oral, IV	6–18 h	↓	↓

tients, these risks should probably be discussed with the parents in the child's absence.

    D. Blood transfusions. The need for blood transfusions needs to be mentioned specifically in the preoperative discussion. Jehovah's Witnesses object to blood transfusions on religious grounds, and an increasing number of patients are concerned about transfusion-acquired infection. Even though every effort is made to avoid transfusions in most cases, the need for blood is real and must be described to each patient.

VIII. Premedication. Premedication in any surgical patient is given for one of four reasons: anxiety, amnesia, analgesia, and protection from secretions and noxious reflexes. For pediatric cardiac patients, premedication is required for all of these indications and will be discussed in detail in Chap. 13.

    For adults, analgesia, sedation, and amnesia for the painful preoperative procedures are of greatest importance. Morphine 0.1 mg/kg plus scopolamine 0.3–0.4 mg are used most often with or without supplemental benzodiazepines such as diazepam or midazolam. The dose of scopolamine, however, should be reduced to 0.2 mg for patients over age 70. For the sickest patients, such as those with critical aortic or mitral stenosis and those undergoing cardiac transplantation or artificial heart implantation, it is often wise to administer no preoperative medication and use small doses of intravenous narcotic in the operating room.

    We have found, using continuous measurement of oxygen saturation with pulse oximetry in the patient's hospital room, that premedication in the above doses does not decrease oxygen saturation below that found during normal sleep in most patients about to undergo coronary bypass surgery. The majority of these patients have normal ventricular function and no severe lung disease. However, patients with valvular heart disease and left ventricular failure may be exceptions to this general finding and may require supplemental oxygen. Further, during insertion of monitoring catheters in the operating room, preoperative sedation combined with the Trendelenburg position and in some cases additional intravenous sedation does result in hypoxemia in a significant number of patients undergoing myocardial revascularization procedures. Therefore, premedicated patients must be treated with caution if additional intravenous sedation is added.

Complete preoperative evaluation and proper premedication, including especially the use of beta blockade in appropriate patients with good ventricular function, smooth the patient's transition into the operating room and may reduce the incidence of perioperative ischemia in susceptible patients.

REFERENCES

1. CASS Principal Investigators and Associates. Myocardial infarction and mortality in the Coronary Artery Surgery Study (CASS) randomized trial. *N. Engl. J. Med.* 310:750–758, 1984.
2. Carliner, N. H., Fisher, M. L., Plotnick, G. D., et al. Routine preoperative exercise testing in patients undergoing major noncardiac surgery. *Am. J. Cardiol.* 56:51–58, 1985.
3. Chung, F., Houston, P. L., Cheng, D. C. H., et al. Calcium channel blockade does not offer adequate protection from perioperative myocardial ischemia. *Anesthesiology* 69:343–347, 1988.
4. Detsky, A.S., Abrams, H. B., Forbath, N., et al. Cardiac assessment for patients undergoing noncardiac surgery. *Arch. Intern. Med.* 146:2131–2134, 1986.
5. Eerola, M., Eerola, R., Kaukinen, S., et al. Risk factors in surgical patients with verified preoperative myocardial infarction. *Acta Anaesthesiol. Scand.* 24:219–223, 1980.
6. Goldman, L., Caldera, D. L., Nussbaum, S. R., et al. Multifactorial index of cardiac risk in noncardiac surgical procedures. *N. Engl. J. Med.* 297:845–850, 1977.
7. Kennedy, J. W., Kaiser, G. C., Fisher, L. D., et al. Clinical and angiographic predictors of operative mortality from the collaborative study in Coronary Artery Surgery (CASS). *Circulation* 63:793–802, 1981.
8. Rao, T. L. K., Jacobs, K. H., and El-Etr, A. A. Reinfarction following anesthesia in patients with myocardial infarction. *Anesthesiology* 59:499–505, 1983.
9. Slogoff, S., and Keats, A. S. Does perioperative myocardial ischemia lead to postoperative myocardial infarction? *Anesthesiology* 62:107–114, 1985.
10. Slogoff, S., and Keats, A. S. Does chronic treatment with calcium entry blocking drugs reduce perioperative myocardial ischemia? *Anesthesiology* 68:676–680, 1988.
11. Steen, P. A., Tinker, J. H., and Tarhan, S. Myocardial reinfarction after anesthesia and surgery. *J.A.M.A.* 239:2566–2570, 1978.
12. Warner, M. A., Divertie, M. B., and Tinker, J. H. Preoperative cessation of smoking and pulmonary complications in coronary artery bypass patients. *Anesthesiology* 60:380–383, 1984.

SUGGESTED READINGS

Goldmann, D. R., Brown, F. H., Levy, W. K., et al. *Medical Care of the Surgical Patient*. Philadelphia: J.B. Lippincott, 1982.

Grossman, W. Blood Flow Measurement: The Cardiac Output. In W. Grossman (ed.), *Cardiac Catheterization and Angiography* (3rd ed.). Philadelphia: Lea & Febiger, 1986. Pp. 101–154.

Grossman, W. Profiles in Valvular Heart Disease. In W. Grossman (ed.), *Car-

diac Catheterization and Angiography (3rd ed.). Philadelphia: Lea & Febiger, 1986. Pp. 359–381.

Hurst, J. W., Logue, R. B., Rackley, C. E., et al. *The Heart, Arteries, and Veins* (6th ed.). New York: McGraw-Hill, 1986. Pp. 555–1372.

Mangano, D. T. Preoperative Assessment In J. A. Kaplan (ed.), *Cardiac Anesthesia* (2nd ed.). New York: Grune & Stratton, 1987. Pp. 341–392.

Nabel, E. G., Rocco, M. B., Barry, J., et al. Asymptomatic ischemia in patients with coronary artery disease. *J.A.M.A.* 257:1923–1927, 1987.

The Cardiac Operating Room

Thomas M. Skeehan and Wayne K. Marshall

The care of cardiac surgical patients requires a specialized operating room environment. Though all cardiac rooms are not alike, all have certain common characteristics. The purpose of this chapter is to discuss the unique properties of the cardiac operating room:

1. Its daily function and specialized personnel
2. Preparation of anesthetic equipment for elective and emergency procedures
3. Electrical safety
4. Operating room design—location within the hospital, configuration of the operating room itself, and selection of specialized anesthetic and monitoring equipment

This discussion will allow, first, the resident beginning to care for the cardiac patient to feel at home in this complex environment, and second, the future practitioner or program director to make informed choices in the design of a cardiac operating suite.

I. **Daily operating room function.** A cardiac operating room (OR) is larger than most operating rooms, requiring approximately 700 square feet of floor space. The room should be square, or as close to square as possible, to accommodate the extra equipment and personnel that must be present for a cardiac case. Several important features differentiate the environment of a cardiac operating room from that of other operating rooms. Large surgical, anesthesia, and perfusion teams must work very closely with each other, sharing space and support facilities.

A. **Surgical team.** The surgical team includes at least two surgeons and a scrub nurse. During many coronary bypass procedures, a second surgical team harvests leg veins while the chest is being prepared, thus raising the number on the team to five. Usually two large thoracotomy tables are needed for instruments. In addition, a defibrillator and some type of refrigeration unit for making cold slush to cool the surface of the heart are needed near the surgical field for cardiac procedures.

Nursing personnel provide the greatest amount of minute-to-minute support in a cardiac operating room, not only assisting with the procedure but also providing materials to the operating team. This sometimes demanding job requires at least two, and probably more, people if any difficulties arise during the surgical procedures. The circulating nurse is responsible to the anesthesiologist for the care and well being of the patient and most often provides care and support, especially to pediatric patients before and during induction of anesthesia. During the procedure, the circulating nurse may be needed by the anesthesiologist to provide blood, special medication, or a "second pair of hands."

B. **Anesthesia team.** The anesthesia team for the cardiac operating room requires about one-sixth to one-seventh of the total floor space. This space will contain the equipment that is required to provide anesthesia care for any cardiac procedure. This equipment includes an anesthesia machine equipped with air as well as nitrous oxide and oxygen flowmeters, vaporizers for halothane, enflurane, and isoflurane, a volume ventilator, and capacity to deliver positive and end-expiratory pressure. A drug cart containing a large supply of cardiovascular drugs, and a large number of invasive and noninvasive monitors are required.

This equipment must all be arranged so that it is easily viewed and is within reach from the head of the table (see sec. II for room preparation). Extra space should be present for storage of additional equipment, especially monitoring catheters of all sizes. This type of equipment should be close at hand, since the need for it may be immediate.

In view of the complexity of the invasive monitoring procedures and equipment in the cardiac OR, anesthesia technicians are employed at many institutions to:

1. Prepare invasive monitoring transducers, flush, and intravenous solutions
2. Maintain electronic monitors
3. Prepare airway equipment
4. Prepare medications and drug infusions under the personal supervision of the anesthesiologist
5. Apply noninvasive patient monitors
6. Assist in patient care and monitoring during insertion of invasive monitoring catheters and induction of anesthesia
7. Assist in patient transport to the intensive care unit (ICU)

In the absence of specialized anesthesia assistants, these functions are performed by operating room nurses or perfusionists.

C. **Perfusion team.** There must be adequate room to position the cardiopulmonary bypass (CPB) machine beside the operating room table. The CPB machine is often placed to the patient's left, so it can be viewed by the operating surgeon, and close to the head of the table to facilitate communication between the anesthesiologist and perfusionist. In addition to the room required for the bypass machine itself, floor space is required for other perfusion equipment such as the heat exchanger used to heat or cool the blood passing through the CPB machine and thereby control the patient's temperature, a cell saver apparatus used to concentrate and reinfuse shed blood during and after CPB, and a topical cooling device (if employed). In addition, the one or two perfusionists on the team will require some type of supply cart that is close at hand.

Perfusionists have special training, certification, and expertise in the operation not only of the cardiopulmonary bypass machine but also of other artificial circulatory support devices:

1. Intra-aortic balloon pump (IABP)
2. Cell saver
3. Rapid infusion devices
4. Ventricular assist devices

Thus, depending on the scope of their services, perfusionists may provide services to other rooms as well as the cardiac operating room.

Perfusionists require the direction of the anesthesiologist regarding the

1. Administration of medications, anesthetics, blood, and fluid during CPB
2. Maintenance of vital signs during CPB
3. Maintenance of arterial blood gases and metabolic parameters during CPB

A good working relationship and mutual discussion of patient management between the anesthesiologist and the perfusionist is necessary for patient care during cardiopulmonary bypass and especially during preparation for weaning from bypass.

II. **Preparation of anesthetic equipment.** Patients presenting for cardiac surgery are usually unstable. The need for emergency resuscitation or institution of cardiopulmonary bypass may occur without warning. Therefore, a full range of anesthetics and resuscitation equipment must be prepared and immediately available before the patient enters the operating room. Room set-up will be discussed for elective as well as emergency cases.

A. **Elective surgery**

1. **Airway items.** Checking the anesthesia machine, making sure suction is available, and having airway equipment readily at hand are basics in anesthetic practice that do not change when administering an anesthetic to a cardiac patient.
2. **Medications.** Bolus and continuous infusion medications that should be prepared or available for any case involving cardiopulmonary bypass are listed in Table 2-1.
3. **Intravenous solutions.** Unless a patient is a diabetic or has a history of hypoglycemia, glucose-free solutions should be used in cardiac procedures that will involve cardiopulmonary bypass. Glucose-free solutions will minimize the chance of hyperglycemia developing during the period of bypass, which may be important for protection of the brain in the event of global or focal ischemia. At least two peripheral intravenous infusions should be prepared.

   Prior to bypass, intravenous fluids should **not** be warmed in any way. Rather, the patient's temperature should be allowed to fall during this period. After bypass, intravenous solutions should be warmed as they are given to a patient.
4. **Monitors.** A core of monitors should be employed for a cardiac case. Indications for their use are outlined in Table 2-2.

B. **Emergency surgery**
1. **Airway.** The appropriate airway equipment should be ready to secure the airway rapidly. Two suction apparatuses, laryngoscopes, and endotracheal tubes should be available.
2. **Medications.** In addition to medications prepared for elective surgery, the more potent inotropes listed in Table 2-1 should also be prepared. **Epinephrine** should be prepared for bolus administration.
3. **Intravenous lines.** Two blood administration intravenous sets should be available for emergency cases. Should the patient arrive from another area of the hospital with intravenous lines in place, these can be used for the induction of anesthesia. **The only absolute requirement in providing emergency cardiac anesthetic is adequate intravenous access** with a large-bore intravenous line. A volume line can be placed directly into the right atrium by the operating surgeon should no other intravenous line be available.
4. **Preoperative monitoring lines.** For the patient presenting in shock there will be little or no time to establish any invasive monitoring lines. For the patient who is having an acute myocardial infarction but is hemodynamically stable, noninvasive monitors such as electrocardiography (ECG), blood pressure cuff, capnography, and pulse oximetry can and must be established safely and quickly. The highest priority should be set on obtaining good intravenous access. A femoral arterial line, left atrial line, right atrial line, and transthoracic pulmonary artery (PA) catheter can be established in due course during the procedure while the patient is safely undergoing cardiopulmonary bypass.

   Patients who are coming emergently from a cardiac catheterization laboratory often have invasive monitoring lines in place, including some type of arterial line and a PA catheter. Switching the arterial line to the operating room transducer is a simple task. However, the PA catheter may be in a location inaccessible to the cardiac anesthesiologist. If the PA catheter is located in the subclavian vein, it may be occluded when the sternum is retracted.

   If the PA catheter is located in the groin, proper and rapid preparation of a groin PA catheter can make this catheter extremely useful during an emergency procedure. The two main problems are obtaining accurate cardiac output and pulmonary capillary wedge pressure measurements. For cardiac output measurements using a

Table 2-1. Adult medications

Drug	Concentrations		Doses			
	Bolus	Infusion[a] (mg/250ml)	Bolus	Infusion	Prepared	Available
1. Anesthetics						
Thiopental (induction)	25 mg/ml		1–4 mg/kg		Yes	
Fentanyl	50 µg/ml		25–100 µg/kg		Yes[b]	
Sufentanil	50 µg/ml		5–20 µg/kg			Yes
Alfentanil	500 µg/ml		50–200 µg/kg			Yes
2. Amnestics						
Midazolam	1 mg/ml		1–2 mg			Yes
Scopolamine	0.4 mg/ml		0.2–0.4 mg			Yes
3. Muscle relaxants						
Pancuronium	1–2 mg/ml		0.1 mg/kg		Yes	
Vecuronium	1–2 mg/ml		0.1 mg/kg		Yes	
Succinylcholine	20 mg/ml		1–2 mg/kg		Yes	
4. Cardiovascular medications						
Anticholinergics						
Atropine	0.4 mg/ml		0.4–1.0 mg		Yes	
Robinul	0.2 mg/ml		0.2–0.6 mg			Yes

Inotropes						
Calcium chloride	100 mg/ml		7–10 mg/kg		Yes	
Dopamine		200–800		2–20 µg/kg/min	Yes^c	
Dobutamine		250–1000		0.5–20.0 µg/kg/min		Yes
Amrinone	5 mg/ml	200–1000	0.75 mg/kg^d	5–20 µg/kg/min		Yes
Isoproterenol		1–4		0.5–20.0 µg/kg/min		Yes
Epinephrine	4–8 µg/ml	1–4	2–8 µg (low) 0.5–1 mg (high)	Start 1–16 µg/min, titrate to effect	Yes (bolus)	Yes
Ephedrine	5 mg/ml		2.5–10		Yes	
Vasopressors						
Phenylephrine	1 mg/ml	10–20	50–200 mg	20–500 µg/min	Yes	
Norepinephrine		1–4		1–16 µg/min		Yes
Metaraminol	400 µg/ml	100	100–500 µg	20–500 µg/min		Yes
Vasodilators						
Trimethaphan	1 mg/ml	250	1–3 mg	0.5–6.0 mg/min	Yes	
Sodium Nitroprusside		50		0.1–8.0 µg/kg/min	Yes	
Phentolamine	1 mg/ml		1–5 mg	1–20 µg/kg/min		Yes
Prostaglandin E$_1$α		1–2		0.05–0.40 µg/kg/min		Yes
Antiarrhythmics						
Lidocaine	20 mg/ml	2000	1–2 mg/kg	1–4 mg/min		Yes
Digoxin	0.25 mg/ml		0.25 mg^e			Yes
Verapamil	2.5 mg/ml		5–10 mg^f			Yes
Bretylium	50 mg/ml	500–1000	5–10 mg/kg^g	1–2 mg/min		Yes
Procainamide	100 mg/ml	1000–2000	100 mg^h	2 mg/kg/h		Yes
Antianginals						
Nitroglycerin IV or sublingual (SL)	0.2–0.4 mg/ml	50–100	IV—50–100 µg SL—0.15–0.60 mg	0.1–7.0 µg/kg/min	Yes	Yes

Table 2-1. (continued)

Drug	Concentrations		Doses		Prepared	Available
	Bolus	Infusion[a] (mg/250ml)	Bolus	Infusion		
Nifedipine (SL only)			10–20 mg SL, extracted from capsule			Yes
5. Anticoagulants and reversal						
Heparin (for CPB)	10 mg/ml		3 mg/kg		Yes	
Protamine	10 mg/ml		1.0–1.5 mg per mg heparin[j]			Yes[i]

[a]To obtain μg/ml, multiply milligrams in 250 ml by 4.
[b]Narcotic doses given are for an entire case. One of the potent narcotics should be drawn into syringes if it will be the main agent.
[c]At least one of the inotropes should be prepared because one may be needed immediately.
[d]Bolus over 1 min.
[e]Total digitalizing dose over first 24 h is 1.00–1.25 mg.
[f]In 1- to 2-mg increments.
[g]Repeat to maximum of 30 mg/kg.
[h]Repeat dose every 2–5 min to total of 12 mg/kg.
[i]Should be prepared if routinely given by the anesthesiologist or in case of an emergency.
[j]Should be given slowly over 10–30 min.

Table 2-2. Physiologic measurements during a cardiac anesthetic

Body system	Type of measurement	Parameter measured	Primary indications
Cardiovascular	ECG	Lead II	Cardiac rhythm; myocardial ischemia
		Lead V	Myocardial ischemia
	Arterial catheter	Arterial blood pressure	Blood gas measurement, blood chemistries, continuous blood pressure measurements
	Oscillometric	Arterial blood pressure	Noninvasive blood pressure measurement
	Swan-Ganz catheter	Pulmonary artery pressure	Assessment of pulmonary vascular resistance
		Pulmonary capillary wedge pressure	Assessment of left ventricular filling
		Thermodilution cardiac output	Assessment of stroke volume, stroke work, systemic vascular resistance
		Mixed venous saturation	Continuous indirect assessment of cardiac output
	Left atrial catheter (when needed)	Left atrial pressure	Assessment of left ventricular filling
	Transesophageal echocardiography	Valvular function	Assessment of need and effect of valve surgery
		Left ventricular wall motion	Ventricular failure or ischemia
		Intracardiac air (macrobubbles)	Open cardiac procedure to detect intracardiac air

Table 2-2. (continued)

Body system	Type of measurement	Parameter measured	Primary indications
Respiratory	Mass spectrometry	Inspired O_2 Expired O_2 Inspired CO_2 Expired CO_2 Inspired anesthetic gases Expired anesthetic gases	Prevention of Hypoxia Hypercarbia Anesthetic overdose
	Capnography	End-tidal CO_2	Confirmation of endotracheal tube position, disconnection of monitor, detection of spontaneous ventilation, detection of rebreathing, detection of obstructive pulmonary disease
	Pulse oximeter	Arterial hemoglobin O_2 saturation	Assessment of tissue oxygenation
Central nervous system	Electroencephalogram	Compressed spectral array	Anesthetic depth, detection of embolism, ischemia
	Temperature	Nasopharyngeal Rectal	Core temperature measurement* Shell temperature measurement*

*See Chapters 4 and 7 for definitions of core and shell temperatures.

Table 2-3. Electrical terms

Ampere (amp or A)	Unit of electron flow, or current (I). One amp = 6.24×10^{18} electrons per sec passing a point. Amount of current in a circuit will depend on voltage and resistance
Volt (V)	That potential difference that produces a current of 1 amp in a substance with a resistance of 1 ohm
Resistance (Ω)	Analogous to flow resistance. Related to current and voltage by: Resistance (Ω) = potential (V) · current $(I)^{-1}$
Hertz (Hz)	For alternating current, refers to the frequency with which the current changes polarity each second
Macroshock	Current of > 1mA, which is the perception threshold
Microshock	Current of < 1mA, which bypasses skin resistance to cause hazard
Electrical burn	Thermal injury resulting from the dissipation of electrical energy in the form of injurious heat

PA catheter in the groin, the difficulty lies in obtaining an injection port that is close to the hub of the central venous pressure (CVP) port. This difficulty can be overcome by simply using a point more proximal to the transducer in the flush system as the injection port. The volume injected should be the same whether it is injected distally or proximally. One **must** remember to precede any cardiac output measurement by injecting 2 or 3 ml of fluid that is the **same temperature** as the injectate temperature. This will flush the line of any fluid that has been warmed by the body. Reliable cardiac outputs can be obtained in this way from a femoral PA catheter.

To obtain wedge pressure measurements from the head of the table, a low-volume infusion line can be connected to the balloon port, and a 3-ml syringe can be connected at the head of the table. The volume of these infusion lines is only 300–400 µl. Thus they add little compliance to that present if the syringe is used directly on the balloon port.

If set up this way, the femoral PA catheter remains useful intraoperatively. The only function that is lost is the ability to maneuver the catheter should a wedge pressure measurement be unobtainable.

III. Electrical safety
A. Introduction.
Electrical safety refers not only to patient safety while he or she is in the operating room but also to the safety of the personnel caring for the patient. The major hazards can be classified as macroshock, microshock, and thermal burns. Some general terms are outlined in Table 2-3.

1. Macroshock. Macroshock encompasses the range of electrical currents greater than 1 milliamperes (mA), which represents the perception threshold. Current greater than 6 amperes (A) cause sustained myocardial contraction, respiratory paralysis, and severe shock and burns. Macroshock is an uncommon occurrence in the operating room because of: (1) isolation transformers (sec. **II.E.1.a.**); (2) insulation of electrical equipment; (3) patient isolation from ground; (4) proper grounding of equipment; and (5) line isolation monitoring (sec. **III.E.1.b**).

2. Microshock. The term **microshock** applies to very small amounts of current that are below levels necessary for perception (i.e., 1 mA).

Significant morbidity has resulted from currents as low as 20 µA. Standard operating room isolation transformers provide no protection against currents of this magnitude. **Microshock cannot occur unless the skin resistance has been bypassed.** Morbidity from microshock almost always results from electrically induced ventricular arrhythmias or fibrillation. Because cardiac patients often have indwelling catheters which lead directly to the heart, as well as intracavitary or epicardial pacemaker wires, these patients are more susceptible to microshock hazard from these low-resistance pathways.

   3. **Burns.** Electricity is a form of energy, and dissipation of energy can take the form of heat. With the extremely high amounts of energy used in the operating room, electrical hazard can take the form of burns. Burns are usually secondary to use of the electrocautery unit and will be discussed in sec. **III.F.** below.

B. **Results of Shock**
   1. **Ventricular fibrillation.** Alternating current of 60 Hz can lead to ventricular fibrillation owing to disruption of the normal transmembrane charge flow that determines automaticity and conduction properties of the myocyte. Several reviews of accidents occurring in humans have established the current threshold to be about 100 µA (microshock), but again, this amount depends on the size of the catheter and other factors (sec. **III.C.**).
   2. **Dysrhythmias.** It is noteworthy that in many of the animal studies, rhythm disturbances occur prior to reaching currents needed to produce ventricular fibrillation. It is important to note that these rhythm disturbances can cause severe hypotension and mortality just as severe as that associated with ventricular fibrillation. Pump failure produced by rhythm disturbances occurs at approximately one-half the current threshold needed to produce ventricular fibrillation (Fig. 2-1).

C. **Determinants of electrical hazard**
   1. **Current density.** The total effect of the current depends largely on the current density. The same current applied to a large area will produce much less disruption of physiologic function than when it is applied to the tip of a needle or to the tip of a small fluid-filled catheter. In the case of a small bore central venous catheter placed directly in the right atrium, one can see that the amount of current needed to produce a significant arrhythmia would be small.
   2. **Current duration.** Cardiac muscle can recover quickly from a direct current that is applied for only microseconds but may become completely depolarized if the current is applied for 1 or more seconds.
   3. **Type of current. Direct** current (DC) is the unidirectional, non-oscillating current that results when a constant voltage is applied across a resistor. When direct current passes through skeletal or cardiac muscle, a sustained contraction can result. **Alternating** current (AC) is current that changes polarity at a specified rate. When alternating current is passed through tissues, various effects can result. It is the rate, or **frequency,** of the change in polarity that determines the magnitude of the hazard. The higher the frequency, the larger a current is needed to produce tissue damage or disrupt physiologic function. Low-frequency alternating currents, such as the standard 60 Hz used commonly in the United States, can cause significant tetanic contraction of skeletal muscles as well as ventricular fibrillation with small currents.
   4. **Skin resistance.** Skin resistance is an important concept that has many implications for the patient undergoing cardiac surgery. Resistance across intact skin can be as large as 1 million ohms (Ω), when the skin is dry. This amount can drop by a factor of 1000 when

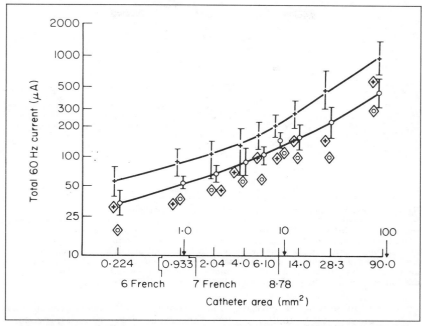

Fig. 2-1. Current thresholds for ventricular fibrillation and pump failure (caused by dysrhythmias) in anesthetized dogs as a function of catheter size. + and ⊕ average and lowest fibrillation thresholds; 0 and ⬦= average and lowest pump failure thresholds. (Modified from O.Z. Roy, J.R. Scott, and G.C. Park. 60-Hz ventricular fibrillation and pump failure thresholds versus electrode area. *IEEE Trans. Biomed. Eng.* 23:47, 1976. With permission).

skin is wet, especially with an electrolyte solution such as saline or perspiration. However, when the skin surface is bypassed, the resistance falls to approximately 500 Ω. Fluid-filled catheters that penetrate the skin place the patient at higher risk of shock or thermal injury.

5. **Current threshold (AC). Current threshold** is a term used by some to quantify that amount of current at 60 Hz needed to cause ventricular fibrillation. There is disagreement about what this current threshold is, and several studies have determined the value to be anywhere between 50 and 1000 μA (microshock range). Differences are no doubt due to species of animals studied, stimulus duration and to differences in the amount of resistance between studies. One group found that catheter size affected this threshold value (Fig. 2-1), stating that size of the catheter affected the current density, which in turn determines threshold value. As catheter size decreases, so also does the total amount of current needed to produce fibrillation (current density increases).

D. **Mechanisms of hazards.** Electrical hazard is possible when (a) there is a path for electric current to flow from an electronic device through a patient to ground, and (b) there is some fault in the electrical grounding of the apparatus. There is always a small amount of leakage of current from the components within a monitoring device and from its metal housing due to limits of insulation, dirt, humidity, and capacitive

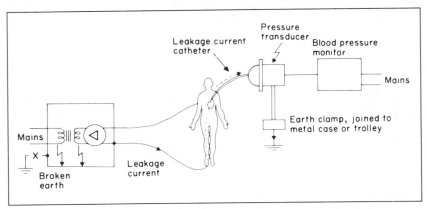

Fig. 2-2. Diagram of a faulty ground wire from an ECG monitor, causing leakage current *(dotted line)* to travel to ground directly through the heart via a central catheter. Note that 3 conditions must be met simultaneously to have a shock situation: (1) the ground lead must be faulty; (2) a leakage current from either main, or isolated circuitry must be present; and (3) an alternative path to ground through the patient must exist. (From C.E.W. Hahn. Electrical Hazards and Safety in Cardiovascular Measurements. In C. Prys-Roberts [ed.], *The Circulation in Anaesthesia: Applied Physiology and Pharmacology.* London: Blackwell, 1980, P. 618. With permission.)

coupling from AC current. This current is usually safely grounded to the hospital ground. If however, this ground circuit is faulty, the leakage current can travel through the patient to the ground, as shown in Fig. 2-2. If the circuit includes an intracardiac monitor such as a CVP line, the leakage current can be transmitted directly to the heart, creating a microshock hazard.

E. **Prevention of electrical hazard**

1. **Macroshock**

a. **Isolation transformers.** The isolation transformer is used in many operating rooms to prevent macroshock. It is simply a transformer that isolates the electrical power supply of the entire operating room from the hospital supply system, which is connected to ground (Fig. 2-3, top). Therefore, there is no path for current to reach ground in a properly isolated operating room. A third connector at each outlet provides a circuit for grounding from the external metal equipment case to the hospital ground while leaving the components isolated (Fig. 2-3, bottom).

b. **Line isolation monitor.** The line isolation monitor (LIM) monitors the electrical isolation of the operating room electrical components from ground, thereby monitoring the proper function of the line isolation transformer. If either limb from the secondary coil of the isolation transformer (Fig. 2-3, top) comes in contact with ground by connection with a piece of faulty equipment, the alarm will sound, indicating a current of more than 2 mA flowing through ground. If the physician or the patient is grounded, and if either of them comes in contact with the other secondary limb of the isolated system, a complete pathway for current flow through the common ground could occur, and the physician or the patient would be shocked. The current necessary to set off the alarm is 2 mA, which is above the threshold for ventricular fibrillation with intact skin resistance.

It is important to note, however, that the LIM will **only**

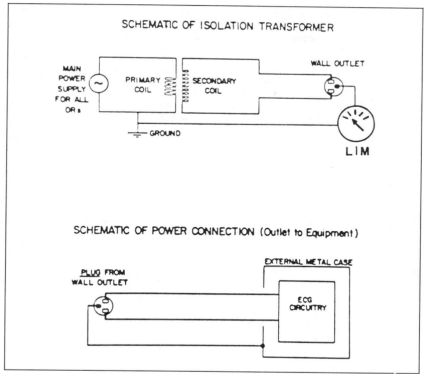

Fig. 2-3. *Top.* Schematic of an isolation transformer used in operating rooms demonstrating the windings of the primary and secondary coils. Current flows in the secondary coil owing to the magnetic field generated from passing alternating current through the primary coil. The primary and secondary coils are physically isolated. The line isolation monitor (LIM) measures the amount of current flowing from the isolated secondary current to ground. *Bottom.* Typical connection of an ECG monitor to the isolated (secondary) circuit. (Modified from L. Litt and I.J. Rampil. Physics and Anesthesia. In R.D. Miller [ed.], *Anesthesia* [2nd ed.]. New York: Churchill Livingston, 1986. P. 108.)

alarm if the leakage current from the internal circuitry to its housing reaches a certain level. It will **not** alarm, for instance, if the ground lead is faulty. The LIM itself does not provide protection from shock but will only provide a warning.

2. **Microshock**

a. **Isolation of individual electronic device.** Microshock hazard can be prevented by using equipment that eliminates all paths for current to flow through a patient to ground. Obviously, this approach not only requires good equipment design but also relies on excellent maintenance and continued testing of equipment once it is placed in use. In this system, each piece of equipment uses its own transformer coupling between the power supply and the patient connections. It is estimated that resistance to abnormal current flow to ground is on the order of 20 MΩ, which would subsequently limit any type of current flow to less than 5 μA. Some manufacturers (i.e., Siemens) use infrared coupling between the patient connection and electrocardiogram and pressure monitors to provide **complete** isolation.

b. Avoidance of a human connection for leakage current to travel directing to the myocardium. This situation could occur when anyone touches a piece of OR equipment with a leakage current of less than 2 mA (remember that the line isolation monitor would not alarm at this current, but a microshock hazard still exists) and simultaneously touches either an exposed epicardial pacer lead or the end of a fluid-filled catheter in the heart.

A similar microshock hazard would occur if the caregiver generated static electricity from walking and then touched a device connected to the heart. This would be unlikely, however, since most operating rooms have conductive flooring and are grounded.

Of course, there is no substitute for vigilance in preventing electrical hazards (macroshock or microshock). Situations in which measuring or recording systems display excess noise in the form of humming or drifting in the baseline may represent a problem with the electronic circuitry. If the line isolation monitor is employed in the operating room, and this alarm demonstrates a low resistance between the isolated power lines and ground, it cannot be ignored. The offending piece of equipment should be identified and sent to be repaired.

E. Surgical cautery hazards. Surgical cautery machines operate at extremely high frequencies, ranging from 0.5–3.0 MHz and therefore represent less of a shock hazard. More significantly, electrocautery machines represent a heating and burning hazard.

1. Principle of operation. Surgical cautery units operate by placing extremely high current densities at the active electrode, or cutting edge, of the diathermy unit. With a current of approximately 1 A, a cautery unit can produce power densities of several thousand watts per cubic centimeter at the tip of the small cutting unit. This power produces a rise in temperature of several thousand degrees centigrade at the very tip of the unit, enough to cause physical rupturing of the cells with which it comes in contact. The current then spreads rapidly as it travels to the indifferent electrode, which is usually a wide conducting pad placed near the surgical site, usually on the underside of the patient. The larger the indifferent electrode, and the better the conduction between skin and electrode, the lower the current density and the less heat produced at the indifferent electrode.

2. Burns. Burns result when current generated by the diathermy unit passes by an alternate route to ground. Again, current density is important in determining whether a burn will exist. The chance of a patient sustaining a burn will be much greater if current passes through a small surface, such as a needle electrode, than through a wide ECG patch.

Even with the isolated electrocautery units in use today, because of the extremely variable range of operating frequencies, it is nearly impossible to eliminate completely all leakage current that will find alternative pathways to ground. That is why, for example, ECG tracings routinely pick up cautery artifacts.

3. Prevention of burns

a. The most important factor is maintaining good contact of the indifferent electrode with the patient's skin. This will maximize the dissipation of current power and prevent heat buildup.

b. Site of ECG electrodes is important in minimizing the cautery current traveling to an electrode. The ECG electrodes should be placed as far away as possible from the incision and cautery ground.

c. The size of ECG electrodes is extremely important. Needle ECG electrodes should never be used. Furthermore, an electrode with as large a patch as possible (preferably 100 mm^2) should be used to lower the current density.

d. All monitoring or measuring equipment should be isolated to protect against cautery burns. Such isolation will greatly increase the resistance to current from the electrocautery unit that might travel to the patient by way of a monitoring catheter.

e. Pressure transducers should not be grounded in any way, such as by using metal clamps to hold them in place.

f. Needle temperature probes should not be used routinely by an anesthesiologist, especially if the probe has any type of metallic tip. The intracardiac temperature probe that is commonly used for cardiac cases should also be used with due caution to prevent any cautery burns.

f. The electrocautery unit should not be used if any alarm or indicator light on the console warns of inadequate patient grounding.

IV. Design of the cardiac operating room

A. Location within the hospital

1. Relation to the OR suite. A viable cardiac surgery program requires several operating rooms dedicated to, or designed for, cardiac surgery. These cardiac operating rooms should be located close to each other and designed as a suite either within or adjacent to the rest of the operating complex. Such a location makes these rooms accessible to nursing and other ancillary services without excessive duplication of resources. Obviously, if the cardiac service is a large one requiring many rooms, its location in approximation with the OR suite becomes less important. A location close to other operating rooms, however, allows nurses, anesthesia assistants, perfusionists, and surgical consultants to be readily available.

2. Relation to the critical care unit. Proximity to the postoperative intensive care unit (ICU) is probably of more concern than the location of the cardiac operating room within the operating suite. Close proximity means that less distance must be covered and less time will elapse between completion of the procedure and initiation of full monitoring and observation in the ICU. The operating room and intensive care unit should be located on the same floor if possible to avoid elevator transport and if possible should be located within the same wing. Elevator transportation poses a particularly difficult situation when the patient is receiving numerous infusions and requires either an intraaortic balloon pump or ventricular assist devices. In terms of distance, simple logic dictates that the longer the distance traveled, the greater the opportunity for the patient to become unstable and require emergency care. This care cannot be rendered properly while the patient is in an elevator or hallway.

3. Relationship to the cardiac catheterization laboratory. Patients must sometimes be transported quickly from the cardiac catheterization laboratory to the operating room. Because an increasing number of therapeutic procedures—coronary angioplasty, valvuloplasty, and intraaortic balloon insertions—are performed in the catheterization laboratory, the number of patients coming to the operating room may increase. Proper care of these patients requires close proximity of the cardiac operating room to the cardiac catheterization laboratory.

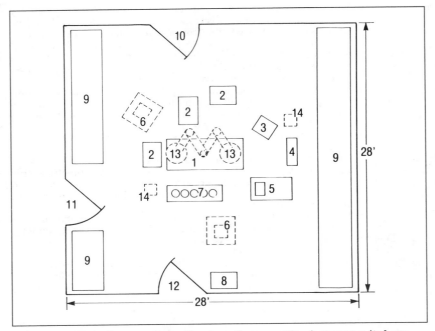

Fig. 2-4. Schematic diagram of a cardiac operating room. Key features are its large, square size, three entry doors, and nonoverlapping anesthesia, surgical, and perfusion space. (1) Operating table, (2) sterile surgical tables, (3) anesthesia machine, (4) anesthetic drug and supply cart, (5) cardiovascular monitor, (6) ceiling-mounted monitor screens, (7) cardiopulmonary bypass machine, (8) perfusionist supply cart, (9) storage cabinets, (10) patient entrance, (11) surgeon entrance, (12) perfusionist entrance, (13) operating lights, (14) medical gas, vacuum, electrical outlets.

B. **Room design.** Several general principles are followed when a cardiac operating room is being designed or remodeled (Fig. 2-4).
  1. **Room access.** Although the number of doors required by a cardiac operating room is probably more than that needed for other rooms, the number of entry doors should be restricted to limit the risk of infection to the patient. There must be a door for patient entry and exit to the outside corridor of the operating suite. There must be a separate door for entry and exit of perfusion equipment and personnel from a perfusion storage area because movement of large machinery through common doors may hinder the movement of other personnel. Last, there should be a separate entry door for personnel who have completed the surgical scrub. It is imperative that this entry be unimpeded by equipment and other personnel in the operating room. One of these entries must be accessible to the anesthesiologist, allowing him to enter close to the head of the table.
  2. **Temperature regulation**
    a. **Range of temperatures.** Room temperature during bypass should be maintained at an extremely low level of approximately 65°F. A low room temperature is needed to provide a cool environment for those parts of the heart most exposed (such as the right ventricle), so that excessive myocardial rewarming does not occur during cardiopulmonary bypass. However, because of hypothermic

Table 2-4. Electrical outlets for the cardiac operating room

Operating room utility	
Operating room table	1
Electrocautery units	2
Topical slush machine	1
Defibrillator[a]	1
Sternal saw	1
Surgical headlight	2
Warming lights	1
Extra outlets	2
	11
Anesthesia	
Anesthesia machine[a]	1
Monitors[a,b]	2
Blood warmers	2
	5
Perfusion	
Bypass machine[a]	2
Heat exchanger	1
Topical cooling pump	1
Cell retrieval system	1
	6
Total	22

[a]Denote those that should have a backup emergency power source.
[b]The monitors should all be incorporated on one self-contained monitoring cart, with strip electrical outlets incorporated for individual monitors. Extra outlets should be supplied for equipment used intermittently, such as transesophageal echocardiograph or electroencephalograph.

bypass, patients may be cool at the end of a cardiopulmonary bypass run, and thus it may be necessary to warm the room to approximately 80°F in the postbypass period to promote rewarming.

   b. Autonomous control. It is imperative that temperature control be regulated from the operating room itself because wide swings in room temperature may be needed for a single case. Further, it is necessary that the heating and cooling systems for the cardiac room be able to provide rapid changes in temperature.

3. Electrical access. The electrical requirements in a cardiac operating room are greater than those in other operating rooms because of the extra equipment that is present.

   a. Number. Twenty or more separate outlets may be needed to supply electricity to equipment in the operating room (Table 2-4).

   b. Emergency outlets. If it is not possible for the entire operating room to be on emergency power, at least 25% of the outlets should have the capability of being switched to emergency power in case of a power failure. These outlets should be prominently labeled. Equipment that is vital to maintenance of a patient's life during a procedure, such as the anesthesia machine and the cardiopulmonary bypass machine, should have reserve emergency outlets.

4. Medical gas supply lines. The supply lines include conduits that provide anesthetic gases, vacuum, and air to the operating room. At least two separate supply line systems must be available—one for the anesthesia machine and one for the bypass machine. The anesthesia machine requires air, oxygen, nitrous oxide, and vacuum, whereas the bypass machine requires oxygen, air, and vacuum.

  a. Location. Ideally, the supply lines should be located on a telescoping ceiling column. They should be movable along a ceiling track so that they can be easily put out of the way if not used during a particular case. In addition, they should be telescoped so that when used, they can be brought down to a convenient location and likewise when not in use can be pushed up out of the way. These movable columns can also be wired to contain additional electrical outlets, thus keeping electrical cords off the floor, where they are a danger to operating room personnel.

C. Design and location of monitoring equipment

  1. Monitoring system

  a. Capabilities. In designing a monitoring system for cardiac surgical anesthesia, the first step is to delineate the physiologic variables the system should measure and the capabilities it should possess. These can be divided into input parameters and output capabilities.

  (1) Input. Input refers to the information collected by the monitor through various patient or machine interface devices (i.e., pressure transducers, temperature probes, electrocardiographic leads, and so on). The number and variety of inputs is determined by the number and type of physiologic or machine parameters to be measured.

  (2) Output. Output refers to the information provided to the anesthesiologist by the monitoring equipment. This information can take several forms, ranging from electronic tones (pulse beeps; alarm) to sophisticated hard copies on calibrated strip chart recorders.

  (a) The most common and the most immediately useful form of output of physiologic information is the **cathode ray tube** (CRT) display. In a properly designed system, all pertinent information is displayed on one CRT (in one location) in easily readable form, and all parameters displayed are easily distinguishable one from another and labeled. A multicolor monitor is necessary to distinguish up to six simultaneous parameters. In addition, all pressure information and information pertaining to the ECG and end-tidal carbon dioxide measurements are displayed in waveform format.

     To display all of these parameters simultaneously a large (19–25 in.) CRT with six-channel waveform and associated digital display capabilities is required. In addition, the CRT display must be configurable as either six separate windows, one common window with six waveforms (common zero baseline), or a combination of the two.

     If each trace is displayed in its own separate window, there is no overlap of traces, and the shape of each waveform is seen most clearly. This format is always used for ECG traces. However, displaying several traces with a common baseline is most useful for displaying pressure gradients or phase relationships between waveforms of intravascular pressure traces (Fig. 2-5).

     The pressure waveforms should be accompanied by the corresponding digital pressures including systolic, diastolic, and mean values. These values are randomly selectable for each pressure.

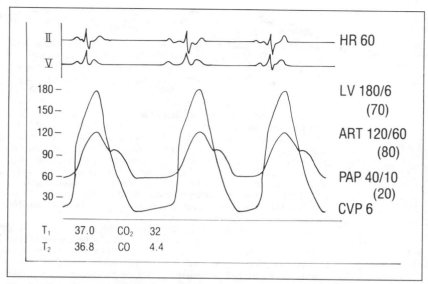

Fig. 2-5. Example of the output from six-channel cathode ray tube (CRT) showing
(1) simultaneous dual electrocardiogram (ECG) leads with heart rate displayed;
(2) calibrated pressure waveforms (only two of possible four shown) with common
baseline to show magnitude of left ventricular-arterial gradient across the aortic
valve; (3) numeric values of systolic, diastolic, and mean pressures for four pressures;
and (4) numeric values of two temperatures (T_1 and T_2), cardiac output (CO), and end-
tidal carbon dioxide (CO_2). HR = heart rate; LV = left ventricle; ART = arterial; PAP
= pulmonary artery pressure; CVP = central venous pressure.

Digital values are also needed for heart rate (determined from the electrocardiogram), pulse rate (determined
from the arterial waveforms), two temperatures, carbon
dioxide values (inspired and expired), respiratory and anesthetic gas values, arterial oxygen saturation (pulse oximetry), and cardiac output.

Even though large CRT displays (25 in.) are available, this amount of simultaneous information leaves no
excess room on the display screen. Therefore, any housekeeping information, such as that necessary for menu-driven
software, should not displace physiologic information but
be displayed on a separate CRT.

(b) **Permanent records** of the collected information should be
readily available, either for use in the permanent medical
record, for archival purposes, or for short-term use of waveform information. Short-term waveform information can be
available on an eight-channel calibrated chart recorder with
configurable speeds as well as waveform selection. Medical
record or archival needs usually involve printing of trended
data over the duration of the procedure.

In view of increasing needs to store data in archival
and trend form, all information, both digital and waveform,
should be available through electronic output for interface
and transfer to suitable computers.

b. Design. In using a monitoring system in a modern cardiac operating room, several characteristics of the design of the machine (i.e., how it functions) are important.

(1) **Modularity.** Modularity refers to the ability to expand a basic machine to fit many different needs. This is economical for surgical suites with a variety of applications in many rooms. A base unit is placed in each operating room, and modules with different capabilities are then added to the base unit to provide an infinitely configurable unit. Of necessity, the base unit must be able to accommodate a sufficient number of modules to allow configuration of all simultaneously monitored parameters (see sec. **Iv.C.1.a.**(1) above) of two electrocardiograms, four blood pressures, two temperatures, carbon dioxide levels, cardiac output, electroencephalographic measurements, pulse oximetry, and respiratory and anesthetic gases. With this type of unit, economy stems from the need to purchase fewer modules than would be needed to outfit all rooms with all capabilities. Further, maintenance and updating of each monitor is simplified by the use of modules.

(2) **Compatibility.** For modularity to be useful, all base units and modules in the operating room suite should be made by the same manufacturer and should be interchangeable. This not only increases economy but also allows flexibility during times of maintenance on a particular unit. Compatibility also applies to peripheral equipment such as transducers.

(3) **Ease of use.** The monitor should be easy to use and understand, even to novice personnel. The controls should be uncluttered and their functions clearly identified, and the unit should require minimal interactions and minimal set-up time.

(4) **Cleaning and maintenance.** The monitor should be relatively fluid resistant and easy to clean. The controls should be flush with the face, and the housing should be flat, facilitating easy cleaning with soap and water. All invasive patient contact devices (i.e., pressure transducers, temperature probes) should be disposable. Routine maintenance should be easily performed without removal or disassembly of the unit. Likewise, repair should be done on-site and should require minimal time. Replaceable circuit boards and modular components in most modern electronic monitors greatly facilitate this process.

(5) The **system at Penn State** was custom designed by the Department of Anesthesia to fit the exact needs of the cardiac anesthesia team. It is based on a commercially available modular system now standard throughout both the operating room and intensive care unit. The system is designed to work with a hospital standard disposable pressure transducer, which is compatible with all monitors including the transport unit.

The system incorporates three additional six-channel CRT displays: two 25-in. slave CRTs suspended from the ceiling and one 19-in. slave in the monitor cart. The three slave CRTs are full color monitor units to allow individual color coding of the four pressure waveforms and the associated digital values. This greatly enhances rapid visual assimilation of physiologic data. The CRTs are also calibrated to allow pressure determinations to be made from the waveform itself.

The two slave displays suspended from the room ceiling are visible to and formatted to serve the surgeon and the perfusionist. The slave CRT on the cart is visible to and formatted to serve the anesthesiologist.

The information continually displayed on the large CRTs includes two electrocardiographic leads, four pressure waveforms, heart rate, two temperatures, digital values for all four blood pressures, end-tidal carbon dioxide, and cardiac output.

Housekeeping functions for the menu-driven software in the base unit appear only on the small monochrome CRT and do not disturb the physiologic displays. In addition, the carbon dioxide waveform is displayed on the monochrome CRT.

Separate electronic devices measure hemoglobin oxygen saturation (pulse oximeter) and respiratory and anesthetic gases (multiplexed mass spectrometer); automatic noninvasive blood pressure measurement and transesophageal echocardiography are also available.

All of this diverse equipment, including an integrated, calibrated, configurable, six-channel chart recorder, is contained on a custom-designed cart. This cart is mobile, has an isolated power supply, and is sufficient to house all monitoring equipment in one place (26 in.D × 52 in.W × 72 in.H) (Fig. 2-6).

2. **Location of monitor.** The location of the patient-monitoring equipment within each operating room is of equal importance as the equipment design. In the ideal circumstance, the monitor should be located as close as possible to the patient and anesthesiologist while still allowing performance of surgery. Several relationships are of concern.

The monitor equipment should be placed at the head of the patient operating table, usually on the patient's left (most anesthesia machines are designed as right-handed machines). The controls must be readily accessible to the anesthesiologist standing at the head of the patient. The CRT should be easily visualized by the anesthesiologist without turning away from the patient and should be at eye level. The CRT also needs to be visualized by the surgeon and the perfusionist (if present) concurrently with the anesthesiologist.

Likewise, the anesthesiologist should be able to manage the patient's airway and reach the controls on both the anesthesia machine and the monitor simultaneously and without moving.

The equipment commercially available today cannot incorporate all of the indicated parameters into one electronic monitoring device. Therefore, every effort should be made to consolidate the various monitoring devices needed into one location (i.e., on one movable cart). This cart should be easily mobile, should have its own isolated power supply, and should be configured to conform to the needs for visualization and access by the anesthesiologist. The alarms for all monitoring devices should be integrated in one display.

The 19-in. color CRT is placed on the cart directly to the anesthesiologist's left at eye level, as are the pulse oximeter and the mass spectrometer. The monitor controls are immediately beneath the CRT, again directly to the anesthesiologist's left. In addition, one of the larger CRT monitors is positioned at the foot of the patient table, directly in front of the anesthesiologist for ease of viewing during crucial aspects of patient care.

A diagram of the location of the patient monitoring and anesthetic equipment in the cardiac operating room at University Hospital, Penn State College of Medicine is shown in Figure 2-4.

Alternative equipment configurations, which are effective in the cardiac operating suite, have also been proposed (see Bazard et al.).

3. **Choosing a manufacturer.** Because an ideal monitoring system may not be available, much care and thought necessarily goes into

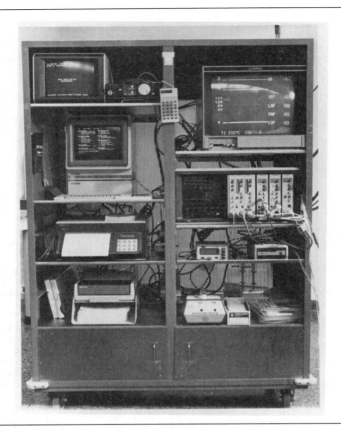

Fig. 2-6. The self-contained anesthesia monitor cart at the University Hospital, Penn State College of Medicine.

choosing which manufacturer to deal with when purchasing monitoring equipment. The practicing anesthesiologist needs to use his expertise in planning the purchase of monitoring equipment for his hospital. Some concerns are specific to the cardiac operating rooms, but certain general aspects should always be kept in mind to ensure compatibility with the remainder of the operating suite.

a. **The product line** that a manufacturer offers is the first item to consider. If a given manufacturer's stated list of equipment for sale does not include at least one suitable item, it is unlikely that the manufacturer will design and produce a unit on request. If the product line is applicable, inquiries should be made about the record of service of the particular model in question. Consideration should also be given to the age of the unit design: old designs are often technologically out of date, and very new designs are untested. In general, a design that has been in operation for 1–2 years is suitable.

b. **The reputation** of the company itself is also important. The length of time the manufacturer has been doing business is often a measure of the reliability of the product. Also, competitors' opinions about a company can be of assistance. The number of units in service is an indication of product demand. Finally, person-to-person contact with existing users is very useful.

c. **The reliability** of the particular model of interest should be determined. The service record of the unit, user contact, an estimate of the average down-time for the particular model, the delineation of the service support structure and service availability in the anesthesiologist's area are imperative. In general, companies that service their own products provide better service.

d. **Compatibility.** The new acquisition should, whenever possible, be compatible with equipment in the remainder of the operating unit and the intensive care unit. This factor is especially important in large institutions, in which economies of scale can greatly reduce the average cost per unit.

e. **Custom-design.** The willingness of the manufacturer to custom-tailor units to a given set of specific needs is crucial if plans are made to create a custom-designed system. In addition, the manufacturer should provide software or hardware updates as technology improves.

f. **Cost.** Last but not least, considerations of cost are often the deciding factor in today's climate of cost containment. However, it should be remembered that cheaper is not necessarily the most economical, and that considerations of standardization, compatibility, and capability are of equal importance.

SUGGESTED READINGS

Bazard, M. G., Petre, J., Cosgrove, D., et al. Operating room design at the Cleveland Clinic Foundation. *Cleve. Clin. J. Med.* 55:267–274, 1988.

Hahn, C. E. W. Electrical Hazards and Safety in Cardiovascular Measurements. In C. Prys-Roberts (ed.), *The Circulation in Anaesthesia, Applied Physiology and Pharmacology.* London: Blackwell Scientific, 1980. Pp. 605–633.

Litt, L.,, and Rampil, I. J. Physics and Anesthesia. In R. D. Miller (ed.), *Anesthesia* (2nd ed.). New York: Churchill Livingstone, 1986. Pp. 75–116.

3

Cardiovascular Drugs

David R. Larach

Numerous potent drugs are used to manage a variety of hemodynamic problems before, during, and after cardiothoracic operations. This chapter reviews the clinical indications, administration, and cautions to be observed in the use of cardiovascular drugs. The package insert or *Physicians' Desk Reference* (PDR) should be consulted before using any unfamiliar drug.

I. Drug dosage calculations

A. Conversions to milligram (mg) or microgram (µg or mcg) per milliliter

1. Drugs are administered in milligrams or micrograms, but unfortunately, not all drugs are labeled in a uniform manner. Conversion of units often is necessary.
2. A drug labeled z% contains z g/dl; $10 \times z$ equals the number of g/liter or the number of mg/ml.
   a. Example: Mannitol 25% solution contains 25 g/dl, which equals 250 g/liter, or 250 mg/ml.
   b. Example: Lidocaine 2% contains 2 g/dl, or 20 g/liter, or 20 mg/ml.
3. Concentrations stated as a ratio are converted to mg/ml or µg/ml, using two rules:

   1:1000 = 1 g/**thousand** ml = 1 **milli**gram/ml

   1:1,000,000 = 1 g/**million** ml = 1 **micro**gram/ml

   a. Example: Resuscitation epinephrine is packaged as 1:10,000. Thus, it is one-tenth as concentrated as 1:1000, which is 1 mg/ml; therefore, 1:10,000 is 0.1 mg/ml (or 100 µg/ml).
   b. Example: A regional anesthetic block is to be performed with epinephrine 1:200,000 added to the local anesthetic. Since 1:1,000,000 would be 1 g/ml, and the desired concentration is 5 times higher (1,000,000/200,000 = 5), a 5-µg/ml epinephrine concentration is needed.

B. Calculating infusion rates using standard drip concentrations (adults)

1. **Step 1. Dose rate (µg/min):** Calculate the desired dose to be infused per minute. Example: A 70-kg patient who is to receive dopamine at 5 µg/kg/min needs a 350 µg/min dose rate.
2. **Step 2. Concentration (µg/ml):** Calculate how many micrograms of drug are in each milliliter of solution. Example: Dopamine 200 mg added to 250 ml fluid = 200/250 mg/ml = 0.8 mg/liter = 800 µg/ml concentration.
3. **Step 3. Volume infusion rate (ml/min):** Divide the **dose rate** by the **concentration** (µg/min / µg/ml = ml/min). The infusion pump should be set for this volume infusion rate. Example: 350 µg/min / 800 g/ml = 0.44 ml/min. Conversion of volume rate from ml/min to ml/hr simply involves multiplying by 60 min/hr (0.44 ml/min × 60 = 26 ml/hr). A rule of thumb: An infusion pump at a rate of 15 ml/hr delivers a number of **micro**grams of drug/minute equal to the number of **milli**grams of that drug dissolved in 250-ml fluid. Example: Dopamine 200 mg is mixed in 250-ml fluid. Thus, at 15 ml/hr, 200 µg is being delivered per minute.

C. Preparation of drug infusions for pediatric patients

1. **Step 1.** Round off **weight** to nearest whole number of kilograms body weight (some approximation is acceptable).
2. **Step 2.** Decide on a **starting dose per kilogram** for the drug; some standard values are as follows:

Dopamine   }
Dobutamine }   5 μg/kg/min
Nitroprusside   0.5 μg/kg/min
Epinephrine   }
Norepinephrine }   0.05 μg/kg/min
Isoproterenol }

3. **Step 3.** Multiply **starting dose** per kilograms and **weight** to give **starting dose rate** in μg/**min.**
4. **Step 4.** Decide on **volume rate** of fluid that should carry this starting dose of drug into the patient:

For most children over 5 kg   0.1 ml/min (6 ml/hr)
For babies   0.05 ml/min (3 ml/hr)

5. **Step 5.** Divide starting dose rate by volume rate to give desired **concentration** of drug. Units cancel: μg/min ÷ (ml/min) = μg/ml. Example: In a 6.3-kg baby:
   a. Round off weight to 6 kg.
   b. Calculate dopamine and isoproterenol at standard starting dosages.
   c. Decide on starting dose rate:
      (1) Dopamine: 5 μg/kg/min × 6 kg = 30 μg/min.
      (2) Isoproterenol: 0.1 μg/kg/min × kg = 0.6 μg/min.
   d. **Choose volume rate: 0.05 ml/min.**
   e. Calculate concentration:
      (1) Dopamine: 30 μg/min ÷ 0.05 ml/min = 600 μg/ml.
      (2) Isoproterenol: 0.6 μg/min ÷ 0.05 ml/min = 12 μg/ml.
   f. **Mix:**
      (1) Dopamine: 600 mg/liter (or 150 mg/250 ml).
      (2) Isoproterenol: 12 mg/liter (or 3.0 mg/250 ml).
II. **Adrenergic receptor pharmacology**
   A. **Receptor activation.** Can responses to a drug dose be predicted? Many factors determine the magnitude of response produced by a certain drug dosage.
      1. **Pharmacokinetics** relate dosage to plasma drug concentration.
      2. **Pharmacodynamics** relate plasma drug concentration to drug effect.
         a. **Concentration of drug at the receptor** is affected by tissue perfusion and by the drug's protein binding, lipid solubility, ionization state, diffusion characteristics, and local metabolism.
         b. **Number of receptors** per end-organ cell may vary owing to physiologic regulation.
            (1) **Up regulation** (increased receptor population) is seen with a chronic *decrease* in receptor stimulation. Example: Chronic beta blockade produces an increased number of beta-adrenergic receptors.
            (2) **Down regulation** (decreased receptor population) is caused by chronic *excess* receptor stimulation. Example: Chronic antiasthmatic therapy with beta agonists produces a reduced number of beta-adrenergic receptors.
         c. **Drug-receptor affinity and efficacy**
            (1) Receptor activation by a drug produces a biochemical change in the cell. Example: Alpha-adrenergic receptor activation may open channels through which calcium ions can enter smooth muscle cells. Beta-adrenergic receptor stimulation may increase adenylate cyclase activity in smooth muscle cells, elevating cyclic AMP levels.

(2) The cell responds. Example: Increased intracellular calcium may cause contraction of smooth muscle. Conversely, increased cyclic AMP relaxes smooth muscle.

(3) Many factors can alter cellular responsiveness to receptor activation. Example: Acidosis and hypoxia can reduce the responsiveness of many tissues to receptor stimulation.

d. Some **clinical implications.**

(1) **β-blocker dosage** must be individualized because patients have varying blood levels of catecholamines and tissue populations of catecholamine receptors as well as varying cellular responsiveness.

(2) **β-blocker withdrawal.** The beta-receptor population is upregulated during chronic β-blocker therapy. Therefore, when β blockers are suddenly stopped, a withdrawal syndrome may occur, manifested as a hyperadrenergic state with tachycardia and hypertension. Myocardial ischemia or infarction may result. **Thus, β-blocker therapy should generally be either continued preoperatively or tapered.**

B. **Adrenergic receptor subtypes** (Fig. 3-1).

1. **Alpha-1 postsynaptic receptors** mediate peripheral vasoconstriction (arterial plus venous), which is especially responsive to neurally released norepinephrine. Cardiac alpha-1 receptors cause positive inotropy while decreasing the heart rate.

2. **Alpha-2 receptors**

(a) **Presynaptic alpha-2 receptors** on nerve terminals decrease norepinephrine release by sympathetic nerve terminals. This negative feedback system conserves neuronal norepinephrine; high norepinephrine concentrations around the nerve terminal thus inhibit further norepinephrine release. Activation of **brain alpha-2** receptors (e.g., with clonidine) exerts an antihypertensive action by decreasing sympathetic nervous system activity and sedation.

(b) **Postsynaptic alpha-2 receptors** mediate constriction of vascular smooth muscle, like alpha-1 receptor response, but these receptors may not be innervated. Stimulating postsynaptic alpha-2 plus alpha-1 receptors simultaneously may cause more vasoconstriction than is produced by either type alone.

3. **Beta-1 postsynaptic receptors** activate the heart to increase heart rate (HR), contractility, atrioventricular node conduction, and automaticity; they also cause lipolysis and increased renin release.

4. **Beta-2 receptors**

(a) **Postsynaptic receptors** mediate peripheral vasodilation (especially skeletal muscle), potassium uptake, insulin release, gluconeogenesis, bronchodilatation, and uterine relaxation. These receptors also are present on cardiac muscle.

(b) **Presynaptic receptors** increase the release of norepinephrine from sympathetic nerve terminals.

5. **Dopaminergic receptors** mediate renal and mesenteric vasodilation, increase renal salt excretion, and reduce gastrointestinal motility.

III. **Beta-adrenergic blocking drugs**

A. **Actions.** These drugs cause competitive antagonism of beta-adrenergic receptors with the following cardiovascular effects:

β Blockers

HR	Decreased
Contractility	Decreased (LVEDP* rises)
BP	Decreased

*Left ventricular end-diastolic pressure.

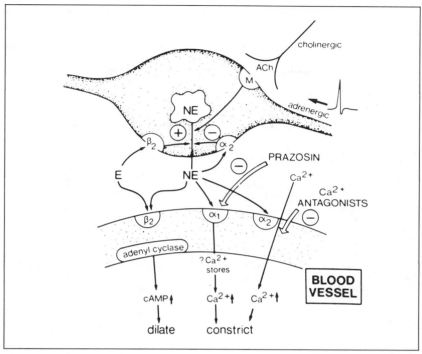

Fig. 3-1. Schematic representation of the adrenergic receptors present on the sympathetic nerve terminal and vascular smooth muscle cell. Norepinephrine (NE) is released by electrical depolarization of the nerve terminal; however, the quantity of NE released is *increased* by neuronal (presynaptic) beta-2-receptor or muscarinic-cholinergic stimulation and is *decreased* by activation of presynaptic alpha-2-receptors.

On the *postsynaptic* membrane, stimulation of alpha-1- or alpha-2-adrenergic receptors both cause vasoconstriction, whereas beta-2-receptor activation causes vasodilation. Prazosin is a selective alpha-1 antagonist drug. Note that NE does not stimulate beta-2-receptors, but epinephrine *(E)* does. (From L.H. Opie. Vasodilators and Vascular Smooth Muscle. In L.H. Opie [ed.], *The Heart.* Orlando: Grune & Stratton, 1984. P. 234. With permission.)

SVR†	Increased (unless drug has ISA‡)
Atrioventricular conduction	Decreased
Atrial refractory period	Increased
Automaticity	Decreased

B. Advantages. Beta-adrenergic blocking drugs
1. Reduce the myocardial oxygen consumption rate $M\dot{V}O_2$ (decrease HR and contractility).
2. Increase diastolic filling time, an important determinant of myocardial oxygen supply.
3. Show synergism with nitroglycerin for myocardial ischemia; blunt the reflex tachycardia and increased contractility caused by nitroglycerin or other vasodilator drugs.

†Systemic vascular resistance.
‡Intrinsic sympathomimetic activity.

4. Have an antidysrhythmic action, especially **atrial dysrhythmias;** also useful against catecholamine-induced ventricular dysrhythmias. Propranolol also possesses a nonspecific local anesthetic (i.e., quinidinelike or "membrane-stabilizing") action that may suppress dysrhythmias, especially at high doses.
5. Decrease left ventricular ejection velocity (useful in patients with septal hypertrophy or aortic dissection).
6. Have antihypertensive action.
7. To maintain beta blockade, continue drug PO (per os) dose preoperatively or give intravenously (IV) intraoperatively or postoperatively (for propranolol IV, use one-tenth PO dosage or less; see sec. III.E.2.)

C. **Disadvantages**
  1. Severe bradydysrhythmias.
  2. Heart block (first-, second-, or third-degree, especially if prior cardiac conduction abnormalities are present, or if IV β blockers **and** IV calcium channel blockers are co-administered).
  3. Bronchospasm.
  4. Congestive heart failure (CHF), which exacerbates preexisting failure.
  5. Masking of signs of hypoglycemia (except sweating).
  6. SVR increased due to inhibition of beta-2 vasodilation; use with care in patients with severe peripheral vascular disease.
  7. Coronary artery spasm through unopposed alpha vasoconstriction (only in susceptible patients).

D. **Distinguishing features of beta blockers.** See Table 3-1.
  1. **Selectivity (beta-1).** Selective β blockers possess a higher potency at beta-1 than at beta-2 receptors. They are less likely to cause bronchospasm or increased SVR than a nonselective drug. However, beta-2 antagonism is **not** eliminated, only reduced; selectivity is dose dependent (drugs lose selectivity at higher dosages). Great care must be exercised when an asthmatic patient receives **any** β blocker.
  2. **Intrinsic sympathomimetic activity.** These drugs possess "partial agonist" activity. Thus, drugs with intrinsic sympathomimetic activity (ISA) will **block** beta-receptors (preventing catecholamines from combining with a receptor) but will also cause mild **stimulation** of the same receptors. A patient receiving a drug with ISA would be expected to have a higher resting HR and cardiac output (CO) but show no change with exercise; also, lower SVR secondary to beta-2 stimulation would be expected, compared to a drug without ISA. Finally, the beta effects produced by a full agonist such as isoproterenol will be diminished in the presence of a β blocker with ISA because the latter will competitively inhibit the more potent full agonist from combining with beta receptors.
  3. **Duration of action.** In general, the β blockers with longer durations of action are eliminated by the kidneys, whereas propranolol and the 4–6 hour duration drugs undergo hepatic elimination. **Esmolol,** the ultra-short-acting β blocker (plasma half-life, 9 minutes), is eliminated within the blood by a red blood cell esterase. After abrupt discontinuation of esmolol infusion, most drug effects are eliminated within 5 minutes. The duration of esmolol is not affected when plasma pseudocholinesterase is inhibited by echothiophate or physostigmine.

E. **Clinical use**
  1. Always begin with a low dosage and increase slowly, titrating dosage to effect.
  2. For propranolol IV dosage use 0.5–1.0-mg increments every 2–5 minutes as needed while constantly monitoring ECG, pulmonary capillary wedge pressure (PCWP; if pulmonary artery [PA] catheter in place), BP, and lung sounds. IV dosage is **much smaller** than PO

Table 3-1. Beta-adrenergic blocking drugs

	Propranolol (Inderal)	Timolol (Blocadren)	Nadolol (Corgard)	Metoprolol (Lopressor)	Atenolol (Tenormin)	Pindolol (Visken)	Labetalol (Trandate)	Esmolol (Brevibloc)
Bioavailability[b]	33	75	20	50	55	>90	25	
Beta half-life[c]	3.5–6.0 hr	3–4 hr	14–24 hr	3–4 hr	6–9 hr	3–4 hr	3–8 hr	9 min
Elimination	H	H (80%) R (20%)	R (75%)	H	R (85%)	H (60%) R (40%)	H	Blood
Active metabolites	Yes	No	No	No	No	No	No	No
Beta-1 selectivity	No	No	No	Yes	Yes	No	No	Yes
ISA	No	No	No	No	No	Yes	No	No
Alpha antagonist	No	No	No	No	No	No	Yes	No
IV use	Yes	No	No	Yes	No	No	Yes	Yes
Relative PO potency[d]	1.0	6.0	1.0	1.0	1.0	6.0	0.3	
Initial PO dose (mg)[e]	10–20 bid–qid	5–15 qd–bid	40 qd	50 qd	50 qd	5 bid	100 bid	
Maximum PO dose (mg)[e]	80 qid	30 bid[f]	320 qd[f]	200 bid[f]	100 qd[f]	30 tid[f]	1200 bid	
Maximum usual IV dose (mg)[g]	4–8 in 0.5-to 1.0-mg increments	No	No	15 in 5-mg increments	No	No	20 load, then 40–80 q10min to max 300	0.25–0.5 mg/kg load, then 50–200 μg/kg/min

H = hepatic elimination; R = renal elimination.

[a]Timolol eye drops can produce systemic beta blockade.

[b]In percent after oral dose.

[c]Half-life may not be predictive of clinical duration of action.

[d]Ratio of potency when compared with propranolol: 1.0 indicates that drug is equipotent with propranolol.

[e]Usual dosages for adults.

[f]Decrease dosage in renal failure.

[g]IV doses must be given in small, divided doses with careful monitoring. Adult dosages are given.

Source: Modified from D. R. Larach, and W. A. Kofke. Cardiovascular Drugs. In W. A. Kofke and J. H. Levy (eds.), *Postoperative Critical Care Procedures of the Massachusetts General Hospital.* Boston: Little, Brown, 1986. p. 469. With permission.

dosage because first-pass hepatic extraction is bypassed. The usual maximum acute IV propranolol dose is about 0.1 mg/kg.

3. If β blockers **must** be given to a patient with bronchospastic disease, choose a selective beta-1 blocker such as metoprolol and consider concomitant administration of an inhalation beta-2 agonist (such as albuterol).

4. **Treatment of toxicity.** Beta agonists (e.g., isoproterenol, possibly in large doses) are the mainstay. Cardiac pacing, calcium, amrinone, or glucagon may be effective because these agents do not act via beta-receptors.

5. Assessment of beta blockage. If beta blockade is adequate clinically, a patient should not demonstrate an increase in HR with exercise (walking or climbing steps).

6. When agonist drugs with alpha or both alpha and beta actions are administered to patients who are beta-blocked, a greater elevation of BP can be expected owing to alpha vasoconstriction unopposed by beta-2 vasodilation. This may produce deleterious hemodynamic results (increased afterload with little increased cardiac inotropy). See dobutamine in sec. **IV.B.4** below.

7. **Esmolol** is a new selective β blocker with an ultra-short duration of action. Esmolol is given by IV injection (loading dose) followed by continuous infusion. It is of greatest use when the required duration of beta blockade is short (i.e., to attenuate a short-lived stimulus). Another useful application of esmolol is to determine how well a patient tolerates beta blockade. Should deleterious effects occur, they can be quickly reversed by stopping the infusion. Esmolol's ultra-short duration of action plus its beta-1 selectivity and lack of ISA make it a logical choice when it is necessary to administer a β blocker to patients with asthma, heart failure, or other relative contraindication.

8. **Labetalol** is a combined alpha and beta antagonist, which can achieve vasodilation without reflex tachycardia. Labetalol is useful for preoperative or postoperative control of hypertension. During anesthesia, its long duration of action makes it less useful for minute-to-minute control. However, a basal amount of labetalol will reduce the dosage of nitroprusside or other short-acting drug necessary to control the blood pressure.

IV. **Pressor and inotropic drugs**
  A. **Treatment of low cardiac output: summary of pharmacologic principles**
    1. **Goals:** to improve myocardial function and organ perfusion.
       a. Increase CO by increasing stroke volume (SV) to meet body demands.
       b. Increase myocardial oxygen supply (increase diastolic arterial pressure [DAP], decrease LVEDP, and increase diastolic perfusion time) while providing an adequate mean arterial pressure (MAP) for perfusion of other organs.
       c. Minimize myocardial oxygen demand: decrease HR and systolic wall stress (afterload, by appropriately lowering systolic arterial pressure [SAP] and left ventricular end-diastolic volume [LVEDV]), optimize contractility.
    2. **Therapy**
       a. Optimize preload.
       b. Reduce afterload (consistent with adequate BP).
       c. Increase cardiac inotropy (increase free ionized calcium level inside cell) by using one of the following methods:
          (1) Beta-1 adrenergic stimulation.

(2) Calcium salts.
(3) Digitalis.
(4) Phosphodiesterase inhibition (amrinone).
(5) Glucagon (rarely).
(6) Alpha-1- and beta-2-adrenergic stimulation (secondary).
d. Raise heart rate if bradycardia is present.
3. **Monitoring.** Inotropic drugs are used most effectively while monitoring the patient's beat-to-beat BP with an arterial line, cardiac filling pressures with a PA catheter, and CO by thermodilution. Once adequate preload has been obtained (PCWP or left atrial pressure), the inotropic drug dosage is titrated to CO and BP. If SVR is normal or elevated, addition of a vasodilator frequently improves CO. Frequent CO measurements (together with signs of adequate organ perfusion—kidney, brain, heart) are invaluable in permitting rational drug and dosage selection.
B. **Sympathomimetic drugs**
1. **Similarities**

Sympathomimetic Drugs
a. Beta-1-agonist effects

HR	Increased
Contractility	Increased
Conduction velocity	Increased throughout heart
AV block	Decreased
Automaticity	

b. All beta agonists share the following characteristics:
(1) Starling curve shifted up and to left (increased SV at same preload and afterload)
(2) Risk of myocardial ischemia
(3) Risk of dysrhythmias
(4) Risk of drug interactions
c. Most effective benefits occur if any hypovolemia is treated before or during therapy.
d. There is a risk of tissue damage or sloughing if the drug is injected outside of a vein. In general, drugs with alpha-agonist (vasoconstrictor) actions **should not be infused continuously through a peripheral IV** line because of the risk of extravasation or infiltration. Small doses of these drugs are sometimes given in bolus form through peripheral IV lines; this practice is acceptable provided that:
(1) No central venous catheter is available.
(2) The drug bolus is injected only into a **free-flowing** IV line.
(3) The IV site is observed closely during and after the injection.
e. **Diastolic ventricular dysfunction.** Cardiac beta-receptor activation hastens **relaxation** of the myocardium during diastole. Diastolic relaxation is an active, energy-consuming process that pumps free intracellular Ca^{2+} into storage sites. Abnormal relaxation may occur in ischemia or other myocardial disorders, leading to abnormal diastolic stiffness. Drug-induced reduction in diastolic stiffness (by reducing ischemia or activating beta-receptors) will lower LVEDP and LVEDV, improve diastolic filling, reduce left atrial (LA) pressures, and improve the myocardial oxygen supply-demand ratio.
f. **Systolic ventricular dysfunction.** More complete ventricular ejection during systole will reduce the LV end-**systolic** volume.

This shrinks heart size, reduces LV systolic wall tension (by LaPlace's law), and decreases myocardial oxygen consumption.

2. **Differences**
   a. Peripheral vascular effects (alpha, beta-2, dopaminergic receptor activity)
   b. Offset of action (i.e., monoamine oxidase [MAO], catecholamine-O-methyl transferase [COMT], neuronal uptake, tissue uptake)
   c. Tachycardia, induced reflex effects
   d. Direct versus indirect mechanism of action
      (1) **Direct** receptor agonist drugs
      (2) **Indirect-acting drugs** release stored neuronal norepinephrine. These drugs lose their effectiveness when body catecholamine stores become depleted, as is seen with long-term inotropic therapy with indirect-acting drugs, in patients with chronic CHF, and with reserpine or guanethidine use.
      (3) **Mixed direct and indirect** drugs act by a combination of (1) and (2).

3. **Drug interactions**
   a. **Interactions of MAO inhibitors**
      (1) Monoamine oxidase is an intraneuronal enzyme that inactivates (deaminates) norepinephrine, dopamine, and serotonin. The MAO inhibitors increase the concentrations of catecholamines in the neuron and around the receptors by reducing their breakdown. Administration of adrenergic agonists to patients with MAO-inhibition can produce a life-threatening hypertensive crisis. Because the enzyme is irreversibly inactivated by hydrazine-class drugs (phenelzine), 2-3 weeks optimally should elapse between discontinuing phenelzine and performing elective surgery. Return of function requires synthesis of new enzyme. Nonhydrazine MAO inhibitors (pargyline, tranylcypromine) are reversible but are also slow in offset.
      (2) The **greatest risk** of inducing a hyperadrenergic state occurs with the **indirect-acting drugs** such as **ephedrine, metaraminol,** and **amphetamine** because indirect sympathomimetics release the increased intraneuronal stores of norepinephrine that are normally rapidly metabolized by MAO. Because dopamine has an indirect action also, it should be used with extreme care in the MAO-inhibited patient, beginning with very low doses.
      (3) **Preferred drugs** are those with **purely direct activity:** epinephrine, norepinephrine, isoproterenol, phenylephrine, and dobutamine. When exogenously administered in titrated doses, the direct-acting drugs do not "flood" the intracellular MAO as with indirectly released norepinephrine. These drugs also may be more dependent on alternative metabolic pathways for degradation, In MAO-inhibited patients, all pressor drugs should be used cautiously, in small dosages with BP monitoring and observation of the ECG for dysrhythmias.
   b. **Reserpine interactions.** Reserpine depletes intraneuronal catecholamine stores. Thus, with chronic use, a "denervation hypersensitivity" state is induced (probably by postjunctional receptor up-regulation). Indirect-acting sympathomimetic drugs show **less** effect than usual because of depleted stores, whereas direct-acting or mixed-action sympathomimetic drugs may produce **exaggerated** responses because of receptor up-regulation. The best approach is to start with small dosages of direct-acting drugs while carefully monitoring BP.

c. **Tricyclic antidepressant or cocaine interactions.** These drugs (including the tetracyclic drugs) increase the concentration of catecholamine at receptors by **blocking the reuptake of catecholamines by the prejunctional neurons.** This reuptake mechanism is very important in the offset of action of catecholamines. Interactions between these drugs and sympathomimetic agents can be very severe and are frequently more intense than the widely feared MAO-inhibitor reactions. In general, if sympathomimetic drugs are required, small dosages of direct-acting agents with careful monitoring of BP and ECG are most effective.

d. **Treatment of hypertensive sympathomimetic interactions.** Approaches include the following:
   (1) Alpha blockade: phentolamine, labetalol, chlorpromazine
   (2) Direct vasodilation: nitroprusside, hydralazine, trimethaphan
   (3) Ganglionic blockade: trimethaphan

4. **Dobutamine** (Dobutrex)
   a. Dobutamine is a synthetic catecholamine.
   b. **Actions**
      (1) Direct beta-1 plus beta-2 agonist.
      (2) Alpha-1 receptors are also stimulated by dobutamine. On myocardial cells, alpha-1 activation increases contractility *without increasing heart rate.* On vascular cells, alpha-1 activation causes vasoconstriction. There is no alpha-2 effect.
      (3) On the **heart,** dobutamine appears to possess some selectivity for inotropy—the increase in myocardial contractility is greater than the rise in heart rate. Mechanisms include:
            (i) **Inotropy.** The beta-1 and alpha-1 actions are **additive** because both receptors stimulate myocardial contractility.
            (ii) **Heart rate.** The beta-1 and alpha-1 actions are **subadditive** because only beta-1 receptors induce tachycardia, whereas alpha-1 receptors cause either no change or tend to reduce the rate.
      (4) On the **vessels,** dobutamine is predominantly a **vasodilator** drug. Mechanisms for vasodilation include:
            (i) Beta-2 mediated vasodilation that is only partially counteracted by dobutamine's alpha-1 constrictor effects (a "physiologic antagonism"). The drug is devoid of alpha-2 receptor activity, which may limit its vasoconstrictor action.
            (ii) A major metabolite of dobutamine, (+)-3-O-methyldobutamine, is an alpha-1 *antagonist,* which could diminish the amount of alpha-1 mediated vasoconstriction ("pharmacologic antagonism"). Thus, as dobutamine is metabolized, the alpha-1 actions of the drug could diminish over time.
      (5) There is no dopaminergic agonist activity, unlike dopamine.

   Dobutamine

HR	Increased
Contractility	Increased
CO	Increased
BP	May increase, **decrease,** or remain unchanged
SVR	Decreased by dilating **all** vascular beds; slight increase may be seen only at low dosages (alpha)
PVR*	Decreased

*Pulmonary vascular resistance.

    c. Offset. Offset of action is achieved by metabolism by COMT and by conjugation with glucuronide in liver; an active metabolite is generated.

d. Advantages

    (1) Direct agonist only (unlike dopamine).

    (2) Cardiac contractility is increased by stimulating both alpha-1 and beta-1 receptors in the heart.

    (3) Less tachycardia than with isoproterenol or dopamine but only at low doses.

    (4) Potent vasodilator due to beta-2 action and lack of alpha-2 mediated vasoconstriction.

    (5) Peripheral vascular effects are similar to those of isoproterenol, or a combination of dopamine plus nitroprusside: decreased SVR → decreased left ventricular (LV) afterload → increased SV. However, unless the increase in CO outweighs the magnitude of decrease in SVR, BP **falls.** This is true because BP = CO × SVR.

    (6) Heart size decreases owing to improved systolic and diastolic function. This characteristic may improve myocardial oxygen demand-supply ratio, possibly lessening ischemia.

    (7) Renal blood flow **may** increase (due to a beta-2 effect, not because of selective dopaminergic receptor agonism).

    (8) There is no MAO metabolism (probably a good choice for MAO-inhibited patients).

    (9) PVR is decreased (may be beneficial for patients with right ventricular failure).

e. Disadvantages

    (1) Tachycardia and dysrhythmias occur; they are dose-related and often severe at high doses.

    (2) Hypotension may occur; **dobutamine is an inotrope but is not necessarily a pressor.**

    (3) Coronary steal similar to that occurring with isoproterenol is possible, leading to ischemia.

    (4) The drug is a nonselective vasodilator: Blood flow may be shunted from kidney and splanchnic bed to skeletal muscle in some circumstances.

    (5) No dopaminergic renal vasodilation occurs.

    (6) Tachyphylaxis has been reported after prolonged (more than 72 hours) use. This might be related to the alpha-blocking metabolite of dobutamine.

f. Indications. Low CO states (cardiogenic shock), especially with increased SVR or PVR.

g. Administration. IV only (central line is preferable, but dobutamine has little vasoconstrictor activity, making peripheral use less risky).

h. Clinical use

    (1) **Dobutamine dose:** IV infusion, 2–20 μg/kg/min. Some patients may respond to initial doses as low as 0.5 μg/kg/min, and at such low doses heart rate does not usually rise.

    (2) Usually mix 250 mg in 250 ml of IV solution (1000 μg/ml).

    (3) Dobutamine has about half the inotropic potency of dopamine.

    (4) Unless neuronal norepinephrine stores are depleted, dobutamine may not be superior to a combination of dopamine plus nitroprusside.

    (5) Dobutamine increases CO with a lesser increment in myocardial oxygen consumption and higher coronary blood flow compared with dopamine as a single drug. This effect is explained by the vasodilating action of dobutamine. Patients with coro-

nary artery disease may benefit; however, addition of nitro-glycerin or nitroprusside to dopamine may be equally effective.

(6) Dobutamine acts similar to a fixed-ratio combination of an **inotropic** drug and a **vasodilator** drug. These two components cannot be titrated separately.

(7) When dobutamine is given to beta-blocked patients, SVR may increase. Invasive hemodynamic monitoring is required to ascertain the drug's effect on CO and SVR.

5. **Dopamine** (Intropin)
   a. Dopamine is a catecholamine precursor to norepinephrine and epinephrine in nerve terminals and the adrenal medulla (also a central neurotransmitter).
   b. **Actions**
      (1) **Direct action:** alpha (alpha-2 effect possibly is greater than alpha-1), beta-1, beta-2, and dopaminergic agonist.
      (2) **Indirect action:** induces release of stored norepinephrine from nerve terminals.
      (3) Dose response (approximate)

Dopamine **Dose (μg/ kg/min)**	**Receptor-activated**	**Effect**
1–3	Dopaminergic	Increased renal and mesenteric blood flow
3–10	Beta-1 + beta-2 (plus dopaminergic)	Increased HR, contractility, and CO; decreased SVR; PVR may rise; alpha vasoconstriction begins to appear
>10	Alpha (plus beta plus dopaminergic)	Increased SVR, PVR; decreased renal blood flow; increased HR, dysrhythmias. Increased afterload may decrease CO

   c. **Offset** is achieved by uptake by nerve terminals plus metabolism by MAO and COMT. Small quantities of dopamine can be metabolized to norepinephrine in nerve terminals.
   d. **Advantages**
      (1) Increased renal perfusion and urine output at low to moderate dosages (partially due to a specific dopaminergic agonist effect, not blocked by propranolol).
      (2) Less tachycardia than with isoproterenol.
      (3) More "selective" vasodilator than isoproterenol. Blood flow shifts from skeletal muscle to kidney and splanchnic beds.
      (4) Blood pressure response is easy to titrate because of its mixed inotropic and vasoconstrictor properties.
   e. **Disadvantages**
      (1) There is a significant indirect-acting component; response can diminish when neuronal catecholamines are depleted (e.g., in patients with chronic CHF, during reserpine treatment).
      (2) Tachycardia, dysrhythmias (atrial plus ventricular) may occur.
      (3) There is a less potent inotropic effect than with epinephrine or isoproterenol.
      (4) Skin necrosis may result if extravasation occurs.
      (5) Renal vasodilating effects are overridden by alpha-mediated vasoconstriction at high dosages (>10 μg/kg/min) with risk of renal, splanchnic, and skin necrosis. Monitor urine output.

(6) Pulmonary vasoconstriction is possible (due to alpha effect on pulmonary vasculature).

(7) Systemic vasodilation occurs at low dosages. Blood pressure may decrease (afterload reduction may be beneficial).

(8) Drug may reduce respiratory drive in spontaneously ventilating patients.

f. Indications

(1) Hypotension due to low CO or low SVR.

(2) Renal failure or insufficiency.

(3) Temporary therapy of hypovolemia until circulating blood volume is restored.

g. Administration: IV only (by central line)

h. Clinical use

(1) **Dopamine dose:** IV, 1–20 μg/kg/min.

(2) Usually mix 200 mg in 250-ml IV solution (800 μg/ml).

(3) Good first choice for treating hypotension temporarily until intravascular volume can be expanded, or until a specific diagnosis can be made.

(4) Correct hypovolemia if possible before use (as with all pressors).

(5) Switch to or add another drug (preferably a direct-acting agonist such as epinephrine or amrinone) if inotropic response is not adequate at doses of 10–20 μg/kg/min.

(6) Add a vasodilator (e.g., nitroprusside) to counteract vasoconstrictor effects if afterload reduction would be beneficial. Invasive monitoring for measurement of CO and SVR is needed for rational selection of inotrope and vasodilator dosages. For example, a patient with a normal BP may have a low CO and a high SVR and might benefit from a vasodilator and an inotrope.

6. Ephedrine

a. Ephedrine is a plant-derived noncatecholamine

b. Actions

(1) Mild direct alpha plus beta-1 plus beta-2 agonist actions

(2) Important indirect norepinephrine release from neurons

Ephedrine

HR	Small increase
Contractility	Increased
CO	Increased
BP	Increased
SVR	Small increase
Preload	Increased (venoconstriction effect)

c. Offset. 5–10 minutes IV; no metabolism by MAO or COMT; renal elimination

d. Advantages

(1) Mild pressor and inotrope

(2) Short duration IV (3–10 minutes); lasts about 1 hour IM

(3) Generally little tachycardia (prior atropine administration may potentiate HR rise)

(4) No uterine vasoconstriction—safe in pregnancy

e. Disadvantages

(1) There is a blunted effect if norepinephrine stores are depleted

(2) There is a high risk of MAO inhibitor interaction because endogenous norepinephrine is released

(3) Tachyphylaxis with repeated doses may occur

f. Indications

(1) Hypotension due to low SVR or low CO, especially if heart rate is low

(2) Temporary therapy of hypovolemia until circulating blood volume is restored

(3) Hypotension due to regional anesthesia (spinal or epidural)

(4) Transient myocardial depression (anesthetic overdose)

g. **Administration:** IV, IM, SQ, PO

h. **Clinical use**

    (1) **Ephedrine dose.** IV: 2.5–5.0 mg bolus, repeat or increase as needed; IM: 25–50 mg

    (2) Ephedrine is conveniently mixed in a syringe (5–10 mg/ml) and can be given as an IV bolus into a freely running IV line.

    (3) Ephedrine is a useful, quickly acting, titratable IV pressor that can be administered in bolus form when no central line is available for drug infusion (e.g., dopamine).

7. **Epinephrine** (Adrenalin)

a. Epinephrine is a catecholamine produced by the adrenal medulla.

b. **Actions**

    (1) Direct agonist at alpha-1, alpha-2, beta-1, and beta-2 receptors

    (2) Dose response (adult, approximate)

Epinephrine

Dose (µg/min)	Receptors activated	SVR
1–2	Beta	May decrease
2–10	Beta and alpha	Variable
>10	Alpha and beta	Increased

    (3) Increased contractility and HR with all dosages, but SVR may decrease, remain unchanged, or rise dramatically depending on the dosage. Cardiac output usually rises, but at high dosages, peripheral alpha stimulation may cause a lowered SV due to high afterload.

c. **Offset** occurs by uptake by neurons and tissue and by metabolism by MAO and COMT (rapid).

d. **Advantages**

    (1) This drug is direct acting; its effect is not dependent on release of endogenous norepinephrine.

    (2) Potent alpha and beta stimulation results; it may have greater maximal effects than dopamine or dobutamine.

    (3) It is a powerful inotrope with variable (and adjustable) alpha effect.

    (4) If BP rises, tachycardia may be diminished due to reflex vagal stimulation (alpha effect).

    (5) It is a most effective bronchodilator and mast cell stabilizer; useful for primary therapy of severe bronchospasm or anaphylaxis.

    (6) If diastolic BP rises and heart size decreases, myocardial ischemia may be reduced. However, as with any inotropic drug, production of myocardial ischemia is possible.

e. **Disadvantages**

    (1) Tachycardia and dysrhythmia may occur.

    (2) Organ ischemia secondary to vasoconstriction, especially kidney and skin, may result; this may be counteracted by a vasodilator and is dose related. Urine output must be monitored with a urinary catheter.

    (3) Pulmonary vasoconstriction may occur, which can produce pulmonary hypertension and possibly right ventricular failure (addition of a vasodilator may reverse this).

(4) There is a risk of myocardial ischemia. Positive inotropy and tachycardia increase myocardial oxygen demand and reduce oxygen supply.

(5) Skin infiltration can cause necrosis (as with any potent alpha agonist); thus, a central line is preferable.

f. Indications

(1) Cardiac arrest (especially asystole or ventricular fibrillation); electromechanical dissociation. Primary mechanism is thought to be increased coronary perfusion pressure during cardiopulmonary resuscitation.

(2) Anaphylaxis and other systemic allergic reactions; epinephrine is the **agent of choice.**

(3) Cardiogenic shock, especially if a vasodilator is added.

(4) Bronchospasm.

g. Administration: IV (by **central line**); via endotracheal tube (rapidly absorbed by tracheal mucosa); SQ

h. Clinical use

(1) **Epinephrine dose**

(a) **SQ:** 10 μg/kg (maximum of 400 μg or 0.4 ml 1:1000) for treatment of mild to moderate allergic reactions or bronchospasm

(b) **IV**

(i) **Low-to-moderate dose** (for shock, hypotension): 2–8 μg bolus (IV), then infusion at 1–16 μg/min; pediatric, 0.05–0.50 μg/kg/min.

(ii) **High dose** (for cardiac arrest, resuscitation): 0.5–1.0 mg IV bolus; pediatric, 5-15 μg/kg (may be given intratracheally in 1–10-ml volume). One mg epinephrine is 1 ml of 1:1000, or 10 ml of 1:10,000.

(iii) *Warning!* **With high-dose IV epinephrine extreme hypertension with stroke or myocardial ischemia may be produced. A starting dose of more than 10 μg epinephrine IV bolus should not be given to a patient except in extremis!** To facilitate low-dose administration, epinephrine is best diluted (3 mg/250 ml, or 12 μg/ml) and drawn into a 3-ml syringe before it is needed.

(2) Watch for signs of excessive vasoconstriction: Monitor SVR, urine output, extremity perfusion. Addition of a vasodilator may help maintain organ perfusion.

(3) This drug is often used together with a vasodilator drug.

(4) Addition of a vasodilator (e.g., nitroprusside) to epinephrine will counteract the alpha vasoconstriction, leaving positive cardiac inotropy. For example, the epinephrine dosage can be titrated to CO and HR while the nitroprusside dosage is titrated to SVR.

(5) Consider concomitant use of intraaortic balloon pump to improve myocardial oxygen supply-demand ratio if myocardial ischemia occurs.

8. Isoproterenol (Isuprel)

a. Isoproterenol is a synthetic catecholamine.

b. Actions

(1) Direct beta-1 plus beta-2 agonist

(2) No alpha effects

Isoproterenol

HR	Marked increase (direct + reflex effect)
Contractility	Increased

CO	Increased
BP	Frequently decreased
SVR	Markedly decreased; all vascular beds dilated; dose related

c. Offset. Rapid; uptake by liver, conjugated, 60% excreted unchanged; metabolized by MAO, COMT.

d. Advantages

(1) Isoproterenol is a direct beta-receptor agonist.

(2) It is the most potent beta agonist per microgram.

(3) It increases CO by three mechanisms:

(a) Increased HR

(b) Increased contractility → increased SV

(c) Reduced afterload (SVR) → increased SV

(4) It is a bronchodilator (IV or inhaled)

(5) It is a pulmonary vasodilator (reduces PVR unless hypoxemia, hypercapnia, or acidosis is present)

e. Disadvantages

(1) **It is not a pressor!** Blood pressure often falls (beta-2 effect) while CO rises.

(2) Hypotension may produce organ hypoperfusion and ischemia.

(3) Myocardial ischemia may occur. Isoproterenol is a poor drug for patients with coronary artery disease because the combination of tachycardia, positive inotropy, and hypotension often worsens myocardial oxygen supply-demand mismatch.

(4) Tachycardia is associated.

(5) Dysrhythmias occur.

(6) Coronary steal is possible. Nonselective coronary vasodilation can overcome autoregulation, thereby reducing blood flow to ischemic regions of myocardium while flow to nonischemic areas increases.

(7) May unmask preexcitation in patients with an accessory atrioventricular conduction pathway (e.g., Wolff-Parkinson-White [WPW] syndrome).

(8) Dilates all vascular beds and is capable of shunting blood away from critical organs toward muscle, skin, and so on.

f. Indications

(1) Bradycardia unresponsive to atropine, if pacing is not immediately available.

(2) Low CO, especially for situations in which increased inotropy is needed and tachycardia is not detrimental, such as:

(a) Pediatric patients with fixed SV.

(b) After resection of ventricular aneurysm (small fixed SV).

(c) Denervated heart (after cardiac transplantation).

(3) Pulmonary hypertension or right heart failure.

(4) Atrioventricular block: Use as temporary therapy to decrease block or increase rate of idioventricular foci until pacing can be instituted. Use with caution in second-degree Mobitz type II heart block because this block may increase in degree with isoproterenol.

(5) Status asthmaticus: Intravenous use mandates continuous ECG and BP monitoring.

(6) β blocker overdose.

(7) **Important:** Isoproterenol should **not** be utilized for therapy of **cardiac asystole.** CPR with epinephrine or pacing is the therapy of choice because isoproterenol-induced vasodilation results in reduced carotid and coronary blood flow during CPR.

    g. Administration: IV (safe through peripheral line, will not necrose skin); PO

    h. Clinical use

        (1) Isoproterenol dose. Usual starting dose (IV infusion) is 0.05 μg/kg/min. Usual dose range:

            (a) Adults: 0.5–20.0 μg/min.

            (b) Children: 0.05–0.50 μg/kg/min.

        (2) Usually mix 1–2 mg in 250 ml IV solution (4–8 μg/ml).

        (3) Drug can be mixed with epinephrine for additive beta with less alpha stimulation than with epinephrine alone

9. Metaraminol (Aramine)

    a. Metaraminol is a synthetic noncatecholamine.

    b. Actions

        (1) Direct alpha-1 and alpha-2 agonist with some beta activity.

        (2) Indirect norepinephrine release from nerve terminals (activating alpha-1, alpha-2, and beta-1 receptors).

        (3) Actions similar to those of norepinephrine.

Metaraminol

HR	Small increase or decrease
Contractility	Increased
CO	May decrease (due to increased SVR)
BP	Increased
SVR	Markedly increased

    c. Offset is slow (90-minute duration IM) and is terminated by tissue uptake. There is little metabolism by MAO or COMT.

    d. Advantages

        (1) Pronounced increase in SVR in low peripheral resistance states.

        (2) Reflex lowering of HR if BP rises.

    e. Disadvantages

        (1) Preserved cerebral and coronary blood flow at expense of all other organs; may produce renal, splanchnic, or skin necrosis.

        (2) Increased PVR.

        (3) Reduced potency with depletion of norepinephrine stores.

        (4) Action as a **false transmitter** in sympathetic nerve terminals. Metaraminol is taken up by the nerve terminal and stored in place of norepinephrine. Subsequent nerve depolarization causes release of metaraminol, which is **much less potent** than norepinephrine. This is the mechanism producing **tachyphylaxis,** which is seen after several hours of use. Also, sudden discontinuation of long-term metaraminol therapy can result in **profound hypotension** that persists until new norepinephrine is synthesized by nerves. Although no pressor or inotrope should be stopped abruptly, metaraminol in particular must be **tapered slowly.**

        (5) Interaction with MAO inhibitors (releases stored norepinephrine).

        (6) Possibly diminished pressor effect with concomitant tricyclic antidepressant administration. Because metaraminol must be taken up into the nerve terminal, uptake is blocked by tricyclic drugs.

        (7) Some beta-1 effect occurs, which can cause myocardial ischemia or dysrhythmias.

    f. Indications for use

        (1) Hypotension due to low SVR, such as sepsis, vasodilator excess, regional anesthesia.

        (2) Temporary therapy of hypovolemia until circulating blood volume is restored.

g. **Administration:** IV, SQ, IM

h. **Clinical use**

(1) Metaraminol **dose** (usual)

(a) IV infusion: 20–500 µg/min

(b) IV bolus: 100–500 µg

(c) IM and SQ: 1–10 mg

(2) Usually mix 100 mg in 250 ml (400 µg/ml).

(3) Metaraminol is useful in low SVR states that are not responsive to a pure alpha-1 agonist (e.g., phenylephrine). This response may be explained by the combined direct and indirect activation of alpha-1 and alpha-2 receptors by metaraminol, causing greater vasoconstriction.

10. **Methoxamine** (Vasoxyl)

a. Methoxamine is a synthetic noncatecholamine.

b. **Actions.** The drug is a direct alpha-1 agonist, devoid of beta effect.

c. **Offset.** There is a longer duration of action than with phenylephrine (1.0–1.5 hours IM) and no metabolism by MAO or COMT.

d. **Indications for use**

(1) **Hypotension** due to low SVR states: sepsis, regional anesthesia.

(2) Temporary therapy of hypovolemia until circulating blood volume is restored.

e. **Clinical use**

(1) **Methoxamine dose** (adult): IV, 1–5 mg slow bolus: IM, 10–20 mg.

(2) The long duration of action of methoxamine makes it difficult to titrate the dosage to rapidly changing hemodynamic conditions. Phenylephrine often is more useful.

11. **Norepinephrine** (noradrenaline, Levophed)

a. Norepinephrine is the primary physiologic postganglionic sympathetic neurotransmitter; it is also released by adrenal medulla.

b. **Actions**

(1) Direct alpha-1 and alpha-2 actions and beta-1 agonist action.

(2) Virtually **no** beta-2 (vasodilator) effect.

Norepinephrine

HR	Variable; unchanged or may ↓ if BP rises and causes reflex vagotonia; increases if BP remains low
Contractility	Increased
CO	Increase or decrease (depends on SVR)
BP	Increased
SVR	Markedly increased; vasoconstriction unopposed by any beta-2 vasodilation (compared with dopamine or epinephrine)
PVR	Increased
Preload	Increased (due to venoconstriction)

(3) Stroke volume and CO may increase or decrease (markedly elevated SVR and BP reduces ejection fraction), but **BP usually rises.**

c. **Offset** is by neural uptake and metabolism by MAO and COMT (rapid).

d. **Advantages**

(1) Direct adrenergic agonist.

(2) Redistributes perfusion to brain and heart because all other vascular beds are constricted.

(3) Elicits maximal alpha-1 and alpha-2 vasoconstriction; may be effective when phenylephrine (alpha-1 only) is not.

e. Disadvantages
  (1) Reduced organ perfusion: risk of ischemia of kidney, skin, liver, bowel.
  (2) Myocardial ischemia possible; increased afterload, HR, contractility.
  (3) Pulmonary vasoconstriction.
  (4) Dysrhythmias.
  (5) High risk of skin necrosis with subcutaneous extravasation.
f. Indications for use
  (1) Peripheral vascular collapse when it is necessary to increase SVR (e.g., septic shock); temporary therapy only because of risk of organ ischemia.
  (2) Conditions in which a rise in SVR is desired together with cardiac stimulation.
g. Administration: IV only, by central line only.
h. Clinical use
  (1) Usual **norepinephrine** starting infusion doses: IV, 1–2 μg/min (adult); usual range, 0.05–0.30 μg/kg/min.
  (2) Usually mix 3 mg in 250 ml IV solution (12 μg/ml).
  (3) Minimize duration of use; follow urine output closely with urinary catheter.
  (4) Drug can be used with vasodilator (nitroprusside) to counteract alpha stimulation while leaving beta-1 stimulation intact; this will also improve CO by providing afterload reduction. However, if intense vasoconstriction is **not** required, a different drug should generally be used.
  (5) For treating severe right ventricular failure, the simultaneous infusion of norepinephrine into the *left atrium* (through a surgical left atrial catheter) plus the pulmonary vasodilator **prostaglandin E$_1$** (PGE$_1$) into the *right atrium* has proved beneficial in some patients (D'Ambra et al., 1985). The LA norepinephrine reaches the systemic vascular bed first and reduces the systemic vasodilation of PGE$_1$. Much of the LA norepinephrine is metabolized peripherally before it reaches the lung.
12. Phenylephrine (Neo-Synephrine)
  a. Phenylephrine is a synthetic noncatecholamine.
  b. Actions
    (1) The drug is a direct alpha-1 agonist.
    (2) It has no clinically apparent beta effects although some laboratory studies show a small degree of beta stimulation.
    (3) It causes vasoconstriction, arteriolar and venous.

  Phenylephrine

HR	Decreased (reflex, caused by BP elevation)
Contractility	Minimal increase
CO	Decreased (increased afterload reduces SV) or no change
BP	Markedly increased
SVR	Markedly increased
Preload	Small increase (venoconstriction increases venous return to heart)

  c. Offset occurs by rapid metabolism by MAO; there is no COMT metabolism.
  d. Advantages
    (1) Phenylephrine is a direct agonist with a short duration (less than 5 minutes).
    (2) It is a reliable vasopressor.

(3) When used during hypotension, phenylephrine will increase coronary perfusion pressure without increasing myocardial contractility. If *hyper*tension is avoided, myocardial oxygen consumption does not rise substantially. If contractility depressed due to ischemia, drug may cause **rise** in CO.

(4) It increases perfusion pressure for the brain, kidney, and heart in the presence of low SVR states.

(5) It is useful for correcting hypotension in patients with coronary artery disease **without** significant CHF.

(6) For patients with supraventricular tachycardia, reflex vagal stimulation in response to increased BP may terminate the dysrhythmia; phenylephrine treats both the hypotension and the dysrhythmia.

(7) It restores SVR after functional sympathectomy during spinal or epidural anesthesia.

(8) It increases SVR during cardiopulmonary bypass.

(9) Can reduce right-to-left shunt during acute cyanotic spells in Tetralogy of Fallot.

e. Disadvantages

(1) Phenylephrine decreases SV secondary to increased afterload **unless** restoration of coronary perfusion pressure has removed myocardial ischemia.

(2) It increases PVR.

(3) It decreases renal and other organ perfusion; urine output, limb perfusion must be monitored.

(4) Bradycardia can occur, primarily as reflex response to hypertension; usually not severe, frequently desirable (responds to atropine).

(5) In rare, susceptible patients, alpha agonists may induce coronary artery spasm, which may be counteracted by nitrates.

f. Indications for use

(1) Hypotension due to peripheral vasodilation, low SVR states (e.g., septic shock, vasodilator excess).

(2) Temporary therapy of hypovolemia until blood volume is restored.

(3) Supraventricular tachycardia (SVT).

g. Administration: IV infusion (central line preferable) or IV bolus

h. Clinical use

(1) **Phenylephrine dose**

    (a) IV infusion: 10–500 μg/min

    (b) IV bolus: 50–200 μg, increased as needed (some patients with peripheral vascular collapse may require 1000–2000 μg bolus injections to raise SVR)

    (c) Pediatric:; 1 μg/kg bolus

(2) Mixing

    (a) IV infusion: Usually mix 30 mg in 250 ml IV fluid (120 μg/ml)

    (b) IV bolus: Dilute 10 mg in 10 ml IV solution (1 mg/ml = 1000 μg/ml). When placed in a tuberculin syringe, 100-μg boluses are easily administered (0.1 ml).

    (c) Pediatric: Dilute to 0.1 mg/ml so that 0.1 ml = 10 μg.

(3) Nitroglycerin may be added to reduce preload while maintaining arterial BP with phenylephrine. This combination may maximize myocardial oxygen supply while minimizing increases in myocardial oxygen consumption.

(4) Phenylephrine can reduce the vasodilation and hypotension caused by calcium channel blocking drugs such as verapamil.

(5) Phenylephrine is the vasopressor of choice for short-term use in most patients with coronary artery disease or aortic stenosis without severe CHF (see sec. **IV.B.12.d.3** above).

C. Nonsympathomimetic inotropic drugs

1. Amrinone (Inocor)

a. Amrinone is a bipyridine derivative unrelated to known sympathomimetic or other inotropic drugs. It inhibits the enzyme subtype phosphodiesterase-III, causing elevation of cyclic AMP in cardiac muscle (positive inotropy) and vascular smooth muscle (vasodilation).

b. **Actions**

Amrinone

HR   Little change; increased at higher doses
SVR   Decreased
CO   Increased

c. **Offset** occurs by hepatic conjugation and excretion; elimination half-life is 5–8 hours in patients with severe CHF.

d. **Advantages**
   (1) Amrinone demonstrates both inotropic and vasodilator properties, which are both useful in patients with CHF.
   (2) It does not product tachycardia.
   (3) Its inotropic effect is **not** mediated by beta-receptors; retains its effectiveness in beta-blocked patients.
   (4) It may be used in combination with beta-agonist inotropic drugs.

e. **Disadvantages.** Thrombocytopenia may occur after variable duration of therapy (usually more than 24 hours).

f. **Indication for use.** Short-term therapy of severe heart failure, especially when not responsive to conventional therapy.

g. **Administration:** IV infusion only. Do not mix in dextrose-containing solutions. Usually mix 100 mg in 250 ml of normal saline (400 μg/ml). Also may be infused undiluted with syringe pump.

h. **Clinical use**
   (1) Amrinone loading dose: 0.75 mg/kg; may be repeated in 30 minutes.
   (2) Maintenance infusion: 5–20 μg/kg/min.
   (3) Maximal daily dose: 10 mg/kg/day.
   (4) Be prepared for significant vasodilation after loading dose administration. During cardiac surgery, when possible give loading dose *during* cardiopulmonary bypass to maintain blood pressure (may increase loading dose to 1.0–1.5 mg/kg owing to pump circuit dilution).
   (5) May be added to sympathomimetic inotropic drugs.
   (6) Coadministration with disopyramide may cause severe hypotension and should be avoided.

2. Calcium

a. Calcium is an inorganic substance that is physiologically active only as the calcium ion (Ca^{+2}).
   (1) Normally, about 50% of the total plasma calcium is bound to proteins and anions, whereas about 50% remains free as Ca^{2+} and can participate in biologic processes.
   (2) **Factors affecting ionized calcium**
       (a) Alkalosis (metabolic or respiratory) decreases Ca^{2+}.
       (b) Acidosis increases Ca^{2+}.
       (c) Citrate binds (chelates) calcium, causing a reduction in *total* as well as *ionized* calcium concentrations in plasma.
   (3) **Normal plasma concentration:** Ionized calcium = 1.0–1.3 mM/liter.

b. Actions
Calcium

HR	No change or decrease (vagal effect)
Contractility	Increase
BP	Increase
SVR	Variable, often increases
Preload	Little change
CO	Increase

c. Offset. Calcium is incorporated into muscle, bone, and other tissues.

d. Advantages
(1) Calcium causes positive cardiac inotropy without inducing tachycardia.
(2) It has rapid action with a duration of about 10–15 minutes (7 mg/kg dose)
(3) Reversal of myocardial depression, which is caused by the following conditions:
    (a) Halogenated anesthetics
    (b) Calcium-blocking drugs (CBDs)
    (c) Hypocalcemia
    (d) Cardiopulmonary bypass (administer only **after** heart has been well reperfused)
    (e) Beta blockers (watch for bradycardia!)
(4) It reverses cardiac toxicity characteristic of **hyperkalemia** (e.g., dysrhythmias, heart block, and negative inotropy).

e. Disadvantages
(1) Calcium potentiates the effect of digitalis; it can provoke digitalis toxicity in patients who are therapeutically digitalized. This toxicity can present as ventricular dysrhythmias, atrioventricular block, or asystole. Ventricular fibrillation refractory to cardioversion can be precipitated.
(2) Calcium potentiates the effects of hypokalemia on the heart (dysrhythmias).
(3) Severe bradycardia is possible but uncommon; the vagal mechanism is seen most frequently in children.
(4) When extracellular calcium concentration is increased while the surrounding myocardium is being reperfused or is undergoing ongoing ischemia, increased cellular damage or cell death occurs.

f. Indications for use
(1) Hypocalcemia
(2) Hyperkalemia (to reverse atrioventricular block or myocardial depression)
(3) Hypotension due to decreased myocardial contractility
(4) Anesthetic overdose
(5) Increased Mg^{2+} plasma levels

g. Administration
(1) Calcium chloride: IV, preferably by central line (causes vein inflammation and sclerosis).
(2) Calcium gluconate: IV, by peripheral or central line.

h. Clinical use
(1) **Calcium dose**
    (a) Calcium chloride: adult, 250–1000 mg slow IV; pediatric, 10–20 mg/kg slow IV.
    (b) Calcium gluconate: 30–60 mg/kg slow IV.
(2) During **massive blood transfusion** (more than 1 blood volume replaced), a patient receives a large load of **citrate,** which binds calcium. In normal situations, hepatic metabolism quickly

eliminates citrate from plasma, and hypocalcemia does not occur. However, in the presence of hypothermia, shock, positive pressure ventilation, or alpha-agonist therapy, hepatic extraction may be decreased with resultant **severe hypocalcemia** (also, reduced bone perfusion decreases bone Ca^{2+} release). Under these conditions, administration of calcium salts may be necessary. Ionized calcium levels should be followed frequently to guide therapy.

(3) Some critically ill patients with low CO may require very high doses of calcium chloride (up to 1.5 mg/kg/min) to raise Ca^{2+} levels to normal.

(4) Calcium was formerly used to treat asystole, but there is **no evidence** that calcium has any beneficial effect on asystole. It is **not recommended** for treating asystole or electromechanical dissociation unless hypocalcemia or hyperkalemia may be present.

(5) Calcium should be used with care in situations in which ongoing myocardial ischemia may be occurring or during reperfusion of ischemic tissue. "Routine" administration of calcium to all patients at the end of cardiopulmonary bypass for coronary revascularization is best avoided, especially if the heart has been reperfused only minutes earlier.

3. **Digoxin** (Lanoxin)
   a. Digoxin is one of many glycosides derived from the foxglove plant.
   b. **Actions**
      (1) **Mechanism of action.** Digoxin inhibits membrane sodium-potassium ATPase, causing Na^+ accumulation in cells, leading to increased intracellular ionized calcium, which leads to increased Ca^{2+} release from the sarcoplasmic reticulum into the cytoplasm with each heartbeat, thus causing increased myocardial contractility
      (2) **Hemodynamic effects**

Digitalis	
Contractility	Increase
Myocardial oxygen consumption rate ($M\dot{V}O_2$)	Increase (in nonfailing heart)
Atrioventricular conduction	Decrease (nonlinear dose response: may need near toxic levels to achieve a change in conduction, especially in patients with high sympathetic tone)
Ventricular automaticity	Increase ($\uparrow$ rate of phase 4 depolarization)
Refractory period	Decrease (in atria and ventricles); increase in atrioventricular node

      (2) Digitalis hemodynamics in CHF

HR	Decrease
SV	Increase
SVR	Decrease
$M\dot{V}O_2$	Decrease

   c. **Offset.** Digoxin elimination half-life is 1.7 days; it is handled by renal elimination. In anephric patients, elimination half-life is more than 4 days.

d. Advantages

  (1) Supraventricular antidysrhythmic action.

  (2) Reduced ventricular rate in atrial fibrillation or flutter.

  (3) Improved ventricular function in chronic CHF; digitalis currently is the only positive inotropic drug that is given orally.

e. Disadvantages

  (1) Digoxin has an extremely **low therapeutic index;** 20% of patients show toxicity at some time.

  (2) Increased MVO_2 and SVR occur in patients without CHF.

  (3) The drug has a long half-life, and it is difficult to titrate dosage; toxicity is long-lived.

  (4) There is large interindividual variation in therapeutic and toxic serum levels and dosages; need to correlate levels with clinical signs.

  (5) Toxic manifestations are life-threatening, and toxicity is difficult to diagnose; digoxin can produce virtually any dysrhythmia. For example, digitalis is useful in treating SVT, but digitalis toxicity can also cause SVT.

  (6) Avoid in patients with tachycardia and wide QRS complexes in the **Wolff-Parkinson-White syndrome; conduction in the accessory atrioventricular pathway may be accelerated** in these patients, so atrial fibrillation may rapidly induce ventricular fibrillation. Beta blockers, procainamide, quinidine, or disopyramide is preferred for use in this disorder.

f. Indications for use

  (1) Atrial fibrillation with rapid ventricular rate, especially in patients with CHF.

  (2) Supraventricular tachydysrhythmias (except in patients with Wolff-Parkinson-White syndrome who demonstrate anterograde conduction through the accessory atrioventricular pathway)

  (3) Chronic ventricular contractile dysfunction.

g. Administration: IV, IM PO

h. Clinical use (general guidelines only)

  (1) Digoxin dose (assuming normal renal function; decrease maintenance dosages with renal insufficiency)

    (a) Adult. Loading dose IV and IM, 0.25- to 0.50-mg increments (total 1.00–1.25 mg or 10–15 μg/kg); maintenance dose, 0.125–0.250 mg/day based on clinical effect and drug levels

    (b) Pediatric digoxin (IV administration)

Age	Total digitalizing dose (DD) (μg/kg)	Daily maintenance dose (divided doses, normal renal function)
Neonates	15–30	20–35% of DD
2 mo–2 yr	30–50	25–35% of DD
2–10 yr	15–35	25–35% of DD
>10 yr	8–12	25–35% of DD

  (2) Digoxin has a gradual onset of action over 15–30 minutes or more; peak effect occurs 1–5 hours after IV administration.

  (3) Use with caution in presence of beta blockers, diltiazem, verapamil, and calcium.

  (4) Always consider the possibility of **cardiac toxicity.**

    (a) Anesthesia and surgery can make a normally digitalized patient toxic.

(b) **Signs of toxicity:** dysrhythmias, especially with features of **both increased automaticity and conduction block** (e.g., junctional tachycardia with a 2:1 atrioventricular block). Premature atrial or ventricular depolarizations, atrioventricular block, accelerated junctional tachycardia, ventricular tachycardia or fibrillation (may be unresponsive to countershock), or gastrointestinal or neurologic toxicity may also be apparent.

(5) **Factors potentiating toxicity**

    (a) Hypokalemia, hypomagnesemia, hypercalcemia, hyperventilation, alkalosis, glucose or insulin infusion (with hypokalemia from insulin), lactate infusion (with hypokalemia from metabolic HCO_3^- production), acidosis (decreased intracellular potassium), renal insufficiency, quinidine therapy, hypothyroidism.

    (b) Succinylcholine may cause ventricular dysrhythmias, which may be prevented by defasciculation. The cause is unknown.

    (c) **Beware of calcium salt administration in digitalized patients!** Malignant ventricular arrhythmias (including ventricular fibrillation) may occur, even if the patient has received no digoxin for more than 24 hours. Follow ionized calcium levels to permit use of smallest possible doses of calcium. Use careful monitoring.

    (d) Concurrent quinidine administration impedes clearance of digoxin.

(6) **Therapy for digitalis toxicity**

    (a) Raise serum potassium to upper limits of normal (unless atrioventricular block is present).

    (b) Treat ventricular dysrhythmias with phenytoin or lidocaine.

    (c) Treat atrial dysrhythmias with phenytoin.

    (d) Beta-blockers are effective for dysrhythmias, but ventricular pacing may be required if atrioventricular block develops.

    (e) Beware of cardioversion. Intractable ventricular fibrillation refractory to countershock may be induced. Use low energy sychronized cardioversion and slowly increase energy as needed. Consider prophylactic lidocaine administration to reduce risk of inducing ventricular arrhythmias during cardioversion of supraventricular dysrhythmias.

(7) **Serum digoxin levels**

    (a) Therapeutic: about 0.5–2.5 ng/ml. A serum level of under 0.5 ng/ml rules out toxicity; a level of over 3.0 ng/ml is definitely toxic.

    (b) High serum levels **without** clinical toxicity may occur in children, in hyperkalemic patients, or when digitalis is used as an atrial antidysrhythmic agent.

    (c) Low serum levels **with** clinical toxicity may occur in patients with hypokalemia, hypomagnesemia, hypercalcemia, myocardial ischemia, hypothyroidism, or after cardiopulmonary bypass (increased tissue sensitivity).

(8) Because of the long duration of action, long latency of onset, and risk of toxicity with digoxin, it is difficult to titrate digitalis to treat acute heart failure. Beta-adrenergic drugs, amrinone, or calcium are usually preferred to digoxin as first-line drugs for treating acute heart failure because of their greater efficacy and safety.

4. Glucagon

  a. Glucagon is a polypeptide hormone produced by the pancreas.

b. Actions. Glucagon binds to the cell surface, activates adenylate cyclase, and increases intracellular cyclic AMP. The glucagon receptor is separate from the beta receptor. Thus, beta-blockers do not block the actions of glucagon.

Glucagon

Contractility	Increase
HR	Increase
SVR	Variable
CO	Increase

c. Offset of action of glucagon occurs by proteolysis by the liver, kidney, and plasma. Onset occurs in 3–5 minutes; duration of action lasts 20–30 minutes.

d. Advantages
  (1) There is a low risk of ventricular dysrhythmias unless the drug is given rapidly IV.
  (2) Glucagon has a positive inotropic effect even in the presence of beta blockade.

e. Disadvantages
  (1) Nausea and vomiting.
  (2) Tachycardia, which can be significant.
  (3) Possibly ineffective with chronic CHF.
  (4) Catecholamine release from a pheochromocytoma.
  (5) Glycogenolysis, which can lead to hyperglycemia, insulin release, and hypokalemia.
  (6) Potentiation of oral anticoagulants in high dosages.
  (7) Anaphylaxis possible.
  (8) Increased atrioventricular conduction, which can produce increased ventricular rate during atrial fibrillation.

f. Indications for use
  (1) Refractory CHF (this indication has not been approved by the Food and Drug Administration (FDA)).
  (2) Beta-blocker toxicity (not FDA approved).
  (3) Spasm of sphincter of Oddi.
  (4) Hypoglycemia (especially if no IV access and the agent is administered IM).

g. Administration: IV, IM, SQ
h. Clinical use
  (1) **Glucagon dose:** 1–5 mg IV slowly; 0.5–2.0 mg IM/SQ
  (2) Infusion: 25–75 μg/min
  (3) Rarely used in modern clinical practice owing to gastrointestinal side effects and severe tachycardia; also, it may be difficult to titrate the dosage.

V. Vasodilator drugs
  A. Comparison
    1. Sites of action

Venous (decreased preload)	Arterial (decreased SVR)	Both
All nitrates	Calcium blockers	Angiotensin-converting enzyme (ACE) inhibitors
	Chlorpromazine	Nitroglycerin (IV high dose)
	Hydralazine	Nitroprusside
	Minoxidil	Prazosin
	Phentolamine	Doxasosin
	Trimethaphan	

  2. Mechanisms of action

    a. Direct vasodilators: calcium blockers, hydralazine, minoxidil, nitroglycerin, nitroprusside, trimethaphan

    b. Alpha-adrenergic blockers: chlorpromazine, droperidol, labetalol, phentolamine, prazosin, terazosin

    c. Ganglionic blockers: trimethaphan

    d. Angiotensin-converting enzyme (ACE) inhibitor: captopril, enalapril, lisinopril

    e. Central alpha-2-agonists (reduce sympathetic tone): clonidine, guanabenz, guanfacine, methyldopa

3. Indications for use

    a. Hypertension, increased SVR states. Use arterial or mixed drugs.

    b. Controlled hypotension. Short-acting drugs are most useful (e.g., nitroprusside, nitroglycerin, trimethaphan).

    c. Valvular regurgitation. Reducing SVR with any drug will tend to improve forward CO.

    d. Congestive heart failure

Type of CHF	Preferred vasodilator class
Elevated filling pressures	Venous
Elevated SVR	Arterial
Both	Mixed (or combination)

4. Cautions

    a. Hyperdynamic reflexes. All vasodilator drugs decrease SVR and BP with resultant baroreceptor activation. This cardiac sympathetic stimulation produces **tachycardia** and **increased contractility.** Myocardial ischemia due to increased myocardial O_2 demands can be additive to ischemia produced by lowering BP, which reduces coronary blood supply. Addition of a beta blocker can attenuate these reflexes.

    b. Ventricular ejection rate. Reflex sympathetic stimulation will also increase the rate of ventricular ejection of blood (dP/dt) and raise the systolic **aortic** wall stress. This may be detrimental with aortic dissection. Thus, addition of beta blockade or use of a ganglionic blocker is beneficial in patients with aortic dissection, aortic aneurysm, recent aortic surgery, or idiopathic hypertrophic subaortic stenosis.

    c. Stimulation of the renin-angiotensin system is implicated in the "rebound" increased SVR and PVR when some vasodilators are abruptly discontinued. Renin release can be attenuated by concomitant beta blockade, and renin's actions are attenuated by ACE inhibitors.

B. Chlorpromazine (Thorazine)

1. Actions

    a. Alpha-1 blockade

    b. Decreased SVR

    c. Neuroleptic antipsychotic, major tranquilizer

2. Offset occurs by hepatic metabolism.

3. Disadvantages and advantages

    a. It is difficult to titrate dosage to degree of vasodilation. A **profound sudden decrease in SVR and BP** may occur, especially with larger dosages or when the drug is given in combination with other vasodilators.

    b. Central nervous system (CNS) depression may occur, which may be desirable during cardiac anesthesia.

    c. The drug has a long duration of action (several hours).

    d. Blockade of dopaminergic receptors may result in extrapyramidal CNS manifestations with dystonia, akathisia, dyskinesia, or pseudoparkinsonism.

e. This agent can help terminate hiccups.

4. Clinical use. Chlorpromazine dose: 1–2 mg given as IV bolus, repeated every 2 minutes to maximum dose of 25 mg in acute cases. Chlorpromazine has relatively few beneficial attributes in cardiac surgical patients.

C. Clonidine (Catapres)

1. Actions

a. CNS: Clonidine reduces sympathetic outflow to body, secondary to central inhibitory alpha-2-agonist effect.

b. It reduces norepinephrine release by peripheral sympathetic nerve terminals.

c. Clonidine is a partial agonist (activates receptor submaximally after binding but also will antagonize effects of other alpha-2 agonists).

d. There is some direct vasoconstrictor action at alpha-2 receptors on vascular smooth muscle, but this effect is outweighed by the vasodilation induced by **a.** and **b.** above.

2. Offset. One-third of the drug is offset by renal elimination; half-life for elimination is 13 hr.

3. Advantages

a. Alpha-2-agonists potentiate **general anesthetics and narcotics** through a central mechanism. This effect can substantially reduce doses of anesthetics and narcotics required during surgical anesthesia and has been used during myocardial revascularization surgery.

4. Disadvantages

a. No parenteral preparation can be done; must be administered by gastric tube or transcutaneous patch to unconscious patient.

b. Rebound hypertension may occur on abrupt withdrawal, which can be severe, life-threatening, and difficult to treat.

c. Clonidine may potentiate opiate drug effects on CNS.

d. Sedation can occur.

5. Clinical use

a. Clonidine dose usual: 0.2–0.8 mg/day PO; maximum, 2.4 mg/ day.

b. Rebound hypertension frequently follows abrupt withdrawal. Clonidine should be continued until immediately before the operation and either resumed soon postoperatively (by skin patch, nasogastric tube, or when patient is taking drugs PO) or another type of antihypertensive drug substituted. Alternatively, clonidine can be replaced by another drug 1–2 weeks preoperatively.

c. It may be administered preoperatively to reduce anesthetic requirements. However, excessive hypotension may occur with such use, requiring vasopressor therapy.

d. Transdermal clonidine patches require 2–3 days to achieve therapeutic plasma drug levels.

e. Guanabenz is a related drug with similar effects and hazards.

D. Diazoxide (Hyperstat)

1. Action. Diazoxide is a direct vasodilator; it has primarily arteriolar action with little venodilation.

2. Offset occurs by renal filtration, plus a small degree of hepatic metabolism.

3. Advantages

a. Rapid onset.

b. Diazoxide often does not lower BP below normal range because preload is kept almost unchanged; CO usually rises as BP falls.

4. Disadvantages

a. It is difficult to titrate the dosage to effect unless the drug is given slowly. However, because of high protein binding, slow IV administration may attenuate its hypotensive response. Lack of minute-to-minute control makes diazoxide less popular for perioperative BP control than nitroprusside or trimethaphan.
b. Coronary artery steal may be produced.
c. Salt and water retention may occur.
  5. **Clinical use**
a. Diazoxide dose: Rapid IV injection of 1–3 mg/kg over 30 sec (maximum, 150 mg), repeated q5–15 min, produces rapid vasodilation and lowering of BP that can persist for 3–15 hours. Alternatively, a continuous infusion may be administered (7.5–30.0 mg/min) with constant BP measurement.
b. Pediatric dose: 1–3 mg/kg IV in increments.
E. Droperidol (Inapsine)
  1. **Actions.** Droperidol produces alpha-1 blockade and decreases SVR. It is a shorter duration analog of haloperidol and a neuroleptic major tranquilizer with dopaminergic receptor antagonistic activity.
  2. **Advantages and disadvantages**
a. This drug is similar to chlorpromazine (see sec. **IV.B.3**).
b. It produces somewhat less sedation than chlorpromazine. Patients appear quiet and relaxed. However, they may feel extremely anxious or dysphoric without verbalizing these emotions. Direct questioning and reassurance are warranted.
c. The drug potentiates narcotic-induced respiratory depression.
d. It is a potent antiemetic, even in low dosages.
e. It is long acting (3–8 hours).
  3. **Clinical use. Droperidol dose:** 1.25–5.00 mg IV bolus or IM. Droperidol is useful for sedation during awake intubation of cardiac patients.
F. Guanabenz (Wytensin) is similar to clonidine
  1. **Actions**
a. This drug is an alpha-2 agonist similar in actions to clonidine (see sec. **IV.C.**
  2. **Guanabenz dose:** 4 mg PO bid, maximum 32 mg bid.
G. Guanfacine (Tenex)
  1. **Actions**
a. Guanfacine is an alpha-2 agonist similar in actions to clonidine (see sec. **IV.C.**)
b. It has a longer duration of action due to renal elimination (half-life 15–20 hours).
  2. **Guanfacine dose:** 1 mg PO qd, maximum 3 mg/day.
H. Hydralazine (Apresoline)
  1. **Actions**
a. This drug is a direct vasodilator; it may also inhibit peripheral conversion of dopamine to norepinephrine.
b. It produces primarily arteriolar dilatation, with little venous (preload) effect.

Hydralazine

HR	Increased (reflex)
Contractility	Increased (reflex)
CO	May increase
BP	Decreased
SVR and PVR	Decreased
Preload	Little change

  2. **Offset** occurs by acetylation in the liver. Patients who are slow acetylators (up to 50% of the population) may have higher plasma

hydralazine levels, and may show a longer effect, especially with oral use.

3. **Advantages**
   a. **Selective vasodilation.** Hydralazine produces more dilation of coronary, cerebral, renal, and splanchnic beds than of vessels in the muscle and skin. This is generally a beneficial blood flow distribution pattern.
   b. Relatively pure reduction in SVR.
   c. Maintenance of uterine blood flow (if hypotension is avoided).
4. **Disadvantages**
   a. There is a period of latency; after IV administration, little or no effect may be seen for up to 5–15 minutes, and peak effect should occur by 20 minutes. Thus, at least 10–15 minutes should separate dosages.
   b. Hyperdynamic state with reflex tachycardia can precipitate myocardial ischemia.
   c. A lupuslike reaction, usually seen only with chronic PO use, may occur with high doses (>400 mg/day) given for more than 12 months, and in slow acetylators.
   d. Myocardial ischemia due to coronary steal is possible.
5. **Clinical use**
   a. **Hydralazine dose**
      (1) IV: 2.5–5.0 mg bolus q15 min as needed (maximum usually 20–40 mg).
      (2) IM: 20–40 mg q4–6h.
      (3) PO: 10–50 mg q6h.
      (4) Pediatric dose: 0.2–0.5 mg/kg q4–6h, slowly IV.
   b. Latency of onset of action limits its use in acute hypertensive crises.
   c. When patients are receiving substantial doses of nitroprusside or trimethaphan, the doses can be reduced by the addition of hydralazine. This decreases the risk of cyanide toxicity from nitroprusside or prolonged ganglionic blockade from trimethaphan.
   d. Because duration of action is a few hours, administration to hypertensive patients intraoperatively will help control postoperative hypertension also.
   e. Addition of a β blocker attenuates reflex tachycardia.
   f. Patients with coronary artery disease should be monitored for myocardial ischemia because a coronary artery steal may be produced.

I. **Labetalol** (Normodyne, Trandate)
   1. **Actions**
      a. Alpha-adrenergic antagonist
      b. Beta-adrenergic antagonist (nonselective, blocks beta-1 and beta-2 receptors)
      c. See sec. **III** for more details, including dosage
      d. Actions

   Labetalol

BP	Decreased
HR	Decreased
SVR	Decreased
CO	Variable

J. **Methyldopa** (alpha-methyldopa, Aldomet)
   1. **Actions.** A metabolite, alpha-methylnorepinephrine, produces a clonidinelike alpha-agonist effect in the brain, reducing sympathetic outflow. Also, peripheral sympathetic transmission is decreased by

means of generation of a false neurotransmitter and by reduction in catecholamine synthesis.

Methyldopa

HR	Decreased
CO	Decreased
BP	Decreased
SVR	Decreased

2. **Offset** occurs by renal excretion; duration of action is 10–16 hours.
3. **Advantages**
   a. Long duration, slow smooth onset.
   b. Useful for thoracic aortic dissection patients (dP/dt not increased).
   c. No relfex tachycardia.
4. **Disadvantages**
   a. Slow onset; even when given IV, onset is delayed for 4–6 hours.
   b. Sedation, psychosis, or depression.
   c. Positive direct Coombs' test (in 10–20% of chronic therapy patients) occurs with infrequent hemolytic anemia; may interfere with blood crossmatch.
5. **Clinical use**
   a. **Methyldopa dose:** 0.25–1.00 g IV given over 30–60 minutes q6h.
   b. Pediatric dose: 5–10 mg/kg q6h; maximum dose is 3 g/day.
   c. Use of this drug is decreasing owing to the introduction of newer, less toxic drugs.
K. **Nitroglycerin** (glyceryl trinitrate)
   1. **Actions**
      a. Nitroglycerin is a direct vasodilator, venous dilation is much greater than arterial.

Nitroglycerin

HR	Increased
Contractility	Increased (reflex)
CO	Decreased, due to lowered preload (unless ischemia is reduced)
BP	Decreased
Preload	Marked decrease
SVR	Decreased at higher dosages
PVR	Decreased

   b. **Peripheral venous effects.** Venodilation and peripheral pooling reduce venous return to the heart, decreasing heart size and preload. This effect usually reduces myocardial oxygen consumption and increases diastolic coronary blood flow.
   c. **Coronary artery**
      (1) Spasm is relieved.
      (2) **Flow redistribution** provides more flow to ischemic myocardium and increases endocardial-to-epicardial flow ratio.
      (3) Nitroglycerin may increase flow to ischemic regions through collateral vessels.
   d. **Myocardial effects**
      (1) Improved pump function due to reduced ischemia.
      (2) Antidysrhythmic action (ventricular fibrillation threshold in ischemic myocardium is raised because the drug makes the effective refractory period more uniform throughout the heart).
      (3) Possible ischemic protection (less muscle necrosis when heart is ischemic).
   e. **Arteriolar effects** (higher dosages only)

(1) Arteriolar dilatation decreases SVR. As the systolic myocardial wall stress lowers, myocardial oxygen consumption decreases, and ejection fraction and SV may improve.

(2) Arteriolar dilating effects often require very large doses, over **1000 μg/min** in many patients, whereas much lower doses give effective venous and coronary arterial dilating effects. When reliable peripheral arteriolar dilation is needed, nitroprusside is usually a better choice. (It can be used together with nitroglycerin.)

2. **Offset** occurs by metabolism in smooth muscle and liver.
3. **Advantages**
   a. It has a selective preload reduction (lowers left and right ventricular end-diastolic and atrial pressures).
   b. It has virtually no metabolic toxicity (see sec. **IV.K.4.i.** below).
   c. It is effective for myocardial ischemia
      (1) Decreases infarct size after coronary occlusion.
      (2) Useful to give nitroglycerin **before** an ischemia-producing stress.
      (3) Probably avoids coronary steal phenomenon that can be produced by nitroprusside.
   d. It has a short elimination half-life (4 minutes); duration, 3–9 minutes. Dosage can be titrated to ECG, PA pressures, or BP.
   e. It is useful in **acute CHF** to decrease preload and reduce pulmonary vascular congestion.
   f. It is useful for increasing the vascular capacity; it enables the anesthesiologist to reinfuse residual pump blood into the patient after cardiopulmonary bypass is terminated.
   g. It is a light stable drug.
   h. It dilates the pulmonary vascular bed and can be useful in treating acute pulmonary hypertension and right heart failure.
   i. It attenuates biliary colic and esophageal spasm.
   j. It does not inhibit platelet function clinically.
4. **Disadvantages**
   a. It decreases BP as preload and SVR decrease. This may result in decreased coronary perfusion pressure. Monitor BP and ECG, especially when using IV nitroglycerin.
   b. Reflex tachycardia and reflex increase in myocardial contractility are dose related; consider administering IV fluids or β blockers.
   c. It inhibits hypoxic pulmonary vasoconstriction (but to a lesser extent than nitroprusside); monitor PO_2 or supplement inspired gas with oxygen.
   d. It may increase intracranial pressure (ICP, although ICP often decreases with treatment of hypertension).
   e. It is adsorbed by polyvinyl chloride IV tubing. Titrate dosage to effect; increased effect may occur when tubing becomes saturated. Special infusion sets that do not adsorb drug are available.
   f. **Huge** dosages may be needed to produce arteriolar resistance–lowering effects.
   g. Tolerance. Chronic therapy can blunt hemodynamic and antianginal effects.
   h. Dependence. Coronary spasm and myocardial infarction have been reported after removal of patients from chronic industrial exposure.
   i. Methemoglobinemia. Avoid using more than 7–10 μg/kg/min for prolonged periods.
   j. Pancuronium neuromuscular blockade may be slightly prolonged.
   k. Headache.
   l. Tachyphylaxis
5. **Clinical use**

a. Nitroglycerin dose
  (1) IV bolus: A bolus of 50–100 µg may be superior to infusion for acute ischemia; rapidly changing levels in blood may cause more vasodilation than would a constant infusion (and may be more likely to produce hypotension).
  (2) Infusion: dose range, 0.1–7.0 µg/kg/min. Usually 25–50 mg is mixed in 250 ml IV solution (100–200 µg/ml).
  (3) Sublingual: 0.15–0.60 mg.
  (4) Topical: 2% ointment (Nitropaste), 0.5–2.0 inches q4–8h; or controlled release transdermal preparation (Transderm-Nitro, Nitrodisc), 5–10 mg (or more) q24h or as needed.
b. Unless Tridilset (or other nonpolyvinyl chloride tubing) is used, infusion requirements may decrease after the initial 30–60 minutes.
c. Nitroglycerin is better stored in bottles than in bags if storage for more than 6–12 hours is anticipated.

L. Nitroprusside (Nipride)
 1. Actions
  a. Nitroprusside is a direct-acting vasodilator. The nitrate group is believed to be converted into nitric acid (NO) in vascular smooth muscle, which causes increased cyclic guanosine monophosphate (cGMP) levels in cell.
  b. It has balanced arteriolar (precapillary sphincter) and venous dilating effects

Nitroprusside

HR	Increased (reflex)
Contractility	Increased (reflex)
CO	Increased
BP	Decreased
SVR	Markedly decreased
PVR	Decreased

 2. Advantages
  a. Very short duration of action (1–2 minutes).
  b. Pulmonary vasodilator in addition to systemic vasodilator effects.
  c. Highly effective for virtually all causes of hypertension except a high CO state.
  d. Greater decrease in SVR (afterload) than preload is produced at low dosages.
 3. Disadvantages
  a. Cyanide and thiocyanate toxicity.
  b. Unstable in light. Solution must be protected from light. Photodecomposition inactivates nitroprusside but does **not** release cyanide ion.
  c. Tachycardia and increased inotropy are reflex effects that respond to beta blockade.
  d. Hypoxic pulmonary vasoconstriction blunted. This effect produces arterial hypoxemia in patients with atelectasis or ventilation-perfusion mismatch.
  e. Vascular steal. All vascular regions are dilated equally. Although total organ blood flow may increase, flow may be diverted from ischemic regions (previously maximally vasodilated) to non-ischemic areas that have been appropriately vasoconstricted. Thus myocardial **ischemia may be worsened.** However, severe hypertension is clearly dangerous in ischemia, whereas a steal may only **possibly** occur. Nitroprusside, therefore, may be highly beneficial in patients with hypertension and myocardial ischemia, especially if they are closely monitored.

f. Rebound systemic or pulmonary hypertension may occur if nitroprusside is abruptly stopped (especially in patients with CHF). This effect is possibly due to elevated angiotensin II levels, which can be prevented from rising by adding beta blockade to nitroprusside therapy. Nitroprusside should be tapered.

g. Mild preload reduction due to venodilation occurs; fluids may need to be infused if CO falls.

h. Risk of increased ICP exists (although it often decreases with resolution of hypertension).

i. Platelet function inhibited (clinical consequences are uncertain).

4. **Toxicity**

   a. Chemical formula of nitroprusside is $FeCN_6$. Nitroprusside reacts with hemoglobin to release highly toxic free cyanide ion (CN^-).

   b. Nitroprusside + oxyhemoglobin → four free cyanide ions + cyanomethemoglobin (nontoxic).

   c. Cyanide ion: pharmacologic effects

   (1) Inhibition of cytochrome oxidase, preventing mitochondrial oxidative phosphorylation. This produces tissue hypoxia despite adequate PO_2.

   d. Cyanide detoxification

   (1) Cyanide + thiosulfate (and rhodanase) → **thiocyanate.** Thiocyanate is much less toxic than cyanide ion (see sec. **IV.L.d.5**). Availability of thiosulfate is the rate-limiting step in cyanide metabolism. Thus, **thiosulfate administration is of critical importance in treating cyanide toxicity.** Rhodanase is an enzyme found in liver and kidney that promotes cyanide detoxification.

   (2) Cyanide + hydroxycobalamin → cyanocobalamin (vitamin B_{12}).

   e. Patients at increased risk of toxicity

   (1) Those resistant to vasodilating effects at low dosages (if an initial dose of > 3 μg/kg/min is necessary for effect)

   (2) Those receiving a high-dose infusion (> 8 μg/kg/min). Whenever the dosage approaches this value, frequent blood gas measurements must be performed, and consideration must be given to the following:

   (a) Use a PA catheter to monitor mixed venous oxygenation (see sec. **IV.L.d.2** below).

   (b) Decrease dosage by adding a different vasodilator (such as labetalol, hydralazine, or trimethaphan) or a β blocker.

   (3) Those receiving a high total dose (> 1 mg/kg) over 12–24 hours.

   (4) Those in whom Leber's optic atrophy, tobacco amblyopia, or severe renal or hepatic dysfunction is present.

   f. Signs of nitroprusside toxicity

   (1) **Tachyphylaxis** in response to vasodilating effects of nitroprusside (larger doses are necessary to produce the same effect).

   (2) **Elevated mixed venous PO_2** (due to decreased cellular oxygen utilization) in the absence of a rise in CO.

   (3) **Metabolic acidosis.**

   (4) **No cyanosis** is seen with cyanide toxicity (cells cannot utilize O_2; therefore, blood O_2 saturation remains high).

   (5) **Chronic toxicity** is due to elevated **thiocyanate** levels and is a consequence of long-term therapy. Thiocyanate is excreted unchanged by the kidney (elimination half-life, 1 week). Elevated thiocyanate levels (> 5 mg/dl) can cause fatigue, nausea, anorexia, miosis, psychosis, hyperreflexia, and seizures. Hypothyroidism has been reported.

   g. Therapy of cyanide toxicity

(1) Cyanide toxicity should be suspected when a metabolic acidosis or unexplained rise in mixed venous PO_2 appears in any patient receiving nitroprusside, especially at high dosages.

(2) As soon as toxicity is suspected, **nitroprusside must be discontinued;** lowering the dosage is not sufficent because clinically evident toxicity implies a marked reduction in cytochrome oxidase activity.

(3) Ventilate with 100% oxygen.

(4) Treat metabolic acidosis with bicarbonate.

(5) **Mild toxicity** (base deficit < 10, stable hemodynamics when nitroprusside stopped) can be treated by **sodium thiosulfate, 150 mg/kg IV bolus** (hemodynamically benign).

(6) **Severe toxicity** (base deficit > 10, or worsening hemodynamics despite discontinuation of nitroprusside:

    (a) **Create methemoglobin** that can combine with cyanide to produce nontoxic cyanomethemoglobin, removing cyanide from cytochrome oxidase:

        (i) **Give sodium nitrite, 5 mg/kg IV slow push. (Repeat one-half dose 2–48 hours later as needed),** or

        (ii) **Give amyl nitrite:** Break 1 ampule into breathing bag. (Flammable!)

    (b) **Sodium thiosulfate,** 150 mg/kg IV, should also be administered to facilitate metabolic disposal of the cyanide.

    Note: These treatments should be administered **even during CPR;** otherwise, oxygen cannot be utilized by body tissues.

5. Clinical use

  a. Nitroprusside dose: 0.1–8.0 μg/kg/min IV infusion. Titrate dose to BP and CO.

  b. The usual mix is 50 mg nitroprusside in 250 ml IV solution (200 μg/ml).

  c. Supplement inspired gas with oxygen or monitor PaO_2.

  d. Solution in bottle or bag must be protected from light by wrapping in metal foil. Solution stored in the dark retains significant potency for 12–24 hours. It is usually **not** necessary to cover the administration tubing with foil.

  e. Because of the high potency of nitroprusside, it is best administered by itself into a central line using an infusion pump. If other drugs are being infused through the same line, use a carrier flow so that changes in drug infusion rates do not affect the quantity of each drug entering the patient per minute (the "bolus effect").

  f. Blood pressure should be monitored frequently (every minute), preferably with an arterial catheter. Concurrent use of a PA catheter permits titration of dose not only to BP but also to SVR and filling pressures.

  g. Infusions should be gradually tapered—not abruptly stopped—to avoid rebound increases in systemic and PA pressures.

  h. Use this drug cautiously in patients with concomitant hypothyroidism or severe liver or kidney dysfunction.

M. Phentolamine (Regitine)

  1. Actions

    a. Competitive antagonist at alpha-1 and alpha-2 receptors.

    b. Relatively pure arterial vasodilation with little venodilation.

Phentolamine

HR	Increased
Contractility	Increased
BP	Decreased
SVR	Decreased

     PVR   Decreased
     Preload   Little change

2. **Offset** occurs by hepatic metabolism, some by renal excretion. Offset after IV bolus occurs after 10–30 minutes.
3. **Advantages**
   a. Good for norepinephrine overdose states such as pheochromocytoma.
   b. Antagonizes undesirable alpha stimulation. For example, deleterious effects of norepinephrine extravasated into skin can be treated by local infiltration with phentolamine, 5–10 mg in 10 ml saline.
4. **Disadvantages**
   a. Tachycardia, which can be significant, arises from two mechanisms:
      (1) **Reflex** via baroreceptors.
      (2) **Direct effect of alpha-2 blockade.** Blockade of presynaptic receptors eliminates the normal feedback system controlling norepinephrine release by presynaptic nerve terminals. As alpha-2 stimulation decreases norepinephrine release, blockade of these receptors allows increased presynaptic release. This results in increased **beta-1** sympathetic effects only, since the alpha receptors mediating postsynaptic alpha effects are blocked by phentolamine. Myocardial ischemia or dysrhythmias may result. Thus, the tachycardia and positive inotropy are beta effects that will respond to β blockers.
   b. Gastrointestinal stimulation.
   c. Hypoglycemia.
   d. **Epinephrine may cause hypotension in alpha-blocked patients ("epinephrine reversal") via a beta-2 mechanism.**
5. **Clinical use**
   a. **Phentolamine dose**
      (1) **IV bolus:** 1–5 mg
      (2) **IV infusion:** 1–20 μg/kg/min
   b. When administered for pheochromocytoma, beta blockade generally is also instituted.
   c. This is not the ideal drug for patients with CHF because of the risk of tachycardia.
   d. Beta blockade will attenuate tachycardia.
   e. Phentolamine promotes uniform cooling of children during CPB.
N. **Prostaglandin E₁** (PGE₁, Prostin VR, alprostadil)
   a. **Actions.** This drug is a direct vasodilator acting through specific prostaglandin receptors on vascular smooth muscle cells.
   b. **Offset** occurs by rapid metabolism to inactive substances by enzymes located in most body tissues, especially the lung.
   c. **Advantages**
      (1) Selectively dilates the **ductus arteriosus** (DA) in neonates and infants. May maintain patency of an open DA for as long as approximately 60 days of age and may open a closed DA up to 10–14 days of age.
      (2) Metabolism by lung endothelium somewhat reduces its systemic vasodilator action compared with its potent pulmonary vascular dilating effect.
   d. **Disadvantages**
      (1) Systemic vasodilation is substantial and may produce hypotension.
      (2) Central nervous system effects: fever, seizures.
      (3) May produce **apnea** in infants (10–12%), especially if birth weight is less than 2 kg.

(4) Extremely expensive (synthetic drug).

(5) Inhibits platelet function (reversible).

e. Administration: Infused IV or through umbilical arterial catheter.

f. Indications for use

(1) Cyanotic congenital heart disease with reduced pulmonary blood flow.

(2) **Severe pulmonary hypertension** with right heart failure.

g. Clinical use

(1) **Prostaglandin E_1 dose:** Usual IV infusion starting dose is 0.05 μg/kg/min. The dose should be titrated up or down to the lowest effective value. Doses as high as 0.4 μg/kg/min may be required.

(2) PGE_1 is used to open or maintain the patency of the **ductus arteriosus** to preserve adequate pulmonary blood flow.

(3) Intravenous PGE_1 is used in combination with left atrial norepinephrine for treatment of **severe pulmonary hypertension** with right heart failure: PGE_1 may be infused into the **right atrium** (RA), from which point it proceeds directly to the pulmonary artery, where it can attenuate pulmonary vasoconstriction. Due to lung metabolism, relatively less of the drug passes on to the systemic vasculature. Usually, **norepinephrine** is infused into the **left atrium** simultaneously in doses sufficient to reverse the **systemic** vasodilation of PGE_1 (see D'Ambra et al.).

O. Trimethaphan camsylate (Arfonad)

1. Actions

a. Ganglionic blocker: sympathetic and parasympathetic

b. Direct vasodilator: arterial and venous effects

Trimethaphan

HR	No change or increase
CO	Little change
BP	Decreased
SVR	Decreased
Preload	Decreased

2. Offset occurs partially by renal elimination and partially by cholinesterase; it is rapid, occurring 5–10 minutes after small doses.

3. Advantages

a. Trimethaphan produces relatively pure vasodilation in low doses (with little change in HR or CO).

b. Vasodilation is of short duration in low doses.

c. This drug preserves **autoregulation** in cerebral and perhaps also coronary vascular beds. This effect may be related to trimethaphan's site of arterial action on the larger conducting vessels (less at precapillary sphincters). With trimethaphan (similar to nitroglycerin), conducting vessel dilation increases total blood flow to a region; autoregulation of the precapillary sphincters can then continue to distribute flow to those areas that require it most (ischemic areas). Thus, a steal of blood flow from ischemic to nonischemic areas is less likely.

d. Administration is convenient; it can be used as intermittent IV bolus injections, and protection from light is not required.

e. There is no activation of the renin-angiotensin system and lower plasma catecholamine levels compared with nitroprusside. There is less risk of rebound hypertension than with nitroprusside.

f. Trimethaphan may cause less increase in **intracranial pressure** during controlled hypotension than nitroprusside.

4. Disadvantages
a. Persisting effects are possible for about 1 hour after discontinuation of prolonged high-dose ($> 100–300$ mg) administration.
b. Histamine release occurs at high doses
c. High doses or long duration of infusion can produce the following:
  (1) Tachyphylaxis
  (2) Tachycardia
  (3) Pupillary dilation, which may confuse neurologic examination
  (4) Decreased cardiac inotropy due to sympathetic withdrawal (usually not clinically important)
d. Interaction with aminoglycoside antibiotics at the neuromuscular junction may produce blockade in vitro. This effect occurs at drug concentrations that separately do not affect transmission.
e. Respiratory arrest of uncertain mechanism may occur with high doses, possibly related to neuromuscular blockade (see **d** above).
f. Noncompetitive inhibition of pseudocholinesterase occurs, which may prolong the action of succinylcholine.
g. Use with caution in presence of pheochromocytoma because histamine release may stimulate catecholamine secretion.

5. Clinical use
a. Trimethaphan dose
  (1) IV bolus:; 0.5–20.0 mg is used for acute hypertension. One method of administration involves starting with a 1.0-mg IV bolus, then doubling the dose every minute until the desired fall in BP is produced. Maximal hypotension usually occurs about 1–2 minutes after IV administration and has a duration of action of 5–10 minutes.
  (2) IV infusion: 0.5–6.0 mg/min.
b. Usually mix 500 mg of drug in 500 ml of solution.
c. Trimethaphan can be combined with nitroprusside to decrease dosage of both drugs or to treat refractory hypertension. The effects appear to be synergistic, not just additive, so begin at low dosages and titrate upward carefully.
d. High dosages, which cause complete ganglionic blockade, may be used to reduce the rate of rise of pressure in the aorta in patients with acute **aortic dissection.**
e. High dosages with complete ganglionic blockade can prevent or treat **autonomic hyper-reflexia** in patients with thoracic or cervical spinal cord lesions.
f. Treatment of **acute hypertension.** It is especially useful to prevent or control the sympathetic response (tachycardia and hypertension) that occurs with intubation of the trachea.
g. Trimethaphan is a convenient drug for control of perioperative hypertension. As long as the dosage is limited to less than about 100 mg administered over a few hours, the adverse effects listed in sec. **IV.O.4** are usually avoided.

VI. Calcium-blocking drugs (CBDs)
A. General considerations
1. Tissues utilizing calcium. Calcium is required for many cellular functions, including cardiac contraction and conduction, smooth muscle contraction, neuromuscular transmission, and hormone secretion.
2. How calcium enters cells. Calcium ions (Ca^{2+}) can interact with the intracellular machinery in two ways, by (1) entering the cell from outside, or (2) being released from intracellular storage sites. These two mechanisms are related because Ca^{2+} crossing the sarcolemma acts as a **trigger,** releasing sequestered Ca^{2+} from the sar-

coplasmic reticulum (SR) into the cytoplasm. These processes can raise intracellular free Ca^{2+} concentrations 100-fold.

3. **Myocardial effects of calcium.** The force of myocardial contraction is directly related to the cytoplasmic ionized calcium concentration ($[Ca^{2+}]$), high levels causing contraction and low levels permitting relaxation. At the end of systole, energy-dependent pumps transfer Ca^{2+} from the cytoplasm back into the SR, causing free cytoplasmic Ca^{2+} to decrease. If ischemia prevents sequestration of cytoplasmic Ca^{2+}, diastolic relaxation of myocardium is incomplete. This abnormal **diastolic stiffness** of the heart causes raised ventricular filling pressures and pulmonary wedge pressures and can produce symptoms similar to those of left heart failure.

4. **Myocardial effects of CBDs.** CBDs owe much of their usefulness to their ability to reduce the transmembrane "trigger" current of Ca^{2+}. This reduces the amount of Ca^{2+} released from intracellular stores with each heartbeat. Therefore, all CBDs in high enough doses reduce the force of cardiac contraction, although this effect may be counterbalanced by reflex actions in patients. The presence of afterload reduction and active cardiovascular reflexes (e.g., sympathetic activation) accounts for the major differences seen when CBDs are studied in isolated tissues in the laboratory and compared with their clinical effects. Clinical dosages of some CBDs, such as nifedipine, do not produce myocardial depression in humans.

5. **Other tissues.** The ability of CBDs to decrease Ca^{2+} flow across cell membranes explains other drug actions. For example, **vascular smooth muscle** and myocardial **conduction-system** tissues (especially sinoatrial [SA] and atrioventricular nodes) depend on transmembrane calcium flux to permit vasoconstriction and cardiac impulse conduction, respectively.

6. **Tissue selectivity.** CBDs affect certain tissues more than others. Thus, verapamil in clinical dosages depresses cardiac conduction, whereas nifedipine does not. However, **all CBDs cause vasodilation.**

7. **Direct vs. indirect effects.** Selection of a particular CBD for clinical use is based primarily on its relative potency for **direct cellular effects** in the target organ and its relative potency for inducing **cardiovascular reflexes.**

B. **Clinical effects common to all CBDs**

1. **Peripheral vasodilation**

   a. **Arterial effects.** Calcium-blocking drugs cause primarily **arterial** vasodilation. This effect reduces LV **afterload** and may improve ventricular ejection. Thus, vasodilation helps offset the direct negative cardiac inotropic effects of CBDs.

   b. **Venous effects. Preload** (reflected by central venous pressure [CVP] or PCWP) usually changes little because venodilation is minimal, and negative inotropy is often offset by reduced afterload. However, if CBDs reduce myocardial ischemia and diastolic stiffness, filling pressures may decrease.

   c. **Regional effects.** Most vascular beds are dilated, including the cerebral, hepatic, pulmonary, splanchnic, and musculoskeletal beds. Renal blood flow autoregulation is known to be abolished by nifedipine, making flow pressure dependent.

   d. **Coronary vasodilation** is induced by all CBDs. These drugs are all highly effective for coronary vasospasm. Diltiazem in particular has a selective coronary vasodilating effect, with a given dosage producing a proportionately greater rise in coronary flow than that in other beds. Thus, coronary arteries are dilated at doses causing little decrease in BP. Nifedipine may induce a coronary steal in susceptible patients, causing an exacerbation of ischemia.

  e. **CBDs versus nitrates.** Vasodilation by CBDs differs in several ways from that produced by **nitrates.**

    (1) **Magnitude of relaxation.** Complete vascular relaxation is not produced by nitrates; even with high nitrate concentrations, 20–40% of basal contraction (in potassium-contracted preparations) remains, whereas this is abolished by CBDs.

    (2) **Tachyphylaxis.** Nitrate vasodilation is usually transient, vascular tone being restored in the presence of constant nitrate concentrations. CBD-induced vasodilation persists while the drug is present.

    (3) **Type of vessels.** Nitrates dilate the venous system predominantly, whereas CBDs are primarily arterial vasodilators.

    (4) **Size of vessels.** Nitrates dilate predominantly the large coronary arteries, whereas CBDs dilate both large coronary arteries and small arterioles.

  f. **Reversal of vasodilation.** Vasodilation induced by CBDs can be difficult to reverse. Alpha-adrenergic agonists such as phenylephrine appear to be the most effective agents, although very large doses may be required. Calcium salts (e.g., calcium chloride) are usually ineffective in reversing CBD-induced vasodilation, although they effectively reverse CBD-induced myocardial depression.

2. Depression of myocardial contractility. The myocardium has a marked dependency on Ca^{2+} for contraction. However, the degree of **myocardial depression** that occurs following administration of a CBD is highly variable, depending on the following factors:

  a. **Selectivity.** The **relative potency** of the drug for myocardial depression compared with its other actions is an important factor. Nifedipine is much more potent as a vasodilator than as a myocardial depressant; clinical dosages that cause profound vasodilation have minimal direct myocardial effects. Conversely, vasodilating dosages of verapamil may be associated with significant myocardial depression in some patients.

  b. **Health of the heart.** A failing ventricle will respond to afterload reduction with improved ejection. An ischemic ventricle will pump more effectively if ischemia is reversed. As CBDs reduce afterload and ischemia, CO may rise with CBD therapy in certain situations. Direct negative inotropic effects may not be apparent.

  c. **Compensatory reflexes.** Profound vasodilation will activate the baroreceptor reflex, causing sympathetic stimulation. The released norepinephrine stimulates the heart and peripheral blood vessels, which tends to counteract direct myocardial depression and vasodilation.

  d. **Reversal of myocardial depression.** Calcium chloride, beta-agonists, and amrinone all can be used to help improve excessive negative inotropy. These agents may also help to improve myocardial impulse conduction, as will pacing.

3. Improving myocardial ischemia

  a. **Oxygen supply** can be improved by

    (1) Reversing coronary artery spasm.

    (2) Vasodilating coronary artery, increasing flow to both normal and poststenotic regions. Diltiazem and verapamil appear to preserve coronary autoregulation, but nifedipine may cause a coronary steal.

    (3) Increasing flow through coronary collateral channels.

(4) Decreasing HR (prolonging diastolic duration during which subendocardium is perfused) with verapamil and diltiazem.
   b. **Oxygen consumption** can be reduced by
      (1) Diminishing contractility.
      (2) Decreasing peak LV wall stress (by afterload reduction).
      (3) Decreasing HR (by verapamil and diltiazem).
   c. **Myocardial protection** during reperfusion is being studied. Following a period of ischemia, increased calcium entry into myocardial cells appears to be related to cell death. Studies are in progress to determine whether CBDs may be beneficial in reducing infarct size following injury.
4. **Electrophysiologic depression**
   a. **Spectrum of impairment of atrioventricular conduction**
      (1) **Verapamil.** At one end of the spectrum, clinical doses of verapamil usually produce significant electrophysiologic effects. Thus, verapamil has a high relative potency for prolonging atrioventricular node refractoriness compared with its vasodilating potency.
      (2) **Nifedipine.** On the other hand, nifedipine in dosages that produce profound vasodilation causes no changes in atrioventricular conduction because of its minimal intrinsic electrophysiologic potency and induced sympathetic reflex activation.
      (3) Diltiazem is intermediate between nifedipine and verapamil.
   b. **Atrioventricular node effects.** The depression of atrioventricular nodal conduction by CBDs may be beneficial. Thus, verapamil is a useful antidysrhythmic drug with actions against a broad range of supraventricular and atrioventricular nodal reentrant dysrhythmias. Verapamil often can convert SVT, whereas in atrial flutter and atrial fibrillation the associated ventricular rate is generally slowed. On the other hand, unwanted **atrioventricular block** may complicate antianginal or antihypertensive therapy with verapamil or diltiazem, especially in conjunction with beta blockade.
   c. **SA node effects.** The depressant actions of the CBDs on the SA node differ from those on the atrioventricular node. Thus, diltiazem causes the greatest SA node slowing, while verapamil produces only slight sinus slowing. Nifedipine is often associated with a small increase in sinus rate.
   d. **Ventricular ectopy** may be induced by calcium channel–dependent mechanisms in mitral valve prolapse, atrial or atrioventricular nodal disease, halothane-epinephrine interactions, and some types of digitalis toxicity. Verapamil is often useful in treating these conditions, together with other antidysrhythmic agents.
C. **Verapamil** (Calan, Isoptin)
   1. Verapamil is a papaverine derivative.
   2. **Actions**

Verapamil

HR	Slight decrease in sinus rate
Contractility	Decreased (usually mild unless severe LV failure)
BP	Decreased (unless improved cardiac function offsets decreased SVR)
Preload	May increase slightly
SVR	Decreased
Atrioventricular conduction	Depressed; first-, second-, or third-degree heart block may be produced

3. **Antidysrhythmic spectrum**
   a. Supraventricular tachycardia
   b. Premature atrial depolarizations
   c. Atrial flutter
   d. Atrial fibrillation
   e. Ventricular dysrhythmias due to halothane-epinephrine interaction
4. **Offset** occurs by hepatic metabolism; the plasma elimination half-life is 3–10 hours, and the active metabolite is norverapamil.
5. **Advantages**
   a. Verapamil has high efficacy for treating many atrial dysrhythmias (it is 95% successful in converting reentrant SVT), including those refractory to other modes of antidysrhythmic therapy (e.g., mitral valve prolapse).
   b. Slows ventricular heart rate reliably in atrial fibrillation or flutter.
   c. It has high electrophysiologic potency compared with other actions. Relatively moderate myocardial depression and vasodilation are usually seen in dosages that produce significant atrioventricular nodal and supraventricular antidysrhythmic actions.
   d. Clinically significant myocardial depression is seen only with severe LV dysfunction. In patients with an acute tachydysrhythmia that is impairing pumping, BP and CO usually rise when verapamil restores sinus rhythm.
   e. Duration of vasodilation and myocardial depression is relatively short (approximately 5–15 minutes after administration of IV bolus dose), whereas antidysrhythmic action (IV) may last 30 minutes or more.
   f. Effective antianginal agent, especially when used with a nitrate.
   g. Verapamil is the only CBD currently available for IV use. Unlike β blockers, CBDs have no bronchospastic activity and can be safely used to treat atrial arrhythmias or myocardial ischemia in asthmatic patients.
6. **Disadvantages**
   a. Verapamil carries a risk of causing severe atrioventricular block. Verapamil IV should be used cautiously in patients who are beta-blocked or digitalis-toxic, and facilities for temporary cardiac pacing should be immediately available.
   b. Hypotension secondary to peripheral vasodilation may occur. The risk of hypotension is minimized by the following:
      (1) Use of small (1- to 2-mg) incremental IV doses.
      (2) Administration of a small dosage of an alpha agonist such as phenylephrine (50–100 μg) together with verapamil, giving additional doses as needed.
   c. There is a risk of acute LV failure, which is uncommon except with preexisting, poorly compensated CHF.
   d. Atrioventricular conduction in the presence of aberrant conduction pathways (e.g., Wolff-Parkinson-White syndrome) is either unchanged or **increased.** Thus, verapamil is often avoided in treatment of atrial fibrillation or flutter when anterograde aberrant conduction (wide QRS complexes or delta waves) is present.
   e. Verapamil (given chronically) reduces digoxin elimination and can raise digoxin levels, producing toxicity.
   f. May increase intracranial pressure at time of anesthetic induction.
7. **Indications**
   a. Dysrhythmias, especially atrial or atrioventricular nodal reentrant dysrhythmias.
   b. Ventricular rate control in atrial fibrillation or atrial flutter.
   c. Myocardial ischemia, both classic and vasospastic forms.

d. Hypertension

As the only CBD available for IV use, verapamil may be useful in treating acute hypertensive crisis, especially if (1) it is caused by acute withdrawal of chronic calcium-blocker therapy, (2) there is concomitant myocardial ischemia, or (3) SVT coexists.

8. Clinical use

a. Verapamil dose

(1) IV bolus (adults): **5–10 mg;** administer in 1- to 2-mg increments in unstable patients. Dose may be repeated after 30 minutes (may be given by buretrol after dilution).

(2) IV infusion **(maximum 5 μg/kg/min)** can be started after bolus loading if a continiuous effect is desired.

(3) PO (adults): 40–80 mg tid–qid, maximum 480 mg/day.

(4) Pediatric dose: 75–200 μg/kg IV, may repeat.

b. Verapamil IV is most frequently administered for its **electrophysiologic** actions.

c. Patients must be monitored with ECG and frequent BP determinations during IV verapamil administration. In general, patients will demonstrate a prolongation of the PR interval and peripheral vasodilation at dosages lower than those needed to produce significant myocardial depression.

d. Consider concomitant phenylephrine administration to counteract excessive peripheral vasodilation. Myocardial depression can be counteracted by calcium salts or beta agonists. High-grade atrioventricular block can be treated with atropine, beta agonists, or ventricular pacing.

e. Use extreme caution in treating beta-blocked patients. In general, combined administration of IV verapamil and IV propranolol or IV digoxin should be avoided owing to additive atrioventricular node depression unless pacing equipment is immediately available.

f. Elimination half-life **increases** with chronic therapy, so dosage may need to be reduced after 5–7 days of therapy.

D. Nifedipine (Procardia)

1. Nifedipine is a dihydropyridine calcium blocker.

2. Actions

Nifedipine

HR	Increased (reflex)
Contractility	Increased (reflex)
BP	Decreased
Preload	No change, or slight decrease
SVR	Markedly decreased
Atrioventricular conduction	Increased (reflex)

3. Offset occurs by hepatic metabolism; plasma elimination half-life is 1.5–5.0 hours, and there are no active metabolites.

4. Advantages

a. Profound vasodilation is the predominant effect.

(1) Coronary vasodilation and relief of coronary vasospasm reduce myocardial ischemia.

(2) Peripheral vasodilation can improve CO.

b. Virtually no myocardial depression occurs in clinical dosages. Therefore, it can be used (with close monitoring) in patients with poor ventricular function.

c. Generally this drug is devoid of conducting system toxicity and antidysrhythmic effects.

      d. It may be combined with β blockers without increased risk of atrioventricular block, or with nitrates provided that the patient is monitored for excessive vasodilation.

      e. Nifedipine can relieve esophageal spasm.

5. Disadvantages

      a. It is extremely light-sensitive; thus, no IV preparation is available.

      b. Administration must be PO or via mucosa of the nose or mouth.

      c. Severe hypotension is possible due to peripheral vasodilation.

      d. No significant antidysrhythmic effect occurs unless relief of myocardial ischemia decreases ischemia-induced dysrhythmias.

      e. Gastrointestinal upset or peripheral edema is possible (the latter not due to heart failure).

6. Indications

      a. Myocardial ischemia, both classic and vasospastic

      b. Acute coronary artery spasm

      c. Left ventricular failure with elevated SVR, as an unloading agent (not FDA-approved)

      d. Hypertensive crisis (not FDA-approved), especially with concomitant myocardial ischemia

7. Clinical use

      a. Nifedipine dose: PO, 10–40 mg tid; sublingual, 10–20 mg liquid (extracted from capsule).

      b. Nifedipine is generally selected for its **vasodilator and antianginal** properties.

      c. Sublingual (or intranasal) route is useful in emergency situations, especially in anesthetized or unconscious patients; rapid absorption (1–5 minutes) occurs with this route.

      d. If excessive vasodilation with hypotension is produced, alpha-agonist drugs such as phenylephrine may be used. However, very high dosages of the latter drugs are sometimes required.

      e. In a small proportion of patients angina is exacerbated with nifedipine. This may be related to hypotension or to a coronary steal phenomenon. In this circumstance hypotension should be treated, or another antianginal drug should be added or substituted.

E. Diltiazem (Cardizem)

    1. Diltiazem is a benzothiazepine calcium blocker.

    2. Actions

Diltiazem

HR	Slight decrease
Contractility	No change or small decrease
BP	Decreased
Preload	No change
SVR	Decreased
Atrioventricular conduction	Decreased

      a. Diltiazem has a **selective** coronary vasodilating action, causing a disproportionately greater increase in coronary flow than that seen in other vascular beds.

    3. Offset occurs by hepatic metabolism (60%) and renal excretion (35%); plasma elimination half-life is 2–7 hours; active metabolite is desacetyldiltiazem.

    4. Advantages

      a. Diltiazem often decreases HR during sinus rhythm, which is advantageous in patients with coronary artery disease.

      b. Highly effective in treating and preventing classic or vasospastic myocardial ischemia.

      c. This drug has the fewest side effects and often is best tolerated for chronic use among the three CBDs currently available.

5. Disadvantages

    a. Conduction-system depression with development of atrioventricular block is possible. However, this occurs less frequently than with verapamil.

    b. Sinus bradycardia is possible and may necessitate lowering the dosage or stopping the drug. Diltiazem should be avoided in patients with sinus node dysfunction. Conduction system interactions with digoxin or β blockers may occur. Diltiazem combined with these drugs should be used with caution.

    c. Oral preparations are the only forms of this drug available.

6. Indications

    a. Myocardial ischemia: classic angina and coronary artery spasm.

    b. Stable supraventricular tachycardia or atrial fibrillation in patients who cannot tolerate verapamil (unstable patients should receive cardioversion or other immediate therapy).

7. Clinical use

    a. Diltiazem dose: PO (adult), 30–120 mg tid or qid.

    b. Diltiazem is most frequently utilized for its **antianginal** properties.

    c. No parenteral preparation is available.

    d. Duration of action is longer than its plasma half-life, probably due to its active metabolite.

VII. Therapy of acute cardiac dysrhythmias

A. Overview of dysrhythmias

1. The ECG should be quickly identified as belonging to one of three groups:

    a. Lethal dysrhythmias

        (1) Ventricular tachydysrhythmia. Ventricular fibrillation or ventricular tachycardia

        (2) Bradydysrhythmia. Asystole, complete heart block, HR under 30 (adults)

    b. Potentially dangerous dysrhythmias

        (1) Ventricular ectopy. Premature ventricular contractions (PVCs, unifocal or multifocal), R-on-T phenomenon, coupled ectopy (bigeminy)

        (2) Supraventricular tachycardia. Atrial fibrillation, atrial flutter, junctional tachycardia, sinus tachycardia; paroxysmal atrial tachycardia, Wolff-Parkinson-White syndrome

        (3) Second-degree heart block—Mobitz type 2 (usually wide QRS complexes)

        (4) Bradycardia with heart rate over 40

    c. Generally benign dysrhythmias. Sinus, accelerated junctional (rate < 100), isolated atrial ectopic beats

2. The type of therapy will depend on how well the patient is tolerating the dysrhythmia. If the blood pressure or cardiac output is low, or if organ hypoperfusion exists (e.g., angina), immediate therapy is required.

B. Lethal tachydysrhythmias: Ventricular fibrillation

1. Overview

    a. Therapy must be immediate, since CO is zero or minimal.

    b. Countershock is almost always necessary to restore cardiac rhythm. Pharmacologic agents are used to make the heart more responsive to countershock.

    c. If a patient is not responding to therapy, the differential diagnosis explained in sec. **VII.G** must be considered immediately.

    d. In some cases, bretylium may convert ventricular fibrillation to a stable rhythm. If a defibrillator is not immediately available, bretylium should be the initial antidysrhythmic therapy of ventricular fibrillation.

2. Electrical therapy of ventricular fibrillation: defibrillation. Applying an electrical shock to the heart is **the only reliable therapy for ventricular fibrillation.** Defibrillation should be performed immediately on diagnosing ventricular fibrillation. Defibrillation should **not** be delayed by any other procedures (i.e., starting IV, tracheal intubation). Mechanism of action is simultaneous depolarization of the entire heart, thereby terminating a circus rhythm.

    a. Energy setting (1 joule = 1 watt-second)

        (1) Adults   Initial shock: 200 joules

        (2) Children   2 joules/kg

    b. If unsuccessful, repeat countershock immediately

        (1) Adults   200–300 joules

        (2) Children   Double to 4 joules/kg

    c. If still unsuccessful, increase energy to maximum (360–400 joules), and use this maximum energy for all subsequent defibrillation attempts.

    d. Synchronization: During ventricular fibrillation, ensure that the synchronization **switch is off.** With the synchronization switch on, the defibrillator will **not** deliver any power until a QRS is detected (in ventricular fibrillation, none will ever arrive!). This means that **synchronization will prevent delivery of a countershock if the patient is in ventricular fibrillation!** Synchronization should be used only when attempting to convert a rhythm in which QRS complexes are already present (i.e., ventricular tachycardia, SVT, atrial fibrillation, atrial flutter).

3. Pharmacologic therapy is used if initial defibrillation attempts are unsuccessful. Useful drugs include epinephrine, lidocaine, bretylium, and procainamide.

C. Lethal tachydysrhythmias: Ventricular tachycardia

  1. Overview

    a. Ventricular tachycardia may be sustained (ongoing) or nonsustained (runs of variable length that terminate spontaneously). Either type may degenerate without warning into ventricular fibrillation.

    b. Certain patients with ventricular tachycardia can maintain sufficient cardiac output to remain conscious. In such patients, it may be feasible to attempt pharmacologic therapy prior to electrical therapy. The potential lethality of this dysrhythmia must be recognized.

    c. Torsade de pointes is a form of polymorphic ventricular tachycardia in which the envelope of the ECG has a sine wave appearance. Procainamide and other type 1A antidysrhythmic drugs must **not** be used because they may induce or exacerbate the dysrhythmia. Magnesium sulfate may be effective pharmacologic therapy.

  2. Electrical therapy of ventricular tachycardia: countershock

    a. If pulse is absent, treat the same way as ventricular fibrillation (see sec. **VII.B.2.** above).

    b. For unstable ventricular tachycardia (hypotension, symptoms), provide sedation or analgesia if appropriate and initiate cardioversion using **50 joule** energy initially. If unsuccessful, increase energy for subsequent shocks as follows: **100, 200, and then 360 joule.**

    c. For stable ventricular tachycardia, use pharmacologic therapy first; if unsuccessful, use cardioversion as above.

  3. Use pharmacologic therapy if initial countershocks are unsuccessful. Useful IV drugs include lidocaine, procainamide, and bretylium.

D. Lethal bradydysrhythmias
1. Asystole
  a. CPR with cardiac compressions should be instituted immediately.

  b. Asystole is sometimes actually a very fine (low-amplitude) form of ventricular fibrillation and thus may respond to countershock.

  c. Definitive therapy consists of **ventricular pacing** (see Chap. 16).

  d. For pharmacologic therapy, useful drugs include atropine and epinephrine. Do not use isoproterenol for asystole because of reduced coronary perfusion pressure during CPR.

2. Heart rate below 40 beats/minute
  a. If the heart is still beating, do not touch it (i.e., do not perform CPR)! Cardiac compressions may induce ventricular fibrillation in such patients.

  b. Use pharmacologic agents or pacing to accelerate the HR.

  c. Certain persons may tolerate sinus or junctional bradycardia (i.e., trained athletes) with heart rates near 40 and not require therapy.

  d. For pharmacologic therapy, useful drugs include atropine, isoproterenol, and epinephrine. **Avoid lidocaine** or other antidysrhythmic agents because asystole may result.

E. Ventricular ectopy
1. Overview
  a. Ectopic ventricular beats may progress to ventricular fibrillation or ventricular tachycardia, especially if myocardial ischemia is present. High-risk PVCs include multifocal, coupled (bigeminy), runs of two or more consecutive beats and R-on-T phenomenon.

  b. Ventricular ectopic beats can be produced by bradycardia (escape beats), myocardial ischemia, or blood gas or electrolyte abnormalities. These problems should be sought when PVCs are present.

  c. Occasionally, no cause for PVCs can be determined, and myocardial ischemia is not present. In such cases, the choice of whether or not to treat the PVCs is controversial.

2. **Pharmacologic therapy.** Useful drugs include lidocaine, procainamide, propranolol, bretylium, and quinidine.

3. **Pacing** (atrial or ventricular) may stop PVCs by overdrive suppression. Atrial pacing is preferred unless heart block is present.

F. Supraventricular tachycardia
1. Overview
  a. Therapy is determined largely by how well the patient is **tolerating** the dysrhythmia.

  b. **Countershock of SVT.** If the dysrhythmia is tolerated poorly, with hypotension, angina, or CNS changes, it must be immediately reversed, usually using **synchronized** countershock. Lower energies are needed than with ventricular dysrhythmias: Start at 5 joules if chest is open or 10–20 joules (closed chest, adults), and double the energy until conversion is achieved.

  c. If the dysrhythmia is tolerated fairly well, there is time to try pharmacologic or mechanical therapy. If the patient is already intubated, cardioverison under IV sedation or anesthesia may be the best initial treatment in some cases.

2. Methods of increasing vagal tone
  a. Mechanical induction of a **reflex** vagal discharge can be achieved by carotid sinus massage (unilateral—avoid massage in the presence of carotid atherosclerosis), Valsalva maneuver, sustained lung inflation, or eyeball pressure (avoid in the presence of ocular disease).

  b. Pharmacologic induction of a reflex vagal discharge occurs when IV **phenylephrine** raises BP.

c. **Edrophonium** causes a direct stimulation of cardiac muscarinic cholinergic receptors.

3. **Pacing** (atrial) may stop SVT by overdrive suppression.

4. **Pharmacologic therapy.** Other useful IV drugs include verapamil, beta-adrenergic blockers, and digoxin.

F. **Specific antidysrhythmic drugs**

1. **Amiodarone** (Cordarone)

a. **Actions.** Amiodarone is an iodinated benzofuran that markedly prolongs the action potential duration and QRS, QT, and PR intervals. It impairs sinus node function, is a potent vasodilator, and is an alpha- and beta-receptor noncompetitive antagonist. It acts on the atria and ventricles.

b. **Offset** occurs by hepatic elimination; very high lipid solubility results in marked tissue accumulation. Half-life is *20–100 days.*

c. **Advantages.** This drug may be effective for arrhythmias refractory to all other therapy.

d. **Disadvantages**

(1) It is highly toxic. **Pulmonary fibrosis** may be fatal, as may hepatitis or cirrhosis. Neurologic or gastrointestinal side effects are common. Photosensitivity, corneal microdeposits, hypothyroidism or hyperthyroidism may occur.

(2) Exacerbation or induction of dysrhythmias, including torsade de pointes, may occur.

(3) Heart block may occur.

(4) It may interact with general anesthetics to produce heart block, profound vasodilation, or myocardial depression. Extremely high doses of catecholamines may be required to reverse these effects during anesthesia.

(5) Extremely long duration of action (many weeks) makes toxicity long-lived even if the drug is stopped abruptly.

(6) This drug may increase the effect of oral anticoagulants, phenytoin, digoxin, diltiazem, quinidine, and other drugs.

e. **Administration:** Oral only.

f. **Clinical use**

(1) **Amiodarone dosage:** 800–1600 mg/day for 1–3 weeks, gradually reducing dosage to 400–600 mg/day for maintenance.

(2) Amiodarone should be utilized only by a qualified cardiologist. Frequent pulmonary, thyroid, and hepatic evaluations must be performed.

2. **Atropine**

a. Atropine is a belladonna alkaloid.

b. **Actions.** This drug is a competitive antagonist at muscarinic cholinergic receptors.

c. **Offset,** when given IV, occurs in 15–30 minutes; when given IM, SQ, PO, offset occurs in 4 hours. There is minimal metabolism of the drug, and 77–94% of it undergoes renal elimination.

d. **Advantages:** Rapid onset.

e. **Disadvantages**

(1) Tachycardia (undesirable with coronary disease).

(2) Exacerbation of bradycardia by low dosages ($\leq$0.2 mg in an adult).

(3) Sedation (elderly patients).

(4) Urinary retention.

(5) Increased intraocular pressure in patients with closed-angle glaucoma. Atropine may be safely given, however, if miotic eye drops are given concurrently.

f. **Indications:** Bradydysrhythmias.

g. **Administration:** IV, IM, SQ, PO, via endotracheal tube.

    h. Clinical atropine use: IV bolus. In adults, use 0.4–1.0 mg (may repeat); in children, use 0.02 mg/kg (minimum 0.1 mg, maximum 0.4 mg, may repeat).

3. Beta-adrenergic blockers (see sec. **III** above).

4. Bretylium (Bretylol)

    a. Bretylium is a bromobenzyl quaternary ammonium compound.

    b. Actions

        (1) Markedly prolongs action potential duration and refractory period.

        (2) Makes action potential duration more uniform throughout myocardium, thus decreasing stability of circus rhythms. It is especially useful for reentrant rhythms with **random conduction** over multiple anatomic pathways (i.e., tachydysrhythmias in which each depolarization is different such as ventricular fibrillation).

    c. Offset. Duration of action is 6–24 hours after IV loading dose. Elimination occurs with almost 100% renal excretion of unchanged drug; there are no metabolites. Maintenance dosages must be reduced with renal insufficiency.

    d. Advantages

        (1) Rarity of serious **cardiac** toxicity in suggested dosages makes bretylium relatively safe.

        (2) Bretylium may convert some cases of ventricular fibrillation to a regular rhythm without shock! It also facilitates electrical cardioversion.

        (3) Bretylium raises the threshold for inducing ventricular fibrillation by electrical shocks.

        (4) It has a transient initial positive inotropic effect, which is probably due to release of norepinephrine from adrenergic nerve terminals.

    e. Disadvantages

        (1) Transient initial hypertension, increased HR, and possibly increased ectopy may occur. These effects are due to release of norepinephrine from the nerve terminals.

        (2) Postural hypotension due to decreased SVR may result, probably related to inhibition of neural norepinephrine release. Patients should be kept supine. Hypotension may be severe but should respond to phenylephrine.

        (3) Bradydysrhythmias (including sinus arrest) following IV use may occur but is very uncommon.

        (4) There may be delayed onset, up to 10–20 minutes after IV bolus injection.

    f. Indications. Ventricular dysrhythmias, especially ventricular fibrillation or ventricular tachycardia, which are refractory to therapy.

    g. Administration: IV, IM

    h. Clinical use.

        (1) Bretylium dose. For life-threatening ventricular dysrhythmias, use bretylium IV by rapid injection, 5–10 mg/kg q15–30min as needed, to a maximum of 30 mg/kg (administered undiluted).

        (2) Dose for other ventricular dysrhythmias

            (a) Loading dose: IV 5–10 mg/kg injected slowly over 10 minutes; dose is repeated once after 1–2 hours as needed.

            (b) Maintenance dose: IV 5–10 mg/kg infused over 10–20 minutes q6h, or as a constant infusion, 1–2 mg/min (adults, rarely needed due to long duration); IM 5–10 mg/kg q6–8h (undiluted).

5. Calcium-blocking drugs (see sec. **VI**).
6. Calcium (see sec. **IV.C.2**).
7. Disopyramide (Norpace)
  a. Actions
    (1) Disopyramide action is similar to that of procainamide (see sec. **VII.F.16.b** below).
    (2) It has a marked anticholinergic effect.
  b. Advantages
    (1) It is effective for ventricular and supraventricular dysrhythmias.
    (2) Atrioventricular nodal conduction is not depressed (and is possibly improved because of its anticholinergic effect); thus disopyramide may be used in patients with bundle branch block without producing high-grade atrioventricular block.
  c. Disadvantages (see sec. **VII.F.16.e.** and **17.e.** below).
    (1) Negative inotropy may produce acute heart failure.
    (2) Dose-dependent anticholinergic effects prevent its use in patients with urinary retention or some types of glaucoma.
    (3) It is available only in an oral preparation.
  d. Indications
    (1) Ventricular dysrhythmias, including recurrent ventricular tachycardia
    (2) Supraventricular dysrhythmias
  e. Administration: PO only
  f. Clinical use
    (1) Disopyramide dose
      (a) Load: 300 mg
      (b) Maintenance: 150–200 mg q6h
    (2) Use with extreme caution in the presence of LV dysfunction.
    (3) Toxicity is increased with hyperkalemia or with amrinone therapy.
8. Edrophonium (Tensilon)
  a. Action. This drug is an acetylcholinesterase inhibitor; its action is reversible.
  b. Offset occurs in 5–10 minutes in low dosages and at 1.1 hours at high dosages given for reversal of neuromuscular blockade; elimination half-life is 1.8 hours.
  c. Advantages. Rapid and short-lived.
  d. Disadvantages
    (1) Sinus arrest or complete heart block is possible.
    (2) In higher dosages (without opposing antimuscarinic anticholinergic therapy), edrophonium can produce cholinergic crisis (e.g., weakness, increased oralpulmonary secretions, gastrointestinal hypermotility).
  e. Indications. Supraventricular tachycardia.
  f. Administration: IV
  g. Clinical use
    (1) Edrophonium dose. Give 1 mg IV as test dose, then 9 mg IV (total 10 mg).
    (2) Use only with continuous ECG monitoring, with atropine and pacing equipment nearby.
9. Encainide (Enkaid)
  a. Action. Encainide is a local anesthetic drug (Na^+ channel blocker) with effects similar to those of flecainide; it acts primarily on the ventricle. It prolongs the QRS duration in low doses but does not change the interval from the end of the QRS to the end of the T wave substantially.

   b. Offset occurs by hepatic metabolism. In 90% of patients, extensive metabolism produces active metabolites that produce more effect than the unchanged drug. Half-life 3–12 hours.
   c. Advantages
      (1) Does not reduce myocardial contractility or cardiac output, unlike flecainide.
      (2) Is not likely to induce torsade de pointes.
      (3) Does not interact with digoxin, unlike flecainide.
   d. Disadvantages
      (1) It is less effective than other drugs for sustained ventricular tachycardia.
      (2) It may exacerbate dysrhythmias (as may any antidysrhythmic drug).
      (3) It may produce heart block.
      (4) IV preparation is not available.
      (5) It may cause visual changes, dizziness, or headache.
   e. Indications. Oral therapy of PVCs or nonsustained ventricular tachycardia.
   f. Administration. PO only.
   g. Clinical use
      (1) Encainide dose: 25 mg tid, increasing no more frequently than every 3–5 days to a maximum of 75 mg qid.
      (2) Decrease dosage in patients with renal insufficiency.
      (3) Because of the possibility that this drug may increase the incidence of myocardial infarction or mortality, it may be appropriate to restrict its use to patients with life-threatening dysrhythmias.
10. Epinephrine (see sec. **IV.B.7**).
11. Flecainide (Tambocor)
   a. Action. Flecainide is a local anesthetic drug that acts primarily on the ventricle, decreases intracardiac conduction, and prolongs the ventricular refractory period.
   b. Offset. It is eliminated by combined hepatic and renal mechanisms; its long half-life (13 hours) may be further increased in geriatric patients or those with renal insufficiency.
   c. Advantages. It is more effective in suppressing PVCs than quinidine or disopyramide.
   d. Disadvantages
      (1) It may exacerbate dysrhythmias or induce new dysrhythmias.
      (2) It can produce sinus node dysfunction or atrioventricular block.
      (3) It impairs myocardial contractility in patients with LV dysfunction.
      (4) No IV preparation is available.
   f. Administration. Oral use only.
   e. Clinical use
      (1) Flecainide dosage: 100 mg PO bid, increasing every 4 days to a maximum of 400 mg/day.
      (2) Plasma concentrations should be monitored.
      (3) Because of the possibility that this drug may increase the incidence of myocardial infarction or mortality, it may be appropriate to restrict its use to patients with life-threatening dysrhythmias.
12. Isoproterenol (see sec. **IV.B.8**).
13. Lidocaine (lignocaine, Xylocaine)
   a. Lidocaine is a tertiary amine amide-type local anesthetic that blocks Na^+ channels.
   b. Actions

      (1) Activity is localized to ventricles, with no significant atrial or atrioventricular nodal antidysrhythmic actions.

      (2) Lidocaine decreases automaticity, especially in ischemic ventricular tissue.

      (3) Reentrant dysrhythmias may be abolished by **improving conduction** in areas of the heart that previously demonstrated unidirectional conduction block.

    c. Offset. Duration of action is 15–30 minutes after administration of bolus dose; offset occurs by hepatic metabolism (95% metabolites are not active). Factors that reduce hepatic blood flow will prolong the duration of action (e.g., CHF, alpha agonists, liver disease).

    d. Advantages. Since moderate toxicity does not cause adverse **cardiac** effects, lidocaine is very safe.

    e. Disadvantages

      (1) CNS excitation may result from mild to moderate overdose, producing confusion or seizures.

      (2) CNS depression may result from a severe overdose, producing sedation or respiratory depression.

      (3) Lidocaine can convert idioventricular rhythm to asystole. **Do not administer for complete heart block!**

      (4) Hypotension may occur but is rare with suggested dosages.

      (5) Lidocaine is probably safe for use during **malignant hyperthermia,** based on recent information.

    f. Indications: Ventricular dysrhythmias.

    g. Administration: IV or via endotracheal tube.

    h. Clinical use

      (1) **Lidocaine dose**

        (a) Loading dose: IV, 1 mg/kg twice (second dose is give 20–30 minutes after first dose).

        (b) Maintenance dose: 15–50 μg/kg/min (i.e., 1–4 mg/min in adults).

      (2) Lidocaine is most effective for **orderly types of reentrant dysrhythmias,** such as ventricular tachycardia and coupled ventricular ectopy (e.g., bigeminy).

      (3) It is helpful in facilitating conversion of ventricular fibrillation.

      (4) When given prior to endotracheal intubation, it may help to blunt sympathetic stimulation. This is especially useful in patients with coronary artery disease.

14. Mexiletine (Mexitil)

    a. Actions. Mexiletine is a local anesthetic related to lidocaine but is orally active. It shortens the action potential duration and refractory period without prolonging QRS or QT duration.

    b. Offset occurs mostly by hepatic metabolism; half life is 9–11 hours.

    c. Advantages. It is usually effective for PVCs or nonsustained ventricular tachycardia.

    d. Disadvantages

      (1) No IV preparation is available.

      (2) It may be less effective for sustained ventricular tachycardia than for PVCs.

      (3) It may exacerbate dysrhythmias or sinus node dysfunction.

      (4) It may cause atrioventricular block.

      (5) It has frequent side effects, primarily gastrointestinal, neurologic, rheumatologic, hepatic, and hematologic.

    e. Administration. Oral only.

    f. Clinical use

      (1) **Mexilitine dosage:** 100–200 mg PO tid; increase every 2–3 days to a maximum dosage of 1200 mg/day.

(2) It may interact with rifampin or phenytoin to reduce plasma concentrations; alkalinization of the urine may increase plasma levels.

(3) Plasma levels should be monitored.

15. Phenytoin (diphenylhydantoin, Dilantin)

a. Phenytoin is an antiepileptic drug structurally related to the barbiturates but lacking sedative effect.

b. **Actions.** Similar to those of procainamide (see sec. **VII.F.16.b**).

c. **Offset.** Elimination half-life is 6–24 hours (variable), increasing as plasma levels increase; metabolism is more than 95% hepatic. Dosage should be guided by plasma drug levels.

d. **Advantages.** Phenytoin is effective in treating dysrhythmias (especially ventricular dysrhythmias) due to digitalis toxicity.

e. **Disadvantages**

(1) Phenytoin has disadvantages that are similar to those of procainamide (see sec. **VII.F.16.d**).

(2) Rapid IV administration may cause hypotension and dysrhythmias, atrioventricular block, and respiratory depression.

(3) Hepatic microsomal enzyme induction alters metabolism of phenytoin, as does Coumadin.

(4) Hyperglycemia may occur.

f. **Indications.** Phenytoin is usually reserved for **digitalis toxic** dysrhythmias that are unresponsive to potassium replacement therapy and lidocaine.

g. **Administration.** IV, PO.

h. **Clinical use**

(1) **Phenytoin dose**

(a) **Loading dose:** Adult: 100-mg IV increments are given until dysrhythmia is abolished or a dose of 1000 mg is reached (10–15 mg/kg). Give slowly (25–50 mg/min) while monitoring BP and ECG data. Pediatric dose: 5–20 mg/kg given slowly (<1–3 mg/kg/min).

(b) **Maintenance dose.** Long duration of action makes infusion unnecessary; one to two bolus doses per day are adequate for maintenance of drug levels. Adult: 300–400 mg/day; children 5 mg/kg/day.

(2) IM absorption is erratic.

(3) Therapeutic plasma level is 7.5–20.0 µg/ml.

16. Procainamide (Pronestyl)

a. Procainamide is an amide local anesthetic drug.

b. **Actions**

(1) Procainamide stabilizes membranes, thereby decreasing automaticity and conduction in all cardiac tissue, both normal and ischemic.

(2) Myocardial depressant effects convert regions of unidirectional conduction block into bidirectional conduction block, explaining the drug's beneficial effect on reentrant dysrhythmias.

(3) Procainamide's ability to reduce automaticity explains beneficial effects on enhanced-automaticity dysrhythmias, especially in the atria and atrioventricular node.

c. **Offset.** Duration of action is 2–4 hours; metabolism is both hepatic (50% of drug is metabolized to N-acetylprocainamide, the active metabolite) and renal (50%). Slow acetylators are more dependent on renal elimination. Reduce maintenance dosages in patients with renal insufficiency.

d. **Advantages**

(1) This drug has a wide spectrum of antidysrhythmic activity and is effective against atrial, atrioventricular nodal, and ventricular dysrhythmias.

(2) It slows conduction through accessory conduction (e.g., Kent) pathways.

(3) It is safe for use during malignant hyperthermia.

e. Disadvantages

(1) Toxicity is first manifest in the heart, at drug levels that cause no other toxicity.

(2) It can induce torsade de pointes, a form of ventricular tachycardia (especially in patients with a long QT interval).

(3) Electrophysiologic depression may occur. With sufficiently high dosage, procainamide will cause atrioventricular nodal block and intraventricular conduction delay. Pacing or beta-adrenergic agonist therapy may be necessary if overdose is given.

(4) Decreased myocardial contractility can induce CHF.

(5) Vasodilation may occur.

(6) Central nervous system excitability may occur, with confusion and seizures.

(7) Lupuslike syndrome is seen only with long-term therapy.

(8) This drug can increase ventricular response rate with atrial tachydysrhythmias.

f. Indications for use

(1) Ventricular dysrhythmias

(2) Supraventricular dysrhythmias

(3) Accessory conduction pathway dysrhythmias such as Wolff-Parkinson-White syndrome

g. Clinical use

(1) **Procainamide dose**

(a) **Loading dose**

(i) IV: 10–50 mg/min (100 mg q2–5min) until toxicity or desired effect occurs up to 12 mg/kg

(ii) IM: 6–12 mg/kg

(iii) Pediatric IV: 3–6 mg/kg given slowly

(b) **Maintenance dose**

(i) Adult. IV infusion: 2 mg/kg/h; IM: 6 mg/kg q3–8h; PO: 250–1000 mg q3h.

(ii) Children. IV infusion, 20-50 μg/kg/min; PO: 30–50 mg/kg/day divided in four to six doses.

(2) **Stop drug administration** before maximal dose in the following situations:

(a) More than 50% increase in QRS duration

(b) PR interval prolongation

(c) Hypotension

(d) Disappearance of dysrhythmia

(3) Procainamide is not a first-line drug for acute life-threatening dysrhythmias because of its high potential for cardiac toxicity. It must be administered with extreme care.

17. Quinidine

a. Quinidine is structurally similar to quinine; it is found in the bark of the cinchona tree.

b. Actions are similar to those of procainamide (see sec. **VII.F.16.b** above).

c. Offset. Duration of action is 4–6 hours; metabolism is hepatic (60–85% of drug) to inactive metabolites. Prolonged effect occurs with hepatic or renal failure or CHF; shortened effect occurs with hepatic enzyme induction.

d. Advantages

(1) It is useful for both atrial and ventricular dysrhythmias.

(2) Greater dosing interval is possible than with procainamide.

e. Disadvantages

(1) Quinidine may induce life-threatening ventricular dysrhythmias, including the torsade de pointes form of ventricular tachycardia.

(2) Vagolytic effect may cause tachycardia and can increase the ventricular response rate in atrial tachydysrhythmias.

(3) It interacts with digoxin to increase digoxin plasma levels, leading to digitalis toxicity.

(4) It is dangerous given IV (see **h** below).

(5) It shares the other adverse effects of procainamide (except that there is no lupuslike reaction).

(6) It may potentiate the action of oral anticoagulants.

(7) It may exacerbate myasthenia gravis.

f. Indications: Ventricular dysrhythmias, supraventricular dysrhythmias.

g. Administration: PO; rarely IV.

h. Clinical use

(1) **Quinidine dose. Important note: IV use is *not recommended.***

(a) IV adult dose (quinidine gluconate) is 4–10 mg/kg at less than or equal to 0.3–0.4 mg/kg/min with careful monitoring; maximum dose is 600 mg. *Consultation with a cardiologist is recommended prior to IV quinidine administration. Use of IV quinidine in pediatric patients is not recommended. See sec.* (2) *and* (3) *below.*

(b) PO adult dose (sulfate): 200–600 mg q6–8h; adult dose (gluconate): 324–648 mg q8–12h; pediatric dose (sulfate): 3–6 mg/kg q3h (maximum, 12 mg/kg).

(2) Use IV very cautiously. Stop IV infusion for the following reasons:

(a) Increase in QRS duration of more than 25-50%.

(b) Loss of P waves.

(c) Disappearance of dysrhythmia.

(d) Hypotension.

(3) Quindine is not recommended for IV use except in special circumstances owing to the high incidence of hypotension, vasodilation, myocardial depression, and **increased** frequency of ventricular dysrhythmias.

(4) Intramuscular injection is painful with erratic absorption.

(5) Other uses are similar to those of procainamide (see sec. **VII.F.16.g**).

18. Tocainide (Tonocard)

a. Tocainide is an analog of lidocaine but is orally active; it is an amide local anesthetic.

b. Actions

(1) This drug has ventricular effects only.

(2) Like lidocaine, it has no significant depressant effect on conduction, so that PR, QRS, and QT intervals remain unchanged.

c. Offset is by renal excretion of unchanged drug (40%) and hepatic metabolism. Elimination is prolonged in patients with renal failure, hepatic failure, or alkaline urine. Normal half-life is 11–17 hours.

d. Advantages

(1) Unlike lidocaine, oral administration is effective.

(2) Antidysrhythmic spectrum of action resembles that of lidocaine.

(3) No significant depression of contractility occurs.

   e. Disadvantages
      (1) Central nervous system excitation may occur, with tremor, paresthesia, confusion, and seizures.
      (2) There may be allergic reactions.
      (3) Coadministration with propranolol may produce psychosis.
   f. Indications: Ventricular dysrhythmias.
   g. Administration: PO only.
   h. Clinical use
      (1) Tocainide dose: 400–600 mg PO tid. Maximum dose, 800 mg tid.
      (2) Tocainide may be safer for treating chronic ventricular ectopy than procainamide, quinidine, or disopyramide and may be effective for treating dysrhythmias refractory to those agents.
H. Refractory dysrhythmias: differential diagnosis. Lethal dysrhythmias that continue despite treatment may be caused by nondelivery of drugs, metabolic abnormalities, inadequate systemic perfusion, myocardial ischemia, drug toxicity, or mechanical abnormalities. If blood pressure is absent, CPR should be instituted immediately. Always remember the "ABCs" of CPR: airway, breathing, circulation.
1. Drug delivery problems
   a. IV patency. Infiltrated peripheral IVs. Can blood be withdrawn from central lines? **Alternative routes** may be used when IV access is not available, especially the intratracheal route (lidocaine, epinephrine, atropine)
   b. Dosage error
   c. Outdated drug
2. Metabolic abnormalities
   a. Oxygen (hypoxemia)
      (1) Pneumothorax (tension?)
      (2) Endotracheal tube problem (e.g., esophageal intubation, kink or plug in tube, endobroncheal intubation—ventilating only one lung)
      (3) Patient not receiving **oxygen** in **adequate volumes**
      (4) Lung disease (bronchospasm, pulmonary edema, atelectasis, aspiration of gastric contents)
   b. Potassium
      (1) Hyperkalemia
         (a) Effects: heart block, asystole, dysrhythmias, negative inotropy
         (b) Diagnosis: ECG (e.g., peaked T waves, loss of P waves, heart block, dysrhythmias, ventricular tachycardia, ventricular fibrillation)
         (c) Treatment
            (i) Alkalosis shifts potassium ions from the vascular space into cells. Give bicarbonate or hyperventilate the patient; either works immediately as a temporary measure
            (ii) Insulin plus glucose shifts potassium ions into cells. Adult doses: regular **insulin,** 10 units IV, plus **dextrose** 50% × 50 ml (25 gm), which works in 10–30 min
            (iii) Calcium salts reduce adverse cardiac effects of hyperkalemia (see sec. **IV.C.2** for dosage) and work immediately as a temporary measure
            (iv) Diuretic increases renal K^+ elimination. **Furosemide,** 0.1–1.0 mg/kg IV, works over 30 min to many hours
            (v) Dialysis eliminates K^+ from body rapidly
            (vi) Ion-exchange resin eliminates K^+ from body, acting slowly over hours

  (2) Hypokalelmia. Dysrhythmias constitute the most important effect, especially in patients receiving digitalis. Avoid respiratory or metabolic alkalosis, both of which will exacerbate hypokalemia. Therapy is K$^+$ replacement by slow infusion (never by bolus IV)

 c. Acid-base. Arterial blood gas analysis is indicated, looking for respiratory or metabolic acidosis or alkalosis. Avoid treating **respiratory acidosis** with bicarbonate. The only effective therapy is **ventilation.**

 d. Calcium, magnesium

  (1) Hypocalcemia: negative inotropy, treat with IV calcium

  (2) Hypomagnesemia may cause dysrhythmias. **Magnesium sulfate,** 1–2 gm (8–16 mEq), can be administered by slow IV infusion. Normal plasma magnesium level is 0.7–1.2 mM/liter, and levels should be monitored to avoid toxicity

 e. Hypothermia. A cold patient will have marked cardiac irritability and will tend to develop ventricular fibrillation that may be refractory to countershock until the temperature is normalized. Rewarm patient using passive or active techniques. A patient is never dead until warm and dead.

3. Inadequate perfusion: ineffective CPR.

 a. Assessment of perfusion during CPR. The adequacy of CPR should be assessed continuously by several means:

  (1) Palpation of a central pulse (femoral or carotid)

  (2) Blood pressure (arterial line, if available)

  (3) Blood gases (especially noting worsening of metabolic acidosis); examination of venous blood gases is valuable in addition to the standard arterial analysis

  (4) End-tidal CO_2 concentration (indicating delivery of metabolic CO_2 to the lungs)

  (5) Urine output (Foley catheter)

 b. Causes of inadequate perfusion during CPR

  (1) Inadequate preload

   (a) Hypovolemia: blood loss, dehydration

   (b) Pericardial tamponade

   (c) Tension pneumothorax

   (d) Pulmonary embolus

   (e) Venodilation

   (f) Vena cava compression

  (2) Inadequate afterload (SVR)

   (a) Inappropriate **vasodilation**

   (b) Sepsis

   (c) Drug effect

  (3) Inadequate contractility

   (a) Myocardial ischemia

   (b) Preexisting cardiomyopathy

   (c) Metabolic abnormalities

   (d) Drug effects

  (4) Valvular heart disease

   (a) Aortic stenosis

   (b) Mitral stenosis

   (c) Aortic regurgitation

   (d) Mitral regurgitation

  (5) Mechanical impairment

   (a) Pericardial tamponade. Therapy: pericardiocentesis or pericardiotomy

   (b) Tension pneumothorax. Therapy: pleural aspiration or tube thoracostomy

   (c) Aortic dissection

(d) **Myocardial rupture** (free wall or septum)

(e) **Electromechanical dissociation:** diagnosis of exclusion only. Prognosis is poor. Little benefit from administration of calcium. Epinephrine is sometimes helpful.

4. **Myocardial ischemia.**

a. **Coronary artery disease** (fixed stenoses)

b. **Coronary artery spasm** (reversible with therapy of nitroglycerin or nifedipine)

c. **Dysrhythmogenic focus** of tissue following myocardial infarction

d. If antianginal medication and elevation of coronary perfusion pressure do not help, consider insertion of intraaortic **balloon pump**

5. **Drug toxicity.** Many pharmacologic agents can product dysrhythmias. In approximately 10% of patients receiving an antidysrhythmic drug, the dysrhythmia will be exacerbated. Sympathomimetic agents with beta-1 activity, tricyclic antidepressants, some phenothiazine drugs, cocaine, and others may all induce dysrhythmias. Eliciting a drug history may be helpful.

6. **If all else fails,** consider **open cardiac massage** because this may be the only means of supporting the circulation (in patients with critical aortic stenosis, for example).

VIII. **Diuretics**

A. **Actions.** Modern IV diuretics act at the loop of Henle in the kidney to block reabsorption of electrolytes from the tubule. This action increases excretion of water and electrolytes (Na, Cl, K, Ca, Mg) from body.

B. **Effects shared by all loop diuretics**

a. **Hypokalemia**

2. **Metabolic alkalosis**

3. **Increased serum uric acid**

4. **Ototoxicity.** Deafness, temporary or permanent, is rare with ethacrynic acid but has also been reported with furosemide or bumetanide. Coadministration with an aminoglycoside antibiotic may increase risk. One possible mechanism for this is drug-induced changes in endolymph electrolyte composition.

C. **Specific drugs**

1. **Furosemide** (Lasix)

a. **Offset** is by renal tubular secretion of unchanged drug and of glucuronide metabolite; half-life of 1.5 hours is increased in patients with renal failure.

b. **Clinical use**

(1) **Furosemide dosage.**

(a) **Adults.** The usual IV starting dose for patients not currently receiving diuretics is 2.5–5.0 mg, increasing as necessary to 200-mg bolus. Patients already receiving diuretics usually require 20- to 40-mg initial doses to produce a diuresis. A continuous infusion (0.5–1.0 mg/kg/hr) may be more effective in producing a sustained diuresis than intermittent bolus injections.

(b) **Pediatric dosage.** 1mg/kg initially; maximum dose is 6 mg/kg.

(2) Because furosemide is a sulfonamide, allergic reactions may occur in sulfonamide-sensitive patients (rare).

(3) Furosemide often causes transient vasodilation of veins and arterioles, with reduced cardiac preload.

2. **Bumetanide** (Bumex)

a. **Offset** is by combined renal and hepatic elimination; half-life is 1–1.5 hours.

b. **Clinical use**

(1) **Bumetanide dosage:** 0.5–1.0 mg IV. It may be repeated every

2–3 hours to a maximum dose of 10 mg/day. IM dose is identical.

(2) Myalgias may occur.

3. **Ethacrynic acid** (Edecrin)

   a. **Offset** is by combined renal and hepatic elimination.

   b. **Clinical use**

      (1) **Ethacrynic acid dose:** 50 mg IV (adult dose), titrated to effect.

      (2) Use of this drug is usually reserved for patients who fail to respond to furosemide or bumetanide.

4. **Mannitol**

   a. **Mechanism of action.** Mannitol is an osmotic diuretic that is eliminated unchanged in urine; it is also a free-radical scavenger. Not a loop diuretic.

   b. **Advantages**

      (1) Unlike the loop diuretics (e.g., furosemide), mannitol retains its efficacy even during *low glomerular filtration* states (e.g., **shock**).

      (2) It *protects* the kidney against development of acute renal failure.

      (3) As an osmotically active agent in the bloodstream, it will pull free water out of organs (e.g., reducing **cerebral edema**).

   c. **Clinical use**

      (1) Mannitol dosage. Initial dose is 12.5 g to a maximum of 0.5 g/kg acutely.

      (2) It may produce hypotension if administered as a rapid IV bolus.

      (3) It may induce transient congestive heart failure because intravascular volume will expand before diuresis begins.

      (4) It is useful for prevention of renal failure due to poor renal perfusion, hemoglobinuria, or nephrotoxins.

      (5) It is used in treatment of cerebral edema.

SUGGESTED READINGS

Antonaccio, M. J. (ed.). *Cardiovascular Pharmacology* (2nd ed.). New York: Raven, 1984.

D'Ambra, M. N., LaRaia, P. J., Philbin, D. M., et al. Prostaglandin E_1. A new therapy for refractory right heart failure and pulmonary hypertension after mitral valve replacement. *J. Thorac. Cardiovasc. Surg.* 89:567–572, 1985.

Ewy, G. A., and Bressler, R. L. (eds). *Cardiovascular Drugs and the Management of Heart Disease.* New York: Raven, 1982.

Gilman, A. G., Goodman, L. S., Rall, T. W., et al. *The Pharmacological Basis of Therapeutics* (7th ed.). New York: Macmillan, 1985.

Kaplan, J. A. (ed.). *Cardiac Anesthesia* (2nd ed.). Orlando: Grune & Stratton, 1987.

Kaplan, J. A. (ed.). *Cardiac Anesthesia. Vol. 2, Cardiovascular Pharmacology.* New York: Grune & Stratton, 1983.

Ream, A. K., and Fogdall, R. P. *Acute Cardiovascular Management, Anesthesia and Intensive Care.* Philadelphia: Lippincott, 1982.

Roberts, N. K., and Gelband, H. *Cardiac Arrhythmias in the Neonate, Infant, and Child* (2nd ed.). Norwalk, CT: Appleton-Century-Crofts, 1983.

Ruffolo, R. R., Jr. Review: The pharmacology of dobutamine. *Am. J. Med. Sci.* 294:244–248, 1987.

Smith, N. T., Miller, R. D., and Corbascio, A. N. *Drug Interactions in Anesthesia.* Philadelphia: Lea & Febiger, 1981.

The Medical Letter (New Rochelle, N.Y. 10801) is an excellent source of up-to-date drug information.

This chapter is a revision of D. R. Larach and W. A. Kofke, Cardiovascular Drugs. In W. A. Kofke and J. H. Lerry (eds.), *Postoperative Critical Care Procedures of the Massachusetts General Hospital.* Boston: Little, Brown, 1986. The contribution of W. A. Kofke is acknowledged with thanks.

Monitoring the Cardiac Surgical Patient

Thomas M. Skeehan and Daniel M. Thys

I. Cardiovascular monitors
  A. Electrocardiogram
  B. Noninvasive blood pressure monitors
  C. Intravascular pressure measurements
  D. Arterial catherization
  E. Central venous pressure
  F. Pulmonary artery catheter
  G. Left atrial pressure
  H. Cardiac output
  I. Transesophageal echocardiography
II. Pulmonary system
  A. Pulse oximetry
  B. Capnography
III. Temperature
  A. Indications
  B. Types of measuring devices
  C. Sites of measurement
  D. Risks of bleeding
  E. Recommendations for temperature monitoring
IV. Renal function
  A. Indications for monitoring
  B. Urinary catheter
  C. Electrolytes
V. Neurologic function
  A. Indications for monitoring the EEG
  B. Processed versus raw EEG
  C. Evoked potentials

Patients presenting for cardiac surgery require extensive monitoring because of (1) severe, often unstable cardiovascular disease, (2) coexisting multisystemic diseases, and (3) the unphysiologic conditions associated with cardiopulmonary bypass.

Monitoring techniques have been developed to provide early warning of conditions that may lead to potentially life-threatening complications. This chapter will provide a system by system discussion of the indications, applications, and techniques of currently available monitoring modalities as well as their advantages, disadvantages, and complications.

I. Cardiovascular monitors

A. **Electrocardiogram.** The intraoperative use of the electrocardiogram (ECG) has increased during the last several decades. Originally, this monitor was used during anesthesia for the detection of dysrhythmias only in high-risk patients. However, since then its importance as a standard monitor has been recognized, and its use during the conduct of any anesthetic is now recommended. Its usefulness for the intraoperative diagnosis of myocardial ischemia is now well established owing to the efforts of many cardiovascular anesthesiologists.

1. **Indications**

   a. **Diagnosis of dysrhythmias**

   b. **Diagnosis of ischemia** (see Chap. 11). In the anesthetized patient, the detection of ischemia by ECG becomes even more important because the usual symptom, angina, cannot be elicited. See Fig. 11-5 for characteristic patterns of ECG detection of ischemia.

   c. **Diagnosis of conduction defects**

   d. **Diagnosis of electrolyte disturbances**

2. **Techniques**

   a. **The three-electrode system.** This system utilizes only electrodes on the right arm, left arm, and left leg. The potential difference between two of the electrodes is recorded while the third electrode serves as a ground. One pair of electrodes can be selected for monitoring at one time; three ECG leads (I, II, III) can therefore be examined.

      The three-lead system has been expanded to include the augmented leads, which identifies one of the three leads as the exploring electrode and couples the remaining two at a central terminal with zero potential. This creates leads in three more axes (aVR, aVL, aVF) in the frontal plane (Fig. 4-1). Leads II, III, and aVF are most useful for monitoring the inferior wall, and leads I and aVL for the lateral wall; however, the anterior wall cannot be monitored using these leads.

   b. **The modified three-electrode system.** Numerous modifications of the standard bipolar limb lead system have been developed. Both standard and modified bipolar limb leads are described in Table 4-1. Modified leads can be used to maximize P-wave height for the diagnosis of atrial dysrhythmias or to increase the sensitivity of the three-lead ECG for the detection of anterior myocardial ischemia. In clinical studies, these modified three-electrode systems have been shown to be as sensitive as the standard V_5 lead system for the intraoperative diagnosis of ischemia.

   c. **The five-electrode system.** The use of five electrodes (one lead on each extremity and one precordial lead) allows the recording of the six standard frontal limb leads as well as one precordial unipolar lead. All limb leads act as a common ground for the precordial unipolar lead. The unipolar lead is usually placed in

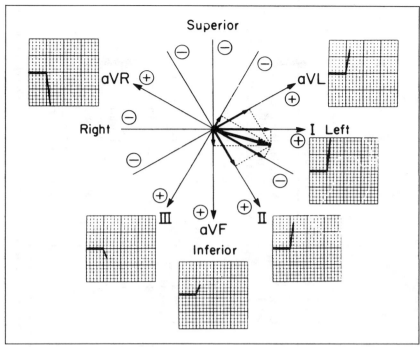

Fig. 4-1. The six frontal plane axes that are available from three leads (R arm, L arm, and L leg) are shown. I, II, and III are bipolar leads, meaning that the potential between two electrodes (one positive, one negative) is monitored. The augmented leads (aVR, aVL, and aVF) are unipolar leads; one lead is the exploring electrode (the positive terminal), and the other two are connected and set at zero potential (indifferent, or neutral). The potential difference is then the absolute difference between the exploring and zero terminals. Connecting the two indifferent leads together produces the augmented lead axes that are between the bipolar lead axes. A sample electrical vector is shown *(heavy arrow)*, with its projections to the six frontal axes. The direction of the electrical vector, then, is dictated by the degree of the deflection seen on the axis of each particular lead of the surface ECG. (From D.M. Thys, and J.A. Kaplan. *The ECG in Anesthesia and Critical Care.* New York: Churchill Livingstone, 1987. P. 5. With permission.)

the V_5 position, along the anterior axillary line in the fifth intercostal space.

(1) **Advantages.** With the addition of only two electrodes to the ECG system, seven different leads can be monitored simultaneously. More important, all but the posterior wall of the myocardium can be monitored for ischemia. In patients with coronary artery disease it has been shown that 90% of ischemic episodes will be detected by ECG if multiple leads, and particularly the V_5 lead, are analyzed[5]. Therefore, a correctly placed V_5 lead in conjunction with limb leads should enhance the diagnosis of the vast majority of intraoperative ischemia events. Multiple ECG leads will also be useful in the diagnosis of atrial versus ventricular dysrhythmias.

(2) **Disadvantage.** The V_5 electrode should not interfere with the operative field for a median sternotomy, although it will cer-

Table 4-1. Bipolar and augmented leads for use with three electrodes

Lead identifier	Right arm electrode	Left arm electrode	Left leg electrode	Lead select	Advantages
Standard					
I	Right arm	Left arm	Ground	I	Monitoring lateral ischemia
II	Right arm	Ground	Left leg	II	Monitoring for (1) dysrhythmia (good P-wave and QRS height) (2) inferior ischemia
III	Ground	Left arm	Left leg	III	Monitoring for inferior ischemia
Augmented					
aVR	Right arm	Common ground	Common ground	aVR	Monitoring lateral ischemia
aVL	Common ground	Left arm	Common ground	aVL	Monitoring lateral ischemia
aVF	Common ground	Common ground	Left leg	aVF	Monitoring inferior ischemia
Special					
MCL_1	Ground	Under left clavicle	V_1 position	III	Monitoring for dysrhythmia (good P-wave and QRS height)
CS_5	Under right clavicle	V_5 position	Ground	I	Monitoring anterior ischemia
CM_5	Manubrium sternum	V_5 position	Ground	I	Monitoring anterior ischemia
CB_5	Center of right scapula	V_5 position	Ground	I	Monitoring for (1) anterior ischemia; (2) dysrhythmia (good P-wave)
CC_5	Right anterior axillary line	V_5 position	Ground	I	Monitoring ischemia

Source: Modified from R. M. Griffin and J. A. Kaplan. ECG Lead Systems. In D. Thys and J. Kaplan (eds.), *The ECG in Anesthesia and Critical Care.* New York: Churchill Livingstone, 1987, p. 20. With permission.

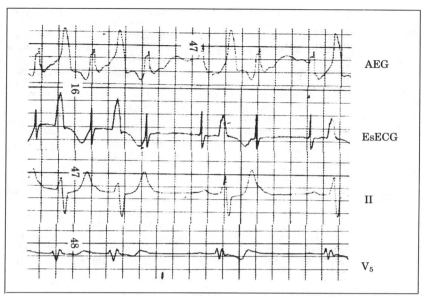

Fig. 4-2. Esophageal electrocardiogram (EsECG) clearly identifying progression of first-degree heart block (PR = 0.24 seconds) to second-degree block (Mobitz type II). P waves appear as spikes in the EsSCG, and the diagnosis is verified by the intra-atrial electrocardiogram (AEG). Because of the long PR interval, P waves are buried in the T wave in both leads II and V_5, leading to the possibility of an incorrect diagnosis of sinus bradycardia. (From R.A. Kates, J.R. Zaidan, and J.A. Kaplan. Esophageal lead for intraoperative electrocardiographic monitoring. *Anesth. Analg.* 61:783, 1982. With permission.)

tainly interfere with a left thoracotomy incision. The four limb leads should be placed on the back of the shoulders and hips, where they will be disturbed the least during median sternotomy. The V_5 lead, as well as the two leg leads, should be well protected with waterproof tape, since surgical preparation solutions will loosen electrode patches and interfere with the electrical signal.

d. Invasive ECG

    (1) Esophageal. Esophageal leads can be incorporated into the esophageal stethoscope and are very useful for the diagnosis of atrial dysrhythmias (Fig. 4-2). The relative ease and safety of the esophageal ECG lead has been demonstrated. Although 100% of the atrial dysrhythmias were correctly diagnosed with the esophageal lead (using intracavitary ECG as the standard), lead II led to a correct diagnosis in 54% of the cases and V_5 in 42% of the cases[4]. In addition, the esophageal lead is sensitive for the detection of posterior wall ischemia.

    (2) Endotracheal. ECG leads have been incorporated into the endotracheal tube. Although such endotracheal tubes are presently not available commercially, they may be useful in pediatric cardiac patients for the diagnosis of atrial dysrhythmias.

    (3) Multipurpose pulmonary artery (PA) catheter. The multipurpose PA catheter has all the features of a standard PA catheter (see sec. **I.F.**). In addition, three atrial and two ventricular electrodes have been incorporated into the catheter. These electrodes allow not only recording of intracavitary ECGs but also atrial or atrioventricular pacing. A selective ECG can be recorded to diagnose atrial, ventricular, or atrioventricular nodal dysrhythmias or conduction blocks.

(4) Epicardial electrodes. It is common practice for cardiac surgeons to place ventricular or atrial epicardial pacing wires prior to weaning the patient from cardiopulmonary bypass or before sternal closure. Although the primary intent of these wires is to allow atrioventricular pacing in the postbypass period, they can also be utilized to record atrial and ventricular epicardial ECGs. These leads are most useful in the postoperative diagnosis of complex conduction problems and dysrhythmias (see Chap. 10).

3. Recording and interpretation. To fully utilize the capabilities of ECG monitoring, particular attention must be paid to the elimination of major sources of artifact and error.

a. Patient-electrode interface. The electrical signal generated by the heart and monitored by the ECG is very weak, amounting to only 0.5-2.0 mV at the skin surface. It is therefore imperative that the skin be prepared optimally to avoid signal loss at the skin-electrode interface. The skin should be clean and free of all dirt, and it is best to abrade the skin lightly to remove part of the stratum corneum, which can be a source of high resistance. Skin resistance can be as great as 1,000,000 Ω (ohms). To avoid the problem of muscle artifact, electrodes should be placed over bony prominences whenever possible.

b. Electrodes. Electrodes should all be of the silver chloride type to avoid a resistance mismatch between various kinds of electrodes. Needle electrodes should be avoided at all times because of the risk of thermal injury related to cautery use.

c. Leads and connecting cables

(1) Insulation. The main source of artifact from ECG leads is loss of integrity of the insulation on leads and connecting cables.

(2) Motion artifact. Lead movement will lead to artifact, which can be minimized by twisting the leads on themselves.

(3) Crossing cables. Crossing other monitoring cables (especially the pulse oximeter cable, which transmits an amplified signal) over the ECG leads will cause significant interference.

d. Electronic filtering system. Most ECG monitors have filters to decrease environmental artifacts. They can usually operate in two modes, each with a different frequency response:

(1) Monitoring mode (0.5–40.0 Hz). The monitoring mode eliminates both low- and high-frequency artifacts such as wandering baseline but also distorts the height of the QRS complex and the degree of ST-segment depression or elevation.

(2) Diagnostic mode (0.05–100.00 Hz). This mode does not filter the higher frequency signals but is more subject to artifact. The ECG in diagnostic mode will accurately reflect abnormal (i.e., ischemic) changes.

e. Display. Most ECG displays are of the cathode-ray, oscilloscope type. Calibration of the trace with the 1-mV calibration signal is necessary to interpret ST-segment changes properly. A calibrated strip chart recording of the ECG should be available so that a more careful analysis of dysrhythmias and ST-segment abnormalities can be performed.

      f. Computer-assisted ECG interpretation. Computer programs for on-line analysis of dysrhythmias and ischemia are currently available (see Chap. 12).

    4. Risks associated with ECG. Patient risk with skin electrodes should be minimal as long as needle electrodes are not utilized. Even the more invasive forms of ECG monitoring such as esophageal, endotracheal, and intracavitary recordings are safe provided proper patient isolation is ensured and monitors with leakage currents are avoided. The concept of microshock hazard is addressed in Chap. 12.

    5. Recommendations for ECG monitoring. It is recommended that for cardiac surgical anesthesia, a five-electrode surface ECG monitor be used in the diagnostic mode. Ideally, this monitor should be able to display at least two leads simultaneously. The use of two simultaneous leads to monitor two different areas of myocardium supplied by two different coronary arteries facilitates the diagnosis of dysrhythmias and increases the ability to detect ischemia. If a more detailed ECG is required postoperatively, the epicardial atrial and ventricular wires can be used. If these wires are not available, other methods of invasive ECG monitoring should be considered. A hard copy of ECG patterns should be available for more accurate diagnoses.

B. Noninvasive blood pressure monitors

    1. Indications in the cardiac patient. Usually, noninvasive methods for measuring blood pressure are not adequate for monitoring hemodynamic parameters during a cardiac surgical procedure, especially one that involves cardiopulmonary bypass. Because of the following limitations they often are used merely as adjuncts to invasive blood pressure monitoring.

      a. Inaccuracy. Inaccurate measurements occur, especially at extremes of hyper- or hypotension.

      b. Intermittent data. Blood pressure measurements are provided only every 1–2 minutes.

      c. Requirement for pulsatile flow. These methods cannot be used during nonpulsatile cardiopulmonary bypass.

    2. Techniques. Noninvasive blood pressure detection relies on the principle of pulsatile flow. If a cuff is applied to a limb and inflated to a pressure greater than systolic, flow to the arteries distal to the occlusion is reduced to zero. As the cuff pressure is slowly released through the systolic and then diastolic pressure, characteristic changes occur in pressure or flow distal to the cuff. These changes can be detected by one of four methods:

      a. Auscultation (Korotkoff sounds). The cuff pressure at which the first sounds are heard distally with a stethoscope has been shown to correlate with systolic pressure, and the pressure at which these sounds become muffled and then disappear has been shown to correlate with the diastolic pressure.

      b. Oscillometric method. A microprocessor interprets oscillations within the occluding cuff to determine systolic, mean, and diastolic blood pressure, using changes in oscillation amplitude (Fig. 4-3). This is the most commonly used method for automated devices.

      c. Ultrasonic detection. An ultrasound beam is directed at the wall of the brachial artery. Blood pressure is derived from the shift in the frequency of the reflected ultrasound waves resulting from changes in the movement of the arterial wall as the cuff deflates.

      d. Plethysmographic method. In this method, a small cuff is placed on the index finger, not on the upper arm. The skin is illuminated by a weak light source, and a photosensor is stimulated by the reflected light. With pulsatile blood flow the density of the tissue changes (as its volume changes), and the intensity of the sensed

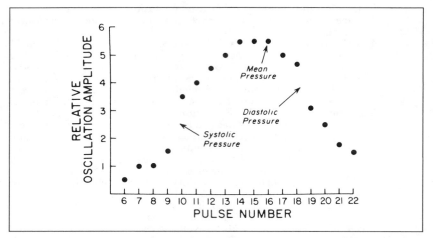

Fig. 4-3. The noninvasive oscillatory blood pressure technique measures the amplitude of oscillation in the cuff pressure itself during the time the cuff is cycling. The cuff is first inflated to suprasystolic pressures; during this time, only weak pressure fluctuations in the proximal portion of the cuff are sensed from the proximal, nonoccluded segment of the artery. As the pressure is decreased, oscillations in cuff pressure increase in amplitude as distal portions of the artery begin to pulse. A sudden, large increase in the oscillation amplitude has been correlated with systolic pressure. As mean arterial pressure is reached, the oscillation amplitude reaches a peak and thereafter declines. As the pressure on the cuff is decreased, a sudden decrease in oscillation amplitude occurs, which correlates with diastolic pressure. This system can be microprocessor controlled and automated and can function in a noisy environment. (Modified from H.P. Apple. Automatic Noninvasive Blood Pressure Monitors: What Is Available. In J. S. Gravenstein, R. S. Newbower [eds.], *Essential Noninvasive Monitoring in Anesthesia.* New York: Grune & Stratton, 1980. P. 11. With permission.)

light varies accordingly. By applying a known pressure to the finger, a self-calibrated estimation of blood pressure is obtained.

3. **Risks of noninvasive BP measurement.** Three types of risks are associated with noninvasive BP measurements.

   a. Venostasis or ischemia from prolonged cuff inflation.

   b. Ulnar neuropathy from direct compression.

   c. Inaccurate pressure determinations leading to treatment error.

      No matter what detection technique is used, the accuracy of the measurement will be markedly influenced by the size of the cuff and how it fits the limb (or finger). Using a cuff that is too large tends to underestimate blood pressure, whereas using a cuff that is too small tends to overestimate blood pressure. The width of a properly sized cuff is equal to two-thirds of the circumference of the limb on which it is placed.

      In general, it is recommended that any unexpected abnormally high or low blood pressure obtained by an indirect method be repeated immediately before a treatment is undertaken.

4. **Recommendations for noninvasive BP measurement.** The advantages and disadvantages of the various noninvasive techniques are outlined in Table 4-2. The availability of an indirect blood pressure measurement is desirable during all cardiac surgical procedures. It can serve as a back-up for the intraarterial system and may prove very useful before invasive monitoring is established and in the immediate postbypass period when the direct **radial** arterial

Table 4-2. Noninvasive techniques of blood pressure determination

A. Auscultation of Korotkoff sounds
  1. Reliable and easy to use
  2. May underestimate low pressures
  3. Has not been satisfactorily automated
  4. Not practical in noisy operating room
B. Oscillometric
  1. Most commonly used
  2. Can be automated
  3. Can be used in noisy environment
  4. Subject to motion artifact
  5. Underestimates high pressures and overestimates low pressures
C. Ultrasonic
  1. Can be automated
  2. Requires precise positioning of Doppler crystal
  3. Subject to motion artifact
D. Plethysmographic
  1. Provides a measure of blood flow as well as pressure
  2. Less useful in vasoconstricted, hypotensive patients

pressure measurement may be falsely low. In order not to interfere with a direct form of measurement, noninvasive blood pressure should be obtained in the contralateral limb.

C. **Intravascular pressure measurements.** In cardiac anesthesia it is very common to measure pressures within blood vessels directly. Arterial pressure is often measured by placing a catheter in a peripheral artery while other catheters are placed within the central circulation to measure the central venous or intracardiac pressures. The components of a system of intravascular pressure measurement are the intravascular catheter, fluid-filled connector tubing, a transducer, and an electronic analyzer and display system.

  1. **Characteristics of a pressure waveform.** Pressure waves in the cardiovascular system can be characterized as complex periodic sine waves. These complex waves are a summation of a series of simple sine waves of differing amplitudes and frequencies, which represent the natural harmonics of a fundamental frequency. The first harmonic, or fundamental frequency, is equal to the heart rate (Fig. 4-4), and the first ten harmonics of the fundamental frequency will contribute significantly to the waveform.

  2. **Properties of a monitoring system**
    a. **Frequency response** (or **amplitude ratio**) is the ratio of the measured amplitude versus the input amplitude of a signal at a specific frequency. In a good monitoring system, the frequency response should be constant over the desired range of input frequencies—that is, the signal is not distorted (amplified or diminished). The ideal amplitude ratio is close to 1. The signal frequency range of an intravascular pressure wave response is determined by the heart rate. If a patient's heart rate is 120 bpm, the fundamental frequency is 2 Hz. Because the first ten harmonics contribute to the arterial waveform, frequencies up to 20 Hz will contribute to the morphology of an arterial waveform at this heart rate.

    b. **Natural frequency** (or **resonant frequency**), a property possessed by all matter, refers here to the frequency at which the monitoring system itself resonates and amplifies the signal. The

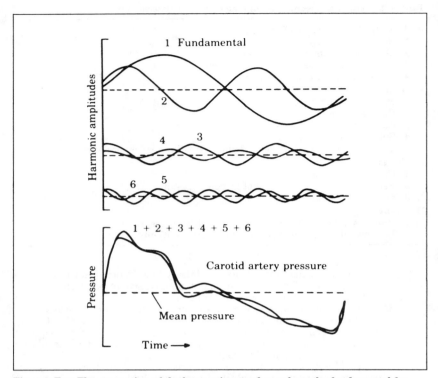

Fig. 4-4. *Top.* The generation of the harmonic waveforms from the fundamental frequency (heart rate) by Fourier analysis. The first six harmonics are shown. *Bottom.* The addition of the six harmonics to reproduce an actual blood pressure wave. The first six harmonics are superimposed, showing a likeness to, but not a faithful reproduction of, the original wave. The first ten harmonics of a pressure wave must be sensed by a catheter-transducer system, if that system is to provide an accurate reproduction of the wave. (From J.P. Welch, and M.N. D'Ambra. Hemodynamic Monitoring. In W. A. Kofke, and J. H. Levy [eds.], *Postoperative Critical Care Procedures of the Massachusetts General Hospital.* Boston: Little, Brown, 1986. P. 146. With permission.)

natural frequency (f_n) of a monitoring system is directly proportional to the catheter lumen diameter (**D**), inversely proportional to the square root of the tubing connection length (**L**), inversely proportional to the square root of the system compliance ($\Delta V / \Delta P$), and inversely proportional to the square root of the density of fluid contained in the system (δ). This is expressed as follows:

$$f_n \propto D \cdot L^{-2} \cdot (\Delta V/\Delta P)^{-2} \cdot \delta^{-2}$$

Therefore, to increase the natural (resonant) frequency and reduce distortion, it is imperative that a pressure sensing system be composed of short, low compliance tubing with as large a diameter as possible, filled with a low-density fluid such as water.

Ideally, the natural frequency of the measuring system should be at least 10 × the fundamental frequency to reproduce the first 10 harmonics of the pressure wave without distortion. In

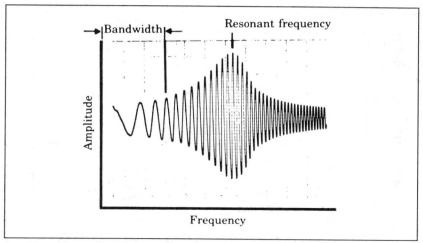

Fig. 4-5. Pressure recording from a pressure generator simulator, which emits a sine wave at increasing frequencies (horizontal axis). The frequency response (ratio of signal amplitude$_{OUT}$ to signal amplitude$_{IN}$) is plotted on the vertical axis for a typical catheter-transducer system. The useful band width (range of frequency producing a "flat" response) and the amplification of the signal in the frequency range near the natural frequency of the system are shown. (From J.P. Welch, and M.N. D'Ambra. *Hemodynamic Monitoring.* In W. A. Kofke, and J. H. Levy [eds.], *Postoperative Critical Care Procedures of the Massachusetts General Hospital.* Boston: Little, Brown, 1986. P. 148. With permission.)

clinical practice, the natural frequency of most measuring systems is in the range of 10–20 Hz. If the input frequency is close to the system's natural frequency (which is usually the case in clinical situations), the system's response will be amplified (Fig. 4-5). Therefore, these systems require the correct amount of **damping** to minimize distortion.

c. The **damping coefficient** reflects the rate of dissipation of the energy of a pressure wave. This property can be altered to decrease the erroneous amplification of an underdamped system or increase the frequency response of an overdamped system. Figure 4-6 describes the relationship between frequency response, natural frequency, and damping coefficient.

When a pressure monitoring system with a certain natural frequency duplicates a complex waveform with any one of the first ten harmonics close to the natural frequency of the system, amplification will result if correct damping of the catheter-transducer unit is not performed. The problem is compounded when the heart rate is fast (as in a child or a patient with a rapid atrial rhythm), which increases the demands of the system by increasing the input frequency (Fig. 4-7). **Correct damping of a pressure monitoring system should not affect the natural frequency of the system.**

The damping coefficient of a system can be estimated by measuring the time required for the system to settle to baseline after a high-pressure flush while observing the amplitude of successive waves as the system settles to zero (Fig. 4-8).

After a rapid pressure change, an underdamped system will

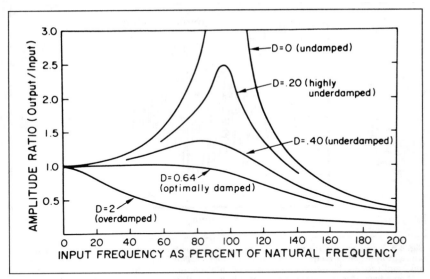

Fig. 4-6. The amplitude ratio (or frequency response) on the vertical axis is plotted as a function of the input frequency as a percent of the natural frequency (rather than as absolute values). In the undamped or underdamped system, the signal output is amplified in the region of the natural frequency of the transducer system; in the overdamped system, a reduction in amplitude ratio for most input frequencies is seen. This plot exhibits two important points: (1) If a catheter-transducer system has a high natural frequency, less damping will be required to produce a flat response in the clinically relevant range of input frequencies (10–30 Hz); (2) for systems with a natural frequency in the clinically relevant range (usual case), a level of "critical" (optimal) damping exists that will maintain a flat frequency response. (From W. Grossman. *Cardiac Catheterization* [3rd ed.]. Philadelphia: Lea & Febiger, 1985. P. 122. With permission.)

continue to oscillate for a long period of time. In terms of pressure monitoring, this translates to an overestimation of systolic and an underestimation of diastolic BP. An overdamped system will not oscillate at all but will settle to baseline slowly, thus underestimating systolic and overestimating diastolic pressures. A critically damped system will settle to baseline after only one or two oscillations and will reproduce systolic pressures accurately. An optimally or "critically" damped system will exhibit a constant (or "flat") frequency response in the range of frequencies up to the f_n of the system (Fig. 4-6). If a given system does not meet this criterion, components should be checked, especially for air, or the system replaced. Even an optimally damped system will begin to distort the waveform at higher heart rates because a greater number of the first ten harmonics will cluster around the system's natural frequency (Fig. 4-7).

3. **Strain gauges.** The pressure monitoring transducer can be described as a variable resistance transducer. A critical part of the transducer is the diaphragm, which acts to link the fluid wave to the electrical input. When the diaphragm of a transducer is distorted by a change in pressure, voltages are altered across the variable resistor of a Wheatstone bridge contained in the transducer. This in turn pro-

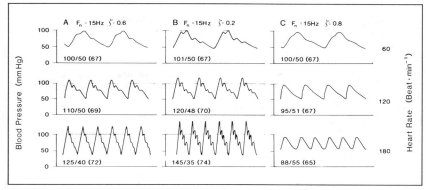

Fig. 4-7. Comparison of three catheter-transducer systems with the same natural frequency (15 Hz) under different conditions of heart rate. Pressures are displayed as systolic/diastolic (mean). The reference blood pressure for all panels is 100/50. *A*. A critically damped system ($\zeta = 0.6$) provides an accurate reproduction until higher heart rates (>150) are reached. *B*. An underdamped system ($\zeta = 0.2$) shows distortion at lower rates, leading to overestimation of systolic and underestimation of diastolic pressures. *C*. An overdamped system ($\zeta = 0.8$) demonstrates underestimation of systolic and overestimation of diastolic pressures. Note also that diastolic and mean pressures are affected less by the inadequate monitoring systems. (f_n = natural frequency; ζ = damping coefficient)

duces a change in current, which is electronically converted and displayed (Fig. 4-9).

4. Sources of error in intravascular pressure measurement

a. Low transducer frequency response. Low-frequency response refers to a low-frequency range over which the ratio of output to input amplitude is constant (i.e., no distortion). If the natural frequency of the system is low, its frequency response will be low also. Most transducer systems used in clinical anesthesia can be described as underdamped systems with a low natural frequency. Thus, any condition that decreases f_n response any further should be avoided. Air within a catheter-transducer system represents the most common cause of monitoring errors. Because of its compressibility, air not only decreases the response of the system but also leads to overdamping of the system. Therefore, the commonly held belief that an air bubble placed in the pressure tubing decreases artifact by increasing the damping coefficient is simply incorrect. The bubble will also decrease the natural frequency of the system below a critical level and can lead to inaccurate pressure measurement. A second common cause of diminution of frequency response is failure of the flush device with formation of a partial clot in the catheter.

b. Catheter whip. Catheter "whip" is a phenomenon in which the motion of the catheter tip itself produces a noticeable pressure swing. This artifact is usually not observed with peripheral arterial catheters but is more common with PA or left ventricular catheters.

c. Resonance in peripheral vessels. The systolic pressure measured in a radial arterial catheter may be up to 20–50 mm Hg higher than the pressure measured in the central aorta. This is due to many complex interactions of the blood as it is ejected from

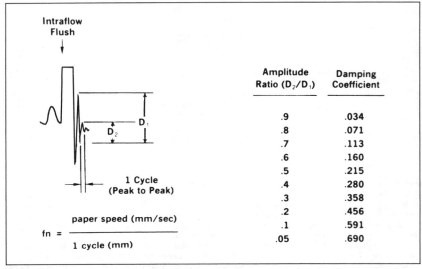

Fig. 4-8. The "pop" test allows one to derive f_n and ζ of a catheter-transducer system. The test should be done with the catheter in the artery in order to test the system in its entirety, since all components contribute to the harmonics of the system. The test involves a rapid flush (with the high pressure flush system used commonly), followed by a sudden release. This produces a rapid decrease from the flush bag pressure, and, owing to the inertia of the system, an overshoot of the baseline. The subsequent oscillations about the baseline are used to calculate f_n and ζ. For example, the arterial pulse at the far left of the figure is followed by a fast flush and sudden release. The resulting oscillations have a definite period, or cycle, measured in millimeters. The natural frequency, f_n, is the paper speed divided by this period, expressed in cycles·second^{-1}, or Hz. If the period were 2 mm and the paper speed 25 mm/second, f_n = 12.5 Hz. For determining f_n, a faster paper speed will give better reliability. The ratio of the amplitude of one induced resonant wave to the next, D_2/D_1, is used to calculate damping coefficients (right column). A damping coefficient of 0.2-0.4 describes an underdamped system, 0.4-0.6 an optimally damped system, and 0.6-0.8 an overdamped system. (From R.F. Bedford. Invasive Blood Pressure Monitoring. In C. D. Blitt [ed.], *Monitoring in Anesthesia and Critical Care Medicine.* New York: Churchill Livingstone, 1985. P. 59. With permission.)

the left ventricle into the aorta. The characteristics of the pressure wave as it travels down the arterial tree are modified as a result of narrowing of the arteries, the decrease of elastic tissue in distal vessels, and the addition of reflected waves to the arterial waveform as it progresses distally in the arterial system (Fig. 4-10).

d. **Changes in electrical properties of the transducer.** Electrical balance, or electrical zero, refers to the adjustment of the Wheatstone bridge within the transducer so that zero current flows to the detector at zero pressure. Transducers should be electronically balanced periodically during a procedure because the zero point may drift if, for instance, the room temperature changes. This drift can be due to a membrane-dome coupling phenomenon or to a drift in the pressure amplifier circuitry. Calibration of transducers to a mercury standard should be carried out periodically to verify the electronic calibration. In the presence of a baseline drift in the transducer system, a pressure waveform may not be

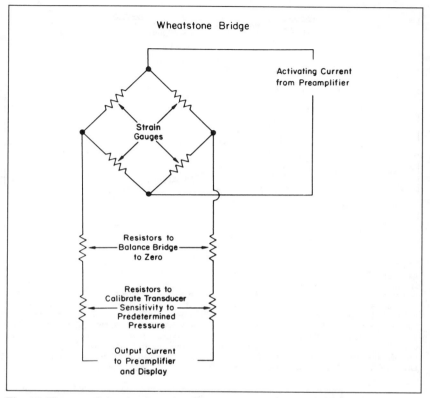

Fig. 4-9. Diagram of the circuitry of a pressure transducer. The diaphragm (not shown) is labeled *strain gauges* in the figure and is linked to the resistors as shown. A distortion in diaphragm shape caused by pressure changes in the system alters the electrical resistance in the strain gauges, resulting in a small current or input signal. The transducer preamplifier has three functions: (1) supplying an activating current (also termed an *excitation bridge*) across the circuit; (2) providing proper electrical balancing to calibrate the transducer to zero and to calibrate its sensitivity on exposure to a known pressure; and (3) receiving the input signal from the transducer, produced when the resistance of the bridge changes. Only the Wheatstone bridge and the diaphragm are contained in the transducer. (From R.F. Bedford. Invasive Blood Pressure Monitoring. In C. D. Blitt [ed.], *Monitoring in Anesthesia and Critical Care Medicine.* New York: Churchill Livingstone, 1985. P. 45. With permission.)

altered at all, and aggressive treatment could conceivably be started on the basis of erroneous values.

e. **Transducer position errors.** By convention, the reference position for hemodynamic monitoring is the right atrium. With the patient supine, the right atrium lies at the level of the midaxillary line. Once its zero level has been established, the transducer must be maintained at the same level as the right atrium. If the transducer position changes, falsely high or low pressure values will result. This is less of a concern when measuring relatively high arterial pressures but can be quite significant when monitoring

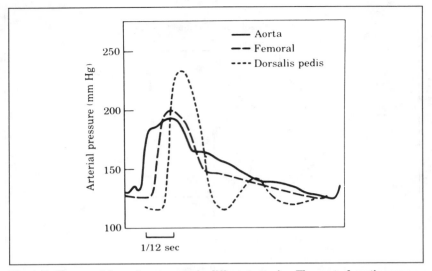

Fig. 4-10. Change of the pulse pressure in different arteries. The central aortic wave-form is more rounded and has a definite dicrotic notch. The dorsalis pedis and, to a lesser extent, the femoral artery show a delay in pulse transmission, sharper initial upstrokes (and thus higher systolic pressure), and slurring (femoral) and loss (dorsalis) of the dicrotic notch. The dicrotic notch is better maintained in the upper extremity pressure wave (not shown). The small second "hump" in the dorsalis wave is probably due to a reflected wave from the arterial-arteriolar impedance mismatching. (From J. P. Welch, and M. N. D'Ambra. Hemodynamic Monitoring. In W. A. Kofke, and J. H. Levy [eds.], *Postoperative Critical Care Procedures of the Massachusetts General Hospital.* Boston: Little, Brown, 1986. P. 144. With permission.)

lower pressure such as central venous pressure (CVP), pulmonary arterial, or pulmonary capillary wedge pressures.

5. **Transducer-tipped catheters.** Currently, catheters are available with pressure-sensing transducers at their tip. These catheters reduce artifacts and errors related to the many linkages in the fluid-filled transducer systems (stop cocks, tubing, air bubbles, clots, etc.). With a flat frequency response of up to 40 Hz they provide extremely accurate blood pressure measurements. The major drawback of these transducers, however, is their expense, as well as their relative fragility. Another transducer-tipped catheter that employs fiberoptic rather than electrical transduction of the pressure signal may reduce the cost of the catheters to the point that they can be manufactured for single use.

D. **Arterial catheterization**

1. **Indications.** For several reasons, arterial catheterization has become standard in the monitoring of the cardiac surgical patient:

   a. Direct arterial pressure measurement is possible during nonpulsatile extracorporeal circulation.

   b. Cardiac surgical patients are usually hemodynamically unstable in the perioperative period.

   c. Close surveillance of arterial blood gases and other blood chemistries is indicated in these patients.

2. **Sites of cannulation.** A wide variety of sites used for cannulation of the arterial tree are described in their approximate order of frequency of use:

Table 4-3. Steps for radial arterial catheter placement

Description of steps	Rationale and possible complications
1. Immobilize and dorsiflex at wrist	Too much dorsiflexion or tape too tight—occludes artery
2. Immobilize thumb with tape	Stabilize the artery against the radial head
3. Palpate artery 3–4 cm along its course	Increases the likelihood of a central puncture
4a. Make small skin wheal with 0.5% Xylocaine after sterile preparation	Keep volume small for this and deeper infiltration to avoid altering anatomy
4b. Infiltrate deeper planes on either side of artery	Decreases the incidence of spasm
5. Make skin nick with 18-gauge needle	Facilitates maneuvering of the catheter
6. Introduce 20-gauge, 2-in. catheter-over-needle unit	Larger bore possibly associated with increased thrombogenesis
7. Advance in rapid, short, 1-mm increments until flashback is seen	Rapid advance increases chance of arterial wall puncture
Three options available:	These three methods are not mutually exclusive but describe three different depths of needle and catheter tip placement:
a. Advance unit 0.5 mm; slide catheter off needle into artery	a. Placement in the arterial **lumen**
b. Advance unit until flashback stops, then withdraw needle (holding catheter stationary); when flashback returns, advance catheter into artery	b. Placement of needle in the **back wall** of the artery (catheter tip will remain in lumen with this method)
c. Advance unit several millimeters, remove needle completely, back catheter until good flow returns, advance catheter into artery either directly or after passing flexible wire	c. Placement of needle and catheter **through** back wall—also termed **transfixing** the artery. Wire should be advanced through lumen of catheter only if pulsatile flow via catheter is present; forcing wire may result in arterial dissection
8. De-air the tubing	Prevents arterial air emboli

a. **Radial artery.** This site is most commonly used for arterial catheterization because catheter insertion is easy and the radial artery provides a reasonably accurate estimation of the true aortic pressure.

(1) **Technique.** Table 4-3 summarizes the steps used for radial arterial cannulation. One technique, that of transfixing the radial artery for catheter insertion, is shown in Fig. 4-11.

(2) **Contraindications.** Inadequate collateral flow to the hand is a relative contraindication to the use of a radial artery catheter.

(a) **Modified Allen's test.** This test screens for patients with inadequate palmar collateralization from the ulnar artery. Originally described by Allen in 1927 and modified by Bedford, it is performed as follows: Apply firm pressure over both radial and ulnar arteries simultaneously and ask the patient to squeeze his hand several times to promote exsan-

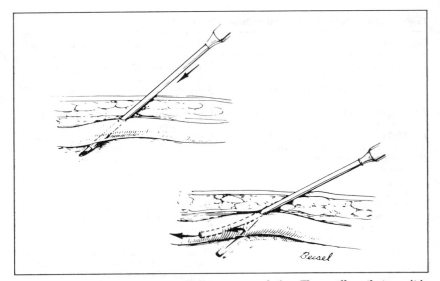

Fig. 4-11. One technique used for radial artery cannulation. The needle-catheter unit is advanced through the artery, as shown in the upper drawing. The lower drawing shows the needle removed and the catheter withdrawn until pulsatile flow is obtained (indicating that the catheter tip is in the lumen); the catheter is then advanced into the artery. (From E.S. Freis. Vascular Cannulation. In W. A. Kofke, and J.H. Levy [eds.], *Postoperative Critical Care Procedures of the Massachusetts General Hospital.* Boston: Little, Brown, 1986. P. 137. With permission.)

guination. Then release the pressure on the ulnar artery, keeping the radial artery compressed, and measure the time needed to refill the nail bed capillaries. If refill time is greater than 15 seconds the test is considered **positive,** suggesting **inadequate collateral flow** from the ulnar artery. Especially in patients with peripheral vascular disease, it is wisest to consider other monitoring and catheter placement options before cannulating the radial artery in the presence of a positive modified Allen's test.

b. Femoral artery. The femoral artery offers two advantages over the radial site. First, the artery is not only superficial but also allows excellent access to the central arterial tree. Second, the femoral artery catheter provides appropriate access to the descending aorta should the placement of an intra-aortic balloon pump (IABP) become necessary during the surgical procedure. Placement of a femoral artery catheter should be considered for any patient in whom difficulty in weaning from cardiopulmonary bypass is expected (e.g., those with depressed ejection fraction, severe wall motion abnormalities, or significant coronary disease).

    (1) Technique. The femoral artery is most easily entered using a Seldinger technique after sterile preparation and draping.

    (2) Contraindications. Cannulation of the femoral artery should be avoided in any patient who has had prior vascular surgery involving the femoral arteries or who has a skin infection of the groin.

c. Aortic root. Aortic root cannulation is of course not an option at the beginning of a cardiac case but should always be considered in the patient whose chest is open and in whom difficulties are encountered in obtaining a reliable blood pressure. A pressure tubing can be handed to the anesthesiologist from the sterile field after a needle or catheter is inserted by the surgeon.

   d. Axillary artery. The axillary artery, like the femoral, provides the anesthesiologist with a superficial, large artery that has good access to the central arterial tree.

     (1) Technique. The axillary artery is most easily entered using a Seldinger technique. Placement of the axillary catheter in the left axilla somewhat reduces the likelihood that any air or debris flushed from the catheter could cause an embolus in a cerebral vessel.

     (2) Contraindications. Cannulation of the axillary artery should be avoided in the presence of any localized skin irritation in the axilla. The increased risk of cerebral embolus of air or debris must be recognized.

   e. Brachial artery. The brachial artery is an easily accessible artery located medially in the antecubital fossa.

     (1) Brachial artery cannulation is similar to that described for the radial artery. A 20-gauge catheter can easily be placed in the brachial artery. The elbow must be immobilized with a long arm board for stability.

     (2) Contraindications. Because the brachial artery is an "end artery," its cannulation is relatively contraindicated. In prospective studies, however, the incidence of brachial artery thromboembolism with an 18-gauge or smaller catheter was low, and this incidence can be minimized by using the shortest and smallest gauge catheter possible.

   f. Ulnar artery. The ulnar artery can be used in the rare circumstances when the radial artery cannot be entered easily. Prior to insertion of an ulnar artery catheter, however, the Allen's test should be repeated as described previously, except that pressure over the radial artery should be released to check for adequate radial artery collateral flow.

   g. Dorsalis pedis and posterior tibialis arteries. In general, these two sites of cannulation are not commonly used because they present difficult management problems in the postoperative period. Further, the distal location increases distortion of the arterial wave (Fig. 4-10).

3. Interpretation of arterial tracings. The arterial pressure waveform contains much information about the patient's hemodynamic status.

   a. HR and rhythm. The heart rate can be determined from the arterial pressure wave. This is especially helpful if the patient is being paced or if electrocautery is being used because pacer spikes or cautery interference can distort the ECG. In the presence of numerous atrial or ventricular ectopic beats, the arterial trace can provide useful information on the hemodynamic consequences of these dysrhythmias.

   b. Pulse pressure. The difference between the systolic pressure and the diastolic pressure provides useful information about fluid status and valvular competence. Life-threatening emergencies such as pericardial tamponade are accompanied by a narrow pulse pressure on the arterial waveform. A sudden increase in pulse pressure may be a sign of worsening aortic valvular insufficiency.

   c. Respiratory variation–volume status. Hypovolemia is suggested by a decrease in arterial systolic pressure with positive pressure ventilation. Positive intrathoracic pressure impedes ven-

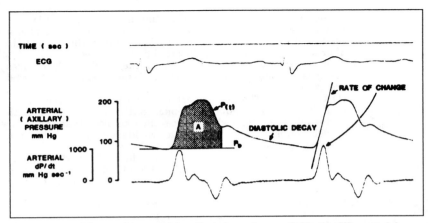

Fig. 4-12. Arterial trace demonstrating the information available from the arterial pressure waveform. Time marker and ECG trace are at top, arterial pressure versus time trace and first derivative (dP/dt) are at bottom. Systolic ejection area *(shaded area A)*, rate of change of pressure during systole (dP/dt), and decay of diastolic pressure are marked as shown (for more explanation, see text). P_d = diastolic pressure, $P_{(t)}$ = instantaneous pressure at time t. (From C. Prys-Roberts. Cardiovascular monitoring in patients with vascular disease. *Br. J. Anaesth.* 53:770, 1981. With permission.)

ous return to the heart and will have a more pronounced effect in the hypovolemic patient. Because this finding is not uniformly seen in patients with hypovolemia, correlation with other findings can help in making the diagnosis.

   d. **Qualitative estimates of hemodynamic indices can be inferred from the central arterial pressure wave (central aorta, femoral artery** (Fig. 4-12).

   (1) **Contractility.** Observation of the upstroke of the central aortic waveform, unlike the peripheral waveform, provides information about the contractile state of the left ventricle. It is well recognized that the first derivative of the pressure-time curve, dP/dt, correlates with the contractile state of the ventricle. A differentiator amplifier is required to quantify dP/dt, which is itself dependent on other factors such as preload and afterload. Nevertheless, a qualitative assessment of contractility can be gained by simple visual observation of the waveform. If the rate of rise is rapid, the contractile state of the ventricle is probably good; a sluggish upstroke in the absence of aortic stenosis or extreme vasoconstriction probably denotes a poorly functioning ventricle.

   (2) **Systemic vascular resistance.** The position of the dicrotic notch as well as the slope of the diastolic decay gives the anesthesiologist some additional information. The decay of the diastolic portion of the central aortic trace is exponential under normal circumstances and is a function of arterial compliance and systemic vascular resistance. With increased systemic vascular resistance, for example, one would expect a dicrotic notch to appear high on the downsloping portion of the arterial trace as well as a steep diastolic decay. Low resistance would present a low-placed dicrotic notch and a shallow diastolic decay.

   (3) **Stroke volume.** The area under the systolic ejection portion of the central aortic arterial pressure curve, denoted by the

difference in measured pressure (P(t)) and diastolic pressure (PD), integrated over the time period for the first positive deflection to the appearance of the dicrotic notch, has been shown to correlate well with stroke volume (Fig. 4-12). With current computerized technology, this type of analysis can be done on-line, yielding information about the patient's stroke volume. Again, central arterial, not peripheral, pressure tracings are usually required for accurate stroke volume determination.

4. Complications of arterial catheterization

a. Ischemia. The incidence of ischemic damage after radial artery cannulation is reportedly low. A study by Slogoff et al,[8] in which the Allen's test was not performed, showed that although abnormal flow patterns were present in up to 25% of patients between 1 and 7 days after radial artery catheterization, there were no adverse signs of ischemia with these findings. Nonetheless, the possible complication of distal ischemia should always be considered, especially in the presence of abnormal results from the Allen's test. If the radial artery is cannulated under these conditions, the hand should be monitored carefully for signs of ischemia.

b. Thrombosis. Although the incidence of thrombosis from radial artery catheterization is high, studies have not demonstrated adverse sequelae, and recanalization of the radial artery occurs in a majority of cases. Patients with significant morbidity from radial cannulation include those with diabetes or severe peripheral vascular disease; in these patients, arterial cannulation should be avoided if results of the Allen's test are positive.

c. Infection. With proper sterile technique, the risk of infection from cannulation of the radial artery should be minimal. In Slogoff's series of 1700 reported cases, no catheter site was overtly infected[8]. Other studies demonstrate a higher infection rate among femoral arterial lines.

d. Bleeding. Although transfixing the artery will put a hole in its back wall, the layers of the muscular media will seal it with minimal bleeding. In the patient with a bleeding diathesis, however, the tendency to bleed from this high pressure system is greater. Unlike central venous catheters, arterial catheters should not be heparin bonded.

e. False lowering of radial artery pressure immediately after CPB. In a large number of patients (up to 72% in one series) the radial artery pressure was significantly lower than the aortic pressure at the completion of cardiopulmonary bypass[10]. Vasoconstriction was **not** found in this series to be the primary reason for this phenomenon. Forearm vasodilation secondary to rewarming may lead to arteriovenous AV shunting, resulting in a steal phenomenon of 5 to 30 minutes or longer in duration. Other studies have suggested that the inaccuracy of radial pressure is due to hypovolemia and vasoconstriction[6]. Whatever the mechanism, if suspicion arises that a peripheral arterial trace is dampened (owing to slow up-stroke or loss of the dicrotic notch, for example), a direct pressure measurement should be obtained from a central site.

5. Recommendations for BP monitoring. Under most circumstances, the radial arterial pressure measurement will be accurate before and after cardiopulmonary bypass. In the patient with poor left ventricular function, addition of a femoral arterial catheter prior to cardiopulmonary bypass is warranted, not only to obtain a second comparable blood pressure but also to ensure arterial access should intraaortic balloon counterpulsation become necessary. If an internal mammary artery (IMA) is dissected to be used as one of the coronary bypass vessels, the radial artery catheter should be placed in the side opposite the IMA harvest, since retraction of the chest wall and compression of the subclavian artery can dampen or obliterate the radial artery traces. If bilateral IMA grafts are planned, a femoral artery catheter may be helpful.

E. **Central venous pressure.** Classically, the central venous pressure (CVP) measures right atrial pressure, and is affected by one or all of the following: (1) circulating blood volume, (2) venous tone, and (3) right ventricular function.

1. **Indications**

   a. **Monitoring.** Monitoring of ventricular preload, and at least CVP, is indicated for any cardiac patient requiring cardiopulmonary bypass, for surgery in which large blood losses or large volume shifts are expected, or for patients in whom pre-existing hypovolemia is suspected.

   b. **Fluid and drug therapy.** The CVP can be used to infuse fluid or blood products, as a port for administering vasoactive drugs, and for postoperative hyperalimentation.

   c. **Special uses.** One may elect to place a CVP catheter in a patient who would ordinarily require a PA catheter when the latter cannot be placed either easily or safely. Placement of a PA catheter can be difficult in patients with numerous congenital cardiac disorders, in those with anatomic distortion of the right-sided venous circulation, or in those requiring surgical procedures of the right heart or implantation of a right heart mechanical assist device.

2. **Techniques.** There are numerous routes by which a catheter can be placed in the central circulation.

   a. **Internal jugular.** The internal jugular vein is the most common access route for the cardiac anesthesiologist.

      (1) **Techniques.** Cannulation of the internal jugular vein is relatively safe and convenient and various approaches exist for its cannulation (Table 4-4, Fig. 4-13). The process of cannulation, regardless of the approach, involves the steps outlined in Table 4-5.

      (2) **Contraindications and recommendations.** Internal jugular vein cannulation is recommended in preference to other approaches to the central circulation in the absence of relative contraindications such as:

         (a) Presence of carotid disease.

         (b) Recent cannulation of the internal jugular vein (with the concomitant risk of thrombosis).

         (c) Contralateral diaphragmatic dysfunction.

         (d) Thyromegaly or prior neck surgery.

            In these cases, the internal jugular vein on the contralateral side should be considered. It should be remembered that the thoracic duct lies in close proximity to the left internal jugular vein and that laceration of the left brachiocephalic vein or superior vena cava by the catheter is more likely with the left-sided approach. This risk is due to the more acute angle taken by the catheter to enter the superior vena cava from the left side.

   b. **External jugular.** The external jugular vein courses superficially across the sternocleidomastoid muscle to join the subclavian vein close to the junction of the internal jugular and subclavian veins. Its course is more tortuous, and the presence of valves makes central access via the external jugular more difficult.

      (1) **Techniques.** The head down position is needed to distend the vein. Traction is also necessary to introduce an 18-gauge cath-

Table 4-4. Sites for internal jugular cannulation

Approaches	Landmarks	Complications
Central	Apex of triangle formed by lateral (clavicular) and medial (sternal) head of sternocleidomastoid muscle (SCM). Aim needle caudally and laterally toward ipsilateral nipple.	Low incidence of pneumothorax; medial direction has higher incidence of carotid puncture
Posterior	Intersection of lateral border of lateral (clavicular) head of SCM and line drawn laterally from cricoid ring. Aim needle caudally and ventrally (anteriorly) toward sternal notch	Higher incidence of carotid puncture; low incidence of pneumothorax
Anterior	Medial border of medial head, 5 cm above clavicle. Direct needle toward ipsilateral nipple.	Carotid puncture more likely unless retracted medially
Supraclavicular	Interscalene groove 2 cm above clavicle. Direct needle caudally and medially	Higher chance of pneumothorax and subclavian artery puncture

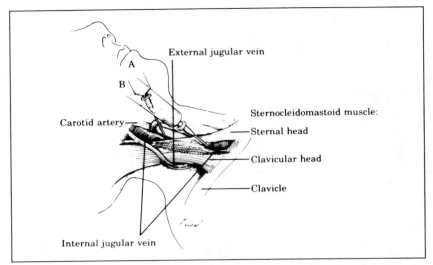

Fig. 4-13. Drawing demonstrating two methods for internal jugular cannulation. *A.* **The anterior approach.** *B.* **the central approach (see text for further details). (From E.S. Freis. Vascular Cannulation. In W. A. Kofke, and J.H. Levy [eds.],** *Postoperative Critical Care Procedures of the Massachusetts General Hospital.* **Boston: Little, Brown, 1986. P. 130. With permission.)**

eter into the external jugular vein. A flexible J guide wire is used to negotiate the tortuous course of the vessel. Central passage of the catheter is usually easier from the left jugular vein. The remainder of the insertion is similar to that already described for the internal jugular.

(2) **Advantages and disadvantages.** The external jugular provides safe access to the central circulation and can be cannulated in a patient receiving heparin or in whom internal jugular cannulation is unsuccessful or contraindicated. The central circulation was successfully cannulated in 75–90% of patients in some reports.

The tip of the external jugular catheter can pass into the subclavian vein or up the internal jugular on the same side or may cross over to the contralateral side. Although drug infusions can be given through a catheter so placed, monitoring of the CVP under these conditions will lead to incorrect values. The position of the catheter should be confirmed by a chest x-ray before drug therapy based on a central venous pressure reading from an external jugular catheter is given.

c. **Subclavian.** The subclavian vein is also readily accessible and thus has been popular for use during cardiopulmonary resuscitation.

(1) **Techniques.** The patient is placed in a head down position to distend the vein. Optimal positioning can be obtained by placing a roll vertically under the patient's spine to move the clavicle out of the way during cannulation.

(2) **Advantages.** The main advantage to subclavian vein cannulation is its relative ease and the stability of the catheter during long-term cannulation.

Table 4-5. Steps for right internal jugular (IJ) cannulation

Description of steps	Rationale and possible problems
1. Verify functioning ECG	Critical for monitoring dysrhythmias
2. Remove pillow, rotate head completely to left. Ask patient to raise head off bed and note position of tensed sternocleidomastoid muscle	Optimizes visualization of landmarks
3. Place patient in Trendelenberg position	Distends IJ and reduces risk of air embolism—may worsen symptoms due to congestive or right ventricular failure
4. Perform careful sterile preparation and drape	Mandatory for central venous cannulation—full glove and gown may be used
5. Recheck landmarks, skin wheal, and deeper infiltration with 1% Xylocaine	IJ is often superficial and may be found during infiltration—withdraw on syringe before injecting local anesthetic
6. Remove local anesthetic from syringe, replace infiltration needle with 19- or 21-gauge 1.5-in. "finder" needle	Not necessary if vein has been found previously, presence of local anesthetic will make any aspirated blood appear bright red
7. Once vein has been located: a. Leave finder needle in place *or* b. Remove finder, remember direction	Serves as reminder of vein location Finder needle may interfere with subsequent cannulation
8. Insert 18-gauge 1¾-in. catheter over needle unit into IJ, following same line	Constant aspiration as unit is advanced is required to see flashback
9. When flashback is seen, advance unit ≈ 1 mm, then advance catheter over needle into vein	Once IV placement is established, end of catheter is capped with finger or syringe to avoid air embolism
10. If blood is not freely aspirated: a. Remove needle b. Replace syringe and aspirate c. Withdraw catheter until free flow of blood occurs d. Advance catheter slowly into vein, or a wire can be inserted through catheter	Catheter is probably through back wall Patient may be hypovolemic, and IV fluid bolus will increase success Increased head-down position may be needed

148

Table 4-5. (continued)

Description of steps	Rationale and possible problems

11. Confirm IV placement by
  a. Lack of pulsatile flow
  b. Measure pressure in the 18-gauge catheter and simultaneous arterial pressure, comparing absolute values and pressure waveforms
  c. Compare IJ and arterial blood samples, visually or by oximetry
	If arterial cannulation is diagnosed, remove catheter and hold pressure for at least 5 min to avoid hematoma

12. Pass flexible wire through catheter, remove catheter	
13. Place central venous pressure catheter over wire or dilator-introducer assembly (pulmonary artery catheter)	ECG should be monitored because arrhythmias can result Skin nick needed if larger introducer will be placed
14. Place sterile dressing	

(3) Disadvantages
  (a) Subclavian vein cannulation carries the highest rate of pneumothorax of any approach. If subclavian vein cannulation is unsuccessful on one side, an attempt on the contralateral side is contraindicated without first obtaining a chest x-ray; bilateral pneumothoraces can be lethal.
  (b) The subclavian artery is easily entered instead of the vein.
  (c) In a left-sided cannulation, the thoracic duct may be lacerated.
  (d) The left subclavian approach may also make threading the catheter into the right atrium difficult because an acute angle must be made by the catheter in order to enter the innominate vein.

d. Arm vein
  (1) Techniques. Central access can be obtained through the veins of the antecubital fossa. The basilic vein, which is located more medially than the cephalic vein, provides the most direct venous route to the central circulation. The best approach for this type of insertion is to insert a short 14-gauge intravenous catheter into the basilic vein and then insert a 16-gauge, 30-cm CVP catheter through the lumen of the 14-gauge catheter. This approach not only allows threading of a central venous catheter but also, in the event that the CVP catheter **cannot** be threaded, ensures the existence of a large-bore catheter for IV access.
  (2) Advantages. The main advantage of placement of a CVP catheter through the peripheral veins is that bleeding can be well controlled in the anticoagulated patient.
  (3) Disadvantages. The disadvantage of this route is the low rate of success in gaining reliable access to the central circulation. Maneuvers that can aid in placing the catheter are the following:
    (a) Rapid advancement of the catheter so that venous spasm will not halt its placement.
    (b) Traction on the arm as the catheter is threaded.
    (c) Abduction of the arm at the shoulder while threading.
    (d) Rotation of the head toward the arm that is being cannulated.

3. Complications. The site-specific complications of central venous catheter insertion are outlined in Table 4-6. The most severe complications of CVP insertion are usually preventable.

4. Interpretation
  a. Normal waves. The normal CVP trace contains three positive deflections, termed the A, C, and V waves (Fig. 4-14).
  b. Abnormal waves. A common abnormality in the CVP trace occurs in the presence of atrioventricular dissociation, when right atrial contraction occurs against a closed tricuspid valve. This produces a large "cannon A wave" that is virtually diagnostic of this condition. Abnormal V waves can occur with tricuspid valve insufficiency, in which retrograde flow through the incompetent valve produces an increase in right atrial pressure during systole.
  c. Right heart function. The CVP offers a direct measurement of right ventricular filling pressure.
  d. Left heart filling pressures. The CVP is a reasonable indicator of left ventricular filling in the presence of good left ventricular function and in the absence of pulmonary hypertension or mitral valvular disease. In patients with coronary artery disease with good ventricular function (ejection fraction greater than 40% and no regional wall motion abnormalities), the CVP correlates well with the pulmonary capillary wedge pressure.

E. Pulmonary artery catheter

Table 4-6. Complications of central venous cannulation

Complication	Internal jugular	Subclavian	Femoral	External jugular
Infection	×	×	×	×
Air embolism	×	×	×	×
Catheter shearing and embolization	×	×	×	×
Thrombophlebitis	×	×	×	×
Local extravasation of fluid and drugs	×	×	×	×
Pneumothorax	×	×		
Hemothorax	×	×		
Pericardial tamponade	×	×		
Tissue trauma				
Nerve	Brachial plexus Carotid Subclavian	Brachial plexus Subclavian	Femoral Femoral	
Artery				
Vein	Superior vena cava (SVC) Thoracic duct (L) Cervical nerve roots	SVC Thoracic duct (L)	Inferior vena cava	SVC
Other				
Sites of fluid infusion with malpositioned catheter	Mediastinum, pericardium, pleural cavity	Pleural cavity, mediastinum	Retroperitoneum, peritoneal cavity	Retrograde up ipsilateral or contralateral internal jugular

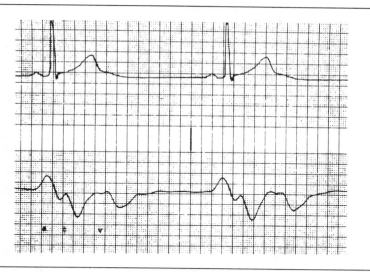

Fig. 4-14. Relationship between ECG *(above)* and CVP *(below)*. The normal CVP trace contains three positive deflections, known as the A, C, and V waves. The A wave occurs in conjunction with the P wave on the electrocardiogram and represents atrial contraction. The C wave occurs in conjunction with the QRS wave and represents the bulging of the tricuspid valve into the right atrium with right ventricular contraction. The final wave, the V wave, occurs in conjunction with the T wave on the ECG and represents right atrial filling before opening of the tricuspid valve. (From J. A. Kaplan, Hemodynamic Monitoring. In *Cardiac Anesthesia* [2nd ed.]. Philadelphia: Saunders, 1987. P. 186. With permission.)

1. **What parameters it measures**
   a. **Pulmonary artery pressure** reflects right ventricular function, pulmonary vascular resistance, and left atrial filling pressure.
   b. **Pulmonary capillary wedge pressure (PCWP)** is a more direct measure of left atrial filling pressure. With the balloon inflated and "wedged" in a distal pulmonary artery, a valveless hydrostatic column exists between the distal port and the left atrium (**LA**).
   c. **Central venous pressure.** A sampling port of the PA catheter is located in the right atrium and allows measurement of the CVP.
   d. **Cardiac output.** A thermistor located at the tip of the PA catheter allows measurement of the output of the right heart by the thermodilution technique. In the absence of intracardiac shunts, this measurement equals left heart output.
   e. **Blood temperature.** The thermistor can provide a constant measurement of blood temperature which is an accurate reflection of core temperature.
   f. **Derived parameters.** Several indices of ventricular performance and cardiovascular status can be derived from parameters measured by the PA catheter. Their formulas, physiologic significance, and normal values are listed in Table 4-7.
2. **Indications for pulmonary artery catheterization.** In some institutions, cardiac surgery with cardiopulmonary bypass represents a universal indication for PA pressure monitoring in adults. Particular indications are described in Table 4-8. Many of the indications for use of the PA catheter for cardiac procedures reflect the necessity

Table 4-7 Derived hemodynamic indices

Parameter	Physiologic significance	Formula	Normal value
Systemic vascular resistance (SVR)	Reflects impedance of the systemic vascular tree—assumes laminar flow of homogeneous fluid	$80 \cdot (MAP - CVP)/CO$	$700-1600$ dynes·sec·cm^{-5}
Pulmonary vascular resistance (PVR)	Reflects impedance of pulmonary circuit	$80 \cdot (PAM - PCWP)/CO$	$20-130$ dynes·sec·cm^{-5}
Cardiac index (CI)	Indexes flows to body surface area (BSA), allows for meaningful comparison between patients	CO/BSA	$2.5-4.2$ L·min^{-1}·m^{-2}
Stroke volume index (SVI)	Reflects fluid status and ventricular performance	$CI/HR \cdot 1000$	$40-60$ ml·beat^{-1}·m^{-2}
Left ventricular stroke work index (LVSWI)	Estimates work of left ventricle, reflects contractile state	$(MAP - PCWP) \cdot SVI \cdot 0.0136$	$45-60$ g·m·m^{-2}
Right ventricular stroke work index (RVSWI)	Estimates work done by right ventricle and RV performance	$(PAM - CVP) \cdot SVI \cdot 0.0136$	$5-10$ g·m·m^{-2}

MAP = mean arterial pressure, CVP = central venous pressure, CO = cardiac output, PCWP = pulmonary capillary wedge pressure, HR = heart rate, PAM = pulmonary artery mean pressure.

Source: Modified from J. A. Kaplan. Hemodynamic Monitoring. In J. A. Kaplan (ed.), *Cardiac Anesthesia* (2nd ed.). Philadelphia: Saunders, 1987. P. 203. With permission.

Table 4-8. Indications for using the pulmonary artery catheter in cardiac surgery

Patients for CABG with
   —Poor LV function (EF < 0.40, LVEDP > 18 mmHG)
   —LV wall motion abnormalities
   —Recent MI (< 6 months) or complication of MI
   —Severe angina
   —Significant (> 75% stenosis) left main coronary disease
Patient with valvular disease
Presence of pulmonary hypertension
Combined coronary stenoses and valvular disease
Complex cardiac lesions
Patient age > 65 years
Patients with other systemic disease

EF = ejection fraction, LVEDP = left ventricular end-diastolic pressure.
Source: Modified from J. A. Kaplan. Hemodynamic Monitoring. In J. Kaplan (ed.), *Cardiac Anesthesia* (2nd ed.). Philadelphia: Saunders, 1987, p. 193. With permission.

to monitor the left ventricle separately from the right ventricle (**RV**), since in many cardiac patients pressures measured on the right side (i.e., CVP) do not adequately reflect those on the left side. The benefits of PA monitoring in these patients include:

a. **Assessing volume status.** In many patients with differences in right and left ventricular function, volume status is difficult to determine because of the large disparity between right (CVP) and left (PCWP) heart filling pressures. Knowing both of these values can aid in the diagnosis of hypovolemia or hypervolemia.

b. **Diagnosing right ventricular failure.** The right ventricle is a thin-walled, highly compliant chamber that can fail during cardiac surgery either because of a primary disease process (inferior myocardial infarction) or as a result of the surgical procedure (inadequate myocardial protection). Right heart failure presents as an increase in the CVP, a decrease in the CVP to mean PA gradient, and a low cardiac output.

c. **Diagnosing left ventricular failure.** Knowledge of pulmonary artery and wedge pressures can aid in the diagnosis of left-sided heart failure if other causes (ischemia, mitral valve disease) are eliminated. Simultaneous readings of high pulmonary artery pressures and wedge pressure in the presence of systemic hypotension and low cardiac output are hallmarks of left ventricular (**LV**) failure.

d. **Diagnosing pulmonary hypertension.** With normal pulmonary vascular resistance, the PA diastolic (**PAD**) and wedge pressure agree closely with one another. A disparity in these parameters, characterized by a higher PAD, suggests the presence of pulmonary hypertension.

e. **Assessing valvular disease**
   (1) Tricuspid and pulmonary valve stenosis can be diagnosed by means of a pulmonary artery catheter by measuring pressure gradients across these valves (**tricuspid:** CVP to RV end-diastolic pressure (RVEDP) gradient; **pulmonic:** RV systolic to PA systolic pressure gradient). These measurements can be accomplished by the "pullback" method, measuring gradients with the distal port, or by employing a Paceport PA catheter with an RV port (see sec. **F.5.** below for types of catheters).

(2) Mitral valvular disease is reflected in the wedge pressure tracing. Mitral insufficiency appears as an abnormal V wave, representing an increase in pulmonary wedge pressure from the regurgitant flow. This abnormal wave appears slightly out of phase from the arterial pulse pressure; the delay is due to slower transit of the regurgitant pulse pressure in the highly compliant pulmonary circuit (see Fig. 12-10). V waves also appear in other conditions, including ischemia, ventricular pacing, and presence of a ventricular septal defect. The presence and degree of V-wave abnormalities also depends on the compliance of the left atrium. In patients with chronic mitral valve insufficiency, for example, the left atrium has a higher compliance, and a large regurgitant volume will not always result in a dramatic V wave. Measuring a gradient in mitral stenosis requires simultaneous measurement of LVEDP, which is not routinely performed in the operating room.

f. Early diagnosis of ischemia. Although the ECG is the cornerstone for the diagnosis of ischemia, it is not always sensitive, particularly in the case of subendocardial ischemia. Usually, significant ischemia (transmural or subendocardial) is associated with development of a decrease in ventricular compliance, which is reflected in either an increase in pulmonary artery pressures or an increase in pulmonary capillary wedge pressure. In addition, the development of pathologic V waves may occur secondary to ischemia of the papillary muscle (Fig. 4-15).

3. Interpretation of PA pressure data

a. Effects of ventilation. The effects of ventilation on PA pressure readings can be significant in the low pressure system of the right-sided circulation because airway or transpleural pressure is transmitted to the pulmonary vasculature.

(1) When a patient breathes spontaneously, the negative intrapleural pressure that results from inspiration can be transmitted to the intravascular pressure. Thus, "negative" PA diastolic, wedge, and central venous pressures may occur with spontaneous ventilation.

(2) Positive airway pressures can be transmitted to the vasculature during positive pressure ventilation, leading to false elevations in pulmonary pressures with controlled ventilation.

(3) The established convention is to read pulmonary pressures at **end-expiration.** This is best done by reading the data directly from a calibrated screen or from a hard copy of the trace. The digital monitor numerical read-out may give incorrect information because these numbers reflect the absolute highest (systolic), lowest (diastolic), and mean (area under pressure curve) values for **several seconds,** which may include one or more breaths.

b. Location of catheter tip. PA pressure measurements depend on where the tip of the catheter resides in the pulmonary vascular tree. In areas of the lung that are well ventilated but poorly perfused (West's zone I), the readings will be more affected by changes in airway pressure. Likewise, even when the tip is in a good location in the middle or lower lung fields, large amounts of PEEP (greater than 10 mm Hg) will cause erroneous PA values.

4. Timing of placement. A debate exists whether PA catheter insertion pre-induction is indicated in adult patients with good left ventricular function. Opponents to pre-induction insertion argue that the discomfort associated with PA catheter placement may cause deleterious hemodynamic changes. Another argument against pre-

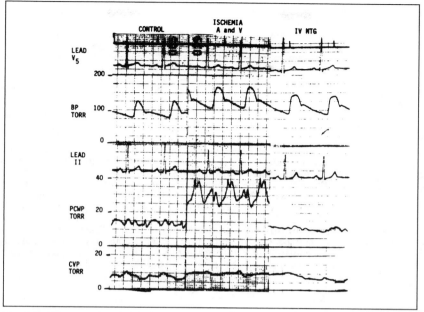

Fig. 4-15. Hypertension from incision leading to an ischemic episode, demonstrated by the appearance of significant A, C, and V waves in the pulmonary capillary wedge pressure (PCWP) trace. These resolve with the institution of IV nitroglycerin. Note the lack of significant changes in the ECG (V₅) during this episode. BP = blood pressure; CVP = central venous pressure. (From J.A. Kaplan, and P.H. Wells. Early diagnosis of myocardial ischemia using the pulmonary arterial catheter. *Anesth. Analg.* 60:792, 1981. With permission.)

induction insertion is that in the vast majority of patients recent hemodynamic information based on the cardiac catheterization data is available; therefore, additional preoperative information is not necessary. In the appropriately medicated patient, however, placement of a PA catheter is not associated with any significant hemodynamic changes[13]. Also, the hemodynamic data collected in the catheterization laboratory may not be an accurate reflection of the current hemodynamic status, especially if the patient was sedated to a different level or was experiencing discomfort during the catheterization. The patient may also have had episodes of myocardial ischemia during the catheterization or may be experiencing ischemia when entering the operating room. If a patient is not sufficiently sedated, the deleterious effects of the anxiety related to the placement of the catheter should be weighed against the benefits expected from its placement. Proper sedation can be achieved in most adult patients so that pre-induction insertion can be performed safely.

5. **Types of PA catheters.** A variety of PA catheters are currently available for clinical use. The thermodilution catheter has a PA port for pressure monitoring and a thermistor for cardiac output measurements at its tip, an RA port for CVP monitoring and for injection of cold saline at 30 cm from the tip, and a lumen for inflation of the balloon (Fig. 4-16). In addition, PA catheters are available that provide:

a. A venous infusion port. This catheter supplies a third port 1 cm proximal to the CVP (31 cm from the tip), for infusion of drugs and fluids.

b. Pacing. Some pulmonary artery catheters have the capacity to provide intracardiac pacing in one of three ways.

   (1) Pulmonary artery catheters with permanently installed atrial and ventricular bipolar pacing electrodes can be used to establish atrial or ventricular pacing or to perform electrophysiologic studies of atrial, ventricular, and atrioventricular nodal electrical activity.

   (2) In other PA catheters, a lumen terminates 19 cm from the catheter tip. When the catheter tip lies in the PA with a normal-sized heart, this port is positioned in the RV. A separate sterile, prepackaged pacing wire can be placed through this port to contact the right ventricular endocardium for RV pacing.

   (3) A newer catheter (Swan-Ganz Thermodilution, A-V Paceport, Baxter Edwards Critical Care) provides atrial or atrioventricular pacing with two separate bipolar pacing probes. This catheter has been shown to provide stable pacing before and after CPB.[12]

c. Mixed venous oxygen saturation. Special fiberoptic PA catheters can be used to monitor mixed venous oxygen saturation (S_vO_2) continuously during surgery by the principle of absorption and reflectance of light through blood. The normal S_vO_2 is = 75%, a 5–10% increase or decrease being considered significant. A significant decrease in S_vO_2 may have several causes.

   (1) A decrease in perfusion (cardiac output), with a higher O_2 extraction ratio.

   (2) An increase in metabolic rate (increased O_2 extraction).

   (3) A decrease in arterial oxygen saturation (S_aO_2) from a decreased O_2 supply.

       Changes in saturation usually precede hemodynamic changes by a significant period of time, making this a useful adjunct to other monitors in the cardiac operating room.

d. Ejection fraction catheter. Newer catheters with faster thermistor response times can be used to determine the right ventricular ejection fraction in addition to the cardiac output.

e. Transthoracic. PA catheters are available that can be placed surgically. These are useful in the patient with difficult IV access and also in emergency situations when time does not allow placement of a transvenous PA line. These are available as two separate catheters. The first acts as a probe that contains a thermistor at the tip and a lumen that ends at the tip for PA pressure monitoring. This catheter is placed directly into the RV outflow tract and guided into the PA. This probe **is not** balloon tipped and therefore cannot be wedged. The second catheter is placed in the RA and is used for injecting the thermal indicator. An existing CVP line can be used to inject the indicator as well.

6. Techniques of insertion. Certain general guidelines should be followed when placing a PA catheter. The steps are outlined in Table 4-9. Placing the introducer is accomplished in a manner similar to that described for CVP insertion. However, special care should be observed with PA catheter placement, noting especially the following points:

   a. Sedation. As mentioned previously, proper sedation is an important part of PA catheter insertion. Because the patient is under a large drape for a longer period of time, he or she should be asked questions periodically to check for oversedation. A clear drape

Table 4-9. Steps for pulmonary artery catheter insertion

Steps	Reasoning/comments
1. Establish monitoring: BP cuff, ECG, pulse oximetry	Monitor for ischemia, hypoxemia, arrhythmia
2. Place nasal cannula	Avoids hypoxemia in sedated patient in head-down position
3. Cannulate central circulation, place dilator/introducer	See Table 4-5
4. Remove catheter from package, place sheath over catheter	This can damage balloon
5. Hand off proximal end to assistant. Flush appropriate ports of catheter with heparinized saline. Monitor at least the distal port.	Placing a PA catheter requires a nonsterile assistant, to connect ports to transducer tubing
6. Check balloon for competence	Should be done after sheath placed over catheter
7. While watching monitor and holding 30-cm mark fixed, raise the distal tip from horizontal to vertical position	This ensures that the correct monitor channel is connected to the distal port. **Only** the pressure channel for the distal port should reflect a rise in pressure
8. Insert PA catheter to 20 cm with balloon **down**	Puts balloon past end of introducer—inflation before this point may damage balloon
9. Inflate balloon with 1.5 cc of air or CO_2	Do not force air into balloon; there is a small amount of resistance before the opening pressure is reached
10. Advance slowly, monitoring the distal port	Look for progressive pressure changes from RA to RV, PA, and PCWP (Fig. 4-17)
11. When RV reached, advance more rapidly	Avoids arrhythmia but advancing slowly may be required to reach the pulmonary outflow tract
12. If RV or PA is difficult to enter:	
a. Have patient take deep breath	Increases pulmonary blood flow
b. Place in head-up position or tilt table to left or right	Places the RV or PA outflow at highest point, where balloon will float
c. Flush PA port with 1–2 ml of cold sterile saline	Stiffens catheter, making threading easier
12. When PA entered, advance slowly	Look for phase shift of V wave or damping of phasic pulse, or both
13. Release balloon	PA trace should return
14. "Size" the PA by inserting gas in 0.5-cc increments, watching PA trace	If PCWP is seen before full 1.5 cc is inserted, the lesser amount should be used **each time** to avoid PA rupture
15. Do not withdraw the catheter at any time with the balloon inflated	Avoids rupture of pulmonic or tricuspid valves

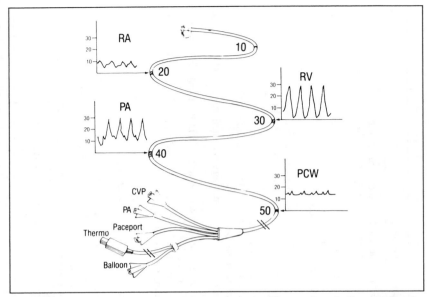

Fig. 4-16. Figure demonstrating pressure waves that will be encountered as a PA catheter is inserted into the wedged position from the right internal jugular vein. Distances on the catheter correspond to insertion distances read at the diaphragm of the introducer and are approximate. Actual distances may vary by ±5 cm. PA catheters should not be advanced more than 60 cm from this approach because this increases the risk of PA rupture or catheter knotting. RA = right atrium; RV = right ventricle; PA = pulmonary artery; PCW = pulmonary capillary wedge; Thermo = thermistor connection for cardiac output determination.

allows visual inspection of the patient's color and may cause a less suffocating feeling.

b. **ECG monitoring during placement.** It is essential to monitor the ECG during placement of the catheter because dysrhythmias are the most common complication associated with this procedure.

c. **Pulse oximetry.** This simple form of monitoring is essential when the patient is under the sterile drapes (where the color of the mucous membranes cannot be observed) and in a head-down position, which renders breathing more difficult. Pulse oximetry also gives the anesthesiologist an **audible** signal of rhythm and may alert him or her to an abnormal rhythm.

d. **Preferred approach.** The right internal jugular vein approach offers the most direct route to the right atrium and thus results in the highest rate of successful PA cannulation.

e. **Balloon inflation.** Air may be used for balloon inflation, although carbon dioxide is safer because it is 20 times more soluble in blood and will be resorbed faster in the event of balloon rupture. If any suspicion exists about balloon competency, no gas injections should be made through the balloon port.

f. **Waveform.** PA catheter placement can be accomplished without the use of fluoroscopy if the pressure at the distal tip of the catheter is measured as it passes from the RA to RV to PA to PCWP position. Representative waveforms are displayed in Fig. 4-16.

Table 4-10. Complications associated with pulmonary artery monitoring

A. Vascular access complications
    1. Inability to gain access
    2. Hemorrhage
    3. Damage to the vessel or associated structure(s)
    4. Pneumothorax
B. Catheter placement complications
    1. Dysrhythmias
    2. Catheter coiling/knotting
    3. Damage to the tricuspid or pulmonary valve(s)
    4. Endocarditis/sepsis
    5. Cardiac perforation
    6. Intracardiac thrombus formation/pulmonary embolus
    7. Paradoxical (systemic arterial) embolus
    8. Pulmonary artery rupture
    9. Pulmonary infarction
    10. Balloon rupture
    11. Thrombocytopenia
C. Monitoring complications
    1. Incorrect data collection
    2. Data misinterpretation/misapplication
    3. "Mesmerism" by pulmonary artery catheter data to the exclusion of other monitoring data and/or clinical factors
    4. Expense

Source: Modified from A. J. Schwartz, and T. J Conahan, III. Pulmonary artery catheters: There are still concerns with their routine use. *J. Cardiothorac. Anesth.* 1(1):7–9, 1987. With permission.

7. **Complications.** Complications can be divided into vascular access, catheter placement, and monitoring problems and are outlined in Table 4-10.

8. **Conclusions.** Pulmonary artery catheters provide a wealth of information about the right and left sides of the circulation. For this reason, they are used for every cardiac surgical procedure in some institutions because their benefits are perceived to outweigh their risks. Studies that show low morbidity rates with use of the PA catheter support this viewpoint. In other institutions, however, their use is much more selective. At present, their role in determining patient outcome has not been incontrovertibly demonstrated.

G. **Left atrial pressure.** In some patients, direct left atrial pressure can be measured after surgical insertion of a left atrial catheter. LA catheters are also used in corrective surgery for congenital lesions when PA catheter insertion is not possible. The left atrial pressure tracing is comparable to the CVP tracing, with A, C, and V waves occurring at identical points in the cardiac cycle. LA catheters are used to monitor valvular function (post-mitral valve replacement or mitral valvuloplasty) or to monitor left ventricular filling pressures whether a PA catheter is available or not. Left atrial pressure measured directly is more accurate than when measured with a pulmonary artery catheter because the effects of airway pressure on the pulmonary vasculature are removed. However, LA pressure does not necessarily reflect left ventricular end-diastolic pressure in the presence of mitral valvular disease. Air should be meticulously removed from LA lines.

H. **Cardiac output**
   1. Methods

a. Fick method. In the classic application of the Fick principle, oxygen is used as the "indicator," using the formula:

$$Q = 10 \times [V\ O_2/(a\text{-}v)\ O_2]$$

The arterial-to-venous difference (a-v) in oxygen content can be estimated closely by using the oxygen content of arterial blood minus the oxygen content of mixed venous blood. Oxygen consumption can be calculated from the inspired and expired oxygen concentrations and the volume of a sample expired gas. This method, however, does not lend itself to easy application in the operating room.

b. Indicator dilution method. In this method an indicator that is not metabolized is injected into the central circulation.

  (1) Dye dilution. A nontoxic dye such as indocyanine green or methylene blue is used. After total mixing in the pulmonary circuit, the dye is carried to the arterial circuit, where blood is continually sampled for the dye and its concentration measured. For most indicators, such as indocyanine green or methylene blue, the concentration is calculated by using spectrophotometric analysis of blood as it is drawn past an infrared light source. The usefulness of this method is limited by the inability to repeat the measurement frequently owing to the increasing background dye concentration.

  (2) Thermodilution. This method is the most commonly utilized cardiac output technique because of its ease of use. The indicator is an aliquot of saline, which is at a lower temperature than the temperature of blood, injected into the right atrium. The change in temperature produced by the injection of this indicator is measured in the pulmonary artery by a thermistor and is integrated over time to generate a value for right ventricular output, which is equal to systemic cardiac output if no intracardiac shunts are present. This method requires no withdrawal of blood and no arterial line, employs an inexpensive indicator, and is not greatly affected by recirculation.

c. Doppler ultrasound. Using the change in frequency of an ultrasonic beam as it reflects off a moving object (Doppler shift), blood flow velocity can be measured in the aorta. This method is noninvasive, since the ultrasound crystal is placed in the esophagus, thus making this method an attractive one. To achieve accurate measurements at least three conditions must be met: (1) the cross-sectional area of the aorta must be known, (2) the ultrasound beam must be directed parallel to the flow of blood, and (3) the beam direction cannot move to any great degree between measurements. Variations from these conditions lead to inaccuracies. Clinical use of this technique has produced problems with accuracy and precision, and its place in routine monitoring is uncertain at this point.

d. Echocardiography. End-diastolic and end-systolic dimensions measured by echocardiography can be converted to volumes, allowing stroke volume and cardiac output to be determined. More details about this technique are provided in the following section.

2. Accuracy and precision. Accuracy refers to the capability of a measurement to reflect the true cardiac output. This means that a measurement is compared to a "gold standard" method. Comparisons between various cardiac output methods, however, make use of different gold standards, making interpretation difficult. **Precision**

indicates the reproducibility of a measurement and refers to the variability between determinations. The methods used clinically are summarized in terms of accuracy and precision in Table 4-11.

For the thermodilution method, studies of precision have involved probability analyses of large numbers of cardiac output determinations. Using this approach, it was found that with two injections, there was only a 50% chance that the numbers obtained were within 5% of the true cardiac output[3]. If three injections yield results that are within 10% of each other, it can be assumed that there is a 90% probability that the average value of the three is within 10% of the true cardiac output. Although the precision of thermodilution is not great, variability can be minimized by knowing what factors lead to increase in errors.

3. **Assumptions and errors.** Certain assumptions are made with the use of both Fick and indicator dilution methods that may or may not actually be true. These are outlined in Table 4-12, along with sources of errors in the various measurements. Some specific errors in cardiac output determination are detailed below.

   a. **Thermodilution method**

      (1) **Volume of injectate.** Since the output computer will base its calculations on a particular volume, an injectate volume less than that for which the computer is set will cause a falsely high value and vice versa.

      (2) **Temperature of injectate.** The controversy over iced versus room temperature injectate centers around the concept that a larger difference between the temperature of the injectate and blood temperatures should increase the accuracy of the cardiac output determination. Some studies have not supported this hypothesis, and the extra inconvenience of keeping syringes on ice, together with the increased risk of infection (nonsterile water surrounding the Luer tip), make the iced saline method a less attractive alternative. If the injectate temperature factor is set incorrectly, errors can occur. For example, an increase of 1°C will cause a 3% overestimation of cardiac output.

      (3) **Shunts.** Intracardiac shunts will cause erroneous values for thermodilution cardiac output values, and this technique should not be utilized if a communication exists between the pulmonary and systemic circulations. A shunt should always be suspected when thermodilution cardiac output values do not fit the clinical findings.

      (4) **Timing with the respiratory cycle.** As much as a 10% difference in cardiac output will result depending on when in the respiratory cycle the injection occurs. These changes are most likely due to actual changes in pulmonary blood flow during respiration.

      (5) **Catheter position.** The tip of the pulmonary catheter must be in the pulmonary artery; otherwise, nonsensical curves are obtained.

   b. **Dye dilution method**

      (1) **Shunts.** The normal dye dilution curve appears as a quick upstroke in dye concentration, followed by a smooth, exponential decay. A smaller recirculation peak occurs late in the curve. A left-to-right shunt causes what is known as an early recirculation, which appears as a "hump" in the downstroke of the exponential phase. A right-to-left shunt will cause a small amount of dye to reach the arterial circulation without passing through the lungs, yielding an early small peak during the initial upstroke. The presence of these aberrant peaks can in

Table 4-11. Accuracy and precision of cardiac output measurements

Method	"Gold standard" comparison	Accuracy	Precision
O_2 consumption (Fick method)	Rotameter or electromagnetic flow probe placed in pulmonary artery	Good	Good
Thermodilution	Fick method	Overestimates output by as much as 10%	Poor—repeat measurements needed
Dye dilution	Fick method Thermodilution	Yields lower values compared to both methods	Good
Esophageal Doppler	Thermodilution	Good, if initial estimate of aortic diameter is accurate	Poor—probe can move easily
Transesophageal echocardiography	Ventricular angiography	Good, if ventricular asynergy is not present	Good

Table 4-12. Possible sources of errors in cardiac output determinations

Thermodilution	Dye dilution	Fick method
A. Assumptions Flow is constant Blood volume is constant No significant venous pooling Indicator flow represents total flow	Same as for thermodilution	Steady state exists for the duration of the study O_2 uptake by tissues equals uptake by lungs
B. Disadvantages (sources of errors) Volume of injectate must be correct Temperature of injectate must be accurate Affected by: (1) Intracardiac shunts (2) Coadministration of IV fluids (3) Phase of respiratory cycle (4) Differences in computer algorithms (5) Patient position (6) Position of catheter in pulmonary artery (7) Speed of injection	Affected by: (1) Intracardiac shunts (2) Volume of dye injected (3) Speed of injection	Subject to gas sampling errors Mixed venous sample will be misleading if catheter is wedged
C. Comments Rapid, easy to use Repetitive measurements possible No arterial line required	Arterial line required Dye must be prepared same day Repeated measurements not possible Not affected by respiratory cycle	More time-consuming, repeat measurements not practical Cumbersome to perform in operating room More equipment required

fact be used to diagnose congenital lesions and to test the adequacy of a repair. Typical recirculation peaks for right-to-left and left-to-right shunts are shown in Chap. 13.

> (2) **Repeat measurements.** Buildup of dye in the bloodstream prohibits repeated measurements because the background concentration will cause errors in accuracy.

c. **Oxygen consumption (Fick) method**

> (1) **Sampling errors.** Gas sampling errors can occur, for instance, when a true expired sample is not obtained or when the volume of the exhaled gas is not accurate. Sampling of arterial rather than mixed venous blood occur if the catheter tip is out too far in the pulmonary artery, resulting in withdrawal of capillary blood.
>
> (2) **Oxygen consumption.** Because oxygen consumption by the lungs rather than the tissues is quantified by this method, significant error can be introduced if lung volumes change (as with ventilation mode or the presence of atelectasis or lung collapse).

I. Transesophageal echocardiography

1. **Basic principles of operation.** Echocardiography is based on the use of ultrasonic waves in the range of 2.5—10 MHz to obtain information on the structure and function of the heart. A vibrating piezoelectric crystal both produces and receives the ultrasound waves. The time required for the wave to travel through biologic structures, together with the intensity of the reflected waves, provides information about the size and intensity of the structures. Because the crystals oscillate at a very rapid frequency, signals can be sent out at a rapid enough rate to obtain details about moving structures. In addition, waves can be processed to analyze the frequency shift (Doppler shift) between emitted and reflected waves to provide information about the direction and velocity of blood flow.

2. **Imaging echocardiography.** Although several kinds of ultrasound imaging techniques have been developed, two are used mainly for echocardiography.

a. **M-mode** provides a unidimensional view of structures along a single, narrow beam. By plotting information on distance and intensity together on the y axis and time on the x axis, one can generate on a screen or strip chart a depiction of the cardiac structures as they move during the cardiac cycle.

b. **Two-dimensional (2-D) mode** overcomes a major limitation of M-mode, that is, its unidimensionality. By changing beam direction rapidly along a single plane, a two-dimensional view is obtained. This scanning can be accomplished mechanically by physically rotating a single crystal, or electronically by serially stimulating a row of crystals such that the resultant waves are slightly out of phase with each other (linear phased-array transmission). With the latter method, smaller transducers can be utilized, making this mode an attractive one for esophageal echocardiography.

c. **Doppler echocardiography** takes advantage of the fact that blood cells can act as moving reflectors of ultrasonic waves, and the phase shift between the transmitted and reflected beams can be used to calculate the flow of blood through a structure. Doppler echocardiography can be combined with 2-D and M-mode echocardiography, and the flow data can be translated into differential color imaging to produce color-flow mapping. This information can be useful in identifying abnormal flows, as seen in valvular lesions. The color of the echo image is determined by the average velocity and direction of the blood cells passing through a discrete area during the sampling period.

3. **Transesophageal echocardiography**
   a. **General.** Developments in miniaturization have made possible placement of up to 64 piezoelectric crystals in a small linear phased-array format. Thus, excellent resolution can be obtained with a probe that can be placed in the esophagus. Transesophageal echocardiography (TEE) offers several advantages compared to standard transthoracic echocardiography.
      (1) Better image resolution and image quality due to the fact that ultrasonic waves pass a short distance through esophageal wall and pericardium and not through bone, fat, and lung.
      (2) Secure transducer position in the closed space of the esophagus.
      (3) Continuous monitoring for indefinite periods in the anesthetized patient.
   b. **Probe placement.** The common probes consist of a flexible gastroscope with a 7 to 8 cm maneuverable section (containing the ultrasonic crystals) at the distal end. This distal section is flexible in the horizontal and vertical planes. The probe is first lubricated with gel and is introduced into the esophagus either blindly or with the aid of a laryngoscope. The patient should be paralyzed to facilitate placement and to avoid damage to the probe. Once the thoracic esophagus has been entered ($\approx$30 cm), the probe can be maneuvered while viewing the 2-D echocardiogram. At present, the size of the TEE probe makes its placement somewhat uncomfortable before induction of anesthesia. Also, maintaining a mask airway and performing laryngoscopy become more difficult with the probe in place. If smaller probes are manufactured in the future, this technique will perhaps be a more clinically useful tool.
   c. **Complications.** To date, there have been no complications due to probe placement in a cardiac surgical placement. Two cases of laryngeal nerve damage have been related to TEE used in conjunction with neck flexion in a sitting craniotomy.
   d. **Axes useful to the anesthesiologist** (Fig. 4-17)
      (1) **Aortic valve view.** This is the most superior view obtained, and one can observe the value in cross section. Leaflet thickness and movement can be assessed.
      (2) **Four-chamber view.** With the probe directly behind the heart, a view of the four chambers, atrioventricular valves, and septum is possible. One can not only assess chamber size, atrioventricular valve function, and septal competence but can also detect intracardiac air bubbles (micro- or macrobubbles). This view is extremely valuable when using Doppler and Doppler color-flow techniques to assess mitral valve function. The echodense property of microbubbles also makes this axis a useful one in conventional TEE for injecting sonicated contrast dye microbubbles into the left ventricle to check for dynamic valve competency after mitral valve repair if Doppler capabilities do not exist.
      (3) **Short axis.** (Fig. 4-18). In this cross-sectional view, the left ventricle appears almost circular, and important information about ventricular volume and function can be obtained. The short axis at the midpapillary level displays regions of myocardium supplied by all three coronary artery systems, making it the most useful view for monitoring for ischemia.
4. **Applications of transesophageal echocardiography in the cardiac patient.** M-mode is usually used in conjunction with 2-D TEE because both can be performed simultaneously. Doppler and color

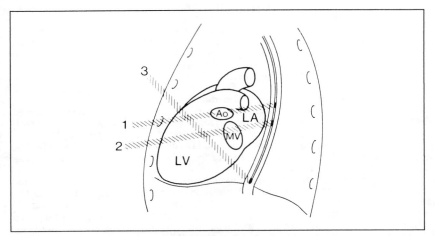

Fig. 4-17. Sagittal section showing the positions of the transesophageal echocardi-ographic (TEE) probe in the esophagus and the three corresponding axes: (1) aortic, (2) four-chamber, (3) mid-papillary short axis. AO = aortic valve, LA = left atrium, MV = mitral valve, LV = left ventricle. (From C.A. Visser, J.J. Koolen, et al. Trans-esophageal echocardiography. *J. Cardiothorac. Anesth.* 2(1):76, 1988. With permission.)

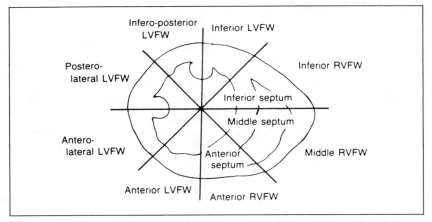

Fig. 4-18. Typical mid-papillary short axis view, with divisions of myocardium into eight segments for examination of regional wall motion. LVFW = left ventricular free wall; RVFW = right ventricular free wall. (From F.M. Clements, and N.P. deBruijn. Perioperative evaluation of regional wall motion. *Anesth. Analg.* 66:255, 1987. With permission.)

Doppler echocardiography is also available on most echo scanners; thus, applications of all three forms of echocardiography follow.

a. **Qualitative estimates of global function**

(1) Changes in 2-D cross-sectional area may signify changes in the contractile state of the ventricle. If contractility is de-pressed, the heart may compensate by increasing end-diastolic volume to place myofibrils under greater stretch.

(2) Wall motion patterns can be used during systole to estimate LV function. During normal systole, the endocardial surfaces of the LV move toward a central point, and the LV wall thickness increases. If function is reduced owing to prior infarction or cardiomyopathy, one or more areas of LV wall will not move properly, or the wall thickness will not increase and may in fact become thinner.

(3) Echocardiographic cardiac output can be obtained by converting diastolic and systolic LV areas to volume parameters to obtain stroke volume and multiplying by the heart rate. The results correlate well with thermodilution methods, but this analysis has to be performed off-line.

b. **Quantitative estimate of global function.** Echocardiography can be useful in determining the contractile state of the myocardium by virtue of its ability to measure changes in left ventricular cavity size. Most commonly, ejection phase indices of contractility are used.

(1) M-mode echocardiography can be used to obtain measurements of left ventricular diameter at end diastole and end systole. The **fractional shortening (FS)** can be calculated as:

$$FS\ (\%) = 100 \times (LVID_d - LVID_s)/LVID_d$$

Where $LVID_d$ = left ventricular end-diastolic dimension and $LVID_s$ = left ventricular end-systolic dimension. This type of unidimensional analysis, however, is inaccurate if significant ventricular asynergy exists.

(2) **Mean rate** of **circumferential fiber shortening** (mean **Vcf**) is simply the FS divided by the duration of left ventricular ejection.

(3) In 2-D mode, ejection fraction (EF) can be assessed by comparing the change in cross-sectional area during systole with the end-diastolic area.

$$EF\ (\%) = (LVEDA - LVESA)/LVEDA$$

Where LVEDA = left ventricular end-diastolic area
LVESA = left ventricular end-systolic area
One study has shown that the ejection fraction area was more sensitive than cardiac output in determining cardiac function[7]. Alternatively, area can be used to estimate volumes using any of several equations, and the EF can be expressed as a ratio of volumes in a manner similar to the above equation. The presence of septal deviations, abnormal wall motion movements, and anatomic abnormalities (aneurysms) will introduce errors into the estimation of EF; however, several studies show good correlation between echocardiographic EF and angiographic values. To decrease error, one can perform several area measurements at different short-axis levels (using Simpson's rule), but this is impractical for continuous monitoring.

(4) **Maximum aortic flow acceleration** can be measured using Doppler flow echocardiography. This is a sensitive indicator of contractility.

c. **Estimating preload.** The end-diastolic area (EDA) as an estimation of end-diastolic volume is a good predictor of preload, since it provides a direct view of the ventricular cavity. This has been supported by several studies. In one, the correlation between EDA and cardiac output was better than that between PCWP and cardiac output[11].

d. Regional wall motion abnormalities. TEE is a sensitive indicator of regional wall motion abnormalities (RWMA), whether they are of chronic or acute origin. Chronic RWMA is usually due to prior infarction, although several rare infiltrative processes can produce this condition also. Acute changes in wall motion were shown to correlate with changes in blood flow to a wall segment in classic studies done years ago. Although a full discussion is impossible here, excellent reviews of this subject are available[1].

(1) Types of ischemic RWMA

(a) Asynchronous. A disruption in the usual orderly progression of movements of various elements of the myocardial wall that combine to produce ventricular contraction.

(b) Hypokinesis. A decrease in the motion of the affected wall segment.

(c) Akinesis. Total lack of contraction.

(d) Dyskinesia. Paradoxical outward movement of the wall segment.

(2) Endocardial motion can be assessed visually or by outlining the endocardial borders at end diastole and end systole. Because translational and rotational movement of the heart can introduce errors if a fixed central point is used for reference, a floating central reference point is used. In this method, the endocardial borders at end diastole and end systole are superimposed on each other, and concentric motion of the endocardium can be evaluated.

(3) The degree of wall thickening is a sensitive monitor of RWMA that is easier to perform than endocardial movement. Although both types of analysis can be done quickly, at present, one must be off-line to analyze either method.

(4) RWMA have been shown to be more sensitive indicators of myocardial ischemia than ECG changes[9] as well as better predictors of progression to myocardial infarction.

e. Valvular function. In addition to the uses of TEE mentioned previously, valvular disease can be identified by conventional and color Doppler TEE.

f. Other clinical uses

(1) Intracardiac air. TEE is especially useful in detecting not only air emboli but also paradoxical air crossing an incompetent ventricular or atrial septum. It has been shown to be the most sensitive of cardiac air compared with precordial the Doppler stethoscope and changes in end-tidal CO_2 and with PA pressures.

(2) Diagnosing congenital heart defects. Although TEE per se would appear to be limited to use in adults, it has been adopted for diagnostic purposes in the pediatric population[2]. As microtechnology becomes better, smaller probes with equal resolution will make TEE an important tool for pediatric cardiac anesthesia and surgery.

g. Future uses. TEE is currently a relatively untapped resource that has the possibility of delivering tremendous clinical advances, some of which follow:

(1) End-systolic indices of contractility. These indices are obtained by combining LV cavity dimensions and the pressure generated by the ventricle. These indices have the advantage of providing load-independent measures of contractility.

(a) **End-systolic pressure-volume relation.** When the end-systolic arterial pressure is plotted against the end-systolic volume, a straight line results, the slope of which is proportional to the contractile state. A steeper slope reflects enhanced contractility.

(b) **End-systolic stress-volume relation.** When wall thickness data are known, the end-systolic wall stress can be estimated and plotted against volume to yield an even more sensitive indicator of contractility.

(2) **Afterload.** Estimates of afterload can be made echocardiographically, using the end-systolic wall stress measurement.

(3) **Diastolic function.** The relaxation phase can be characterized by quantitating the relationship between the decay in pressure postejection ($-dP/dt$) and the ventricular volume. Also, mitral valvular flow can be quantified to investigate ventricular filling during diastole.

(4) **Myocardial perfusion.** By injecting sonicated contrast dye into the aortic root during echocardiography, an echocardiogram of myocardial perfusion can be obtained. The heart is divided into radial endocardial and epicardial domains, so that flow to regions of the myocardium can be correlated with the degree of coronary stenoses. At present, signals must be digitized and analyzed off-line, but technical improvements that would allow rapid, on-line determinations will make this aspect of TEE extremely useful.

II. Pulmonary system
A. Pulse oximetry
1. Indications
a. **Preoperative uses.** Pulse oximetry can help in the general assessment of a patient preoperatively and can be easily used during the preoperative visit. Baseline oxygen saturation before premedication can alert the clinician to possible intraoperative or postoperative respiratory problems. In the patient with preexisting pulmonary hypertension, preoperative oximetry will alert one to the need for supplemental oxygen if premedication is given.

b. **Assessment of oxygenation intraoperatively.** Continuous oximetry will diagnose airway or pulmonary complication rapidly. This capability is of special importance in cardiac patients because hypoxia will lower myocardial oxygen supply and may contribute to myocardial ischemia.

c. **Assessment of perfusion.** The pulse oximeter works on the principle of infrared absorbance of blood as it traverses the capillary bed, and the sensing of a pulse is part of its basic operation. Thus, adequacy of perfusion is likely when the oximeter shows a saturation reading.

d. **Pulse rate.** In the patient with a dysrhythmia, not every beat will lead to adequate perfusion, and this will be sensed by the pulse oximeter. Thus, an audible monitor of the heart rhythm is also available.

2. Advantages and disadvantages are listed in Table 4-13.
B. Capnography
1. Indications
a. **All patients.** End-tidal capnography offers evidence of endotracheal intubation on an immediate, noninvasive basis and thus can corroborate other signs of successful intubation. It also provides continuous monitoring of the expired carbon dioxide.

b. **Patients with lung disease.** The capnograph provides evidence of the severity of small airway obstruction. Obstructive disease

Table 4-13. Pulse oximetry in cardiac procedures

Advantages	Disadvantages
Ease of use	Poor perfusion states (shock, hypothermia) make the saturation unobtainable
Continuous monitor	
Noninvasive	
Some models (Nellcor) have a variable pitch that correlates with the degree of saturation (obviates the need to view the screen)	Some dyes (methylene blue) interfere with the light absorbance
	Electocautery causes interference
Accuracy	Despite shielding, the oximeter cable can cause interference on other monitors if wires cross
	Requires pulsatile flow to operate
	Extraneous lights (e.g., Piling operating room lights) cause interference

causes an upsloping rather than a plateau or constant level of alveolar carbon dioxide.

  c. **Patients with pulmonary hypertension or reactive pulmonary vasculature.** These patients are often asked to hyperventilate voluntarily just prior to induction (to prevent a deleterious rise in arterial carbon dioxide and worsening PA pressures). A capnograph can provide noninvasive evidence that an acceptable level of arterial PCO_2 has been attained. It will also guide the anesthesiologist in providing an effective, safe level of relative hyperventilation, which is essential in the management of these patients on weaning from cardiopulmonary bypass.

 2. **Types**
  a. **In-line models.** An infra-red sensor detects carbon dioxide in the respiratory gas passing through the endotracheal tube.
  b. **Sampling models.** These models continuously withdraw gas from the circuit and analyze it in a remote apparatus.

III. Temperature
 A. **Indications**
  1. **Assessment of evenness of cooling and rewarming**
  2. **Diagnosing hazardous hypothermia or hyperthermia.** Below 32°C the myocardium is irritable and subject to complex arrhythmias, especially ventricular tachycardia and fibrillation. Likewise, significant enzyme desaturation and cell damage can occur with temperatures much above 41°C.
 B. **Types of measuring devices**
  1. **Thermistor.** Commonly used because of their accuracy, thermistors use thermal-sensitive semiconductors. Resistance through the conductor changes with changes in temperature. This type of probe is used in PA catheters and nasal probes to sense temperature.
  2. **Thermocouple.** These probes are made by joining two strips of metals with different specific heats. As temperature changes in the strips, the metals expand or contract to different degrees, producing an electromotive force that is compared to a reference junction in a remote unit. This type of probe is used commonly in tympanic membrane probes.
 C. **Sites of measurement.** Considering the numerous possible sites in which to measure temperature, the question immediately arises as to which is the most accurate. The answer depends on which compartment one desires to measure. At least two exist:

1. Core temperature

a. General. The core temperature represents the temperature of the vital organs. The term **core temperature** used here is perhaps a misnomer because gradients exist even within this vessel-rich group during rapid changes in blood temperature.

b. PAC thermistor. This is the best estimate of the core temperature when pulmonary blood flow is present, i.e., before and after cardiopulmonary bypass. Most cardiac output monitors will display the thermistor temperature.

c. Nasopharyngeal temperature. Nasopharyngeal temperature provides an accurate reflection of brain temperature during cardiopulmonary bypass, although there may be a lag between it and the actual brain temperature. The probe should be inserted into the nasopharynx to a distance equivalent to the distance from the nare to the tip of the earlobe.

d. Tympanic membrane temperature. This temperature also will reflect brain temperature, with the same limitations of lagging behind the actual brain temperature.

e. Bladder temperature. This modality has also been used to measure core temperature, although it may be inaccurate in instances when renal blood flow and urine production are decreased.

f. Esophageal temperature. Because the esophagus is a mediastinal structure, it will be greatly affected by the temperature of the blood returning from the extracorporeal pump and should not be used routinely for cases involving cardiopulmonary bypass.

g. CPB arterial line temperature. This is the temperature of the heat exchanger, i.e., the lowest temperature during active cooling and the highest temperature during active rewarming. During either of these phases, a gradient always exists between the arterial line temperature and any other temperature.

h. CPB venous line temperature. This is the "return" temperature to the oxygenator and probably best reflects core temperature during cardiopulmonary bypass when no active warming or cooling is occurring.

2. Shell

a. General. The shell compartment represents the majority of the body (muscle, fat, bone), which receives a smaller proportion of the blood flow, thus acting as an "energy sink" that can significantly affect temperature fluxes. Shell temperatures will react more slowly than core temperatures. Shell temperature lags behind core temperature during cooling and also during rewarming. At the point of separation bypass, the core temperature will be significantly higher than shell temperature. The final equilibrium temperature with rewarming will probably be closer to the shell temperature than the core temperature measured at the time of separation from bypass.

b. Rectal temperature. Although traditionally thought of as a core temperature, during cardiopulmonary bypass procedures the rectal temperature most accurately reflects muscle mass temperature. If the tip of the probe rests in stool, a significant lag will exist with changing temperatures.

c. Skin temperature. Skin temperature is affected by local factors (warming blanket, topical cooling device, and so on) and will lead to errors in gauging temperature.

D. Risks of bleeding. If the nasal mucosa is disrupted during probe placement, nasal bleeding can result, especially when the patient is heparinized. Similar problems have been reported after placement of probes in the external ear canal. Otherwise, the risks of temperature monitoring are minimal.

E. Recommendations for temperature monitoring. Monitoring temperature at two sites is recommended, one at a core site and one at a shell site. Arterial and venous line temperatures are available directly from the cardiopulmonary bypass apparatus. Nasal temperature monitoring is recommended for core temperature because it will most rapidly reflect changes in the arterial blood temperature. Because rectal temperature monitoring is simple to establish, this is recommended for monitoring shell temperature.

IV. Renal function

A. Indications for monitoring

1. **Incidence of renal failure post-CPB.** Acute renal failure (ARF) is a recognized complication of cardiopulmonary bypass, occurring in from 2.5–31% of cases. ARF is related to preoperative renal function as well as to the presence of coexisting disease. CPB may also affect renal function adversely because the unphysiologic state of nonpulsatile flow may upset the normal autoregulatory mechanisms of renal blood flow.

2. **Use of diuretics in CPB prime.** Mannitol is routinely used during CPB for two reasons:

   a. **Hemolysis** occurs during cardiopulmonary bypass, and serum hemoglobin levels rise. Urine output should be maintained to avoid damage to renal tubules.

   b. **Deliberate hemodilution** is induced with the onset of hypothermic CPB. Maintenance of good urine output during and after CPB allows removal of excess free water.

B. Urinary catheter.
This monitor is the single most important monitor of renal function during surgical cases involving CPB. Establishing a urinary catheter should be a priority in emergencies as well.

1. **Anuria on bypass.** Not uncommonly, little urine will be made while the patient is on cardiopulmonary bypass. Hypothermia and the reduction of arterial flow will also cause a diminution in renal function. Therefore, anuria should not usually be treated aggressively with additional diuretic therapy, especially while the patient is hypothermic.

2. **How much urine is adequate?** Post-CPB, adequacy of urine output depends on several factors; all of which should be optimized:

   a. Volume status
   b. Cardiac output
   c. Hematocrit
   d. Amount of surgical bleeding

C. Electrolytes.
Serum electrolytes, especially potassium, should be checked toward the end of CPB and after bypass. Cardiac patients receive large amounts of potassium if cardioplegia is used, and elimination of this agent depends in part on satisfactory urine output. A low serum ionized calcium level may be the cause of diminished pump function, and can be checked easily before separation from bypass.

V. Neurologic function

A. Indications for monitoring the electroencephalogram (EEG)

1. Associated carotid disease
2. Diagnosis of embolic phenomenon
3. Diagnosis of aortic cannula malposition
4. Diagnosis of inadequate arterial flow on CPB
5. Confirmation of adequate cooling
6. Hypothermic circulatory arrest. Refer to chapter 24.

B. Processed versus raw EEG (see Chapter 24)

C. Evoked potentials

1. **Somatosensory evoked potentials (SSEP).** SSEP can be used to monitor the integrity of the spinal cord. It is most useful in operations such as surgery for a thoracic aneurysm, in which the blood flow to the spinal cord may be compromised. A stimulus is applied to a peripheral nerve (usually the tibial nerve), and the resultant brainstem and brain activity are quantified. Specific uses are discussed further in Chap. 16.
2. **Visual evoked response (VER) and brainstem audio evoked responses (BAER).** These techniques do not have routine clinical application in cardiac surgical procedures, and are not discussed.

REFERENCES

1. Clements, F.M., and deBruijn, N.P. Perioperative evaluation of regional wall motion by transesophageal two-dimensional echocardiography. *Anesth. Analg.* 66:249–261, 1987.
2. Cyran, S.E., Meyer, R.A., Bailey, W.W., et al. Efficacy of intraoperative transesophageal echocardiography in children. Am. J. Cardiol. (in press, 1989).
3. Hoel, B.L. Some aspects of the clinical use of thermodilution in measuring cardiac output. *Scand. J. Clin. Lab Invest.* 38:383–388, 1978.
4. Kates, R.A., Zaidan, J.R., and Kaplan, J.A. Esophageal lead for intraoperative electrocardiographic monitoring. *Anesth. Analg.* 61:781–785, 1982.
5. Kaplan, J.A., and King, S.B. The precordial electrocardiographic lead (V_5) in patients who have coronary artery disease. *Anesthesiology* 45:570–574, 1976.
6. Mohr, R., Lavee, J., and Goor D.A. Inaccuracy of radial artery pressure measurement after cardiac operations. *J. Thorac. Cardiovasc. Surg.* 94:286–290, 1987.
7. Roizen, M.F., Beaupre, P.N., Alpert, R.A. et al. Monitoring with two-dimensional transesophageal echocardiography. Comparison of myocardial function in patients undergoing supraceliac, suprarenal-infraceliac, or infrarenal aortic occlusion. *J. Vasc. Surg.* 1:300–305, 1984.
8. Slogoff, S., Keats, A.S., and Arlund, C. On the safety of radial artery cannulation. *Anesthesiology* 59:42–47, 1983.
9. Smith, J.S., Cahalan, M.K., Benefiel, D.J., et al. Intraoperative detection of myocardial ischemia in high-risk patients: Electrocardiography versus two-dimensional echocardiography. *Circulation* 72:1015–1021, 1985.
10. Stern, D.H., Gerson, J.I., Allen, F.B., et al. Can we trust the direct radial artery pressure immediately following cardiopulmonary bypass? *Anesthesiology* 62:557–561, 1985.
11. Thys, D.M., Hillel, Z., Goldman, M., et al. A comparison of hemodynamic indices derived by invasive monitoring and by two-dimensional echocardiography. *Anesthesiology* 67:630–634, 1987.
12. Trankina, M.F., and White, R.D. Perioperative cardiac pacing using an atrioventricular pacing pulmonary artery catheter. *J. Cardiothorac. Anesth.* 3:154–162, 1989.
13. Waller, J.L., Zaidan, J.R., Kaplan, J.A., et al. Hemodynamic responses to preoperative vascular cannulation in patients with coronary artery disease. *Anesthesiology* 56:219–221, 1982.

SUGGESTED READINGS

Blitt, C.D. *Monitoring in Anesthesia and Critical Care Medicine.* New York: Churchill Livingstone, 1985.

Kaplan, J.A. (ed.) *Cardiac Anesthesia* (2nd ed.). Philadelphia: Saunders, 1987.
Saidman, L.J., and Smith, N.T. *Monitoring in Anesthesia* (2nd ed.). Boston: Butterworth, 1984.

Induction of Anesthesia

George W. Rung and Thomas J. Conahan III

I. Introduction. The induction of anesthesia is one of the most critical periods of the cardiac patient's perioperative course. The goal is to render the patient unconscious, analgesic, amnestic, and motionless to allow passage of an endotracheal airway while maintaining stable hemodynamics. To attain this goal, the anesthesiologist must anticipate the interaction between the patient's pathophysiology, anesthesia, and the planned surgical procedure. Additional factors that may complicate anesthetic induction include normal reflex responses and abnormal patient airway anatomy.

A. Patient pathophysiology

1. Cardiac surgical patients may have multiple causes for their cardiac complaints, including poor ventricular function, valvular dysfunction, myocardial ischemia, dysrhythmias, structural defects, and cardiac tamponade.

2. Systemic pathophysiology may be associated with, cause, or compound preexisting cardiac dysfunction. Specifically, cerebral vascular disease, renal dysfunction, hepatic dysfunction, pulmonary disease, endocrine abnormalities, hypovolemia, hypoxia, hypercarbia, and acidosis complicate anesthetic care for patients undergoing cardiac surgery.

B. Side effects of anesthetic agents. The central nervous system depression (loss of consciousness) associated with induction of general anesthesia may be accompanied by depression of other vital organ systems. Cardiovascular effects of anesthetic induction are often prominent. These effects may be minimized by choosing anesthetic agents with actions favorable for the patient's cardiac pathophysiology. In many cases, circulatory parameters improve after induction of anesthesia.

C. Reflex responses. The "stress response" to surgery and anesthesia may not be beneficial for the cardiac patient. The induction of anesthesia, laryngoscopy, and intubation stimulate elevations in serum catecholamines, cortisol, antidiuretic hormone, glucose, and acute phase proteins. These contribute to hypertension, tachycardia, total body salt and water retention, and postoperative intravascular hyperviscous states. Attenuation of the stress response should be considered prior to anesthetic induction.

D. Abnormal airway anatomy. A patient's airway management may be complicated by two mechanisms. An adequate anesthetic face mask seal, and therefore effectiveness of positive pressure ventilation, may be impaired by the presence of facial hair or absence of teeth. Additionally, intubation of the trachea may be difficult owing to limited jaw or neck motion, an anterior larynx, prominent teeth, a large tongue, or other abnormality.

The design of an appropriate induction sequence depends on the patient's medical condition, the cardiac lesion, the pharmacology of the induction agents, and individual airway abnormalities. The formulation of an anesthetic plan preoperatively is useful as a general guide but must be altered as the anesthetic progresses if indicated by acute changes in pathophysiology. Careful analysis of all available preoperative information enables the anesthesiologist to anticipate possible problems and take steps to avoid them.

II. Induction agents

A. Opioids

1. Pharmacology of opioids

a. Mechanism of action. Opioids exert their effect by activating stereospecific receptors in the central nervous system and gastrointestinal tract. Molecules that fully activate receptors are termed agonists (e.g., morphine, meperidine, fentanyl, and so on), those that partially activate receptors are termed agonist-antagonists (e.g., pentazocine, butorphanol, buprenorphine, nalbuphine), and those attaching to but not activating the receptor are termed antagonists (e.g., naloxone, naltrexone). Activation of opioid receptors interferes with transmembrane calcium ion transport, inhibits adenylate cyclase activity, and inhibits release of neurotransmitters. In clinical doses, opioids do not have direct neurologic or cardiovascular effects independent of receptors. Opioids do not affect peripheral nerve conduction velocity or responsiveness of afferent nerve endings.

b. Pharmacokinetics. Lipid solubility, degree of protein binding, rate of metabolism, and receptor affinity determine the clinical characteristics of an opioid. Pharmacokinetic parameters for commonly used opioids are given in Table 5-1.

c. Side effects. Opioids share similar side effects, differing only in severity. Common side effects are listed in Table 5-2.

d. Reversal. Opioid actions may be antagonized at the receptor site by specific antagonists or agonist-antagonists. An antagonist such as naloxone reverses not only undesirable effects (e.g., respiratory depression) but also analgesia, which may increase sympathetic nervous system activity and possibly cause hypertension, tachycardia, increased myocardial oxygen consumption ($M\dot{V}O_2$), angina, and pulmonary edema. An agonist-antagonist such as nalbuphine offers the advantages of partial reversal of opioid actions (decreased respiratory depression but persistent analgesia) and a longer elimination half-life than most opioids (unlike naloxone), making recurrence of respiratory depression less likely. Even partial reversal of opioid activity may be dangerous in the cardiac patient, who may not tolerate the increased level of sympathetic activity.

2. Morphine
a. Clinical uses
(1) **Premedication** (0.1–0.2 mg/kg IM). Sedation is a desirable side effect in adult and pediatric patients. The dose may be decreased or omitted for patients with preload-dependent lesions (e.g., critical aortic stenosis or mitral stenosis) or reactive pulmonary vasculature.

(2) **Postcardiopulmonary bypass** (0.25–0.5 mg/kg IV). This intraoperative regimen provides a longer duration of action of analgesia with sedation and also lowers blood pressure.

(3) **Intrathecal administration** (0.5–2.0 mg IT). This route has been used experimentally for cardiac surgery in some centers combined with inhalational techniques.

(4) **Sole anesthetic agent** (1-3 mg/kg IV). This method is no longer popular because of its side effects, including venodilation with increased perioperative fluid requirement and need for prolonged postoperative mechanical ventilation.

b. Advantages
(1) Profound analgesia

(2) Minimal myocardial depression when used as sole anesthetic agent

(3) Longer duration of action that allows smooth transition to postoperative period

(4) Decrease in blood pressure may be desirable

(5) Does not sensitize heart to catecholamines

c. Disadvantages
(1) **Histamine release.** The amount of histamine released is related to the speed of morphine administration. There is a large

Table 5-1. Pharmacokinetics of opioid analgesics

	Protein Binding (%)	Volume of distribution (liters/kg)	Clearance (ml/kg/min)	Half-life (min)	Intravenous potency ratio
Morphine	30	3.2	14.7	114	1
Meperidine	60	3.8	15.1	180-264	0.53
Fentanyl	84	4.1	11.6	185-219	292
Sufentanil	93	1.7	12.7	148-164	4,531
Alfentanil	92	0.9	6.4	70-98	73

Source: Modified from R. K. Stoelting. *Pharmacology and Physiology in Anesthetic Practice.* Philadelphia: Lippincott, 1987. Pp. 76. With permission.

Table 5-2. Side effects of opioids

Cardiovascular

Histamine release
   Decreased arteriolar resistance
   Increased venous capacitance
Decreased central sympathetic outflow
Increased vagal tone
Direct action on vascular smooth muscle?

Respiratory

Decreased carbon dioxide responsiveness
Depressed cough reflex
Bronchial smooth muscle spasm (histamine release)

Central nervous system

Dose-dependent depression of consciousness
Nausea and vomiting
Miosis
Chest and abdominal wall rigidity

Gastrointestinal

Biliary smooth muscle spasm that may be difficult to distinguish from angina
Decreased peristaltic activity (ileus)
Constipation

Genitourinary

Urinary retention

---

interpatient variability in the amount of histamine released. Increased plasma histamine may cause venodilation, hypotension, bronchospasm, and anaphylactoid reactions. These effects may be blocked by prior administration of H_1- and H_2-blocking drugs (e.g., diphenhydramine and cimetidine), although histamine release per se is not reduced.

(2) **Tachycardia and hypertension.** With any opioid technique but especially with morphine, there may be an inadequate plasma level of opioid for a given level of surgical stimulation, with resultant sympathetic outflow ("breakthrough"). Once this occurs, it is very difficult to treat using additional opioid.

(3) **Awareness.** Because opioids are relatively impotent amnestics, there is a higher incidence of awareness during surgery when they are used as the sole anesthetic agent.

(4) **Increased volume requirements.** Venodilatation due primarily to histamine release is probably responsible for the increased perioperative fluid requirements.

(5) **Relatively slow onset.** Even with intravenous administration, the onset of action is 5–10 minutes, and cerebrospinal fluid levels are still increasing 20 minutes after injection.

3. **Fentanyl**
   a. **Clinical uses**
      (1) **Anesthetic** (50–150 µg/kg IV). These doses induce unconsciousness, provide analgesia, and obtund reflex responses to surgery and anesthesia. Is high-dose fentanyl a potent anes-

thetic? The thousands of cases done successfully with fentanyl as the sole agent and the fact that the electroencephalographic (EEG) pattern of patients anesthetized with high-dose fentanyl is consistent with deep anesthesia (high-amplitude, low-frequency activity) support its potency as an anesthetic. High-dose opioid "anesthesia" has been associated with reports of intraoperative awareness, however, and it is interesting to note that in animal studies fentanyl can reduce the minimal alveolar concentration (MAC) of a coadministered halogenated agent by a maximum of 65%.

  (2) **"Balanced" technique** (10–25 µg/kg IV). The advantages of adding other central nervous system depressants, including nitrous oxide, halogenated agents, or benzodiazepines, include a reduction in the fentanyl dose required and the beneficial effects of the second drug. Additional drugs may also have undesirable effects that are additive or synergistic with opioids, such as reduction in arteriolar resistance or increase in venous capacitance, resulting in hypotension.

  (3) **Sedation during line placement** (0.5–2 µg/kg IV). These small doses provide effective analgesia and are usually well tolerated by most patients during invasive line placement, but hypoxemia has been reported in this setting.

  (4) **Treatment of pulmonary hypertension.** Fentanyl doses (5–10 µg/kg IV) may attenuate pulmonary hypertensive responses in ventilated neonates with reactive pulmonary vasculature.

b. Advantages

  (1) Profound analgesia

  (2) No myocardial depression—even at plasma concentrations 100 times greater than those attained after clinical doses

  (3) No histamine release

c. Disadvantages

  (1) Long duration of action with high doses due to accumulation in tissues

  (2) Prolonged respiratory depression

  (3) Bradycardia more severe than morphine

  (4) Increased incidence and severity of chest wall rigidity compared with morphine

  (5) Possible exaggeration of cardiovascular effects (myocardial depression, reduced systemic vascular resistance) of other anesthetic agents (e.g., nitrous oxide, diazepam)

4. Sufentanil

a. Clinical uses

  (1) **Anesthetic** (10–20 µg/kg IV). Sufentanil may be used as the sole anesthetic agent at these high doses. In an animal study, it was found that sufentanil could reduce the MAC of a coadministered potent inhalation agent by 80%.

  (2) **"Balanced" technique** (1–5 µg/kg IV).

  (3) **Sedation** (0.05–0.10 µg/kg IV).

  (4) **"Preinduction"** (1.5–3.0 mg/kg intranasal). This technique may be useful for selected pediatric patients who will not cooperate with insertion of an intravenous cannula or application of a face mask, although its use in pediatric cardiac surgery has not been reported. Chest wall rigidity may result.

b. Advantages

  (1) Most potent commercially available opioid—approximately 7–10 times more potent than fentanyl

  (2) Highest µ receptor specificity—approximately 90%

(3) Faster sedation and induction of anesthesia compared with fentanyl or alfentanil is probably related to higher lipid solubility and potency and shorter injection time (owing to lower volume of injectate)

(4) No histamine release

(5) Lower incidence of "breakthrough" hypertension found by some investigators

c. Disadvantages

(1) Bradycardia

(2) Decreased systemic vascular resistance

(3) Chest wall rigidity

(4) Long duration of action at high doses

5. Alfentanil

a. Clinical uses

(1) **Sole anesthetic** (100–200 μg/kg IV for induction). Because elimination half-life is short, a variable rate continuous infusion is recommended. This added complexity may limit its use to shorter cardiovascular procedures, such as exploratory thoracotomy for postoperative hemorrhage or removal of a transthoracic intraaortic balloon pump.

(2) "Balanced" technique (25–75 μg/kg IV).

b. Advantages

(1) Shorter duration of action compared with fentanyl or sufentanil

(2) Notable hemodynamic stability but probably no more stable than fentanyl or sufentanil

(3) Faster recovery of spontaneous ventilation and tracheal extubation compared with fentanyl anesthesia

a. Disadvantages

(1) Lower lipid solubility compared with fentanyl, contributing to longer onset time

(2) Short duration of action suggests use of a constant infusion, complicating care

(3) High incidence of chest wall rigidity (up to 50%)

(4) High incidence of bradycardia

(5) Postoperative nausea and vomiting more common

(6) It has been suggested that there is a population of patients who are hypometabolizers of alfentanil (debrisoquin type)

B. Intravenous nonopioids (Table 5-3)

1. Thiopental

a. **General pharmacology.** Thiopental is an ultra-short-acting barbiturate well suited for the induction of general anesthesia but is not an ideal maintenance anesthetic because it lacks analgesic properties and accumulates with high doses or prolonged administration. Maximum brain concentration is achieved within 1 minute after an intravenous bolus, and its action is terminated by redistribution to other tissues. Brain concentration falls below that required for unconsciousness within 5–10 minutes after injection, but slow hepatic metabolism yields an elimination half-life of 5–12 hours. As thiopental concentration in depot tissues (adipose and muscle) increases, the rate of decline of brain concentration decreases, prolonging the duration of action. The predominant cardiovascular effect is a dose-related decrease in contractility.

b. Clinical uses

(1) Induction of anesthesia if ventricular function is adequate

(2) Rapid sequence induction (full stomach)

(3) May be the induction agent of choice for patients with elevated intracranial pressure or severe cerebrovascular disease be-

Table 5-3. Hemodynamic effects of nonopioid induction agents

Agent	HR	MAP	SVR	PAP	PVR	CVP	LA	CI
Thiopental	↑	↓	—	—	—	—	↑	↓
Diazepam	↑	↓	—/↓	↓	↓	—	—	—
Midazolam	↑	↓	↓	—	—	—	↓	↓
Ketamine	↑	↑	↑	↑	↑ *	↑	—	↑
Etomidate	↑	↓	↓	↓	↑	—	↓	—
Propofol	↑	↓	↓	—	—	—	↑	↓

Note: Drug effect is dependent on individual patient characteristics (e.g., intravascular volume status, ventricular function, sympathetic "tone," beta blockade, etc.).
HR = heart rate, MAP = mean arterial pressure, SVR = systemic vascular resistance, PAP = pulmonary artery pressure, PVR = pulmonary vascular resistance, CVP = central venous pressure, LA = left atrium, CI = cardiac index, ↑ = increased, ↓ = decreased, — = no effect.
*Ketamine does not increase PVR in neonates.
Source: Modified from J. G. Reves, P. Flezzani, and I. Kissin. Pharmacology of Intravenous Anesthetic Induction Drugs. In J. A. Kaplan (ed.), *Cardiac Anesthesia* (2nd ed.). New York: Grune & Stratton, 1987. Pp. 128, 130 and 131. With permission.

cause thiopental lowers intracranial pressure and increases cerebral perfusion pressure if systemic blood pressure is preserved
   (4) Offers brain protection during cardiopulmonary bypass for open heart procedures in high-risk patients
   (5) Can be used as an adjunct to hypothermia for brain protection during deep hypothermic circulatory arrest (DHCA)
 c. **Advantages**
   (1) Rapid onset of action
   (2) Short duration of action unless high doses are used
   (3) Lowers intracranial pressure (ICP) and cerebral oxygen consumption
   (4) Good amnestic properties
 d. **Disadvantages**
   (1) Potent myocardial depression
   (2) Dilates venous capacitance vessels, lowering venous return to the heart and cardiac output
   (3) Exaggerated decrease in cardiac output in patients with hypovolemia, constrictive pericarditis, or cardiac tamponade
   (4) Reflex tachycardia is undesirable for patients with coronary artery disease
   (5) Prolonged duration of action at high doses
   (6) Lack of analgesic activity, even "anti-analgesic" action
2. **Benzodiazepines**
 a. **General pharmacology.** Benzodiazepines have hypnotic, anxiolytic, muscle relaxant, and amnestic properties. The mechanism of action is thought to be potentiation of gamma aminobutyric acid (GABA), an inhibitory neurotransmitter. Metabolism is by hepatic demethylation and hydroxylation (to some active metabolites) and renal excretion. Differences between benzodiazepines are primarily in onset time and duration of action.
 b. **Diazepam**
   (1) Clinical uses
     (a) Premedication (0.05–0.20 mg/kg PO)
     (b) Sedation during line placement (0.05–0.10 mg/kg IV)
     (c) Anesthetic induction (0.3–0.5 mg/kg IV)

      (d) Adjunct for induction (0.10–0.25 mg/kg IV)

      (e) Amnestic agent with opioid technique (0.02–0.10 mg/kg IV)

    (2) Advantages

      (a) Hemodynamic stability during induction with doses of 0.3–0.5 mg IV used as the sole induction agent

      (b) Maintains systemic vascular resistance

      (c) Amnestic action

      (d) Reduces inhalation agent or opioid dose

      (e) Decreases cerebral and myocardial oxygen consumption

    (3) Disadvantages

      (a) Interpatient response is variable.

      (b) Lack of analgesic activity requires additional agent(s) to prevent hyperdynamic response to endotracheal intubation.

      (c) Venodilatation and decreased venous return contribute to lower cardiac output in patients with hypovolemia or cardiac tamponade.

      (d) Pain occurs on intravenous injection, and there is a significant incidence of peripheral vein thrombophlebitis.

      (e) Long terminal half-life and active metabolites favor accumulation in tissue stores.

      (f) Intramuscular injection is painful and poorly absorbed.

  c. Midazolam

    (1) Clinical uses

      (a) Anesthetic induction (0.2–0.4 mg/kg IV)

      (b) Adjunct for induction (0.01–0.10 mg/kg IV)

      (c) Amnestic agent (0.01–0.10 mg/kg IV)

      (d) Premedication (0.05–0.075 mg/kg IM)

      (e) Sedation during line placement (0.01–0.05 mg/kg IV)

    (2) Advantages

      (a) Duration of action shorter than that of diazepam

      (b) Rapid onset of action secondary to high lipid solubility

      (c) Potent amnestic

      (d) Water soluble, less venous irritation, intramuscular injection less painful than diazepam

    (3) Disadvantages

      (a) No analgesic activity

      (b) May decrease systemic vascular resistance at high doses or when combined with opioids

      (c) Reflex tachycardia

      (d) Dysrhythmias

3. Ketamine

  a. General pharmacology. Ketamine is a "dissociative" anesthetic agent that produces unconsciousness, analgesia, and amnesia. Airway reflexes are largely maintained, respiratory depression is minimal, and bronchial smooth muscle is dilated by a direct mechanism. Central sympathetic nervous system activity is preserved or increased. Myocardial contractility is depressed, but compensation often occurs by increased sympathetic activity in normal patients. Myocardial depression becomes evident with high doses of ketamine, in patients with preexisting high sympathetic tone, or in the presence of sympathetic blockade (i.e., pharmacologic or conduction nerve block). Pulmonary artery pressure may be increased by ketamine in adults, but an increase has not been demonstrated to occur in neonates, even those with prior pulmonary hypertension. This important difference may be explained by the immaturity of the sympathetic nervous system at birth.

  b. Clinical uses

(1) "Preinduction" (1–2 mg/kg IM). This is useful for patients (usually children) who cannot or will not cooperate with intravenous catheter insertion or face mask application.

(2) Induction (1–4 mg/kg IV). Anesthetic induction with ketamine maintains sympathetic tone and tends to increase heart rate, systemic arterial pressure, systemic vascular resistance, and cardiac output. These changes are desirable in the setting of hypovolemia, pericardial tamponade, and some congenital lesions (e.g., pulmonary stenosis).

(3) Sedation (0.1–0.5 mg/kg IV). Provides analgesia and sedation with minimal respiratory depression and maintenance of airway reflexes.

c. **Advantages**

(1) Rapid acting

(2) Maintains systemic vascular resistance during induction

(3) Supports blood pressure and heart rate in hypovolemic patients by central sympathetic stimulating mechanism

(4) May be given intramuscularly to induce anesthesia in uncooperative patients

(5) Minimal respiratory depression (may depress respiration in neonates)

(6) Bronchodilation

d. **Disadvantages**

(1) Myocardial depression may not be compensated by increase in sympathetic tone in patients with limited sympathetic nervous system reserve.

(2) Myocardial oxygen consumption is increased.

(3) Emergence delirium and "bad dreams" may be a problem but may be minimized by limiting dose and supplementing this drug with a benzodiazepine.

(4) Ketamine may cause excessive airway secretions.

(5) Increase in myocardial contractility is undesirable in patients with asymmetric septal hypertrophy or tetralogy of Fallot with infundibular spasm. This effect may be attenuated by coadministration of benzodiazepine.

4. **Etomidate**

a. **General pharmacology.** Etomidate is a sedative-hypnotic with a rapid onset and short duration of action after intravenous administration. Its short duration of action is due to rapid redistribution to a large volume of distribution. Metabolism is primarily by hepatic degradation. For prolonged sedation, a continuous infusion is recommended. Its hemodynamic stability has been advocated, even in the setting of acute myocardial infarction. Only small decreases, if any, in systemic and pulmonary arterial pressure, cardiac index, filling pressures, and vascular resistance have been reported in experimental animal and human studies using doses of 0.15–0.60 mg/kg IV.

b. **Clinical uses**

(1) Anesthetic induction (0.3 mg/kg IV)

(2) Sedation (0.01–0.10 mg/kg IV)

(3) Amnestic (0.01–0.10 mg/kg IV)

c. **Advantages**

(1) Rapid onset of action due to lipid solubility

(2) Short duration of action (rapid redistribution)

(3) Hemodynamic stability at doses ranging from 0.2–0.4 mg/kg

(4) Depression of cerebral and myocardial metabolic rate

(5) No decrease in hepatic or renal perfusion

(6) Less hypotension in hypovolemic patients than thiopental

d. Disadvantages
(1) May cause hypotension in hypovolemic patients or those with depressed ventricular function.
(2) Pain on injection (propylene glycol) and increased incidence of thrombophlebitis if injected into a peripheral vein
(3) Myoclonic activity on injection
(4) Inhibition of adrenal steroidogenesis, especially with continuous infusion but may occur after single doses
(5) Lack of analgesic activity; addition of an analgesic is required prior to intubation

5. Propofol
a. General pharmacology.
Propofol is a highly lipid soluble intravenous induction agent with a rapid onset and short duration of action. It is rapidly redistributed and then eliminated by hepatic and nonhepatic routes.
b. Clinical uses
(1) Anesthetic induction (2–4 mg/kg IV)
(2) Maintenance of anesthesia (50–200 µg/kg/min IV)
c. Advantages
(1) Onset is rapid, similar to thiopental.
(2) Recovery time is short compared with barbiturates and benzodiazepines due to its large volume of distribution.
d. Disadvantages
(1) Dose-dependent cardiac depression similar to that of thiopental
(2) No analgesic activity
(3) Duration of apnea longer than with thiopental
(4) Pain on injection into peripheral vein

C. Inhalational agents
1. General pharmacology.
The effects of these drugs are dependent on their tissue tension. Tissue tension is proportional to blood tension, which is proportional to alveolar tension. Therefore, factors that increase alveolar and blood partial pressure contribute to a higher brain tension and faster anesthetic induction.
a. Factors that affect alveolar and blood partial pressure
(1) **Inspired gas partial pressure.** The higher the partial pressure of inspired gas, the greater the resultant alveolar tension.
(2) **Alveolar ventilation.** The greater the ventilation, the faster the rate of rise of alveolar tension.
(3) **Blood/gas solubility.** The more soluble the gas in blood, the slower the rate of rise of alveolar tension.
(4) **Cardiac output.** The higher the cardiac output, the slower the rate of rise of alveolar tension.
(5) **Alveolar-mixed venous blood gradient.** As this difference increases, anesthetic uptake is greater.
The effects of left-to-right and right-to-left shunts are discussed in Chap. 13.

2. Nitrous oxide
a. Clinical uses
(1) Coadministration with a halogenated agent to speed induction and decrease the dose of the halogenated agent
(2) Integral part of a nitrous oxide/opioid technique
b. Advantages
(1) Rapid onset and offset
(2) Good analgesic properties
(3) Minimal cardiac depression in patients with good ventricular function
(4) Stimulation of the sympathetic nervous system may contribute to hemodynamic stability

Table 5-4. Cardiovascular effects of volatile inhalational anesthetics

	Halothane	Enflurane	Isoflurane
Blood pressure	↓ ↓	↓ ↓	↓ ↓
Vascular resistance	0	0/ ↓	↓ ↓
Cardiac output	↓ ↓	↓ ↓	0/ ↓
Cardiac contraction	↓ ↓	↓ ↓ ↓	↓ / ↓ ↓ [a]
Central venous pressure	↑	↑	0
Heart rate	0/ ↓ [b]	0 ↑	↑ ↑
Sensitization of the heart to epinephrine	↑ ↑ ↑	↑	↑ ↑ [c]

Note: Drug effect is dependent on individual baseline patient characteristics (e.g., intravascular volume status, ventricular function, sympathetic "tone," beta blockade, etc.).
0 = no change, ↑ or ↓ = mild increase or decrease, ↑ ↑ or ↓ ↓ = moderate increase or decrease, ↑ ↑ ↑ or ↓ ↓ ↓ = marked increase or decrease.
[a]All these drugs depress myocardial contractility, and degree of depression may be clinically irrelevant in patients with poor ventricular function.
[b]If baseline heart rate is low, there is little change; if high, heart rate will decrease
[c]Degree of sensitization may be dose dependent.
Source: Modified from A. K. Ream, and R. P. Fogdall. *Acute Cardiovascular Management.* Philadelphia: Lippincott, 1982. P. 257. With permission.

  (5) No increase in pulmonary vascular resistance in neonates
  (6) Weak amnestic activity
  (7) Not a malignant hyperthermia triggering agent
  c. **Disadvantages**
    (1) Sympathetic nervous system stimulating property may contribute to intraoperative ischemia.
    (2) May increase pulmonary vascular resistance in adults.
    (3) High nitrous oxide concentrations limit the concentration of oxygen that may be used.
    (4) The truncal rigidity caused by opioids is potentiated by nitrous oxide.
    (5) Intravascular air bubbles enlarge in the presence of nitrous oxide because nitrous oxide is 35 times more soluble in blood than nitrogen. This increases the deleterious effects of air emboli and contraindicates the use of nitrous oxide after cardiopulmonary bypass.
    (6) Depression of myocardial contractility occurs and is especially evident in patients with poor ventricular function and preexisting high sympathetic nervous system outflow.
 3. **Halothane.** Table 5-4 lists the cardiovascular effects of halothane and other halogenated agents.
  a. **Clinical uses**
    (1) Inhalation induction
    (2) Inhalation induction for suspected difficult intubation
    (3) Maintenance agent
    (4) Adjunct to opioid technique
    (5) May be the agent of choice for asthmatics
  b. **Advantages**
    (1) Halothane causes dose-dependent decreases in myocardial oxygen consumption.
    (2) Depression of sinus node tends to lower heart rate, especially if baseline rate is high, favorably affecting myocardial oxygen supply/demand balance.

(3) Inhalation induction with halothane is usually smoother than with other agents because it is less irritating to the airway.

(4) Halothane has about the same smooth muscle-dilating activity as enflurane or isoflurane in vivo, but it causes less reflex bronchoconstriction (less irritating).

c. Disadvantages

(1) Myocardial depression and decreased cardiac output may not be tolerated by patient with borderline cardiac function.

(2) The myocardium is more susceptible to dysrhythmias caused by catecholamines in the presence of halothane.

(3) Depression of the sinus node predisposes the patient to nodal and ectopic rhythms.

(4) Decreased atrioventricular conduction may combine with other factors to produce heart block.

(5) Hepatic injury ("halothane hepatitis"), probably caused by reductive metabolites of halothane, is a rare complication.

4. Enflurane

a. Clinical uses

(1) Maintenance anesthetic

(2) Inhalation induction

(3) Adjunct to opioid technique

b. Advantages

(1) Dose-dependent depression of myocardial contractility and oxygen consumption

(2) Little or no change in heart rate (heart rate may increase when used as sole agent)

(3) Probably no hepatic toxicity

(4) May suppress ventricular arrhythmias

c. Disadvantages

(1) Enflurane has a lower therapeutic index than halothane or isoflurane.

(2) It may induce seizure activity if inspired concentration is increased rapidly.

(3) It causes more respiratory depression than other halogenated agents.

(4) Renal metabolism liberates free fluoride ion, which may temporarily depress renal function, even at low blood levels.

5. Isoflurane

a. Clinical uses

(1) Maintenance anesthetic

(2) Adjunct to opioid technique

(3) Inhalation induction of anesthesia

b. Advantages

(1) Isoflurane maintains cardiac output in patients with normal ventricular function.

(2) Possibly causes less myocardial depression than with halothane or enflurane.

(3) Isoflurane lowers the systemic vascular resistance.

(4) It is intermediate between halothane and enflurane in its "sensitization" of the heart to circulating catecholamines.

(5) The lower blood solubility of isoflurane compared with other halogenated agents yields faster induction and emergence.

(6) It potentiates the action of neuromuscular blocking drugs.

(7) Minimal biodegradation may cause less organ toxicity.

c. Disadvantages

(1) Reflex tachycardia in response to vasodilation occurs unless blocked by opioids or beta-blocking drugs.

Table 5-5. Pharmacokinetics of neuromuscular blocking drugs

	Volume of distribution (ml/kg)	Clearance (ml/kg/min)	Half-life (min)
Curare	300	2.3	120
Pancuronium	260	1.9	144
Metocurine	510	1.2	348
Vecuronium	270	5.2	71
Atracurium	200	5.5	25

Source: Modified from R. K. Stoelting. *Pharmacology and Physiology in Anesthetic Practice.* Philadelphia: Lippincott, 1987. Pp. 181 and 202. With permission.

       (2) It is a more potent inhibitor of hypoxic pulmonary vasoconstriction than halothane or enflurane, which may contribute to hypoxemia.

       (3) It may produce "coronary steal" if coronary perfusion pressure is not maintained. See Chapter 11 for detailed discussion.

       (4) It may increase right-to-left shunt due to decrease in systemic vascular resistance.

III. Neuromuscular blocking drugs

  A. General pharmacology. Neuromuscular synaptic transmission may be blocked by several drugs to produce clinical skeletal muscle relaxation. Competitive, or nondepolarizing, neuromuscular blocking drugs (e.g., curare, pancuronium, metocurine, and so on) occupy the postsynaptic cholinergic receptor but do not stimulate it. The block may be antagonized by increasing the local concentration of acetylcholine by administering an anticholinesterase. Noncompetitive (depolarizing) neuromuscular blocking drugs (e.g., succinylcholine) occupy and stimulate the acetylcholine receptor but prevent subsequent stimulation. Pharmacokinetic parameters are summarized in Table 5-5. Side effects are largely due to stimulation (or blockade) of muscarinic or ganglionic nicotinic cholinergic receptors. Cardiovascular effects are listed in Table 5-6.

  B. Curare

    1. Clinical doses

      a. Endotracheal intubation 0.5–0.6 mg/kg IV

      b. Maintenance relaxation 0.2–0.3 mg/kg IV

      c. Additional maintenance doses 0.05–0.10 mg/kg IV

    2. Advantages

      a. Histamine release and ganglionic blocking activity attenuate hypertensive response to surgical stimulation.

      b. This drug has multiple routes of excretion—approximately 90% is excreted by the renal route and 10% by the biliary tree (biliary excretion increases to 40% with renal failure).

      c. It is inexpensive.

    3. Disadvantages

      a. Histamine release from mast cells triggered by curare may cause hives, hypotension, wheezing, or, rarely, anaphylactoid reactions.

      b. Curare has a relatively long duration of action.

  C. Pancuronium

    1. Clinical doses

      a. Endotracheal intubation 0.1 mg/kg IV

      b. Maintenance relaxation 0.03–0.05 mg/kg IV

      c. Additional doses 0.005–0.010 mg/kg IV

Table 5-6. Hemodynamic effects of muscle relaxants

Relaxant	HR	BP	SVR	CO	Histamine release	Vagal block	Ganglionic block
Tubocurarine	−	↓	↓	↓	+++	−	+
Metocurine	−	↓	↓	−	++	−	−/+
Pancuronium	↑	↑	−	↑	−	++	−
Pipecuronium	−	−	−	−	−	−	−
Vecuronium	−	−	−	−	−	−	−
Atracurium	−	−/↓	−/↓	−/↑	+	−	−
Alcuronium	↑	↓	↓	↑	−	+	+
Doxacurium	−	−	−	−	−	−	−
Fazadinium	↑	−	↓	↑	−	++	++
Mivacurium	−	−/↓	−	−	−/+	−	−
Gallamine	↑	↑	−	↑	−	+++	−
Succinylcholine	↑↓	↑	↑	−/↓	+	*	*

HR = heart rate, BP = blood pressure, SVR = systemic vascular resistance, CO = cardiac output, ↑ = increases, ↓ = decreases, − = no effect, + = small effect, ++ = moderate effect, +++ = marked effect, * = agonist activity.

Source: Modified from R. P. F. Scott, and J. J. Savarese. New Muscle Relaxants and the Cardiovascular System. In J. A. Kaplan (ed.), *Cardiac Anesthesia* (2nd ed.). New York: Grune & Stratton, 1987. Pp. 158. With permission.

2 Advantages
   a. Vagolytic and sympathomimetic action prevents bradycardia produced by coadministered drugs (e.g., opioids).
   b. It has a relatively rapid onset (1–3 minutes).
   c. It has a long duration of action (30–45 minutes).
   d. It does not release histamine.
3. Disadvantages
   a. It may produce tachycardia and therefore adversely affect the myocardial oxygen balance.
   b. The long duration of action may preclude extubation after unexpectedly short or abbreviated procedures.

D. Metocurine
   1. Clinical doses
      a. Endotracheal intubation 0.3–0.4 mg/kg IV
      b. Maintenance relaxation 0.1–0.2 mg/kg IV
      c. Additional maintenance doses 0.05–0.10 mg/kg IV
   2. Advantages
      a. Less histamine release than curare
      b. Less tachycardia than pancuronium
      c. Less hypotension than curare
      d. Minimal hemodynamic alteration when used in combination with pancuronium
   3. Disadvantages
      a. It may cause mild rises in heart rate at higher doses.
      b. Weak ganglionic blockade may result at higher doses.

E. Vecuronium
   1. Clinical doses
      a. Endotracheal intubation 0.1 mg/kg IV. Time to onset may be shortened by administering a "priming dose" of approximately 0.01 mg/kg IV 3–5 minutes prior to giving the intubating dose
      b. Maintenance relaxation 0.025–0.05 mg/kg IV
      c. Additional maintenance doses 0.01–0.02 mg/kg IV
   2. Advantages
      a. Extremely stable hemodynamically. No change in heart rate or blood pressure occurs at usual doses. There are only rare case reports of flushing and bradycardia.
      b. Significant hepatic metabolism allows use in patients with renal dysfunction.
      c. Intermediate duration of action enables titration to a desired level of relaxation or use of a continuous infusion.
   3. Disadvantages
      a. Vecuronium does not antagonize the vagotonic effect of opioids; thus bradycardia usually results.
      b. There is a slight cumulative effect with multiple doses.
      c. Intermediate duration of action requires frequent redosing or continuous infusion for long procedures.

F. Atracurium
   1. Clinical doses
      a. Endotracheal intubation 0.5–0.6 mg/kg IV. Time to onset may be shortened by administering a "priming dose" of approximately 0.01 mg/kg IV 3–5 minutes prior to giving the intubating dose.
      b. Maintenance relaxation 0.2–0.3 mg/kg IV
      c. Additional doses 0.05–0.10 mg/kg IV
   2. Advantages
      a. Does not require hepatic or renal function for termination of effect. Action is terminated by the "Hoffman elimination" and ester hydrolysis.

b. No cumulative effect with multiple redosing or continuous infusion occurs.

c. There is no vagal or ganglionic blocking activity.

3. Disadvantages

a. Intermediate acting (multiple redosing or continuous infusion required).

b. Hypotension secondary to histamine release may occur.

c. Metabolic products of Hoffman elimination (laudanosine) may cause CNS excitatory activity with high or prolonged doses.

G. Succinylcholine

1. Clinical doses

a. Endotracheal intubation 1.0–2.0 mg/kg IV, 4.0–6.0 mg/kg IM

b. Maintenance relaxation: 0.1–0.3 mg/kg IV intermittently; 0.1 mg/kg/min IV by continuous infusion

2. Advantages

a. Rapid onset of profound skeletal muscle relaxation

b. Short duration of action due to rapid hydrolysis by plasma cholinesterase

3. Disadvantages

a. This drug may cause bradycardia and other dysrhythmias due to cholinergic stimulation, especially in children and when atropine is not given prior to succinylcholine administration.

b. Hyperkalemia may result from potassium release from muscle cells during depolarization. This effect is pronounced in certain circumstances (e.g., burns, paraplegia, denervation injuries).

c. Myalgias secondary to muscle fasciculation occur.

d. Muscle fasciculation causes a rise in gastric and intraocular pressure.

e. Succinylcholine is a potent trigger of malignant hyperpyrexia.

f. Weak ganglionic stimulating activity may cause hypertensive response or dysrhythmias.

g. There is prolonged neuromuscular blockade due to abnormal or insufficient plasma pseudocholinesterase or phase II block.

h. Succinylcholine may release histamine.

H. New muscle relaxants

1. Pipecuronium. Pipecuronium bromide is a new long-acting, non-depolarizing muscle relaxant that is structurally similar to pancuronium. Onset and duration of action is also similar to pancuronium, but there is a lack of hemodynamic side effects. There is no evidence of histamine release or autonomic action at up to three times the ED95. Reports of bradycardia when combined with opioid techniques or halothane probably represent a lack of vagolytic action rather than a direct effect. Primary route of excretion is renal. Intubating dose is 0.08–0.10 mg/kg IV. Maintenance dose after succinylcholine is 0.04–0.05 mg/kg IV, with subsequent doses of one-fifth to one-third of the maintenance dose depending on the anesthetic technique.

2. Doxacurium (BW A938U). Doxacurium chloride is a new long-acting, nondepolarizing muscle relaxant that is structurally similar to atracurium. There seem to be no hemodynamic side effects associated with neuromuscular blockade with this drug. There is no histamine release or muscarinic activity. There is no evidence of accumulation with repeated doses or prolonged administration. Doxacurium 0.05 mg/kg IV (approximately twice the ED95) allows intubation in 5 minutes and a dose of 0.08 mg/kg IV produces intubation conditions in 4 minutes. The duration of action increases from 85 to 165 minutes when increasing the dose from 0.05 mg/kg to 0.08 mg/kg, respectively.

3. Mivacurium (BW B1090U). Mivacurium chloride is a new short-acting, nondepolarizing neuromuscular blocking drug that is metabolized by plasma cholinesterase. The rate of metabolism has been reported to be 88% as fast as succinylcholine metabolism. It has weak histamine-releasing properties, causing minimal arterial hypotension with doses greater than 0.2 mg/kg IV (roughly twice the ED95). The hypotension may be attenuated by slowing the rate of injection. The onset of action (about 2 minutes) is not significantly faster than vecuronium or atracurium when given in doses approximately twice the ED95. These higher doses of mivacurium do not significantly prolong the duration of neuromuscular block as seen with other nondepolarizing drugs.

IV. The preinduction period
A. Sedation in the preinduction period
1. **Premedication.** Additional sedative drugs may not be required prior to induction of anesthesia if the patient was mentally prepared and premedicated. The need for sedation often depends on the psychological and physical condition of the patient and the requirement for preinduction invasive procedures. The risk-benefit ratio of preoperative sedation must be considered for each patient individually prior to administration.
2. **Benefits of sedation**
   a. Decrease in "stress" related sequelae—plasma catecholamines, tachycardia, hypertension, ischemia, total body oxygen consumption.
   b. A calm patient is more able to cooperate with procedures.
   c. Hemodynamic measurements more accurately reflect baseline conditions in a calm patient. Anxiety may cause a hyperdynamic circulation and artificially high baseline measurements.
   d. Anxious or uncooperative patients require the attention of operating room personnel who could otherwise perform other duties.
3. Risks of sedation
   a. Decrease in respiratory response to carbon dioxide accompanies sedation, with a resultant rise in arterial PCO_2 and possible increases in pulmonary artery pressure (risking increase in right-to-left shunting and right ventricular failure in patients with congenital heart disease) and intracranial pressure.
   b. Loss of consciousness may predispose to upper airway obstruction and apnea, acidosis, and hypoxemia.
   c. Obtundation of airway reflexes may predispose to pulmonary aspiration.
   d. Depression of the circulation may lead to underestimation of baseline hemodynamic parameters.
B. Determination and optimization of baseline hemodynamic parameters
1. The risks of invasive monitoring must be balanced against the benefits of having the information provided by the monitors. In experienced hands, radial and pulmonary artery catheterizations involve little risk and supply a wealth of information. It is our practice to utilize systemic and pulmonary arterial pressure monitoring in every adult patient undergoing cardiac surgery requiring cardiopulmonary bypass. The presence of a pulmonary artery catheter prior to induction allows determination of left heart filling pressures, cardiac output, and systemic vascular resistance.
2. **Optimization regimen.** If cardiac performance is determined to be suboptimal in the operating room, it should be improved prior to anesthetic induction by addressing each determinate of cardiac output.
   a. **Adequate cardiac filling volume.** The myocardial "preload" required for optimal cardiac output varies between patients, but general management may be guided by LaPlace's law (a smaller

chamber has less wall tension and therefore requires less energy for ejection). Low filling pressures may be acceptable if cardiac output is adequate, but the vascular effects of anesthetic induction (decreased arteriolar resistance and increased venous capacitance) must be anticipated and treated. High filling pressures may indicate hypervolemia, impedance to venous return (e.g., valvular disease or pulmonary hypertension), or ventricular failure. The underlying cause should be treated if possible.

b. Heart rate and rhythm. Bradycardia contributing to a low cardiac output may be treated with a vagolytic agent (glycopyrrolate 0.2 mg IV), a sympathomimetic agent (ephedrine 5 mg IV), or temporary ventricular pacing. Tachycardia may be treated by administration of an anxiolytic (midazolam 0.5 mg IV), opioid (fentanyl 25 μg IV), or beta blocker (esmolol 500 μg/kg IV over 1 minute). Dysrhythmias may be treated pharmacologically, electrically, or by temporary overdrive pacing.

c. Contractility. Poor contractility is indicated by low cardiac output despite normal or high filling pressures, normal or low vascular resistances, and adequate cardiac rhythm. Inotropic support is indicated.

d. Afterload. If cardiac output is low and systemic vascular resistance is markedly elevated, vasodilation will increase cardiac output if filling pressure and cardiac rhythm are maintained. Trimethaphan 1–2 mg IV or sodium nitroprusside 0.5 μg/kg/min IV may be used.

C. Preinduction checklist. A preinduction checklist such as that shown in Table 5-7 may be a useful tool to ensure that all required equipment, drugs, and personnel are available, especially when problems or unusual circumstances may change the anesthesiologist's usual routine.

V. Typical induction sequences

A. Intravenous opioid technique (Table 5-8)

1. Advantages of opioid technique

a. Anesthetic course is usually very stable.

b. Myocardial depression is minimal.

c. Heart rate remains low.

d. Ventilatory depression and decreased airway reflexes facilitate mechanical ventilation.

e. Postoperative analgesia is provided.

f. The myocardium is not "sensitized" to catecholamines.

g. Operating room environmental pollution from anesthetic waste gases is minimized.

h. There is no hepatic or renal toxicity.

i. An antagonist is available.

j. Malignant hyperpyrexia is not triggered.

2. Disadvantages of opioid technique

a. There is no decrease in myocardial energy consumption.

b. "Breakthrough" tachycardia and hypertension may adversely affect myocardial oxygen balance and cause ischemia.

c. Truncal muscle rigidity and resultant decreased chest wall compliance may make ventilation difficult and may necessitate high airway pressures

d. If nitrous oxide is used as an adjunct, the inspired concentration of oxygen is limited.

e. Prolonged ventilatory depression requires mechanical ventilation postoperatively.

f. There is a higher incidence of intraoperative awareness compared to that associated with halogenated agents.

B. Halogenated agent induction technique (Table 5-9)

Table 5-7. Preinduction checklist

Prior to anesthetic induction, the anesthesiologist must:
1. Ensure safe operation of basic anesthetic and emergency equipment (e.g., pacemaker).
2. Prepare all anesthetic and emergency drugs, including infusions.
3. Review recent entries in the patient's chart, including nursing notes, for any changes in the patient's condition in the previous 8 hours, the results of investigations, and the availability of blood products.
4. Identify the patient, inquire about presence of symptoms, ensure adequate sedation, place noninvasive monitors, and note heart rate and rhythm, ST = segment position, blood pressure, and SaO_2.
5. Administer oxygen by nasal cannula.
6. Insert all planned invasive monitors and dedicate a central venous port to drug infusions only.
7. Place the patient in the operative position, then zero and calibrate pressure transducers.
8. Obtain baseline hemodynamic measurements.
9. Optimize hemodynamics.
10. Avoid antibiotic administration during induction to prevent superimposition of a drug reaction on hemodynamic changes with induction.
11. Ensure the availability of required personnel: surgeon capable of opening the chest, perfusionist with operational bypass pump, and nurses with required instruments. The physical presence of the required personnel in the operating room is especially important for patients with left main coronary artery disease or critical aortic or mitral stenosis.
12. Minimize distractions: All unnecessary noise, conversation, and room traffic must cease.
13. Commence induction sequence.

      1. Advantages of halogenated agent induction
          a. Halogenated agents produce a dose-related depression of myocardial oxygen consumption.
          b. The level of anesthesia may easily be titrated to match the level of surgical stimulation.
          c. Intraoperative awareness is unlikely.
          d. Skeletal muscle relaxation is potentiated.
          e. The patient may be extubated soon after surgery.
          f. The side effects of each agent may be used to the patient's advantage (e.g., isoflurane's vasodilating effect may benefit a patient with mitral regurgitation).
      2. Disadvantages of halogenated agent induction
          a. Hypotension is possible due to direct negative inotropic activity.
          b. These agents do not reduce hemodynamic response to surgical stimulation as predictably as opioids.
          c. The myocardium may be sensitized to catecholamine-induced dysrhythmias.
          d. There is a risk of hepatic (halothane) or renal (enflurane) toxicity.
          e. Postoperative analgesia is not provided.
          f. The operating room environment may be polluted if anesthetic waste gases are not scavenged.
          g. These agents may trigger malignant hyperpyrexia.
    C. Combined technique. Combining opioid administration with a halogenated agent provides the advantages of both techniques while minimizing the disadvantages. The contribution of each agent to the overall anesthetic varies with individual practice.

Table 5-8. Opioid induction sequence

1. Administer 100% oxygen (or oxygen–nitrous oxide up to a 50:50 ratio in absence of ventricular dysfunction or pulmonary hypertension) by face mask to replace nitrogen in the lungs with 100% oxygen.
2. Give one-tenth of the muscle relaxant dose to prevent truncal rigidity caused by high-dose opioids. Pancuronium or metocurine may be preferable to vecuronium or atracurium because the vagolytic side effect attenuates the opioid-induced bradycardia, especially in patients taking β blockers.
3. Keep verbal contact with the patient.
4. Slowly administer the opioid induction dose in aliquots of one-tenth of the total dose until consciousness is lost. Treat hypotension with intravenous fluid administration and then small doses of vasoconstrictor (phenylephrine 25–50 μg IV). Bradycardia may be treated with an anticholinergic (atropine 0.2–0.4 mg IV) or beta-sympathomimetic (ephedrine 5 mg IV). Inotropic support is not usually necessary (unless used prior to induction).
5. With loss of consciousness, attempt to ventilate the patient manually. If unable to ventilate, insert oropharyngeal airway (monitor hemodynamic response) and reattempt ventilation.
6. If the patient remains conscious after the full induction dose of opioid, administer a small dose of benzodiazepine or additional opioid. This will usually produce unconsciousness and decrease awareness (and an attendant further decrease in blood pressure).
7. Give the remainder of the muscle relaxant dose if the lungs are able to be ventilated.
8. Consider administration of lidocaine, β blocker, or additional opioid if blood pressure and heart rate are above awake values.
9. While waiting for full muscle relaxation, the surgeon may insert the urinary catheter and rectal temperature probe (observe hemodynamic response).
10. An increase in heart rate or blood pressure should be treated by deepening anesthesia or administering a β blocker or vasodilator.
11. The trachea may be intubated if there was no hemodynamic response to bladder catheterization. Intubation must be performed as gently and quickly as possible.
12. Hemodynamic response to intubation may be treated as in No. 10 above.
13. The period between intubation and surgical incision is usually hemodynamically stable and may be used to determine cardiac output, place other monitors (nasopharyngeal temperature probe, esophageal stethoscope and transesophageal echocardiography transducer, respiratory gas analyzer, etc.), pass an orogastric tube, obtain blood samples for blood gas and baseline activated clotting time (ACT) determinations, and record the events of induction.

VI. Problems during anesthetic induction

A. Hyperdynamic response to tracheal intubation. The prevention or attenuation of this response is preferred to treatment after it occurs. Successful obtundation of the hemodynamic response to intubation is more likely if several of the following techniques are combined:

1. **Premedication.** Clonidine 0.1–0.2 mg PO at the time of premedication has been shown to decrease intraoperative hemodynamic variability and anesthetic requirement. This regimen may also cause hypotension in some patients.
2. **Nerve block.** Blockade of the afferent nerves from the pharynx, larynx, and trachea will prevent the response of the effector organs (e.g., heart and vasculature). The sensory nerves supplying the airway (glossopharyngeal, vagus, and superior laryngeal nerves) may

Table 5-9. Halogenated agent inhalation induction sequence

1. Administer 100% oxygen (or oxygen–nitrous oxide up to a 50:50 ratio in the absence of ventricular dysfunction or pulmonary hypertension) by face mask to replace nitrogen in the lungs with 100% oxygen.
2. Give small amount of opioid (fentanyl 3–5 µg/kg), benzodiazepine (midazolam 1–2 mg), or thiopental (25–75 mg) to gain patient acceptance of inhalation agent (optional).
3. Maintain verbal contact with the patient. Instruct patient to breathe normally and to expect a sweet smell while adding halothane or isoflurane to the inspired gas mixture. Gradually increase the concentration every three breaths until 2.5–3.0 MAC is reached.
4. Awareness is less likely with this technique than with opioids, but patient excitement is more likely. If the patient becomes excited ("stage two"), opioid, thiopental, or benzodiazepine may be given.
5. When respirations become shallow, gently assist ventilation. This usually occurs before complete loss of consciousness.
6. When consciousness is lost, administer the full muscle relaxant dose. A priming dose may be used but is usually not necessary because there is time to wait for onset of muscle relaxation while ensuring adequate depth of anesthesia prior to intubation.
7. Hypotension may be treated by administrating intravenous fluid, discontinuing nitrous oxide, applying stimulation, or decreasing the inspired concentration of volatile agent.
8. Using a graded stimulus approach, an oral airway may be inserted to improve ventilation. If there is no hemodynamic response, the urinary bladder may be catheterized.
9. The potent agent concentration should be transiently increased and nitrous oxide discontinued prior to intubation. The beginning of a drop in blood pressure signals the time to start intubation.
10. The stimulation of tracheal intubation usually reverses the decrease in blood pressure, with return to baseline being the goal. The inspired potent agent concentration may be decreased to 0.5–0.75 MAC during the period of minimal stimulation between intubation and incision.

be blocked by application of nebulized or topical lidocaine 4% (2–3 ml).

3. **Anesthetics**
   a. **Opioids.** Low doses (5–10 µg/kg IV) of fentanyl attenuate the response to intubation, whereas high doses (50–100 µg/kg IV) virtually eliminate the response.
   b. **Lidocaine.** Intravenous (1.0–1.5 mg/kg) or intratracheal (pre-filled applicator with 4 ml of 4% lidocaine) administration is additive to other anesthetics used and also decreases the incidence of ventricular arrhythmias during intubation.
4. **Technique.** A laryngoscopy technique that avoids touching the posterior aspect of the epiglottis should be less stimulating. Regardless of the specific technique used, the duration of laryngoscopy is directly proportional to the degree of hemodynamic response.
5. **Vasodilators and beta and ganglionic blockers.** The hemodynamic response may be blocked pharmacologically at the efferent limb by one or a combination of the following drugs:
   a. Sodium nitroprusside 1.0 µg/kg IV
   b. Esmolol 500 µg/kg IV given over 1 minute
   c. Trimethaphan 1–2 mg IV
   d. Nitroglycerin 1–2 mg/kg/min IV

Table 5-10. Treatment of hypotension with anesthetic induction

HR	CVP/PCWP	SVR	CO	Treatment
↑	↓	↑	↓	Fluid administration
↓	nl or ↑	nl	↓	Chronotrope or pacemaker
↓, nl, ↑	↑	nl	↓	Inotropic agent
nl or ↓	↑	↑	↓	Vasodilator
↑	↓	↓	↑	Vasoconstrictor

HR = heart rate, CVP = central venous pressure, PCWP = pulmonary capillary wedge pressure, SVR = systemic vascular resistance, CO = cardiac output, ↑ = increased, ↓ = decreased; nl = normal.

B. Hypotension. Hypotension associated with the induction of anesthesia should always be anticipated and should be treated promptly. Treatment depends on the mechanism of hypotension, which may be predicted based on the anesthetic technique.

1. **Opioid technique.** Hypotension using an opioid technique is often caused by bradycardia, or decreased arteriolar resistance and increased venous capacitance secondary to decreased sympathetic nervous system activity. Intravenous fluids and vagolytic (or chronotropic) agents are indicated.

2. **Halogenated agent technique.** Halogenated agents are more likely to cause hypotension by direct myocardial depression or vasodilation (e.g., isoflurane), which may be treated by decreasing the inspired concentration of anesthetic or administering an inotropic agent.

3. **Treatment of hypotension.** The cause of hypotension must be quickly diagnosed using all monitors available. Table 5-10 outlines the treatment indicated for specific circumstances.

C. Pulmonary hypertension. Preexisting pulmonary hypertension may be caused by a left-sided obstructive lesion (e.g., mitral stenosis), left ventricular failure, or pulmonary vascular obstructive disease. Acute pulmonary hypertension may be due to reactive pulmonary vasoconstriction in the presence of hypoxia, hypercarbia, acidosis, or high intrathoracic airway pressure. Patients with preexisting pulmonary hypertension usually have increased pulmonary vascular reactivity.

1. **Clinical features.** Elevated pulmonary artery pressure is often associated with depressed cardiac output, elevated central venous pressure, right heart failure, and, in congenital heart disease, an increase in right-to-left shunting.

2. **Prevention**
   a. Encourage the patient to hyperventilate voluntarily prior to induction.
   b. Use 100% inspired oxygen concentration.
   c. Benzodiazepine induction may avoid chest wall rigidity problems associated with opioids and myocardial depression associated with halogenated agents.

3. **Treatment**
   a. **Alveolar hyperventilation.** Hyperventilation is the mainstay of treatment. End-tidal carbon dioxide concentration may not be an accurate guide for therapy, however, because pulmonary blood flow is decreased.
   b. **High inspired oxygen concentration.** Ventilate with 100% oxygen. Alveolar PO_2 may be a more potent stimulus than arterial PO_2.

   c. **Alkalosis.** Administer bicarbonate according to a formula based
      on base deficit (e.g., for [weight (kg)/3] × base deficit, give one-
      half of calculated dose IV to start).
   d. **Minimize airway pressures.**
   e. **Pulmonary vasodilators.** Give prostaglandin E_1 0.1 μg/kg/min
      IV, or aminophylline 5 mg/kg IV over 20 minutes.
D. **Difficult intubation.** Laryngoscopy and intubation of the trachea ideally should require less than 30 seconds to minimize associated hemodynamic perturbation. Patients who are known or suspected to be difficult
   to intubate are at increased risk of hypertension, tachycardia, myocardial ischemia, and loss of airway control during intubation attempts.
   If they are identified preoperatively, this risk may be minimized. Depending on the reason for intubation difficulty, these patients may be
   managed by using intubation adjuncts with the patient either awake
   or anesthetized.
   1. **Awake intubation**
      a. **Indication**
         (1) **Poor mask airway.** If application of positive pressure using
             an anesthetic face mask is difficult in a patient who is sus-
             pected to be difficult to intubate, the airway should be se-
             cured prior to induction of anesthesia.
         (2) **Poor ventricular function.** A patient with impaired myo-
             cardial function may not tolerate induction with a halogenated
             inhalation agent or short-acting barbiturate, and long-acting
             agents (e.g., opioids) should not be used if the patient is sus-
             pected to be difficult to intubate.
      b. **Preparation**
         (1) **Patient position.** "Sniffing" position (neck flexed and head
             extended) is usually optimal for visualization of the larynx and
             is not uncomfortable for the patient.
         (2) **Sedation.** Fentanyl 1–5 μg/kg IV may be given as required,
             in conjunction with midazolam 1–3 mg IV or droperidol 1.25–
             5.00 mg IV.
         (3) **Anesthesia.** Lidocaine 4% may be applied topically using an
             atomizer, nebulizer, or direct application over the glossophar-
             yngeal nerve.
         (4) **Adjuncts.** An **antisialagogue** is indicated to improve visibil-
             ity and conditions for the topical anesthesia to be absorbed and
             decrease the likelihood of laryngospasm secondary to secre-
             tions. **Oxygen** should be administered by nasal cannula. **Ni-
             troglycerin, vasodilators,** and **ganglionic** and **beta blockers**
             should be used as indicated as outlined in sec. **VI.A.5.**
      c. **Technique**
         (1) **Direct laryngoscopy.** Complete visualization of the larynx is
             not necessary. The endotracheal tube may frequently be in-
             serted "blindly" with the use of a stylet. When the tube is
             determined to be in good position, anesthesia may be induced.
         (2) **Fiberoptic bronchoscope-assisted intubation.** The bron-
             choscope may be inserted via the oral aperture to avoid possible
             nasal mucosal injury and bleeding (which may not be appre-
             ciated until heparinization). The endotracheal tube is fitted
             over the bronchoscope, the larynx is visualized, and the trachea
             is entered, while the endotracheal tube is advanced in a Sel-
             dinger fashion. The bronchoscope may then be used to confirm
             correct tube placement.
   2. **Halogenated agent inhalation induction**
      a. **Indication.** A patient who is suspected or previously documented
         to be difficult to intubate may be anesthetized prior to the intu-

bation attempt if he or she has an airway amenable to ventilation by mask, good ventricular function, and no history of gastroesophageal reflux.

    b. Preparation. The patient position and adjuncts listed for awake intubation apply.

    c. Technique. Direct laryngoscopy and fiberoptic bronchoscope-assisted intubation as detailed above may be utilized after the patient is anesthetized. A predominantly halogenated agent inhalation induction (a small amount of thiopental, benzodiazepine, or opioid may be used to make the inspired gas mixture more acceptable to the patient) has the advantage of maintaining spontaneous ventilation. Halothane in 100% oxygen is used for its low airway-irritating properties. The anesthesia may be "deepened" and the patient intubated without muscle relaxants, or a short-acting relaxant (e.g., succinylcholine) may be used. After intubation is accomplished, long-acting anesthetics and muscle relaxants may be given. Should intubation prove impossible by this method, the anesthetic may be turned off, the patient ventilated with oxygen, and allowed to wake up.

E. Patients with a "full stomach." Patients with a history of gastroesophageal reflux, recent oral intake (emergent surgery), and (rarely) pregnancy are at increased risk of regurgitation and pulmonary aspiration of stomach contents after induction of anesthesia. The risk of pulmonary aspiration must be balanced with the risk of tachycardia, hypertension, and myocardial ischemia that may occur if these patients are treated traditionally (i.e., receive an "awake" intubation or "rapid sequence" induction). It is most likely that the cardiac risk outweighs the pulmonary risk in patients undergoing cardiac surgery, and therefore this should receive the most attention.

    1. Prophylaxis

        a. Sodium citrate 15 ml PO 20–60 minutes preoperatively

        b. Metoclopramide 10 mg IM or IV

        c. Suction stomach, then remove nasogastric tube if present.

        d. H_2 blocker 30–90 minutes preoperatively

            (1) Cimetidine 300 mg IV

            (2) Ranitidine 50 mg IV

            (3) Famotidine 20 mg IV

    2. Technique

        a. Modified rapid sequence induction

            (1) Preoxygenation is performed.

            (2) Cricoid pressure and gentle ventilation are used during induction.

            (3) Position patient with head slightly up if filling pressures are adequate.

            (4) Intubation may be expedited by a small dose of thiopental if ventricular function is adequate or by use of a more potent opioid (e.g., sufentanil) and fast-acting muscle relaxant (e.g., succinylcholine).

        b. Awake intubation. Follow technique described for difficult intubation.

F. Patients with bronchospastic disease. Bronchospasm during induction of anesthesia or intubation of the trachea decreases alveolar ventilation and complicates management by producing hypoxia, hypercarbia, acidosis, and decreased venous return secondary to high intrathoracic pressure. These conditions are not tolerated well in patients with cardiac disease and steps should be taken to prevent their occurrence.

    1. Prophylaxis

    a. Continue chronic bronchodilator therapy. Theophylline (a phosphodiesterase inhibitor) and beta-adrenergic agents are the most common. Both increase intracellular cyclic AMP, which causes smooth muscle relaxation. The incidence of dysrhythmias is increased by both agents.

    b. Provide adequate preoperative hydration. Normal hydration decreases mucous plugging and allows clearance of secretions, but the degree of hydration must be tolerated by the patient's cardiac lesion.

    c. Avoid agents that release histamine. Histamine constricts bronchial smooth muscle. Agents that release histamine include morphine, curare, succinylcholine, thiopental, and atracurium.

    d. Give a preoperative aerosolized bronchodilator. A selective beta-2 adrenergic agonist (e.g., albuterol) is preferred, although beta selectivity is not absolute, and tachycardia may result. Administering these drugs by the inhalational route may limit their systemic effects, but there is significant intravascular absorption.

    e. Provide adequate depth of anesthesia prior to intubation. Patients with bronchospastic disease have increased bronchial reactivity that must be blunted prior to intubation.

    f. Utilize anesthetics with bronchodilating activity. Although all halogenated agents are good bronchodilators, halothane may be preferred because it is the least irritating to the airway. Ketamine is a good choice for an intravenous agent if its hemodynamic actions are not contraindicated.

    g. Extubate "deep". If extubation of the trachea is planned in the operating room, it should be done while the patient is still anesthetized to prevent bronchial reaction to the endotracheal tube as anesthesia is lightened.

    h. Start or continue aminophylline postoperatively. If prolonged airway instrumentation and mechanical ventilation is planned, an aminophylline infusion (0.3–0.6 mg/kg/hour IV) should be considered.

G. Cardiac arrest during induction. This is obviously one of the most serious consequences of anesthetic induction. General supportive treatment must be instituted immediately while diagnostic maneuvers are made and more specific treatment is given (chest tube insertion for tension pneumothorax, epinephrine for anaphylactic reaction, and so on). There are certain conditions that do not respond well to the usual resuscitative measures and therefore require mention.

    1. Critical aortic stenosis. It is impossible to generate an adequate cardiac output through a critically stenotic aortic valve by external cardiac massage. Survival depends on early defibrillation, emergency sternotomy, and institution of cardiopulmonary bypass.

    2. Left main coronary artery disease (or equivalent). Coronary artery blood flow is inadequate with external cardiac massage. Emergency myocardial revascularization is indicated.

    3. Valvular mitral stenosis. Blood flow through the heart and cardiac output is limited as in critical aortic stenosis.

    4. Pregnancy. Venous return to the heart may not be adequate for cardiac resuscitation until the fetus is delivered. Temporizing measures include left lateral uterine displacement or lateral patient position during resuscitation.

    Although patients undergoing cardiac surgery are at increased risk of cardiac arrest on induction of anesthesia secondary to their native disease, chances of successful resuscitation are optimized by the induction environment, in which all necessary drugs, equipment, and personnel are available.

VII. Summary. This chapter suggests basic principles of safe anesthetic induction for patients with cardiac disease. The following points should be re-emphasized:

1. The preoperative evaluation is extremely important. In retrospect, most problems at induction can be anticipated, and steps can be taken to prevent or minimize them.
2. Titration of anesthetics is an important concept. Regardless of agent or technique used, it is always best to proceed in a controlled manner while clinically evaluating patient response and adjusting therapy accordingly.
3. As a general rule, it is preferable to use familiar drugs in critically ill patients, especially in unusual situations, even if a new drug or technique may have theoretical advantages.

SUGGESTED READINGS

Gilman, A. G., Goodman, L. S., Rall, T. W., et al. *The Pharmacological Basis of Therapeutics* (7th ed.). New York: Macmillan, 1985.

Ream, A. K., and Fogdall, R. P. *Acute Cardiovascular Management.* Philadelphia: Lippincott, 1982.

Reves, J. G., Flezzani, P., and Kissin, I. Pharmacology of Intravenous Anesthetic Induction Drugs. In J. A. Kaplan (ed.), *Cardiac Anesthesia* (2nd ed.). Orlando: Grune & Stratton, 1987. Pp. 125–150.

Scott, R. P. F., and Saverese, J. J. New Muscle Relaxants and the Cardiovascular System. In J. A. Kaplan (ed.), *Cardiac Anesthesia* (2nd ed.) Orlando: Grune & Stratton, 1987. Pp. 151–175.

Sebel, P. S., and Bovill, J. G. Opioid Analgesics in Cardiac Anesthesia. In J. A. Kaplan (ed.), *Cardiac Anesthesia* (2nd ed.) Orlando: Grune & Stratton, 1987. Pp. 67–123.

Stoelting, R. K. *Pharmacology and Physiology in Anesthetic Practice.* Philadelphia: Lippincott, 1987.

Wood, M., and Wood, A. J. J. (eds.). *Drugs and Anesthesia.* Baltimore: Williams & Wilkins, 1982.

Anesthetic Management in the Precardiopulmonary Bypass Period

Mark E. Romanoff and George W. Rung

The period of time between induction of anesthesia and institution of cardiopulmonary bypass (CPB) is characterized by widely varying surgical stimuli. Anesthetic management during this high-risk period must strive to:

1. Optimize the myocardial oxygen supply-demand ratio in patients at risk for myocardial ischemia. The incidence of ischemia during this period has been reported to be 7–56%[4,9]. Approximately one-half of all intraoperative ischemic events occur prior to CPB.
2. Optimize the ventricular pressure-volume relationship in patients with valvular dysfunction. Manipulation of myocardial preload and afterload may be necessary to compensate for valvular lesions.
3. Maintain ventricular contractility and cardiac output in patients with impaired ventricular function.
4. Optimize systemic and pulmonary vascular resistance in patients with congenital heart disease to avoid worsening of intravascular shunts.
5. Avoid dysrhythmias, which can have a negative impact on all of the above parameters.

Any adverse hemodynamic changes increase the risk of developing ischemia, heart failure, cyanosis, or dysrhythmias before the benefits of surgical repair can ensue.

I. Management of events prior to cardiopulmonary bypass
   A. The pre-CPB period can be subdivided into stages based on the level of surgical stimulation.
      1. **High levels of stimulation include** incision, sternal split, sternal spread, and sympathetic nerve dissection. Inadequate anesthesia at these times leads to increased catecholamine levels, possibly resulting in hypertension, dysrhythmias, tachycardia, ischemia, or heart failure (Table 6-1).
      2. **Low-level stimulation occurs during** preincision, internal mammary artery dissection, and CPB cannulation. Risks during these periods include hypotension, bradycardia, dysrhythmias, and ischemia (Table 6-1).
   B. **Preincision.** The duration of this period, including surgical preparation and draping, is usually 5–20 minutes. Several parameters should be checked during this time:
      1. **Confirm bilateral breath sounds** after final patient positioning.
      2. **Check pressure points.** Ischemia, secondary to compression and compounded by decreases in temperature and perfusion pressure on CPB, may cause a peripheral neuropathy or damage to soft tissues as follows.
         a. **Brachial plexus injury.** Can occur if the arms are hyperextended or if chest retraction is excessive (e.g., occult rib fracture using the Ankeney retractor)[5]. Proper position: If the arms are placed on arm boards, minimize pectoral major muscle tension to avoid stretching the brachial plexus.
         b. **Ulnar nerve injury.** Can occur from compression of the olecranon against the metal edge of the operating room table. Proper position: Provide adequate padding under olecranon. Do not allow arm to contact the metal edge of the operating room table.
         c. **Radial nerve injury.** Can occur from compression of the upper arm against the ether screen or the support post of the Favalaro retractor used in internal mammary dissection. Proper position: Provide adequate padding of the arm. Do not allow the arm to contact metal.
         d. **Finger injury.** Can occur secondary to pressure from members of the operating team leaning against the operating table if the fin-

Table 6-1. Typical hemodynamic responses to surgical stimulation prior to cardiopulmonary bypass

Surgical stimulation	Preincision	Incision	Sternotomy and sternal spread	Sympathetic dissection	IMA dissection	Cannulation
Surgical stimulation	→	↑	↑↑	↑	→	→
Heart rate	→ or ↓	– or ↑	↑↑	– or ↓	– or ↓	– or ↓*
Blood pressure	→ or ↓	– or ↑	↑↑	↑ or ↑↑	– or ↓	– or ↓
Preload	– or ↓	– or ↑	– or ↑	– or ↓	– or ↓	– or ↓
Afterload	– or ↓	↑↑	↑↑ or ↑↑↑	↑ or ↑↑	– or ↓	→
Myocardial O_2 demand	→	– or ↑	↑↑ or ↑↑↑	↑ or ↑↑	→	→

*Dysrhythmias secondary to mechanical stimulation of the heart are likely.
Note: All values are compared to control (preinduction) values.
IMA = Internal mammary artery, ↑ = slightly increased, ↑↑ = moderately increased, ↑↑↑ = markedly increased, ↓ = slightly decreased, → = moderately decreased, – = unchanged.

gers are positioned improperly. Proper position: Hands should be next to the body, fingers in a neutral position away from the metal edge of the table.

e. Occipital alopecia. Can occur 3 weeks after the operation secondary to ischemia of the scalp. Proper position: Pad head; reposition the head frequently during the operation.

f. Heel of foot skin ischemia and tissue necrosis. Proper position: Heels should be well padded.

3. Adjust fresh gas flow

   a. The use of 100% oxygen maximizes inspired oxygen tension, but the inclusion of a small amount of nitrogen probably will not decrease arterial oxygen content significantly and may prevent absorption atelectasis and reduce the risk of oxygen toxicity. A 70% oxygen/30% air mixture is usually adequate for proper oxygenation.

   b. Nitrous oxide can be used during the pre-CPB period. It will, however,

   (1) Limit concentration of inspired oxygen (FiO_2).

   (2) Increase pulmonary vascular resistance (PVR) in adults.

   (3) Increase catecholamine release.

   (4) Possibly induce left ventricular (LV) dysfunction.

   c. This evidence **suggests** that nitrous oxide should not be used in patients with an evolving myocardial infarct or probably in patients with ongoing ischemia because the decrease in FiO_2 and potential catecholamine release can theoretically increase the risk of ischemia and infarct size. This point remains controversial.

4. Check all lines after final patient position is achieved

   a. Intravenous (IV) infusions should flow freely, and the arterial pressure waveform should be assessed to detect dampening or hyperresonance.

   b. IV injection ports should be accessible.

   c. All IV and arterial line connections (stopcocks) should be taped or secured to prevent their movement to minimize the risk of blood loss from an open connection.

   d. Confirm electrical and patient reference "zero" of all transducers (see Chap. 4).

5. **Check hemodynamic status.** Cardiac index and "filling pressures" should be evaluated following intubation.

6. Check blood chemistry

   a. Once a stable anesthetic level is achieved, and ventilation and FiO_2 have been constant for 10 minutes, an arterial blood gas (ABG) measurement should be determined to confirm adequate ventilation and to correlate these data with noninvasive measurements (e.g., arterial hemoglobin oxygen saturation and end-tidal carbon dioxide concentration).

   b. Electrolytes should be determined as clinically indicated.

   c. A blood sample to determine a baseline activated clotting time (ACT) prior to heparinization may be drawn at the same time as the sample for the ABG. The blood can be taken from the arterial line after withdrawal of 5 ml of blood to clear the line of any residual heparin from the flush solution.

   d. Prior to any manipulation of the arterial line (zeroing, blood sample withdrawal, and so on) it is important to announce your intentions. This avoids alarming your colleagues, who may notice the loss of the arterial waveform.

7. Preparing for saphenous vein excision involves lifting the legs above the level of the heart. The increased venous return raises the myocardial preload. This change is desirable in patients with low filling

pressures and normal ventricular function but may be harmful in someone with borderline ventricular reserve. A gradual elevation of the legs may be useful in attenuating the hemodynamic changes. The reverse occurs when the legs are returned to the neutral position.

8. Maintenance of body temperature is not a concern during the pre-CPB time period. It is preferable to allow the temperature to drift down slowly in preparation for CPB. For this reason, increasing the room temperature, humidifying anesthetic gases, warming intravenous solutions, or using a warming blanket are not necessary prior to CPB. These measures must be available for post-CPB management. The physiologic changes of mild hypothermia (34–36°C) include:

   a. Decrease in oxygen consumption and carbon dioxide production (8% for each degree celsius)
   b. Increase in systemic and pulmonary vascular resistance
   c. Increase in blood viscosity
   d. (1) Decrease in central nervous system (CNS) function (amnesia, decrease in cerebral metabolic rate [$CMRO_2$], decrease in cerebral blood flow)
      (2) Decrease in anesthetic requirement (minimum alveolar concentration [MAC] decreases 5% for each degree celsius)
   e. Decrease in renal blood flow and urine output
   f. Decrease in hepatic blood flow
   g. Minimal increase in catecholamines

9. Maintenance of other organ system function
   a. Renal system
      (1) Inadequate urine output must be addressed immediately:
         (a) Rule out technical problems (kinked urinary catheter tubing, or disconnected tubing).
         (b) Optimize and maintain an adequate intravascular volume and cardiac output.
         (c) Avoid or treat hypotension.
         (d) Maintain proper oxygenation.
         (e) Mannitol (0.25 g/kg IV) may be used to redistribute renal blood flow to the cortex and also to maintain renal tubular flow.
         (f) Dopamine (2.5–5.0 μg/kg/min) infusion may be given to increase renal blood flow by renal vascular dilation.
         (g) Diuretics (furosemide 10–40 mg, bumetanide 0.25–1.00 mg) can be given to maintain renal tubular flow if other measures are ineffective.
      (2) Patients undergoing emergent surgery may have received a large radiocontrast dye load at angiography. Avoidance of acute tubular necrosis from the dye utilizing the techniques mentioned above is crucial.
   b. Central nervous system
      (1) An adequate cerebral perfusion pressure (CPP) must be maintained.
         (a) The patient's lowest and highest mean arterial pressures on the ward should be the limits accepted in the operating room to avoid cerebral ischemia.
         (b) Elderly patients have a decreased cerebral reserve and are more sensitive to changes in CPP.
      (2) Patients at risk for an adverse cerebral event include those with known carotid artery disease, those undergoing open heart procedures, and those with a known embolic focus. Management considerations for these patients are discussed in Chapter 24.
   c. Pulmonary system

(1) Maintain normal pH, $PaCO_2$, and adequate PaO_2.

(2) Treatment of systemic hypertension with a vasodilator may induce hypoxemia secondary to inhibition of hypoxic pulmonary vasoconstriction. FiO_2 may have to be increased.

(3) Use of an air-oxygen mixture may prevent absorption atelectasis.

10. Prepare for incision

a. Is the anesthetic depth adequate for the next level of stimulation?

b. Muscle relaxation is needed to avoid movement with incision and sternotomy.

C. Incision

1. An adequate depth of anesthesia is necessary to avoid tachycardia and hypertension in response to the stimulus of incision.

2. Observe the surgical field for patient movement and blood color. Despite an abundance of monitors, the presence of bright red blood is still one of the best ways to assess oxygenation and perfusion.

3. If the patient responds to incision (tachycardia, hypertension, or other signs of "light" anesthesia), the level of anesthesia must be deepened prior to sternotomy. **Do not** allow sternal split until the patient is adequately anesthetized and hemodynamics are stable.

D. Sternal split

1. A very high level of stimulation accompanies sternal split. The incidence of hypertension has been reported to be as high as 88% during high-dose narcotic anesthesia.

a. A cumulative dose of fentanyl 50–70 µg/kg prior to sternal split should decrease the incidence of hypertension to less than 50%. Fentanyl in total doses greater than 150 µg/kg is necessary for a significant reduction in hypertension.

b. Sufentanil 10–30 µg/kg prior to sternal split should result in an incidence of hypertension of 17–67%.

c. Vasodilators are often required for blood pressure control.

d. Bradycardia secondary to vagal discharge can occur if the patient is not adequately anesthetized.

2. An oscillating power saw is often used to cut the sternum. **The lungs should be "deflated"** during this procedure to avoid damage to the lung parenchyma.

3. The patient must be relaxed during sternotomy to avoid air embolism. If the patient gasps and the right atrium is cut, air can be entrained owing to the negative intrathoracic pressure.

4. This is the most common time period for awareness and recall.

a. If an amnestic agent has not been previously administered, it should be considered prior to sternotomy because no agent will cause retrograde amnesia.

b. Awareness has been reported with fentanyl dosages as large as 150 µg/kg and also with lower fentanyl doses supplemented with amnestic agents (see sec. **c.** below. Awareness is **usually** associated with other symptoms of "light" anesthesia (movement, sweating, increase in pupil size, hypertension, or tachycardia).

c. Amnestic supplements can decrease the incidence of recall but cannot ensure amnesia nor protect against the hemodynamic consequences of awareness. All amnestic supplements can possibly cause cardiovascular instability. Listed below are the most common amnestic agents, their dosages, and side effects:

(1) Scopolamine 0.3–0.6 mg may cause tachycardia if administered rapidly IV.

(2) Benzodiazepines (diazepam 5–15 mg, midazolam 2.5–10.0 mg, lorazepam 1–4 mg) can decrease systemic vascular resistance (SVR) and contractility (in the patient with poor ventricular

function), especially when added to a narcotic-based anesthetic. Midazolam has been reported to induce ventricular irritability.

(3) Nitrous oxide may lead to catecholamine release, left ventricular dysfunction, increases in pulmonary vascular resistance (PVR), and an increased risk of hypoxia.

(4) Inhalational agents can cause myocardial depression, bradycardia, tachycardia, dysrhythmias, or decreases in SVR.

5. **Concerns with a cardiac reoperation ("redo heart").** The heart or a vein graft may be adherent to the sternum and can be torn with sternotomy. A vibrating saw is used to decrease the likelihood of damage to soft tissue.

a. The femoral area should **always** be prepared and draped and consideration given to femoral artery cannulation prior to sternal split.

b. If the right atrium, right ventricle, or great vessels are cut, emergency CPB can be initiated using:

(1) "Sucker bypass" with femoral artery cannula or aortic cannula and the cardiotomy suckers used as the venous return line.

(2) Complete femoral artery–femoral vein bypass.

c. It is mandatory to have all the patient's blood available in the room, checked and ready for immediate administration prior to sternal split.

E. Sternal spread

1. A very high level of stimulation can be expected.

2. Confirm equal inflation of lungs visually after the chest is open.

3. Pulmonary artery catheter malfunction with sternal spread has been reported. Numerous case reports in which external jugular or subclavian routes were used have noted kinking of the pulmonary artery catheter as it exits the introducer sheath. If this occurs, the sheath may be withdrawn, which may rectify the problem but will result in the loss of a route for an intravenous infusion. The possibility of bleeding around the catheter and the potential loss of sterility should also be considered.

4. Innominate vein rupture following aggressive sternal spread is possible.

F. Internal mammary artery dissection

1. This is a period of low-level stimulation.

2. The chest is retracted to one side using the Favaloro retractor, and the table is elevated and rotated away from surgeon. The left internal mammary artery (LIMA) is most commonly grafted to the left anterior descending artery.

a. This procedure can cause difficulties in blood pressure measurement.

(1) **Left**-sided radial arterial lines may not function during LIMA dissection owing to compression of the left subclavian artery with chest retraction.

(2) The use of a **right** radial arterial line or an automated noninvasive blood pressure measurement device is suggested.

(3) Transducers must be kept level with the right atrium.

b. Extubation may occur with patient movement during retraction.

c. Radial nerve injury due to compression by the support post of the Favaloro retractor is possible.

3. **Bleeding** may be extensive but hidden from view in the chest cavity (think of volume replacement to treat hypotension).

4. **Heparin** 5000 units may be given during the vessel dissection process.

5. Papaverine may be injected into the internal mammary artery (IMA) for dilation and to prevent spasm. Systemic effects may include hypotension or anaphylaxis.

6. IMA blood flow should usually be more than 100 ml/min (25 ml collected in 15 seconds) to be considered acceptable for grafting.

G. Sympathetic nerve dissection

   1. After the pericardium is opened, the postganglionic sympathetic nerves are dissected from the aorta to allow insertion of the aortic cannula.

   2. The most overlooked period of high level stimulation. This response is best attenuated with beta blockade or vasodilators because it is related to sympathetic discharge rather than "light" levels of anesthesia.

II. Perioperative stress response

  A. Afferent loop

   1. The body responds to stress with an increase in hormones, causing a catabolic response and an increase in substrate mobilization. This response is primarily accomplished through the hypothalamic-pituitary-adrenal axis.

   2. Stimuli that can trigger this response include:

    a. Psychologic

     (1) Preoperative anxiety

     (2) "Light" anesthesia

    b. Physiologic

     (1) Pain associated with invasive monitor placement

     (2) Intubation

     (3) Surgical stimulation

     (4) Changes in blood pressure (hypotension or hypertension)

     (5) Hypoxia

     (6) Hypercarbia

     (7) Cardiopulmonary bypass

     (8) Aortic cross clamp removal

  B. Humoral mediators involved in the stress response

   1. Antidiuretic hormone (ADH)—increased levels with surgery

   2. ACTH—increased; causes increase in cortisol levels

   3. Cortisol—increased; leads to an increase in glucose level

   4. Catecholamines—epinephrine, norepinephrine, dopamine: increased owing to adrenal medulla stimulation

   5. Insulin—decreased inappropriately for level of glucose

   6. Glucagon—increased; causes increase in glucose level and increased contractility of the heart

   7. Growth hormone (GH)—increased; causes an increased rate of protein synthesis

   8. Renin—increased; converts angiotensinogen to angiotensin I

   9. Prolactin—increased levels may be due to increased levels of endorphins

  10. Endorphins—increased

  C. Efferent loop–organ system responses to humoral mediators

   1. Cardiovascular effects

    a. Catecholamines

     (1) Hypertension

     (2) Tachycardia

     (3) Dysrhythmias

     (4) Myocardial oxygen supply and demand ratio affected adversely

    b. Renin, angiotension, ADH

     (1) Increased blood volume (preload)

     (2) Increased SVR (afterload)

     (3) Coronary perfusion pressure possibly affected

    c. Glucagon

     (1) Increased inotropy

   2. Renal effects

      a. Increased aldosterone levels
      b. Decreased urine output (ADH)
      c. Decreased plasma potassium and increased plasma sodium secondary to aldosterone
      d. Decreased renal blood flow
   3. Metabolic effects
      a. Increased myocardial oxygen consumption
      b. Increased cerebral metabolic rate
      c. Increased lactate and pyruvate levels
      d. Increased blood glucose level
      e. Decreased liver and renal blood flow may decrease clearance and increase the duration of action of medications
      f. Increased free fatty acid levels
   4. Neurologic effects
      a. Decreased minimum alveolar concentration (MAC) of anesthetic agents from endorphin production
   5. Pulmonary effects
      a. Increased conversion of angiotensin I to angiotensin II
      b. Bronchodilation and increased dead space
D. Modification of the stress response
   1. Systemic opioids (high dose)
      a. Fentanyl (50–150 μg/kg). Blunts all responses except for prolactin increase and occasional increase in myocardial lactate production prior to CPB. Not effective in blocking stress response during or following CPB.
      b. Sufentanil (10–30 μg/kg). Similar to fentanyl, but some studies have shown increases in norepinephrine levels with sternotomy. Free fatty acid levels increase with cannulation but may be associated with heparin. Not effective in blocking stress response during or following CPB.
      c. Complications. High-dose narcotics can lead to prolonged mechanical ventilation and delayed extubation.
   2. Inhalational anesthetics
      a. MAC BAR (Minimum alveolar concentration that blocks adrenergic response in 50% of patients
         (1) MAC BAR is approximately equal to 1.5 MAC.
         (2) Cortisol and growth hormone levels will increase with this depth of anesthesia.
         (3) 2.0 MAC is needed to reduce catecholamine responses in 95% of patients.
         (4) MAC BAR is associated with myocardial depression, decrease in blood pressure, and increase in pulmonary capillary wedge pressure.
   3. Systemic medications that decrease catecholamine effects
      a. Beta blockers
         (1) Beta blockers attenuate the increase in heart rate and myocardial oxygen demand.
         (2) Adverse effects include
            (a) Decreased contractility.
            (b) Unopposed alpha-adrenergic effects causing a resultant increase in SVR (hypertension) and potential coronary vasoconstriction.
         c. Bronchospasm.
      b. Clonidine[3] (centrally acting alpha-2 adrenergic agonist)
         (1) Clonidine decreases sympathetic peripheral efferent activity.
         (2) It causes a decrease in all catecholamine levels (reduced norepinephrine levels are most prominent).

(3) It decreases heart rate, blood pressure, and SVR in the pre-CPB period.

(4) No attenuation of adrenergic response during or following CPB is seen.

(5) It may cause bradycardia and hypotension in some patients during levels of low surgical stimulation.

c. Vasodilators

(1) Vasodilators are used for treatment for increases in SVR, often secondary to elevated norepinephrine levels.

(2) Adverse effects include

(a) Reflex increase in catecholamines.

(b) Reflex increase in heart rate.

(c) Inhibition of hypoxic pulmonary vasoconstriction causing hypoxia.

4. Regional anesthetic techniques

a. Epidural/subarachnoid

(1) Local anesthetics

(a) These drugs decrease GH, ACTH, ADH, and catecholamine responses to lower abdominal procedures.

(b) Thoracic epidural anesthesia is inconsistent in blocking the stress response to thoracic surgery. This may be due to insufficient somatic or sympathetic blockade or from unblocked pelvic afferents[6].

(c) Adverse effects include decreased SVR, bradycardia, and decreased inotropy from sympathectomy.

(2) Narcotics

(a) Narcotics block the stress response to surgery poorly.

(b) They provide postoperative analgesia for abdominal and thoracic procedures.

III. **Treatment of hemodynamic changes.** Pressor and vasodilator treatment of any hemodynamic change ideally should involve the use of agents with a very short half-life because:

1. The surgical stimuli and the patient response are usually short lived (e.g., after sternotomy the duration of patient response is usually limited to 10–15 minutes).

2. Many agents (β blockers, calcium channel blockers, and vasodilators) will affect hemodynamic parameters for longer than 15 minutes and have half-lives of several hours. Their actions could affect weaning from CPB. For these reasons the use of short-acting agents (esmolol, nitroglycerin, sodium nitroprusside, trimethaphan camsylate, phenylephrine, and ephedrine) should be encouraged.

A. Hypotension

1. Causes

a. Mechanical causes must first be ruled out prior to treatment, including:

(1) Surgical compression of the heart.

(2) Technical problems with invasive blood pressure measurement (kinked catheter, air bubbles, and so on).

b. The most common cause of hypotension is hypovolemia (Table 6-2).

2. Treatment (Fig. 6-1)

B. Hypertension

1. Hypertension occurs in up to 88% of patients with use of a high-dose narcotic technique during the pre-CPB period.

2. Hypertension is less common in patients with left ventricular dysfunction compared to patients with normal contractility.

Table 6-2. Differential diagnosis of hypotension

1. Hypovolemia
2. "Deep" anesthetic plane for level of stimulation.
3. Mechanical compression of the heart or great vessels
4. Decreased myocardial contractility
5. Ischemia
6. Dysrhythmia:
   a. Bradycardia
   b. Tachycardia (decrease in diastolic filling time)
   c. Dysrhythmia leading to loss of atrial contraction and its contribution to ventricular filling
7. Decrease in systemic vascular resistance
8. Constrictive pericarditis in re-operation cases.

Note: Causes of hypotension are listed in order of frequency of occurrence.

3. The most likely cause of hypertension is "light" anesthesia. This is most often seen in younger patients and in those with preoperative hypertension (Table 6-3).
4. Treatment (Fig. 6-2)

C. Sinus bradycardia
1. The most common cause of sinus bradycardia is vagal stimulation, which often results from the vagotonic effects of narcotics (Table 6-4).
2. Treatment
   a. Treatment is indicated for:
      (1) Any heart rate decrease associated with a significant decrease in blood pressure.
      (2) Heart rate of less than 40 beats/minute even without decrease in blood pressure if it is associated with a nodal or ventricular escape rhythm.
   b. The underlying cause should be treated.
   c. Atropine 0.2–0.4 mg IV can cause an unpredictable response.
      (1) It may cause uncontrolled tachycardia and ischemia.
      (2) It is often ineffective.
      (3) Glycopyrrolate (0.1–0.2 mg IV), another vagolytic agent, may induce less increase in heart rate but is also unpredictable and has a longer half-life than atropine.
   d. Pancuronium 2–4 mg IV is often effective owing to its sympathomimetic activity but can also be unpredictable.
   e. Ephedrine 2.5–10.0 mg IV is indicated if bradycardia is associated with hypotension. The response is unpredictable, and the recommended starting dose is 2.5 mg IV.
   f. Pulmonary artery catheters with pacing capabilities are used in some institutions to provide a safe and predictable means of heart rate increase.
   g. Atropine, isoproterenol, and pacing can be used for life-threatening bradycardia.

D. Sinus tachycardia
1. Sinus tachycardia appears to be the most significant risk factor for intraoperative ischemia. Sinus tachycardia of more than 100 beats/minute has been associated with a 40% incidence of ischemia. A heart rate of more than 110 beats/minute was associated with a 32–63% incidence of ischemia[7,8]. The most likely cause is "light" anesthesia (Table 6-5).
2. Treatment

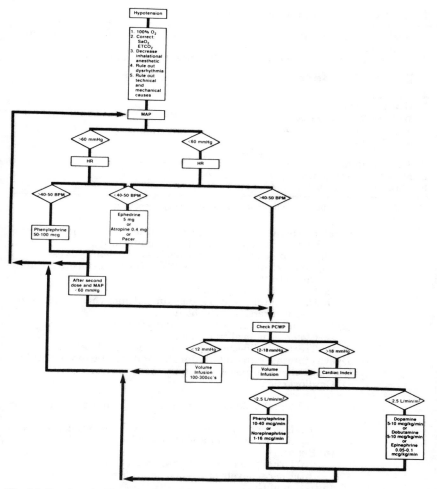

Fig. 6-1. Treatment of hypotension in the prebypass period. SaO₂ = arterial hemoglobin oxygen saturation; ETCO₂ = end-tidal carbon dioxide; MAP = mean arterial pressure; HR = heart rate; PCWP = pulmonary capillary wedge pressure.

      a. Rule out ventilation abnormalities and correct them if present.
      b. Increase anesthetic level if other signs of "light" anesthesia are associated.
      c. Treat the underlying cause.
        (1) Give volume infusion if low preload is evident.
        (2) Address the other causes of tachycardia listed in Table 6-5.
  E. Dysrhythmias
    1. The most likely cause of dysrhythmia in the prebypass period is surgical manipulation of the heart (Table 6-6).
    2. Treatment
      a. Treat the underlying cause. Potassium replacement in the pre-CPB period should be limited to treatment for symptomatic hy-

Table 6-3. Differential diagnosis of hypertension

1. "Light" anesthesia (increased narcotic requirements are noted in patients with chronic tobacco, alcohol, or caffeine use)
2. Dissection of sympathetic nerves from the aorta in preparation for aortic cannulation
3. Hypoxia
4. Hypercarbia
5. Hypervolemia
6. Withdrawal syndromes
   a. β blockers
   b. Clonidine
   c. Alcohol $\left.\right\}$ Rare
7. Thyroid storm
8. Malignant hyperpyrexia
9. Pheochromocytoma

Note: Causes of hypertension are listed in order of frequency of occurrence.

pokalemia because the cardioplegic solution used during CPB may increase the serum potassium level significantly.
  b. **Dysrhythmias causing minor hemodynamic disturbances**
     (1) Supraventricular tachycardia (SVT) (including acute atrial fibrillation/flutter)
        a. Stop mechanical irritation.
        b. Use vagal maneuvers, digoxin, calcium channel blockers, beta blockers, or edrophonium.
     (2) Premature ventricular contractions (PVCs)
        (a) Stop mechanical irritation.
        (b) Treat with lidocaine, procainamide, or β blockers.
  c. **Dysrhythmias causing major hemodynamic compromise.** Continue chemical resuscitation as above concurrent with:
     (1) Cardioversion
        (a) Internal
           (i) Small paddles are applied directly to heart when chest is open.
           (ii) Low energy levels (5–25 joules) are needed for cardioversion (skin impedance is bypassed).
        (b) External
           (i) Usual paddle size is used with chest closed.
           (ii) Energy levels of 25–300 joules are needed.
     (2) Initiation of CPB
IV. Preparation for CPB
  A. Heparinization
     1. Heparin is the preferred agent for anticoagulation. Heparin is a water-soluble mucopolysaccharide with a molecular weight of 15,000 daltons.
        a. Mechanism of action
           (1) Binds to antithrombin III (AT-III), a protease inhibitor.
           (2) Increases the speed of the reaction between AT-III and several activated clotting factors (II, IX, X, XI, XII, XIII).
        b. Onset time—immediate.
        c. Half-life—approximately 2 hours.
        d. Metabolism—by heparinase in the liver.
        e. Potency of different preparations may differ markedly.
           (1) Potency is measured in units (not mg).
           (2) Heparin solutions usually contain at least 120–140 units/ mg, depending on the lot or manufacturer.

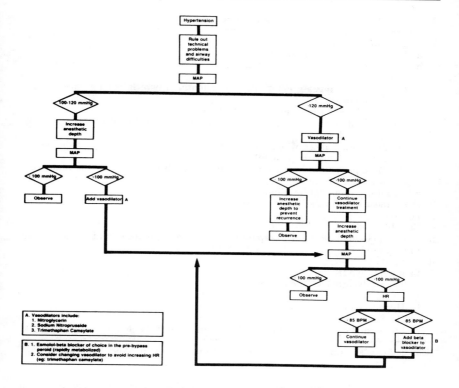

Fig. 6-2. Treatment of hypertension in the prebypass period. MAP = mean arterial pressure; HR = heart rate.

      f. Protamine sulfate rapidly reverses heparin activity by combining with heparin to form an inactive compound.

      g. Dosage

        (1) The initial dosage of heparin for anticoagulation prior to CPB is 300 units/kg.

        (2) This dose has been established by many investigators;[2] however, because many patients may remain inadequately anticoagulated using this dose, subsequent doses of heparin needed for adequate anticoagulation must be established on an individual basis according to the activated clotting time (ACT) see **3.** below).

2. Routes of administration. Heparin must be administered directly into a central vein or into the right atrium with documentation that heparin is being administered into the intravascular space (aspiration to confirm blood return).

3. ACT technique

    a. The ACT monitors the effect of heparin on coagulation. Two milliliters of blood is placed in a tube that contains diatomite (clay),

Table 6-4. Differential diagnosis of sinus bradycardia

1. Vagal stimulation
   a. Vagotonic effects of narcotics
   b. Intense surgical stimulation with "light" plane of anesthesia (e.g., during sternotomy)
      (1) Sufentanil has a greater effect than fentanyl, which has a greater effect than morphine
      (2) Associated with rapid administration
      (3) Associated with initial dose (less bradycardia occurs with subsequent narcotic doses)
      (4) More pronounced when nitrous oxide is not present (nitrous oxide may increase sympathetic tone)
      (5) More pronounced with vecuronium, atracurium, or metocurine compared with pancuronium
   c. Vagotonic effects of halothane
2. Deep anesthetic levels
3. Hypoxia
4. Beta blockade
5. Calcium channel blockers (verapamil and diltiazem produce greater effects than nifedipine)
6. Ischemia
7. Sick sinus syndrome
8. Reflex bradycardia secondary to:
   a. Hypervolemia
   b. Hypertension
      (1) Secondary to vasoconstrictor use
      (2) Secondary to other causes of hypertension (see Table 6-3)

Note: Causes of sinus bradycardia are listed in order of frequency of occurrence.

which causes contact activation of the coagulation cascade. The tube is heated to 37°C, and the mixture is continuously mixed. The time from introduction of blood into the tube until the first clot is formed is the ACT. This measurement can be automated.
   b. Normal automated ACT = 105–167 seconds.*
   c. An ACT of at least 300 seconds is safe for initiating CPB provided that the ACT is rechecked immediately after starting CPB and heparin 3000–5000 units is included in the pump prime.
   d. An ACT of more than 400 seconds is known to prevent fibrin monomer appearance during CPB[10]. Some institutions require an ACT of 480 seconds.
4. Inadequate ACT
   a. Causes of inadequate ACT are listed in Table 6-7.
   b. Treatment of inadequate ACT
      (1) Check ACT before and after heparin administration.
      (2) If the ACT is less than 300 seconds **do not begin CPB.**
      (3) Give more heparin in 5000- to 10,000-unit increments (from different vials or different lots).
      (4) Recheck ACT.
      (5) Fresh frozen plasma (FFP) can be given empirically for treatment of antithrombin III deficiency if an ACT of less than 300 seconds persists despite heparin 800–1000 units/kg and other causes of inadequate ACT are ruled out (old heparin vials, etc.).

*Source: International Technidyne Corporation, 23 Nevsky St., Edison, New Jersey, 08220 1988).

Table 6-5. Differential diagnosis of sinus tachycardia

1. "Light" anesthesia insufficient for level of surgical stimulation
2. Medications
   a. Pancuronium
   b. Scopolamine
   c. Inotropic agents
   d. Isoflurane
   e. Aminophylline preparations
   f. Beta agonists (albuterol, etc.)
   g. Monoamine oxidase inhibitors or tricyclic antidepressants
3. Hypovolemia
4. Ischemia
5. Hypoxia
6. Hypercarbia
7. Congestive heart failure
8. Withdrawal syndromes
   a. β blockers
   b. Clonidine
   c. Alcohol
9. Thyroid storm
10. Malignant hyperpyrexia
11. Pheochromocytoma

} Rare

Note: Causes of sinus tachycardia are listed in order of frequency of occurrence.

Table 6-6. Common causes of dysrhythmias

1. Mechanical stimulation of the heart (e.g., placement of purse-string sutures, cannulation, vent placement, and lifting the heart to study coronary anatomy)
2. Existing dysrhythmias
3. Increase in catecholamine levels
   a. "Light" anesthesia
   b. Hypercarbia
   c. Nitrous oxide use
   d. Halothane (sensitization of myocardium to catecholamines)
   e. Medications
      (1) Pancuronium
      (2) Inotropic agents
      (3) Aminophylline preparations
      (4) Beta agonists (albuterol, etc.)
      (5) Monoamine oxidase inhibitors and tricyclic antidepressants
4. Electrolyte abnormalities including hypokalemia
5. Hypertension
6. Hypotension
7. Ischemia*
8. Hypoxemia

Note: Causes of dysrhythmias listed in order of frequency of occurrence.
*More frequent in patients with severe coronary disease.

        (a) Two to three units of FFP should be given to increase levels of antithrombin III that are presumably depleted or lowered by the causes of heparin resistance listed in Table 6-7.
        (b) Recheck ACT after FFP is given.
  B. Cannulation (Fig. 6-3)

Table 6-7 Causes of inadequate activated clotting time prior to initiating CPB

Technical reasons
  Mislabeled syringe
  Heparin not injected intravascularly (extravasation, not injected into right
    atrium, line disconnection, etc.)
  Heparin of low activity (old or nonrefrigerateed vials)
Heparin resistance
  Heparin use previously or ongoing infusion
  Pregnancy or oral contraceptive use
  Intraaortic balloon pump
  Shock
  Streptokinase use
  Antithrombin III deficiency
  Low-grade disseminated intravascular coagulation (DIC)
  Infective endocarditis
  Intracardiac thrombus
  Elderly patient

Source: Modified from E. F. Anderson. Heparin resistance prior to cardiopulmonary bypass. *Anesthesiology* 64:505, 1986. With permission.

1. A pericardial sling is created prior to cannulation to increase working space and to provide a dam for external cooling fluid and ice slush solution. The sling may lift the heart, which can decrease venous return and lead to hypotension.
2. Purse-string sutures are utilized to keep the aortic and venous cannulae in place during surgery and to close the incisions after decannulation.
3. Nitrous oxide is discontinued to avoid enlargement of air emboli.
4. Heparin is **always** given before cannulation.
5. The aortic cannula is inserted first to allow infusion of volume in case of hemorrhage associated with venous cannulation. Emergency CPB may then be instituted using cardiotomy suckers to deliver venous return ("sucker bypass").
6. The aortic cannula is checked for air bubbles as it is filled with saline and connected to CPB tubing.
7. Prior to infusing volume or initiating CPB all clamps should be removed from the CPB cannula.
8. PEEP may be applied to increase intracardiac pressures to avoid air entrainment during cannulation of the right atrium and left ventricle.
9. Types of cannulae
   a. **Aortic** (Fig. 6-4)
      (1) The aortic cannula should be placed in the ascending aorta proximal to the origin of the innominate artery and distal to the proposed sites of the saphenous vein grafts.
      (2) The straight cannula with a flange prevents the insertion of an excessive length of cannula into the aorta. The flange also serves as an anchoring site for sutures.
      (3) The right angle cannula is most commonly used with the tip directed toward the aortic arch.
      (4) The long tapered cannula is inserted in the ascending aorta and advanced toward the aortic arch. The risk of entering the innominate, carotid, or subclavian arteries is increased using this method. This cannula is frequently used for femoral cannulation.
   b. Venous (Fig. 6-5)

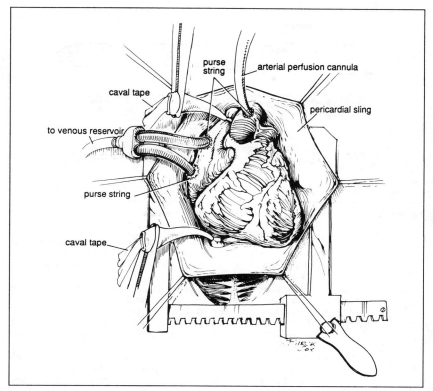

Fig. 6-3. View of an open chest with formation of a pericardial sling (see text). Note arterial and venous cannulation sites. Caval tapes, placed around the superior and inferior vena cava, are tightened to institute complete cardiopulmonary bypass (see Chapter 7 for a discussion of complete and partial cardiopulmonary bypass).

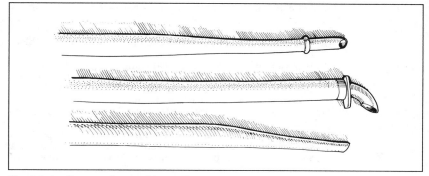

Fig. 6-4. Aortic cannulae used in cardiac surgery (see text).

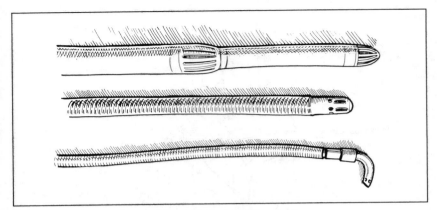

Fig. 6-5. Venous cannulae used in cardiac surgery (see text).

(1) A **single** two-stage cannula (with right atrial and inferior vena caval ports) is usually adequate for coronary bypass and aortic valve surgery. It is placed in the right atrial appendage (see Fig. 6-5, top).

(2) Two cannulae (for the inferior and superior vena cava) (see Fig. 6-5, middle and bottom) can also be used.

    (a) Cannulae are inserted at the respective caval-atrial junctions or at a more convenient location in the atrium. The curved cannulae are frequently used in pediatric cardiac surgery.

    (b) These cannulas are used primarily for situations in which complete bypass (all of the systemic venous return is directed to the heart-lung machine, and none enters the heart) is desired.

        (i) Open heart procedures.

        (ii) Severe right coronary disease to avoid warm blood entering the right atrium.

        (iii) Patients in renal failure. This method allows aspiration of the cardioplegic solution from the coronary sinus to decrease the systemic absorption of potassium.

10. Complications of cannulation

  a. Aortic cannulation

    (1) Embolic phenomena from air or atherosclerotic plaque dislodgment.

    (2) Hypotension.

        (a) Hypotension is usually secondary to hypovolemia (blood loss).

        (b) It may result from mechanical compression of heart.

        (c) A partial occlusion clamp used for cannulation may narrow the aortic lumen (more common in children). Check aortic pressure immediately when the clamp is applied.

    (3) Dysrhythmias. These are most likely due to surgical manipulation.

    (4) Aortic dissection due to cannula misplacement. A pulsatile pressure from the aortic cannula that correlates with the radial mean arterial blood pressure effectively rules out dissection (see Chap. 7).

    (5) Bleeding

         (a) Minor bleeding is not uncommon with cannulation.
         (b) Major bleeding may occur if aorta is torn.
         (c) Treatment consists of infusion of volume as needed, or initiation of CPB.
     b. Venous cannulation
       (1) Hypotension
         (a) If hypotension is due to hypovolemia, give volume in 100-ml increments for adults and 10–25 ml for pediatric patients through the aortic line as needed.
         (b) Mechanical compression of the heart may cause hypotension, especially during inferior vena caval cannulation.
       (2) Bleeding
         (a) Bleeding can occur from a tear of the right atrium or the superior or inferior vena cava.
         (b) Treatment is accomplished by infusing volume or initiating emergency CPB.
       (3) Dysrhythmias
         (a) Dysrhythmias usually result from surgical manipulation.
         (b) No treatment is required if they occur occasionally and are of no hemodynamic significance.
         (c) Cessation of or limitation of mechanical stimulation may be all that is necessary.
         d. Treatment consists in giving medications, cardioversion, or initiating CPB (see sec. **II.E**)
C. Autologous blood removal
   1. If 500–1000 ml of the patient's heparinized blood is removed prior to CPB it can be reinfused after termination of CPB. This blood is spared the rigors of CPB including hemolysis, platelet destruction, and clotting factor degradation. Transfusion with banked blood can be avoided in many cases by this means.
   2. Technique
     a. The patient should have a preoperative hemoglobin at least 12 g/dl to avoid severe anemia post CPB.
     b. Blood (500–1000 ml) is withdrawn from the venous line of the CPB circuit into a blood collection bag prior to initiating CPB.
     c. Anticoagulation is provided by the previously administered heparin.
     d. Clear pump prime is infused through the aortic cannula at the same rate as blood is withdrawn to maintain preload.
   3. Risks
     a. Hypotension
       (1) Hypotension is secondary to a decrease in preload.
         (a) Rate of withdrawal may be too fast.
         (b) Rate of infusion from the bypass circuit may be too slow.
       (2) Treatment consists in decreasing withdrawal rate and increasing infusion rate with transient use of vasoconstrictors.
     b. A decrease in oxygen-carrying capacity leading to ischemia prior to CPB can occur. The hemoglobin concentration will decrease 1–3 g/dl acutely with infusion of the CPB pump prime solution. This will be accentuated at the aortic root and the origin of the coronary vessels. If ischemia occurs, treatment consists of terminating blood withdrawal and beginning CPB immediately.
     c. Infection is a possibility if the sterility of the circuit connections and blood container is not maintained.
     d. Relative contraindications
         (i) Left main coronary artery disease or equivalent
         (ii) Left ventricular dysfunction
        (iii) Emergency surgery

D. Following cannulation and autologous blood withdrawal (if utilized), a checklist is performed and bypass is begun.

REFERENCES

1. Anderson, E. F. Heparin resistance prior to cardiopulmonary bypass. *Anesthesiology* 64:504–507, 1986.
2. Bull, B. S., Korpman, R. A., Huse, W. M., et al. Heparin therapy during extracorporeal circulation. *J. Thorac. Cardiovasc. Surg.* 69:674–684, 1975.
3. Flacke, J. W., Bloor, B. C., Flacke, W. E., et al. Reduced narcotic requirement by clonidine with improved hemodynamic and adrenergic stability in patients undergoing coronary bypass surgery. *Anesthesiology* 67:11–19, 1987.
4. O'Connor, J. P., Ramsey, J. G., Wynands, J. E., et al. The incidence of myocardial ischemia during anesthesia for coronary artery bypass surgery in patients receiving pancuronium or vecuronium. *Anesthesiology* 70:230–236, 1989.
5. Roy, R. C., Stafford, M. A., and Charlton, J. E. Nerve injury and musculoskeletal complaints after cardiac surgery: Influence of internal mammary artery dissection and left arm position. *Anesth. Analg.* 67:277–279, 1988.
6. Rutberg, H., Hakanson, I., and Kehlet, H. Trauma and Stress—The Effect of Neural Blockade. In J. B. Lofstrom, and U. Sjostrand (eds.), *Local Anesthesia and Regional Blockade.* New York: Elsevier Science, 1988. Pps. 259–272.
7. Slogoff, S., and Keats, A. S. Does chronic treatment with calcium entry blocking drugs reduce perioperative myocardial ischemia? *Anesthesiology* 68:676–680, 1988.
8. Slogoff, S., and Keats, A. S. Randomized trial of primary anesthetic agents on outcome of coronary artery bypass operations. *Anesthesiology* 70:179–188, 1989.
9. Sonntag, H., Stephen, H., Lange, H., et al. Sufentanil does not block sympathetic responses to surgical stimuli in patients having coronary artery revascularization surgery. *Anesth. Analg.* 68:584–592, 1989.
10. Young, J. A., Kisker, C. T., and Doty, D. B. Adequate anticoagulation during cardiopulmonary bypass determined by activated clotting time and the appearance of fibrin monomer. *Ann. Thorac. Surg.* 26:231–240, 1978.

SUGGESTED READINGS

Bovill, J. G., Sebel, P. S., and Stanley, T. H. Opioid analgesics in anesthesia: with special reference to their use in cardiovascular anesthesia. *Anesthesiology* 61:731–755, 1984.

Hattersley, P. G. Activated coagulation time of whole blood. *JAMA* 196:436–440, 1966.

Kaplan, J. A. *Cardiac Anesthesia* (vol. 1 and 2). Orlando: Grune & Stratton, 1987.

Lake, C. *Cardiovascular Anesthesia.* New York: Springer-Verlag, 1985.

Ream, A. K., and Fogdall, R. P. *Acute Cardiovascular Management.* Philadelphia: Lippincott, 1982.

Slogoff, S., and Keats, A. S. Does perioperative myocardial ischemia lead to postoperative myocardial infarction? *Anesthesiology* 62:107–114, 1985.

Anesthetic Management During Cardiopulmonary Bypass

David R. Larach

I. Preparations for cardiopulmonary bypass (CPB)

A. The CPB circuit (see Fig. 7-1)

1. **Function.** CPB permits blood to bypass the heart and lungs, draining instead by gravity from the central veins through an artificial lung ("oxygenator") and an external pump that injects oxygenated blood at arterial pressure into one of the great arteries. Thus, CPB sustains systemic blood flow, oxygenation, and ventilation during periods of time when

   a. The heart is asystolic or not ejecting a normal cardiac output.

   b. The lungs are unable to perform physiologic gas exchange owing to inadequate perfusion.

   Even though CPB can provide a normal "cardiac output," a number of important differences exist between the natural and artificial circulations, including nonpulsatile flow, bypass of the lung's endocrine function, and trauma to blood elements. See Chapter 20 for a discussion of the pathophysiology of CPB.

2. **Circuit design.** The **venous conduit** (see Fig. 7-1) drains systemic venous blood to the CPB machine; most commonly, a single cannula is inserted in the right atrium, or separate cannulae are inserted in the superior and inferior vena cavae. The **arterial cannula** returns oxygenated blood from the pump to the aorta, inserting either in the ascending aorta or in a femoral artery. See Chapter 19 for complete details of bypass circuit and design.

   Total (or **complete**) **CPB** occurs when **all** venous blood draining toward the heart is diverted into the pump-oxygenator. **Partial CPB** occurs when only a **portion** of systemic venous blood drains to the pump-oxygenator while the remainder passes through the right heart and lungs and is ejected by the left ventricle (LV). Partial CPB can occur only when the aorta is not cross-clamped, but simply removing the aortic cross clamp does not necessarily mean that total CPB will cease. That depends on whether the heart is filled and is capable of ejecting blood.

B. Preparing the CPB pump for bypass

1. **Composition of bypass perfusate.** In consultation with the anesthesiologist and surgeon, the perfusionist determines the composition of the **pump priming solution**. Generally, this consists of a mixture of electrolytes, buffer, mannitol, and heparin. If the use of a "clear" (i.e., blood-free) prime would result in excessive hemodilution (e.g., [Hb] $< 5–7$ g/dl) given the patient's size and hematocrit, then blood or packed red blood cells are added to the priming solution. See Chapter 19 for a detailed discussion of priming the bypass pump.

2. **Perfusionist's prebypass checklist.** When setting up the CPB pump apparatus and circuit, safe clinical practice requires that the perfusionist take particular care to ensure that at least the following conditions are met: (1) all gas bubbles are expelled from the tubing to prevent arterial air embolism or venous air-lock; (2) all tubing is connected to the pumps for anterograde flow because retrograde flow can cause arterial air injection and lack of perfusion; (3) oxygen is being supplied to the oxygenator; (4) all safety alarms and automatic shut-down sensors are functional and are engaged; and (5) when the arterial perfusion cannula is inserted in the aorta, its transduced pressure shows a **pulsatile** waveform that **correlates** with radial arterial pressure.

C. Anesthesiologist's pre-CPB checklist.
Preparation for CPB by the anesthesiologist begins with a thorough understanding of the proposed sites of cannulation and the bypass procedures to be utilized. Will the heart be arrested? What degree of hypothermia is anticipated? Will

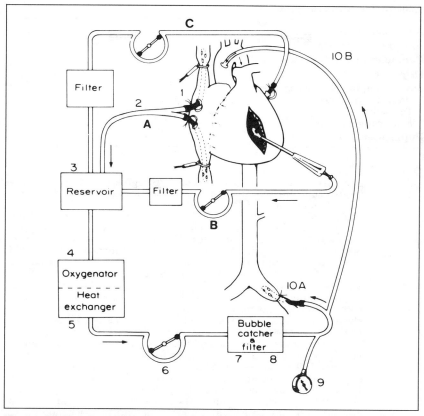

Fig. 7-1. Cardiopulmonary bypass circuit (example). Blood drains by gravity from vena cavae (1) through venous cannula (2) into venous reservoir (3). Blood from surgical field suction and from vent is pumped (B, C) into cardiotomy reservoir (not shown) and then drains into venous reservoir (3). Venous blood is oxygenated (4), temperature adjusted (5), raised to arterial pressure (6), filtered (7-8), and injected into either aorta (10B) or femoral artery (10A). Arterial line pressure is monitored (9). Note that items 3, 4, and 5 are often single integral units. (Modified from Y. Nose. *The Oxygenator.* St. Louis: Mosby, 1973.)

total circulatory arrest be employed? Will special efforts be necessary to provide protection for the heart or other vital organs from ischemia?

The pre-CPB checklist includes (Table 7-1):

1. **Anticoagulation.** Has heparin been given (by the anesthesiologist or surgeon)? Does the patient show **signs** of adequate heparinization? Just because heparin was administered does not guarantee that the patient is anticoagulated! Generally, adequate heparinization requires an activated coagulation time (ACT) of **more than 480 seconds.** The ACT may be accurately measured within 2 minutes of heparin administration.[3] However, when the CPB prime contains additional heparin (e.g., 5000 units), CPB frequently is initiated when the ACT exceeds 300 seconds.

2. **Anesthesia.** Is the patient adequately anesthetized and is adequate muscle relaxation present? Because concentrations of drugs in the

Table 7-1. Prebypass checklist

Anticoagulation—adequate?
Anesthesia—adequate?
Cannulation—proper and patent?
Drips turned off
Monitoring in place and checked
  Pressure transducers
  Temperatures
  Foley catheter
Pupils inspected

blood are diluted by the prime when CPB begins, it is often necessary to give supplemental doses of IV anesthetics and muscle relaxants immediately prior to CPB.

3. **Cannulation.** Is the aortic cannula positioned within the true **lumen** of the aorta? This placement is documented by examining the pressure waveform within the arterial cannula (measured by the perfusionist). The aortic pressure should be **pulsatile** and should **correlate** with the radial arterial pressure after correcting for the vertical height difference between the pump's pressure transducer and the right atrium (1 mm Hg = 1.3 cm H_2O). Are any bubbles evident within the cannula? Check for equality of both **carotid pulses** because the cannula may be obstructing carotid flow (especially if a straight or unflanged aortic cannula is used; see sec. III.A).

4. **Drips.** Once the patient is heparinized, all IV lines may be closed to prevent unnecessary hemodilution. Hypovolemia usually can be managed by infusing prime solution from the CPB pump intermittently in 100-ml boluses once the arterial cannula has been inserted, debubbled, and unclamped. Be aware that pump prime boluses may induce myocardial ischemia or dysrhythmias because the fluid injected into the aortic root enters the coronary arteries without much dilution and may be cold and unoxygenated. Anti-ischemia drugs often are continued until aortic clamping.

5. **Monitoring**
   a. Check the zero and calibration of the arterial pressure transducer.
   b. Insert a nasopharyngeal temperature probe **prior** to heparinization.
   c. Empty the Foley catheter drainage bag or urimeter device because it is important to determine urine output *during* CPB.
   d. If present, the **Paceport** Swan-Ganz pacing wire should be withdrawn out of the right ventricle prior to the surgeon's lifting the heart to prevent ventricular perforation.

6. **Pupils.** Both of the patient's eyes should be examined prior to CPB so that acute **changes** in pupil size or conjunctival chemosis (edema), which may occur on commencing CPB, can be properly interpreted.

II. **Practical aspects of anesthetic management**
   A. **Initial bypass checklist.** During the first 30–60 seconds after initiation of CPB, the anesthesiologist should carefully investigate the items described in Table 7-2.
   B. **The CPB sequence**
      1. **Typical CABG operation.** A typical coronary artery bypass operation proceeds as follows: Hypothermic total CPB is initiated, and when ventricular fibrillation is induced by the cold, the aorta is cross-clamped, and cardioplegic solution is infused through the aortic root to arrest the heart. The distal saphenous vein grafts are placed on

Table 7-2. Initial CPB checklist

Face: Examine for color, temperature, plethora, edema, symmetry

Eyes: Examine pupils for size and symmetry, and conjunctiva for chemosis (edema) and injection

Pump lines: Arteriovenous color difference should be visible

Arterial blood pressure: Normally 30–60 mm Hg initially

Pulmonary artery pressure: If monitored, should be < 15 mm Hg mean

Central venous pressure (CVP): Should be < 5 mm Hg

Examine the heart: Distention, contractility, etc.

Stop ventilation when PA blood flow ceases.

---

the most severely diseased coronary arteries first, to facilitate administration of additional cardioplegic solution (via the vein graft) *distal* to the stenoses. The internal mammary artery anastomosis (if used) is constructed last owing to its fragility and short length. Rewarming begins when the final distal anastomosis is started. The aorta is unclamped, and a partial aortic clamp is applied, permitting construction of proximal vein graft anastomoses during rewarming while cardioplegic solution is being washed out of the heart. When it is sufficiently warm, the heart is defibrillated, and the surgeon continues completing the grafts. Total CPB continues until the heart is reperfused from its new blood supply. Finally, when the patient is adequately rewarmed, the coronary artery grafts are completed, epicardial pacing wires are placed, and CPB is then terminated.

2. **Typical aortic valve replacement/repair operation.** After initiation of CPB and application of the aortic cross clamp, the aortic root is opened, and cardioplegic solution is infused into each coronary ostium under direct vision (to prevent retrograde filling of the LV with cardioplegic solution through an insufficient aortic valve). If regurgitation is minimal, cardioplegia may be administered through the aortic root as described above. The valve is repaired or replaced. Rewarming commences during valve replacement. The heart is irrigated to remove air or tissue debris, and the aortotomy is closed except for a vent. The patient then is placed in steep head-down position, the aortic cross clamp is removed, and the heart is defibrillated. Final de-airing occurs as venous drainage to the pump is retarded, the heart fills and begins to eject (partial CPB), and air is aspirated through the aortic vent, an LV vent, or a needle placed in the apex of the heart. During de-airing, the lungs are ventilated vigorously to help flush bubbles out of pulmonary veins and the heart chambers.

3. **Typical mitral valve replacement/repair operation.** This operation is similar to aortic valve surgery (see **2.** above) except that the left atrium is opened instead of the aorta and the cardioplegic infusion can take place through the aortic root. The valve is replaced or repaired, and a large vent tube is passed through the mitral valve into the LV to prevent ejection of blood into the aorta until de-airing is completed. After thorough irrigation of the field and closure of the atriotomy except for the LV vent, the patient is placed in a steep head-down position, and the cross clamp is removed. The heart is defibrillated, and de-airing occurs as described above. Finally, the LV vent is removed, and de-airing is completed.

4. **Typical combined valve/CABG operation.** Usually the distal vein-graft anastomoses are created first, to permit cardioplegia of the

myocardium distal to severe coronary stenoses. Also, lifting the heart to access the posterior-wall vessels can disrupt myocardium if an artificial valve has been inserted. Next, the valve is operated on, and the operation proceeds as described above.

C. **Maintenance of bypass: checklist.** During CPB the following items should be evaluated intermittently.

1. **Anticoagulation.** The activated coagulation time (ACT) or a similar rapid test of anticoagulation (e.g., Hepcon) must periodically confirm adequate anticoagulation (e.g., ACT > 480 seconds). The ACT should be checked after initiating CPB and every 30–60 minutes thereafter. During periods of **normothermia,** heparin elimination is faster, so prolonged periods of normothermic CPB are much more likely to require heparin supplementation. Additional heparin is usually given in 5000- to 10,000-unit increments, and the ACT is repeated to confirm the response.

2. **Blood-gas and acid-base status** should be checked soon after initiation of CPB and at least every 30–60 minutes thereafter. A continuous blood gas monitoring system should be correlated initially with standard blood gas electrodes during CPB. Arterial oxygen tension (PaO_2) is usually maintained between 100 and 300 mm Hg, and desired mixed venous oxygen tension (PvO_2) values are greater than 30–40 mm Hg (measured at 37°C). For discussion of α-stat and pH-stat acid-base management, see Chapter 20.

3. **Anesthetic depth** should be sufficient (1) to suppress hypertensive or tachycardic responses to surgical stimuli, and (2) to prevent awareness (as assessed ideally by periodic tests of responsiveness, e.g., requesting patient to open eyes). Potent anesthetics (e.g., isoflurane, enflurane) may be administered by connecting a vaporizer to the oxygenator gas inlet. Nitrous oxide is *never* used during CPB because air emboli would enlarge rapidly. Intravenous agents (i.e., narcotics, benzodiazepines, barbiturates, scopolamine) are best administered into the venous blood reservoir. Because hypothermia itself reduces minimal alveolar concentration (MAC) and neuronal activity, additional anesthetic drugs are most commonly required during **warm** periods at the beginning and end of CPB.

4. **Ventilation** of the lungs should cease when **total** CPB begins. This is identified by loss of LV and right ventricle (RV) ejection (flat arterial and pulmonary artery (PA) pressure waveforms). Application of continuous positive airway pressure (CPAP) (2–5 cm H_2O) during total CPB is advocated by some to keep the lungs expanded but probably has little effect. Anesthetic **vaporizers** on the anesthesia machine should be turned off. During **partial** bypass (with ejection), occasional ventilation with 100% oxygen may be needed to ensure that blood traversing the lung is oxygenated, although all of the body's carbon dioxide elimination continues to be performed by the artificial lung. A **pulse oximeter** during partial CPB or pulsatile perfusion can be helpful to identify pulmonary shunting or oxygenator difficulties because arterial blood gases measured at the CPB pump will **not** identify arterial desaturation caused by pulmonary shunt in the patient during partial CPB!

5. **Paralysis** should be sufficient to prevent (1) unconscious movement; (2) respiration (with risk of air entrainment by negative pulmonary venous pressure if cardiac structures are open); and (3) shivering (which increases body oxygen consumption). However, it may be useful to allow retention of a small degree of neuromuscular function sufficient to permit eye opening when testing for intraoperative awareness.

6. **Electrocardiogram (ECG).** Ventricular fibrillation usually occurs at least twice during CPB—once with cooling and once with rewarming of the heart. Onset of **ventricular fibrillation** should be promptly identified and the surgeon informed. When ventricular fibrillation occurs during cooling, appropriate management usually consists in application of the aortic cross clamp with administration of cardioplegia, but sometimes defibrillation is used until an intracardiac vent can be placed. During periods of myocardial arrest, the appearance of electrical activity should be communicated to the surgeon because additional cardioplegia may be indicated. The onset of fibrillation during rewarming usually is treated with defibrillation with or without lidocaine administration because fibrillation depletes myocardial energy stores more quickly than a spontaneous cardiac rhythm. Atrial and ventricular **ectopic beats** occur frequently with cardiac manipulation. Significant ectopy requires therapy only if it persists during unstimulated periods and it is not due to metabolic abnormalities.

7. **Urine production** should be identified and quantitated as a sign of adequate renal perfusion and to assist in appropriate fluid management by the perfusionist. Urine flow rates of 300–1000 ml/hr are commonly seen in hemodilution, especially if mannitol is present in the priming solution. Oliguria ($<$ 1 ml/kg/hr) should prompt an investigation because it may indicate inadequate renal perfusion (see sec. **IV.C.1.b.** below).

8. **Temperature** should be monitored in at least two locations during CPB.

   a. **Core temperature** monitors the well-perfused organs (nasopharyngeal or tympanic membrane probes reflect brain temperature; bladder probe reflects renal temperature **only** if urine flow is adequate and should not be relied on during CPB). Slowed nasopharyngeal cooling could signify impaired cerebral blood flow.

   b. **Shell temperature** monitors the relatively poorly perfused muscle-fat tissues that constitute most of the body's mass and thermal inertia. A rectal probe or skeletal muscle needle sensor measures shell temperature. Because hypothermia induces vasoconstriction in peripheral beds, cooling and rewarming tend to be quite nonuniform during CPB. Thus large gradients (8–10°C or more) often develop between core and shell temperature during cooling.

   c. **Esophageal and pulmonary artery temperature.** A pulmonary arterial thermistor receives little blood flow during total CPB, and esophageal temperature is affected by ice in the pericardial space, making these ineffective sites of temperature monitoring during CPB.

   d. Temperature during initial CPB cooling should decrease faster in the core (i.e., nasopharyngeal temperature) than in the shell (i.e., rectal temperature).

   e. **Rewarming** is usually associated with large gradients between shell and core temperatures due to rapid distribution of warm blood to the well-perfused core organs and reduced flow to peripheral areas owing to vasoconstriction. Administration of vasodilator drugs such as nitroprusside often can hasten rewarming. The perfusionist must not warm the arterial blood too quickly because oxygen becomes less soluble in blood as temperature increases. Thus, rapid rewarming can cause gas bubble formation.

III. **Potential bypass catastrophes.** The safe conduct of perfusion requires vigilance on the part of the anesthesiologist, working in conjunction with the cardiac surgeon and perfusionist, to ensure that perfusion-related problems are diagnosed early and managed quickly. The following complications must be actively searched for during initiation of CPB. They may, however, occur at any time during CPB.

A. Malposition of arterial ("return") cannula. The CPB pump may be expelling blood into undesired locations. Examples include:

1. Aortic dissection

    a. Etiology. Either the cannula orifice is situated within the arterial wall, not in the true lumen, or a dissection was created during the cannulation process.

    b. Prevention is primarily surgical. However, the degree of damage can be markedly reduced if bypass is not initiated into an aortic false lumen. Thus, the perfusionist should always measure the arterial cannula pressure waveform, making sure it is **pulsatile** and that pressure **correlates** with the radial or femoral arterial monitoring line (after correcting for the height difference between the CPB pump and patient) before starting CPB.

    c. Diagnosis

      (1) Occlusion of the arterial true lumen may cause low or zero blood pressure to be measured by the radial or femoral arterial monitoring catheter.

      (2) Perfusionist detects inappropriately high arterial "line" pressure. Ischemia or aortic insufficiency may occur.

      (3) Organ hypoperfusion—oliguria, pupil asymmetry—may be evident.

      (4) Visual inspection or palpation of the aorta may reveal the diagnosis.

    d. Management

      (1) Discontinue CPB.

      (2) Surgeon must reposition or replace the arterial cannula.

      (3) Surgical repair of aortic dissection may be necessary, especially if origin of a critical artery is occluded (e.g., coronary).

2. Carotid or innominate artery hyperperfusion

    a. Etiology. Most or all of the pump outflow can be directed into a carotid artery, usually on the right side (Fig. 7-2). Similar effects may be seen if a jet of blood is directed into a carotid artery. Deleterious effects include cerebral edema or arterial rupture due to high perfusion pressure, or creation of an intimal flap that obstructs arterial flow.

    b. Prevention. Surgeon's vigilance, anesthesiologist's checking for bilateral carotid pulses after cannulation, and use of a short aortic cannula with a flange may help prevent this complication.

    c. Diagnosis

      (1) Ipsilateral blanching of face (transient—not seen if blood is present in CPB priming solution)

      (2) Ipsilateral pupillary dilation

      (3) Ipsilateral conjunctival chemosis (edema)

      (4) Low blood pressure measured by left radial or femoral arterial catheter (a right radial catheter may show **hypertension**).

    d. Management

      (1) Surgeon must reposition the arterial cannula.

      (2) Consider measures to reduce cerebral edema (e.g., mannitol, head-up position)

B. Reversed cannulation

1. Etiology. The pump circuit's venous drainage tubing is accidentally connected to the aorta, and the arterial return pump line is attached to the right atrium or vena cava.

    Blood is sucked out of the aorta, causing arterial hypotension, and is infused into the vena cava at high pressures. High venous pressures and low aortic pressures may allow some organs to be

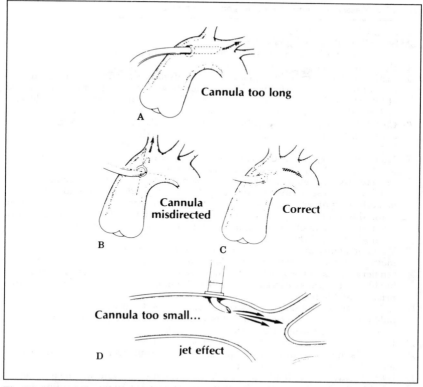

Fig. 7-2. Potential aortic cannulation problems. *A*. Cannula extends into carotid owing to excessive length, causing excessive carotid blood flow. *B*. Angle of cannula insertion is improper, also causing carotid hyperperfusion. *C*. Correct placement. *D*. Cannula diameter is too small; high-velocity jet of blood may damage intima and occlude a vessel. (From W.Y. Moores. Cardiopulmonary Bypass Strategies in Patients with Severe Aortic Disease. In J. R. Utley [ed.], *Pathophysiology and Techniques of Cardiopulmonary Bypass,* Vol. 2. Baltimore: Williams & Wilkins, 1983. P. 190. With permission.)

perfused retrograde, but high pressures may rupture veins. Of greatest risk is bubble formation within the aorta causing air embolization when anterograde perfusion is established.

2. Prevention. Make sure that the arterial cannula shows pulsatile pressure that correlates with the pressure monitoring line. Trace pump lines onto field. Ensure that the tubing is connected properly to the pump and that roller head is not set for "reverse" rotation.

3. Diagnosis
   a. Arterial hypotension, which may be extreme
   b. Facial edema and conjunctival chemosis, which usually is severe
   c. High central venous pressure (CVP) (depending on exact position of CVP line and pump cannulae)
   d. In infants, tense bulging fontanelle
   e. Flaccid aorta and tense vena cava by palpation.

4. Management
   a. Discontinue CPB.

Table 7-3. Massive gas embolism emergency protocol

1. **Stop CPB** immediately
2. Steep **Trendelenburg** position
3. Remove aortic cannula—**vent air** from aortic cannulation site
4. **De-air** arterial cannula and pump line
5. Institute hypothermic **retrograde SVC perfusion** by connecting arterial pump line to the superior vena caval cannula with caval tape tightened. Blood at 20–24°C is injected into SVC at 1–2 liters/min or more, and air plus blood is drained from aortic root cannulation site to the pump (Fig. 7-3)
6. **Carotid compression** is performed intermittently during retrograde SVC perfusion to allow retrograde purging of air from the *vertebral* arteries (see Fig. 7-4)
7. Maintain retrograde SVC perfusion for at least 1–2 min. Continue for an additional 1–2 min if air continues to exit from aorta
8. In **extensive** systemic air injection accidents in which emboli to splanchnic, renal, or femoral circulation are suspected, **retrograde IVC perfusion** may be performed **after** head de-airing procedures are completed. This is performed while the *carotid arteries are clamped* and the patient is in *head-up position* to facilitate removal of air through the aortic root vent but prevent reembolization of the brain
9. When no additional air can be expelled, **resume anterograde CPB,** maintaining hypothermia at 20°C for at least 40–45 min. Lowering patient temperature is important because increased gas solubility helps to resorb bubbles and because decreased metabolic demands may limit ischemic damage prior to bubble resorption
10. Induce **hypertension** with vasoconstrictor drugs. Hydrostatic pressure shrinks bubbles; also, bubbles occluding arterial bifurcations are pushed into one vessel, opening the other branch
11. Express coronary air by massage and needle venting
12. **Steroids** may be administered, although this is controversial; usual dose of methylprednisolone is 30 mg/kg
13. **Barbiturate coma** should be considered if the myocardium will be able to tolerate the significant negative inotropy. Thiopental 10 mg/kg loading dose plus 1–3 mg/kg/hr infusion may be used empirically. If EEG monitoring is available, titration of barbiturate to an EEG burst/suppression (1 burst/min) pattern is preferable.
14. Patient is weaned from CPB
15. Continue ventilating patient with **100% O_2** for at least 6 hrs to maximize blood-alveolar gradient for elimination of N_2.
16. **Hyperbaric chamber** (if locally available) can accelerate resorption of residual bubbles. However, the risk of moving a critically ill patient must be weighed against the potential benefits.

Note: This protocol should be reviewed together by all members of the cardiac team every 3 months.
SVC = superior vena cava, CPB = cardiopulmonary bypass, IVC = inferior vena cava, EEG = electroencephalogram.
Source: Modified from N. L. Mills, and J. L. Ochsner. Massive air embolism during cardiopulmonary bypass: Causes, prevention, and management. *J. Thorac. Cardiovasc. Surg.* 80:712, 1980. With permission.

    b. Place patient in steep Trendelenburg position.
    c. Disconnect and carefully inspect cannulae for air; if air is found, execute **air embolism protocol** (Table 7-3).
    d. After de-airing the aorta and arterial cannula, reverse the tubing connections and resume CPB.

    e. Consider taking steps to reduce cerebral damage (mannitol, steroids, barbiturates, etc.).

C. Obstruction to venous return

  1. Etiology. Reduced blood flow draining into the pump.

    a. Air-lock. The presence of large air bubbles within the venous ("drainage") cannula or tubing prevents blood flow due to surface tension and the low pressure gradient.

    b. Mechanical. Lifting of the heart within the chest by the surgeon often impedes venous drainage. The venous cannulae may be too small. Also, a kinked or malpositioned cannula or the presence of a thrombus or tumor mass will diminish venous blood flow.

    c. Consequences. CPB pump outflow must be reduced immediately to avoid emptying the reservoir. Reduced organ perfusion and organ damage result from reduced perfusion pressure gradient. The brain, liver, and kidneys are particularly vulnerable.

  2. Prevention. Look for large bubbles in the venous pump line and for high regional venous pressures in patient. Always maintain adequate heparinization.

  3. Diagnosis

    a. Decreasing venous blood reservoir volume. If the perfusionist does not reduce the pump flow rate **immediately,** the reservoir may empty with risk of massive arterial air embolism.

    b. Increased CVP. The surgeon may have placed separate superior vena cava (SVC) and inferior vena cava (IVC) cannulae and may tighten the "caval tapes," thereby preventing vena caval blood from entering the right atrium (total CPB). In this case, a CVP monitoring catheter with its orifice within the right atrium will show a **low** CVP pressure even if poor venous drainage conditions exist. If necessary, monitoring of SVC pressures can be easily achieved by attaching the "side-port" of the PA catheter introducer cannula (if used) to a transducer.

    c. Oliguria, conjunctival chemosis, or **injection,** facial plethora, bulging fontanelle. High venous pressures are seen upstream from the obstruction, which can cause organ ischemia by reducing the arteriovenous perfusion pressure. Obstruction may be **regional** (i.e., affecting only the SVC flow), or **global.** It is very difficult to diagnose isolated inferior vena caval flow obstruction.

  4. Management

    a. Reduce pump flow or suspend CPB until cause is found.

    b. Air-lock. Surgeon propels air through tubing by progressively raising and tapping the tubing downstream to the bubble. Search for the source of venous air (is a CVP catheter open to air?).

D. Massive gas embolism. Most massive gas emboli[8] consist of air, although oxygen emboli can be generated by a defective or clotted oxygenator. (For further discussion of this and CPB safety devices see Chapter 19.) The use of a vented arterial line filter on the pump is an important safety device that can help prevent gas embolization; its routine use is strongly recommended. Because of the high risk of stroke, myocardial infarction, or death after massive gas embolism, **prevention** is of utmost importance.

  1. Etiology

    a. Inattention to oxygenator reservoir level: Air is pumped from empty reservoir. Vortexing can permit air embolism when blood level is very low. **This is the most important cause for bypass catastrophes.**

    b. Ejection of blood from heart prior to de-airing procedures; opening a beating heart.

    c. Reversed roller-pump flow in vent line or arterial cannula.

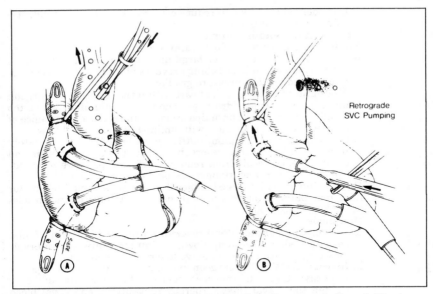

Fig. 7-3. Retrograde perfusion in the treatment of massive gas embolism. *A.* Massive arterial gas embolism has occurred. *B.* Bubbles in the arterial tree are flushed out by performing retrograde body perfusion *into* the superior vena cava by connecting de-aired arterial pump line to superior vena cava (SVC) cannula (and tightening caval tapes). Blood and bubbles exit aorta from the cannulation wound. (From N.L. Mills, and J.L. Ochsner. Massive air embolism during cardiopulmonary bypass: Causes, prevention, and management. *J. Thorac. Cardiovasc. Surg.* 80:713, 1980. With permission.)

    d. Leak or kink in the negative side of the arterial tubing (prior to or **upstream** from roller pump). Negative (suction) pressure at this site may cavitate gas out of solution or entrain room air.

    e. Clotted oxygenator.

    f. Pressurized cardiotomy reservoir (causing retrograde flow of gas through nonocclusive vent line roller head into heart or aorta).

    g. Runaway pump head (switch inoperative, must unplug pump and crank by hand).

    h. Disconnection, breakage, or detachment of oxygenator or lines during CPB.

    i. Suction deep in pulmonary artery branch entrains air from other branches, and air enters left atrium.

    j. Aortic line not clamped at end of CPB; if pump head accidentally restarted, inadvertent air infusion may occur.

        Other etiologies not isolated to CPB include:

    k. Improper flushing technique for arterial or left atrial pressure monitoring lines.

    l. Paradoxical transfer of venous air across atrial or ventricular septal defect.

  2. Prevention. Vigilance; safety devices present must be **turned on.**

  3. Diagnosis. Visual inspection, signs of myocardial or other organ ischemia, withdrawal of air from arterial pressure monitoring line.

  4. Management. See Table 7-3 and Figs. 7-3 and 7-4.

E. Failure of oxygen supply

  1. Etiology. Inadequate gas flow or hypoxic gas mixture.

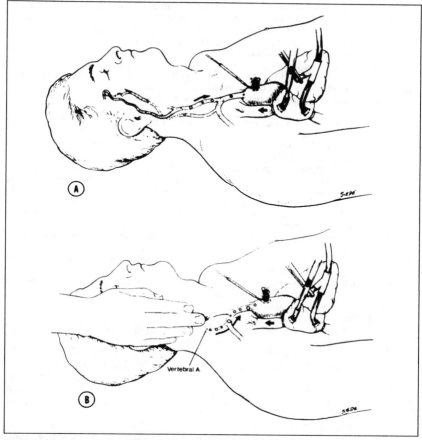

Fig. 7-4. Carotid and vertebral artery de-airing during retrograde perfusion. In the management of massive arterial gas embolism, steep head-down position helps to flush bubbles out of the *carotid arteries*. Application of intermittent pressure to the carotid arteries increases retrograde *vertebral artery* flow, helping to evacuate bubbles. (From N.L. Mills, and J.L. Ochsner. Massive air embolism during cardiopulmonary bypass: Causes, prevention, and management. *J. Thorac. Cardiovasc. Surg.* 80:714, 1980. With permission.)

2. **Prevention.** Vigilance; use of pump arterial line oxygen saturation or PO_2 analyzer; use of oxygen analyzer on pump gas inflow line.

3. **Diagnosis.** Dark blood in arterial cannula (same color as venous cannula blood); blood gas analysis; severe vasodilation.

4. **Management.** Cool patient maximally until oxygen supply is restored; connect a portable oxygen tank to oxygenator if necessary. Remember, **room air or exhaled breath** contains adequate oxygen to help avoid catastrophe if oxygen supply cannot be connected immediately.

F. **Pump or oxygenator failure**

1. **Etiology.** Loss of perfusion can be caused by:

  a. Pump failure. Electrical or mechanical failure, tubing rupture or disconnection, automatic shut-off by bubble or reservoir level detector. "Runaway pump head" may raise pump flow to maximum inappropriately, and pump control switch will be inoperative.

  b. Oxygenator failure may be due to manufacturing defect, clogging due to clot (see sec. **III.G.** below), disruption of shell (trauma, spill of liquid volatile anesthetic), leakage of water from heat exchanger into blood, a too-low occlusion of roller-pump, causing excessive regurgitation and inadequate forward flow, depletion of defoamer.

2. Prevention. Vigilance, availability of backup equipment, adequate heparinization

3. Diagnosis. Blood gas abnormality, acidosis, hypotension, blood leak, excessive hemolysis

4. Management. If body perfusion will be low or absent for more than a minute or two, and if patient cannot be immediately weaned from CPB, then hypothermia to 18–20°C should be induced and consideration given to brain, myocardial, and renal protection, including packing head and heart in ice. Open cardiac massage may be necessary, depending on the stage of the operation.

  a. Pump failure. CPB pumps can be hand-cranked until replacement is obtained or tubing replaced. In case of runaway pump head, the CPB machine must be unplugged and the tubing switched to a different roller head.

  b. Oxygenator failure. For severe failure, oxygenator must be replaced. Attempt to preserve critical organs first.

G. Clotted oxygenator or circuit

  1. Etiology

  a. Inadequate heparinization (heparin must be exerting adequate **effect** regardless of dose or plasma concentration).

  b. Direct administration of fresh frozen plasma to CPB reservoir during CPB (this may present less risk with a bubble oxygenator).

  2. Prevention. This lethal catastrophe should never occur if the patient's coagulation status is assessed prior to initiating CPB and then at frequent intervals thereafter. It can be diagnosed by visual inspection of clot, air exiting from the bubble oxygenator, high arterial cannula pressure (evidence of partially clotted arterial line filter). **Fresh frozen plasma** should be heparinized in the bag (1000 units/250-ml bag) *prior* to administering it into the venous reservoir.

  3. Management

  a. Stop CPB.

  b. If patient is not cold, perform open CPR, apply topical hypothermia.

  c. Reheparinize patient using different lot of heparin.

  d. Replace oxygenator and CPB circuit.

  e. Follow massive gas embolization emergency protocol, if appropriate (Table 7-3).

IV. Differential diagnosis of abnormalities during CPB

  A. Cardiovascular abnormalities

  1. Hypotension. During CPB, systemic vascular resistance (SVR) may be calculated in the usual fashion.

$$\text{SVR (dynes} \cdot \text{sec} \cdot \text{cm}^{-5}) = [\,(\text{MAP} - \text{CVP}) \times 80]/F$$

where F = pump flow rate in liters/min
MAP = mean arterial pressure in mm Hg.

Normally during CPB without venous obstruction, CVP = 0, and this term may be ignored. Always check with the perfusionist before assuming that hypotension is due to a low SVR—the flow rate may have been decreased for some reason!

a. **Low SVR** may be caused by vasodilation due to drugs, anesthetics, metabolic factors, or hyperthermia. Low blood viscosity due to hemodilution will decrease the effective SVR even though blood vessel caliber is unchanged (this often is the cause of the immediate decrease in blood pressure seen on commencing CPB with hemodilution).

b. **Low perfusion flow rate** may be due to an arterial cannula that is clamped or kinked, inadequate roller pump head occlusion causing regurgitation, error in pump flowmeter calibration, or the perfusionist not utilizing a proper "calculated" flow based on temperature and body size.

c. **Cannula disaster** may be due to aortic dissection, carotid or innominate cannulation, or reversed cannulation.

d. **Measurement error** may be due to transducer zero drift, calibration error, clot in monitoring line or transducer, tubing disconnection and so on. (Note: a bubble in the monitoring line should not change the **mean** pressure.)

2. **Hypertension**

a. **High SVR.** Causes include vasoconstriction due to catecholamine release and hypothermia after initiation of CPB and after rewarming begins, light plane of anesthesia, awareness, drugs, hypothermia, metabolic factors (hyperoxia).

b. **Excessive perfusion flow** rate (see sec. **A.1.b.** above).

c. **Innominate artery cannulation** with right radial arterial pressure monitoring.

d. **Measurement error** (see sec. **A.1.d.** above).

3. **High pressure in arterial pump line.** Normally the line pressure is up to three times patient pressure owing to high resistance in tubing and arterial cannula.

a. **Occlusion** may be due to a kinked, clamped, or occluded arterial cannula; carotid or innominate artery cannulation; aortic dissection.

b. **Clotted arterial filter.** Arterial filters should always have a bypass loop for use after restoring adequate anticoagulation.

c. **High SVR in patient.**

d. **Measurement error** (see sec. **A.1.d.** above).

4. **High pressure in pulmonary artery (PA) or left atrium (LA).** Whenever there is doubt about the reason for high PA pressure during CPB, ask the surgeon to palpate the left ventricle because LV distention is the most serious cause of PA hypertension during CPB.

a. **Distention of left ventricle** with retrograde transmission of pressure to the lung vasculature.

(1) **Consequences** of LV distention include

(a) Myocardial ischemia and subendocardial necrosis due to compression by LV cavitary fluid under pressure; this lowers the coronary perfusion pressure to as low as zero.

(b) Warming of the myocardium despite cardioplegia.

(c) Myocardial damage due to stretching; pulmonary edema.

(2) **Etiology** of LV distention includes

(a) Inadequate venous drainage (blood traversing lungs).

(b) Aortic insufficiency with fluid entering LV retrograde across aortic valve (prior to aortic cross-clamping or during cardioplegic solution infusion into aortic root).

          (c) Blood entering LV through bronchial arterial flow, septal defects, pulmonary-systemic shunts, thebesian drainage, coronary sinus effluent, or pericardial collateral vessels.

       (3) Management of LV distention. Improve venous drainage, insert vent in LV or PA or infuse cardioplegic solution into individual coronary ostia. In certain cases deliberate hypotension or total circulatory arrest may be necessary (e.g., for excessive systemic-to-pulmonary collaterals).

    b. Collapse of nonperfused lung around tip of catheter during total CPB may produce an "overwedge" pressure tracing.

      (1) Diagnosis. Inability to withdraw blood from catheter on *gentle* aspiration, or surgeon palpates a flaccid LV.

      (2) Management. Withdraw PA catheter several centimeters or until pressure approaches zero.

    c. Kinked or compressed PA catheter. The PA catheter may be compressed against the clavicle by a sternal retractor (especially when introduced through the subclavian or external jugular route); it may not be possible to withdraw blood from the catheter.

  5. High CVP may be caused by

    a. Poor venous drainage (see sec. **III.C**).

    b. Artifact caused by surgeon tightening "caval tape" around the CVP catheter orifice; this is diagnosed by an inability to withdraw blood from the catheter.

  6. Slowed nasopharyngeal or tympanic cooling may indicate impaired brain cooling. It may be due to

    a. Inadequate carotid artery perfusion due to

      (1) Improper cannulation.

      (2) Carotid occlusion(s).

      (3) Increased intracranial pressure (hematoma?).

      (4) Increased SVC pressure impeding venous drainage and lowering perfusion pressure gradient.

    b. Temperature sensor displaced or calibration error.

  7. Slowed body rewarming may be caused by

    a. Inadequate pump flow rate.

    b. Excessive vasoconstriction—use vasodilator drugs.

    c. Temperature sensor displaced or calibration error.

    d. Failure of heat exchanger.

B. Respiratory and metabolic abnormalities. For a detailed discussion of oxygenation assessment during CPB see Chap. 20.

  1. Hypoxemia of arterial blood may be caused by

    a. Transpulmonary shunt. During partial CPB desaturated blood may be ejected from the LV unless the patient's lungs are ventilated. Systemic arterial hypoxemia may be missed unless the blood sample is drawn from the **patient** instead of from the bypass pump.

    b. Gas supply to artificial lung. Hypoxic gas mixture or inadequate flow rate may be present.

    c. Dysfunction of artificial lung. For bubble oxygenators, excessive filling of the blood reservoir reduces the amount of oxygenation that normally takes place in the debubbling section.

    d. Note: During hypothermia, the diagnosis of hypoxemia should probably be made using the PO_2 calculated for the patient's actual temperature, since this value will be *lower* than the value measured at 37°C by the blood-gas analyzer.

  2. Hypoxemia of mixed venous blood may be caused by

    a. Decreased oxygen delivery causing increased oxygen extraction from blood by tissues. Possible causes include

      (1) Hypoxemia of *arterial* blood.

  (2) Low pump flow rate (see sec. **III.A.2** above).
  (3) Regional hypoperfusion.
  (4) Excessive hemodilution.
  (5) Increased oxygen-hemoglobin affinity reducing oxygen release
   to tissues.
 b. Increased body oxygen consumption rate. Causes include
  (1) Hyperthermia.
  (2) Shivering (may be subclinical).
  (3) Malignant hyperthermia.
  (4) Thyrotoxicosis.
3. Lactic acidosis may be due to
 a. Decreased oxygen delivery to tissues causing anaerobic metabolism of glucose.
 b. Improved perfusion of previously ischemic tissue; tissues receiving little perfusion may accumulate large quantities of lactic acid that is not washed out into the circulation until regional perfusion improves at a later time.
4. Hypercarbia may be due to
 a. Inadequate fresh gas inflow rate to artificial lung.
 b. Use of carbon dioxide-containing gas mixture (pH-stat control).
 c. Increased body carbon dioxide production rate.
 d. Buffering of lactic acid by bicarbonate releases CO_2.
5. Spontaneous respiratory effort is due to
 a. Hypercarbia.
 b. Inadequate narcosis.
 c. Inadequate paralysis.
 d. Awareness.
C. Renal abnormalities
 1. Oliguria may result from
  a. Postrenal problems. These must be ruled out first. Kinked Foley tubing is the most common etiology; ureteral, bladder outlet, urethral, or other Foley tubing obstruction (e.g., blood clots) may be involved.
  b. Decreased renal perfusion with reduced glomular filtration rate. This situation may result from
   (1) Inadequate pump flow rate.
   (2) Relative arterial hypotension due to low SVR (urine output may increase with phenylephrine-induced pressor effect).
   (3) Nonpulsatile perfusion.
   (4) Renal vasoconstriction by drugs.
   (5) Increased IVC pressure.
  c. Hormone-induced free-water retention.
  d. Renal failure.
  e. Hypothermia.
 2. Hemoglobinuria or hematuria. Whenever pink or red urine is noted, a test should be performed to distinguish **hemoglobinuria** (free hemoglobin in urine) from **hematuria** (red blood cells in urine). A laboratory urinalysis can achieve this, or a sample can be quickly centrifuged and the supernatant examined. Clear supernatant implies hematuria; pink supernatant defines hemoglobinuria.
   A quick screening test for red or pink urine may be less accurate: *cloudy* urine is usually hematuria, and *clear* urine is usually hemoglobinuria.
  a. Hemoglobinuria may be caused by
   (1) Hemolysis due to pump-sucker trauma or the CPB pump (most common).
   (2) Blood transfusion reaction.
   (3) Hyperoxia.

(4) Water leak from heat exchanger into blood (hyponatremia also present).

b. Management of hemoglobinuria

(1) Promote a diuresis using mannitol, loop diuretics, dopamine, vasodilators, or vasoconstrictors; consider elevating pump flow.

(2) Measure urine pH and administer systemic sodium bicarbonate if necessary to maintain an alkaline urine pH (avoids acid hematin formation).

c. Hematuria may be due to urinary tract hemorrhage; to manage it, irrigate the Foley tubing.

V. Blood pressure control during CPB

A. Desired blood pressure during various phases of CPB.

Blood pressure management during CPB is controversial. At one extreme, some feel that pressure is irrelevant during CPB as long as the pump provides adequate flow. Others believe, however, that blood pressure should be kept within a certain range by administering vasodilators or vasoconstrictor drugs. This section is written from the viewpoint that provided pump flow is adequate, blood pressure is not important in determining **global** perfusion during CPB but that it may be significant for providing certain **regional** vascular beds with adequate perfusion. Blood pressure control may be especially important during certain periods of CPB.

1. Phase of initial total bypass: warm, aorta not clamped

a. Rationale for regulating MAP: altered regional blood flow autoregulation

(1) **Critical organ stenosis.** In this phase of CPB, the heart is still beating and is still being perfused from the aorta, but the heart is collapsed with low LV systolic wall tension. Although the oxygen consumption of a beating empty heart is less than that of a beating filled heart, myocardial ischemia may still develop given the proper pathology. Thus, if critical coronary stenoses are present, coronary autoregulation may **not** be able to maintain flow to the distal myocardium during hypotension because the distal bed will be maximally vasodilated already. Thus, flow will be pressure dependent. The same mechanism would be active if cerebrovascular or renovascular stenoses were present.

(2) **Chronic hypertension** tends to shift toward higher blood pressures the range of pressures at which blood flow is autoregulated. At pressures lower than these, regional blood flow will become pressure dependent at a value less than the autoregulated flow. This mechanism is particularly important in determining brain and kidney perfusion.

(3) **Myocardial hypertrophy** increases oxygen demand, but muscle growth often advances faster than development of the blood supply, thus altering the ability of coronary artery autoregulation to provide adequate flow at low pressures.

b. Management

(1) **Lower limit of MAP.** Patients with impaired organ flow autoregulation should not be permitted to develop hypotension below a certain critical limit during this phase of CPB. However, it is usually not possible to determine precisely what this lower limit should be.

(2) **Individualization based on cardiac pathology.** Factors to be considered when determining an individual's lower pressure limit include: severity and location of stenoses, collateral flow sources, range of asymptomatic blood pressures preoperatively, extent of hemodilution, heart rate, presence of myocardial hy-

pertrophy, presence of aortic regurgitation, and adequacy of LV drainage.

(3) **Hypothesis testing.** Once an initial value is selected, it should be constantly subjected to hypothesis testing by looking for signs of inadequate regional perfusion at that MAP. Examples include: ischemic electrocardiogram (ECG) changes, loss of urine output, change in electroencephalogram (EEG), or pupil asymmetry.

c. **Practical guidelines.** In the patient without altered flow autoregulation, perfusion generally is maintained at MAP higher than **30–40 mm Hg.** Usually, pediatric patients are permitted to develop even lower MAP without evidence of organ ischemia. However, if evidence of altered flow autoregulation exists (as discussed in sec. **V.A.1.b.** above), then MAP is usually maintained at approximately 70–90 mm Hg during this phase of CPB.

2. **Phase of hypothermic bypass, aorta cross-clamped**

a. **Rationale for regulating MAP.** Because the heart and coronary vasculature are now disconnected from the circulation by the aortic clamp, maintenance of perfusion to other vital organs (brain, kidney) assumes primary importance. **Higher** pressures (MAP>70) often are avoided because of **noncoronary collateral** blood flow into the heart through the pericardium and pulmonary venous drainage. Such collateral flow of relatively warm blood tends to *wash the colder cardioplegic solution out of the heart* and reduces protection against myocardial ischemia.

b. **Practical guidelines.** In patients **without** altered flow autoregulation, blood pressure often is permitted to decrease to as low as 30–40 mm Hg during cold bypass. The presence of **urine production** always is a reassuring sign of renal perfusion, although low or absent urine does not necessarily imply ischemia. If a patient is oliguric at very low perfusion pressures, often raising pressure with a vasoconstrictor will induce a diuresis, presumably as renal perfusion reenters the autoregulatory range. Commonly, **pediatric** patients are permitted to be perfused at pressures as low as 15–20 mm Hg.

3. **Phase of rewarming, aortic side-biting clamp in place**

a. **Rationale for regulating MAP.** A heart with coronary artery disease is **not** receiving any **new** sources of blood during this phase because saphenous vein grafts are not yet connected to the aorta. But flow through the native coronary vasculature has been reestablished. Thus, this situation parallels that of the warm prearrest bypass phase (sec. **V.A.1.** above), and the heart is at risk for ischemia unless an adequate coronary perfusion pressure is supplied. An exception might be patients in whom an internal mammary–coronary connection was created; this connection does not require a proximal anastomosis and provides flow to one coronary artery (and its collateral-linked beds) immediately. The avoidance of high aortic pressures during early **reperfusion** of arrested myocardium may help limit reperfusion damage (see Chap. 21).

b. **Practical guidelines.** As soon as the aortic cross clamp is removed, transient hypotension often occurs (probably due to reopening of the vasodilated coronary bed and washout of metabolites), but this is usually not treated unless it persists for more than several minutes. For patients with significant coronary stenoses not supplied by a patent internal mammary graft or for those with other organs with abnormal flow autoregulation, the MAP during this phase of CPB often is controlled in the 70–90 mm Hg range.

4. Phase of warm bypass, aorta not clamped, heart revascularized
   a. Rationale for regulating MAP. The SVR during warm CPB usually is similar to the SVR in the patient after termination of CPB. Therefore, during this preweaning stage it may be useful to adjust the SVR pharmacologically into the normal range. In this way, very low or high blood pressures can be avoided immediately after CPB termination.
   b. Practical guidelines. During this phase of CPB, the MAP often is adjusted so that it is similar to or slightly lower than values desired after CPB, common adult values being 50–80 mm Hg. Remember that once the heart begins to eject blood prior to weaning, the MAP will rise in relation to the height of the systolic pressure above the mean pressure.

B. Methods of adjusting blood pressure during CPB
  1. Varying pump flow rate. Although it is possible to vary the pump flow rate as necessary to keep blood pressure at desired levels, this is rarely appropriate. Increasing pump flow rate to compensate for low SVR usually is **not** performed because it involves added trauma to blood elements. Decreasing pump flow to compensate for high SVR is not the best form of management because tissue perfusion will suffer and metabolic acidosis will ensue. However, in cases of acute severe vasoconstriction causing mean arterial pressures over 110 mm Hg, it may be useful to reduce pump flow **transiently** until vasodilation can be achieved pharmacologically.
  2. Increasing SVR is the primary means of increasing blood pressure when necessary during CPB. **Alpha-adrenergic agonists** are the drugs most commonly used to raise SVR during CPB. **Phenylephrine** (Neo-Synephrine) is used in 100- to 200-μg bolus doses injected into the oxygenator reservoir and repeated or increased as necessary to achieve the target blood pressure. Rare patients refractory to vasoconstrictor drugs may require 1- to 5-mg boluses to achieve only small rises in SVR. **Methoxamine** (Vasoxyl) and **norepinephrine** (Levophed) are also used occasionally during CPB, although the beta-1 cardiac actions of norepinephrine may be detrimental. Please see Chapter 3 for further details on this and other vasoconstrictor drugs.
  3. Decreasing SVR is the primary means of lowering blood pressure during bypass.
     a. Anesthetics are commonly used to reduce SVR during bypass, even during times when unconsciousness has been ensured by other drugs and hypothermia. **Narcotics** (e.g., fentanyl) and **volatile anesthetics** (e.g., isoflurane) will both achieve vasodilation. However, fentanyl displays tachyphylaxis in its ability to lower SVR; once approximately 100 μg/kg (total dose) has been administered, little or no further effect is produced. Usual adult IV bolus doses during CPB are 250–500 μg. Sufentanil is more effective in lowering SVR than fentanyl; the usual incremental bolus doses during CPB are 2–3 μg/kg with a total dose of 15–20 μg/kg for the entire case.
     b. Volatile anesthetics such as isoflurane produce a reliable dose-dependent vasodilation that is probably a combination of sympatholysis and direct vasodilation. They are administered by calibrated vaporizer in the oxygenator gas inlet line. Usual isoflurane vaporizer settings are 0.5–2.0 vol %. Usually, volatile anesthetics are not administered after aortic cross-clamp removal to ensure adequate time for washout.
     c. Direct vasodilators such as nitroprusside and trimethaphan are useful in controlling SVR and improving perfusion to vasocon-

stricted peripheral vascular beds. **Nitroprusside sodium** (Nipride) is usually administered by infusion into the superior vena cava during bypass. Hypothermia may retard the conversion of cyanide ion to thiocyanate,[9] although production of clinical cyanide toxicity during CPB is rarely seen. Care must be taken to infuse drugs into the bloodstream during CPB and not into the stagnant blood within a cardiac chamber or distal to a caval tape. For example, a drug infused into the RV port of a Paceport catheter will not enter the circulation during total CPB. Usual CPB nitroprusside doses are 1–5 µg/kg/min. **Trimethaphan** (Arfonad) may be administered by IV bolus (1–5 mg) or infusion (0.5–3.0 mg/min).

   d. **Alpha-adrenergic antagonists** will lower SVR and may allow more uniform cooling and rewarming. **Phentolamine** (Regitine) is often used at initiation of pediatric CPB in a bolus dose of 0.5 mg/kg, which appears to last for more than 1 hour.

   e. **Other drugs.** Calcium channel blockers (verapamil IV, nifedipine sublingual) will cause vasodilation, as will the benzodiazepines (diazepam, midazolam) given intravenously. The latter are especially useful in managing hypertensive episodes when awareness cannot be ruled out.

VI. Pharmacology of drugs used during CPB

A. Use of potent anesthetics via pump oxygenator

   a. **Administration.** Potent inhalational anesthetics (e.g., isoflurane) may be administered during CPB using a temperature- and flow-compensating vaporizer placed in the gas inlet line to the oxygenator. Factors affecting the uptake of anesthetic include the gas and blood flow rates, temperature (solubility increases with cold), oxygenator efficiency, and distribution of blood flow. Nitrous oxide should never be used during CPB.

   b. **Filling vaporizers.** Care must be used to avoid spilling liquid anesthetic on the plastic oxygenator shell; rapid dissolution and destruction of the oxygenator have been reported to result.

   c. **Anesthetic washout.** In the near-normothermic patient anesthetic will wash out of the body rapidly because of the relatively high fresh gas flow and blood flow rates. Only 5–15 minutes are usually required to eliminate clinically important anesthetic concentrations unless body stores are unusually large. However, when low gas flow rates are being used (i.e., with membrane oxygenators), the onset and offset of these agents may be slowed[12].

B. Pharmacology of intravenous drugs during CPB

   1. **Pharmacokinetics.** The plasma drug concentrations of numerous drugs can be affected by CPB. CPB factors that are involved include:

   a. **Dilution.** The enlarged circulating blood volume during initiation of CPB dilutes both drugs and plasma proteins and enlarges the volume of distribution. Despite marked decreases in **total** drug concentrations, the pharmacologically active **nonprotein-bound** drug concentration may remain constant because of a decrease in the fraction of drug bound to blood proteins. Example: thiopental.[1]

   b. **Altered elimination.** Due to changes in hepatic, renal, and pulmonary blood flow and enzymatic function, clearance of drugs may be impaired during CPB, especially with hypothermia.

   c. **Extracorporeal absorption.** Drug may be absorbed onto the foreign surfaces comprising the oxygenator and CPB circuit. Examples: fentanyl, nitroglycerin.

   d. **Lung isolation.** During total CPB, the lung is not perfused, making it unavailable for drug or hormonal metabolism. Basic drugs administered during partial CPB may be sequestered in the lung when CPB becomes total. With resumption of pulmonary blood flow at the end of CPB, sudden increases in plasma drug concentrations may occur. Examples: propranolol, fentanyl.

e. **Tissue sequestration.** As blood flow is redistributed during CPB, peripheral tissues binding the drug (e.g., skeletal muscle) become relatively poorly perfused owing to hypothermia. Drugs administered pre-CPB may become "trapped" within tissues and are not released until the peripheral tissues become fully rewarmed. Thus, for drugs given pre-CPB, plasma drug concentrations may decrease, causing the apparent volume of distribution during CPB to rise. Possible examples: dantrolene, digoxin.

2. **Pharmacodynamics.** The **responsiveness** of tissues to a given plasma concentration of a drug may be altered by CPB. Potential causes include hypothermia, electrolyte shifts, and altered hormonal state. Examples: The myocardium may be more sensitive to digoxin after CPB.

3. **Practical considerations.** The pharmacology of most drugs during CPB has not been evaluated sufficiently because knowledge of the nonprotein-bound drug concentrations and their tissue effects is required. Also, there is variability of responses between drugs and for the same drug at different times during CPB. Therefore, the principle of titrating drug dosage to achieve a certain end point is especially important during CPB.

VII. Fluid management during CPB

A. Benefits of hemodilution

1. Hemodilution is defined as a reduction in hemoglobin concentration ([Hb]) caused by addition of nonhemoglobin-containing fluids to the circulating blood volume.

2. Blood viscosity normally increases with cold, causing reduced microcirculatory flow at a constant perfusion pressure during hypothermia. This effect may promote sludging of red blood cells, and could cause organ ischemia.

3. **Hemodilution** lowers **blood viscosity,** counteracting the deleterious viscosity changes caused by hypothermia. Organ blood flow is improved during hypothermia when the [Hb] is kept below approximately 10 g/dl.

4. Blood is not required in the priming solution, avoiding the risks of blood transfusion.

B. Risks of hemodilution

1. **Blood pressure decreases** when CPB commences because dilution markedly reduces blood viscosity.

2. **Lowered colloid oncotic pressure** due to dilution of plasma proteins leads to increased fluid administration requirements and development of tissue edema.

3. **Hemoglobin oxygen saturation** of arterial blood (SaO_2) must be kept near 100% during hemodilution to prevent further decline in blood oxygen transport (O_2 transport = O_2 content × blood flow, where O_2 content = 1.34 × [Hb] × SaO_2 plus a dissolved-O_2 term).

4. **Excessive hemodilution** occurs when blood flow cannot increase further to compensate for the reduction in blood oxygen content; ischemia of critical organs then appears, and signs of anaerobic metabolism may develop. Note that blood oxygen transport should match the normal body oxygen consumption rate ($\dot{V}O_2$).

5. **Increased blood flow.** If [Hb] is reduced by 50% below normal, blood flow must **double** if oxygen transport is to be maintained unchanged. Such a marked rise in flow is not feasible during CPB, hence the importance of combining hemodilution with hypothermia.

6. **Importance of cold.** With hypothermia, body $\dot{V}O_2$ decreases; this means that less oxygen is needed to match body oxygen supply to oxygen demand; once normal body temperature is restored, oxygen transport must also rise, but this may be difficult to achieve when [Hb] is low.

7. **Cold CPB versus warm CPB and post-CPB hemodilution.** Rewarming usually dilates the capacitance vessels in the body, increasing fluid requirements. Often a decision must be made whether to administer additional fluid as blood or blood-free solution. Hemodilution, which is advantageous during hypothermic CPB, may be undesirable during the later normothermic phases of CPB or after termination of CPB (see sec. **C.5.** below). However, despite these concerns, adult patients infrequently receive blood transfusion during CPB.

8. The **limits of hemodilution** cannot be predicted with certainty; most patients with good overall physical status can tolerate hemodilution to [Hb] $\approx$ 7–9 g/dl. Factors that tend to **reduce** the body's ability to tolerate marked reductions include:

    a. **Stenosis** of arteries feeding critical organs; this will prevent blood flow from increasing adequately as [Hb] declines, although the reduction in viscosity accompanying hemodilution helps to increase blood flow past a stenosis.

    b. **Cardiac pump failure** that cannot provide the increased cardiac output necessary to maintain adequate oxygen delivery after CPB.

    c. **Left-shifted oxyhemoglobin dissociation curve** (increased binding of oxygen by hemoglobin). This reduces oxygen release in peripheral tissues; factors contributing to this effect include alkalosis, hypothermia, and decreased 2,3-diphosphoglycerate (DPG) levels.

    d. **Lung disease** that may prevent attainment of 100% SaO_2 following CPB.

C. **Practical fluid management**

1. **"Clear" pump priming solution.** Usually a clear (i.e., nonblood-containing) priming solution is utilized. Typically, this is composed of a buffered electrolyte solution with optional addition of mannitol, heparin, or colloid.

2. **Autotransfusion.** If the [Hb] is sufficiently high, 0.5–1.0 liters of blood may be slowly removed from the patient while the pump prime is being infused to maintain arterial pressure prior to initiating CPB. This anticoagulated autologous blood may be reinfused after CPB, saving platelets and clotting factors. For more details, see Chapter 6.

3. **Blood prime.** Addition of whole blood or packed red blood cells (RBC) to the prime solution is indicated only if use of a clear prime would result in excessive hemodilution. Examples include adults with severe anemia pre-CPB or pediatric patients in whom the pump prime represents a large fraction of the patient's blood volume. For infants receiving a heparinized blood prime, calcium chloride often is added to prevent citrate-induced hypocalcemia on initiating CPB.

4. **Time course of hemodilution.** Hemodilution is usually most severe at the beginning of CPB. As bypass proceeds, free water and electrolytes are filtered by the kidneys and are redistributed by diffusion into interstitial tissue spaces as edema. These effects cause a progressive **rise in hemoglobin concentration** and loss of circulating blood volume. This hemoglobin time course is fortuitous because as oxygen consumption rises with increasing temperature, the increasing [Hb] will allow a concomitant rise in oxygen transport.

5. **Fluid replacement.** Selection of the type of fluid to administer when additional circulating blood volume is required during CPB is based on the following considerations:

   a. **Hemoglobin.** If the [Hb] is less than 4–5 g/dl, it is usually necessary to add RBCs because urinary hemoconcentration is unlikely to raise the [Hb] sufficiently by the end of CPB.

   b. **Decreased reserve for hemodilution.** Incomplete myocardial revascularization during coronary artery bypass (CAB) surgery increases the need for adequate [Hb] post-CPB. In this condition, it may be desirable to maintain Hb at greater than 9–10 g/dl after CPB.

   c. **General medical condition.** Patients who are expected to have difficulty mobilizing edema fluid postoperatively (e.g., those with renal or heart failure) may benefit from colloid (albumin, hetastarch, and so on) instead of crystalloid administration, although this concept remains controversial.

6. **Contracting the blood volume.** When excessive volume is present within the CPB circuit and is not due to venous constriction (cold, vasoconstrictor drugs), then it may be desirable to remove fluid from the patient. Fluid can be removed by one of the following methods.

   a. **Diuresis.** Volume contraction is best accomplished through the kidneys. If urine output is inadequate, administration of 12.5–25.0 g mannitol or 2.5–5.0 mg furosemide to an adult patient not receiving chronic diuretic therapy is usually effective and avoids the marked and prolonged diuresis with hypokalemia caused by larger doses. In patients receiving chronic diuretic therapy the furosemide dose should be 20–40 mg initially, increased as necessary.

   b. **Ultrafiltration.** If adequate diuresis cannot be produced, an ultrafiltration device may be added to the CPB circuit to remove excess water and small ions without significantly affecting plasma electrolyte, blood urea nitrogen (BUN), and protein concentrations. Using a microporous membrane, these devices often can remove 1–2 liters/hr. Since **heparin may be removed** by this method, anticoagulation must be monitored frequently.

   c. **Hemodialysis.** In the presence of renal failure, a hemodialyzer machine can be connected to the CPB pump[10]. The composition of the dialysate is adjusted according to the individual conditions present, and reductions in potassium (K^+), BUN, and creatinine concentrations can be achieved.

D. **Systemic effects of cardioplegia**

   1. **Potassium load.** Cardioplegic solution is designed to produce diastolic cardiac arrest using a combination of high K^+ concentration ($[K^+]$) and profound hypothermia. During the most common adult CPB cases (CAB, aortic valve replacement), the right atrium is usually not opened. Therefore, cardioplegic solution drains from the coronary sinus into the venous cannula, enters the circulating blood volume, and raises the plasma $[K^+]$. Hyperkalemia can cause heart block, negative cardiac inotropy, arrhythmias, and vasoconstriction.

   2. **Avoiding systemic K^+ administration.** In patients with impaired renal function or preexisting hyperkalemia and in children, added K^+ should be avoided. This is accomplished best by cannulating the vena cavae separately, opening the right atrium, and removing the coronary sinus effluent to the wall suction (not recirculated).

   3. **Treatment of hyperkalemia** is accomplished by increasing elimination of K^+ from the body with diuretics or hemodialysis; shifting plasma K^+ into cells by inducing alkalosis with hyperventilation, bicarbonate, or with use of glucose-insulin; or reducing the cardiac

effects of hyperkalemia by administering calcium salts. For more details see Chap. 3.

E. Treatment of hypokalemia. If a patient is hypokalemic, initiating K^+ replacement during CPB is much safer than waiting until after bypass, thus avoiding hypokalemic dysrhythmias during CPB weaning and cardiac arrest during rapid K^+ replacement. K^+ may be administered in bolus doses as large as 8 mEq directed into the venous reservoir without apparent hemodynamic effects; the dose can be repeated as necessary. Larger doses may cause an initial vasodilation followed by vasoconstriction.

VIII. Intraoperative awareness

A. Etiology. Dilution of intravenous anesthetics by the priming solution, absorption of fentanyl onto the pump circuit, and a desire to avoid the negative inotropic effects of volatile and intravenous anesthetics with cardiac depressant actions all may contribute to the return of consciousness during CPB. Because hypothermia itself (below about 30°C) induces unconsciousness, the high-risk periods are when the patient is warm. Because the initial warm CPB period is usually short (except during arrhythmia-mapping procedures), this period is rarely associated with awareness. However, during rewarming the brain and body "core" warm much faster than the body "shell." Patients may be able to recall specific events, conversations, and rarely, pain during and after CPB. It is wise to inform patients of this risk preoperatively.

B. Prevention and diagnosis. Due to interindividual differences in responses to anesthetic and hypnotic drugs, there is no way to guarantee that a patient is unconscious except by avoiding **total** paralysis, asking the patient by name to open his eyes, and observing no response. This awareness test is best performed every 20–30 minutes during rewarming because, in the author's experience, patients rarely recall events if the duration of time during which the patient is arousable is less than about 30 minutes. Administration of muscle relaxants must be skillfully titrated to prevent gross patient movement that increases skeletal muscle oxygen consumption and interferes with surgery. Watching the intensity of body muscle contraction generated by defibrillation is helpful in titrating muscle relaxant doses. However, some practitioners feel that the risk of patient and diaphragmatic motion outweigh the risk of awareness because motion can introduce air into cardiac chambers if the heart has been opened.

Prophylactic administration of additional **narcotic and sedative-hypnotic drugs** on initiation of rewarming will greatly reduce the incidence of awareness. Typical doses are the equivalent of fentanyl 500 μg and scopolamine 0.4 mg (adult doses). Benzodiazepine drugs (e.g., lorazepam 2 mg) are also effective but may induce vasodilation; they are best used if the SVR is high.

C. Treatment. If a patient is found to respond to stimuli, adequate doses of **narcotic, sedative-hypnotic, or anesthetic drugs** must be administered prior to additional **muscle relaxant.** Reassurance should be given. During the postoperative interview, all cardiac surgical patients should be asked to describe (1) the last event prior to loss of consciousness, and (2) the next event. In this fashion, intraoperative awareness can be assessed without prompting. If awareness has occurred, question the patient to make sure operating room and not intensive care unit events are being remembered. Frank discussion of the real nature of intraoperative memories is important to prevent development of neurosis. In certain cases, psychiatric consultation may be indicated.

IX. Total circulatory arrest during bypass. It is necessary to stop CPB and remove the perfusion cannulae during certain surgical procedures includ-

ing repairs of the aortic arch and certain congenital heart lesions. Because all organs are rendered totally ischemic, steps must be taken to preserve vital organs; these include the following procedures (in addition to cardioplegia for the heart).

A. Profound hypothermia (often to 15°C) is the most important factor in preservation owing to its ability to vastly reduce the metabolic rate. Cooling is best performed **during CPB,** when the cold can be supplied to all organs directly through the vasculature **("core cooling").** Alpha-adrenergic blockade with phentolamine (0.2–0.5 mg/kg for infants) is often used to speed cooling and make it more uniform. Alternatively, cold can be applied to the skin, but such "surface cooling" is slower and less even. Commonly, surface cooling is added to core cooling (cooling blanket plus ice around the head) to prevent heat gain from the environment during circulatory arrest.

B. Brain preservation. Frequently, other modalities are added to the effects of cold in an attempt to render the brain less susceptible to ischemic damage[13]. These empirical therapies include **barbiturates** (thiopental titrated to EEG suppression of 1 burst/min, or ≈9–10 mg/kg), **corticosteroids** (e.g., methylprednisolone 30 mg/kg), and **mannitol** (0.25 g/kg, also may provide renal protection). Glucose administration is often avoided to help reduce intracellular acidosis during ischemia. (See Chapter 23 for an in-depth discussion of this subject).

C. Anesthetic management. Large doses of a nondepolarizing muscle relaxant should be given immediately prior to circulatory arrest because CSF acidosis can stimulate respiratory motion, and it is not possible to administer drugs during circulatory arrest. Spontaneous respiration may cause dangerous vascular air entrainment when the heart is open. Maintenance of alpha-stat acid-base status may be beneficial before and after arrest.

X. Management of relevant rare diseases affecting bypass

A. Heparin-associated thrombocytopenia and thrombosis (HATT). During heparin therapy (usually of more than several days' duration), a syndrome of low platelet count and arterial or venous thrombosis may appear. It is believed to be due to an IgG antibody that **induces platelet aggregation** and consumption in the presence of heparin. This syndrome is rare. Any patient receiving preoperative heparin therapy may develop HATT. Signs include unusual bleeding or thrombosis despite heparin. Diagnosis of thrombocytopenia is confirmatory. Administration of large doses of heparin prior to CPB in a patient with HATT is dangerous and may produce more **severe thrombosis** during CPB and marked coagulopathy after CPB.

   1. Management. Pharmacologic inhibition of platelet function may prevent pathologic activation of the platelets by heparin and the antibody. Inhibition may be started preoperatively, using aspirin (600 mg PR) plus dipyridamole, or prostacyclin derivatives. Plasmapheresis may also be effective. Consultation with a qualified hematologist is advised (see Chapter 18).

B. Antithrombin III (AT-III) deficiency. See Chapters 6 and 18.

C. Sickle-cell disease or trait. The congenital presence of abnormal hemoglobin S allows RBCs to undergo "sickle transformation" and occlude the microvasculature or lyse. RBC sickling may be induced by exposure to hypoxia, vascular stasis, hyperosmolarity, or acidosis. Hypothermia produces sickling only by causing vasoconstriction and stasis. CPB may induce sickling by redistributing blood flow, causing stasis, and reducing venous oxygen tensions. Although anesthesia for **noncardiac** surgery is usually well-tolerated in sickle **trait** patients, the situation is different for operations requiring CPB. **Sickle trait** (heterozygous) as well as **sickle disease** (homozygous) patients are both at high risk of developing potentially fatal thromboses during CPB unless appropriate measures are taken. Even with sickle **trait,** 100% of a patient's RBCs contain some amount Hb-S, and a red blood cell containing *any* Hb-S may sickle if the stimulus is sufficiently intense.

1. **Diagnosis. All black patients should undergo hemoglobin S evaluation** prior to surgery with CPB, since sickle **trait** may be completely asymptomatic. The rapid "sickle-dex" test or a "sickle-prep" is appropriate for screening, whereas, an Hb electrophoresis yields important quantitative information if a screening test is positive. Expert preoperative hematologic consultation is advised for sickle **trait** as well as sickle disease patients prior to CPB.

2. **Management.** Reduction of risk of perioperative sickling crisis can be achieved by **RBC transfusion** to dilute the Hb-S RBCs with normal Hb-A RBCs. Despite optimal management including partial exchange transfusion, sickling of 100% of Hb-S-containing RBCs has been observed after CPB in venous blood. Therefore, a key point in management is dilution of the Hb-S cells with Hb-A cells.

   a. Preoperative **partial exchange transfusion** with Hb-A donor blood. Heiner et al.[4] recommended that the proportion of Hb-S-containing RBCs (RBC_s) be reduced from 100% to less than 33% in sickle **trait** or sickle **disease** patients, as follows:

      (1) Measure the percentage of all **hemoglobin** that is Hb-S by Hb electrophoresis (call this Hb-S_{pre}).

      (2) Perform the exchange transfusion and repeat the Hb electrophoresis to obtain Hb-S_{post}.

      (3) Calculate

$$RBC_s = \{\text{percentage of body RBCs that contain Hb-S}\}$$
$$= (\text{Hb-}S_{post})/(\text{Hb-}S_{pre}) \times 100$$

      (4) RBC_s should be decreased below approximately 33% as a result of the exchange transfusion (and will be reduced further with initiation of CPB if a blood-containing prime is used).

   b. Some reports indicate that use of a blood-containing CPB prime with or without preoperative exchange transfusion may provide adequate protection for some sickle **trait** patients provided that Hb-S during CPB is reduced to less than approximately 20%. This theory remains controversial.

   c. Avoid arterial or venous hypoxemia, acidosis, dehydration, and hyperosmolarity. Higher than usual pump flow rates may theoretically raise PvO_2 and reduce sickling.

   d. If hypothermia is used, vasodilator therapy may prevent vascular stasis. Shivering or other factors that increase oxygen consumption when systemic oxygen transport cannot increase will reduce venous oxygen saturation and induce sickling.

D. **Cold hemagglutinin disease**[11]. Autoantibodies against a red cell antigen are activated by cold in these patients, with subsequent hemagglutination, acrocyanosis, and Raynaud's phenomenon. Hemolysis or complement activation may also occur. Cold-induced hemagglutination may cause thrombosis with organ ischemia or infarction. Cold cardioplegic solution contacting coronary blood may cause coronary vascular occlusion with inadequate distribution of cardioplegia and infarction. Diagnosis is made by direct Coombs' test at various temperatures. Cold agglutinins active above 22°C are rare.

   Recommended management includes

1. Do not let blood temperature or patient temperature fall below 22–25°C or critical temperature of antibody.

2. Ensure careful hematologic characterization of the antibody, including titer and critical temperature (highest in vitro temperature at which agglutination persists).
3. Consider preoperative plasmapheresis with fresh frozen plasma replacement.
4. Attempt to maintain patient temperature above critical temperature at all times.
5. Consider alternative techniques of myocardial preservation, including warm crystalloid cardioplegia (to wash out red cells) followed by cold crystalloid cardioplegia, warm blood-potassium cardioplegia, or warm ischemic arrest with intermittent reperfusion.

E. **Cold urticaria.** Patients with this disorder develop systemic histamine release and generalized urticaria in response to cold exposure. Marked histamine release occurs during CPB rewarming and can cause hemodynamic instability. The cardiovascular responses to histamine can be prevented by pretreatment with H_1- and H_2- receptor blockade; concomitant steroid administration may be useful[5].

F. **Malignant hyperthermia**
1. During an acute malignant hyperthermia (MH) crisis, increased skeletal muscle metabolism may cause a mixed metabolic and respiratory acidosis, hyperthermia, rigidity, hyperkalemia, tachycardia, cardiac dysrhythmias, and rhabdomyolysis with myoglobinuria (and late renal failure). MH does not appear to affect cardiac muscle function directly.
2. Known MH **triggering factors** include succinylcholine, halothane, enflurane, isoflurane, and possibly ketamine. There is experimental evidence that rapid heating or therapy with alpha-adrenergic agonists or calcium may trigger MH, but this has not been shown clinically. Blood dantrolene concentration decreased during CPB in one patient, but it is not known whether **additional** dantrolene is necessary during CPB[6].
3. **Management.** Patients with known MH susceptibility should receive prophylactic dantrolene (2.4 mg/kg IV), and additional drug should be given for signs of MH crisis. Recognition of MH crisis can be difficult during the **active rewarming** phase of CPB; monitoring the rate of carbon dioxide elimination or oxygen uptake may permit early diagnosis of MH[7]. It may be prudent to rewarm the patient gradually, avoid calcium administration unless Ca^{+2} concentration is low, and possibly avoid alpha-adrenergic agonists in favor of a pure beta-adrenergic drug such as isoproterenol if this is appropriate for inotropic therapy[2]. Patients may require additional dantrolene during rewarming.

REFERENCES

1. Bjorkstein, A. R., Crankshaw, D. P., Morgan, D. J., et al. The effects of cardiopulmonary bypass on plasma concentrations and protein binding of methohexital and thiopental. *J. Cardiothorac. Anesth.* 2:281–289, 1988.
2. Byrick, R. J., Rose, D. K., and Ranganathan, N. Management of a malignant hyperthermia patient during cardiopulmonary bypass. *Can. Anaesth. Soc. J.* 29:50–54, 1982.
3. Gravlee, G. P., Angert, K. C., Tucker, W. Y., et al. Early anticoagulation peak and rapid distribution after intravenous heparin. *Anesthesiology* 68:126–129, 1988.
4. Heiner, M., Teasdale, S. J., David, T., et al. Aorto-coronary bypass in a patient with sickle cell trait. *Can. Anaesth. Soc. J.* 26:428–434, 1979.
5. Johnston, W. E., Moss, J., Philbin, D. M., et al. Management of cold ur-

ticaria during hypothermic cardiopulmonary bypass. *N. Engl. J. Med.* 306:219–221, 1982.

6. Larach, D. R., High, K. M., Larach, M. G., et al. Cardiopulmonary bypass interference with dantrolene prophylaxis of malignant hyperthermia. *J. Cardiothorac. Anesth.* 1:448–453, 1987.

7. Larach, D. R., High, K. M., Derr, J. A., et al. Carbon dioxide elimination during total cardiopulmonary bypass in infants and children. *Anesthesiology* 69:185–191, 1988.

8. Mills, N. L., and Ochsner, J. L. Massive air embolism during cardiopulmonary bypass: Causes, prevention, and management. *J. Thorac. Cardiovasc. Surg.* 80:708–717, 1980.

9. Moore, R. A., Geller, E. A., Gallagher, J. D., et al. Effect of hypothermic cardiopulmonary bypass on nitroprusside metabolism. *Clin. Pharmacol. Ther.* 37:680–683, 1985.

10. Murkin, J. M., Murphy, D. A., Finlayson, D. C., et al. Hemodialysis during cardiopulmonary bypass: Report of twelve cases. *Anesth. Analg.* 66:899–901, 1987.

11. Park, J. V., and Weiss, C. I. Cardiopulmonary bypass and myocardial protection: Management problems in cardiac surgical patients with cold autoimmune disease. *Anesth. Analg.* 67:75–78, 1988.

12. Price, S. L., Brown, D. L., Carpenter, R. L., et al. Isoflurane elimination via a bubble oxygenator during extracorporeal circulation. *J. Cardiothorac. Anesth.* 2:41–44, 1988.

13. Wickey, G. S., Martin, D. E., Larach, D. R., et al. Combined carotid endarterectomy, coronary revascularization, and hypernephroma excision with hypothermic circulatory arrest. *Anesth. Analg.* 67:473–476, 1988.

SUGGESTED READING

Edmunds, L. H. Jr., and Stephenson, L. W. Cardiopulmonary Bypass for Open-heart Surgery. In W. W. L. Glenn (ed.), *Thoracic and Cardiovascular Surgery.* Norwalk: Appleton-Century-Crofts, 1983. Pp. 1091–1106.

Holley, F. O., Ponganis, K. V., and Stanski, D. R. Effect of cardiopulmonary bypass on the pharmacokinetics of drugs. *Clin. Pharmacokin.* 7:234–251, 1982.

Ream, A. K. Cardiopulmonary Bypass. In A. K. Ream, and R. P. Fogdall (eds.). *Acute Cardiovascular Management. Anesthesia and Intensive Care.* Philadelphia: Lippincott, 1982. Pp. 420–455.

Ionescu, M. I. *Techniques in Extracorporeal Circulation* (2nd ed.). London: Butterworths, 1981.

K. M. Taylor (ed.). *Cardiopulmonary Bypass: Principles and Management.* Baltimore: Williams & Wilkins, 1986.

Tinker, J. H., and Roberts, S. L. Management of Cardiopulmonary Bypass. In J. A. Kaplan (ed.), *Cardiac Anesthesia* (2nd ed.). Orlando: Grune & Stratton, 1987. Pp. 895–926.

Utley, J. R. (ed.). *Pathophysiology and Techniques of Cardiopulmonary Bypass.* Vol. II. Baltimore: Williams & Wilkins, 1983.

Weaning from Cardiopulmonary Bypass

Mark E. Romanoff and David R. Larach

Terminating cardiopulmonary bypass (CPB) requires the anesthesiologist to apply the basic tenets of cardiovascular physiology and pharmacology. The goal is a smooth transition from the mechanical pump back to the heart as the source of blood flow. "Weaning" from the pump involves optimizing cardiovascular variables including preload, afterload, heart rate and conduction, contractility, and the oxygen supply-demand ratio as in the pre-CPB period. However, the time period for optimization is compressed to minutes or seconds and decisions must be made quickly to avoid myocardial injury or damage to the other major organ systems.

I. Preparation

A. The major objectives in preparing for termination of CPB can be remembered with the aid of the mnemonic **CVP:**

C	V	P
Cold	Ventilation	Protamine
Conduction	Vaporizer	Pressure
Calcium	Volume expanders	Pressors
Cardiac output	Visualization	Pacer
Cells		Potassium
Coagulation		Predictors

1. Cold. This is a reminder that core temperature (nasopharyngeal, tympanic membrane, bladder) should be 37°C prior to terminating CPB. Shell, or rectal, temperature should be greater than approximately 32°C. Termination with temperatures less than these will cause hypothermia from equilibration of the cooler, vessel-poor group with the warmer and better perfused vessel-rich group when active rewarming is discontinued. Nasopharyngeal temperature correlates with brain temperature but may be artificially elevated during rapid rewarming (by a large volume of warm CPB blood) and should not be used for determining the temperature at which CPB is discontinued unless it has been stable for 20–30 minutes.

2. Conduction. Cardiac rate and rhythm must be controlled as follows:

a. Rate

(1) A heart rate (HR) of 70–100 bpm is usually necessary for an adequate cardiac output post-CPB owing to the initially lower stroke volume. In coronary artery bypass graft (CABG) procedures the oxygen supply-demand ratio is more favorable following correction, so that a higher rate (70–100 bpm) after CPB will increase cardiac output with less risk of ischemia than prior to correction. Patients with severe limitations of stroke volume (aneurysmectomy) may require even higher rates.

(2) Sinus bradycardia may be treated with atropine or, more predictably, with pacing.

(3) Sinus tachycardia of more than 120 bpm must be treated prior to termination of CPB. Often the act of filling the heart will lead to a reflex decrease in the heart rate to an acceptable level. Other etiologies of increased heart rate must be addressed. **Common etiologies include**

(a) Hypoxia

(b) Hypercarbia

(c) Medications (catecholamines, pancuronium, scopolamine, etc.)

(d) "Light" anesthesia, awareness

(f) Anemia

b. Rhythm

(1) Normal sinus rhythm is preferable. In patients with poorly compliant, thick-walled ventricles (associated with aortic stenosis, hypertension, or ischemia) or large overdistended ventricles (associated with aortic or mitral regurgitation) the artrial "kick" may contribute up to 40% of cardiac output, so that a synchronized atrial contraction (sinus rhythm, atrial or atrioventricular sequential pacing) is **required** before attempting CPB termination.

(2) Supraventricular tachycardia (HR > 120 bpm) should be cardioverted with synchronized internal cardioversion prior to terminating CPB. Lidocaine to prevent ventricular fibrillation following the shock should be considered. The use of short-acting β blockers (e.g., esmolol) or calcium channel blockers may be attempted, but these are usually associated with a decrease in contractility. Digoxin can be effective, but its onset is delayed.

(3) Third-degree atrioventricular block should be treated with pacing, although atropine may occasionally be effective. Beta agonists are effective but may increase inotropy and myocardial oxygen consumption unnecessarily.

(4) Ventricular dysrhythmias are treated as indicated (see Chap. 3).

3. **Calcium.** Calcium salts should be immediately available.

   a. The ionized calcium (Ca^{2+}) level should be evaluated. The routine administration of calcium post-CPB is controversial but is clearly indicated when the ionized calcium level is low and contractility is depressed following CPB.

   b. Calcium levels are affected by pH (decreased pH will increase Ca^{2+} levels, increased pH will decrease Ca^{2+} levels). If an abnormal Ca^{2+} level is measured, correction of pH is necessary, and a recheck of the Ca^{2+} level is required prior to treatment.

   c. Patients taking digoxin may experience life-threatening dysrhythmias following administration of calcium. The use of Ca^{2+} without checking ionized levels should be approached cautiously.

4. **Cardiac output.** The equipment necessary for measuring cardiac output should be available to assess the function of the heart after CPB. This includes a cardiac output computer and saline-filled syringes for thermodilution, or a densitometer and dye for green dye techniques.

5. **Cells**

   a. The hemoglobin concentration should be greater than 7.0 g/dl prior to terminating CPB. If it is not, packed red blood cells or whole blood should be given while the patient is still on CPB to maintain oxygen-carrying capacity. Patients with residual coronary disease or anticipated low cardiac output may benefit from even higher hemoglobin concentrations.

   b. At least one checked unit of blood should be in the room ready to be infused if needed once CPB pump volume is exhausted. Storage of this blood in an ice cooler to prevent spoilage is advocated.

6. **Coagulation.** Anticipate possible coagulation abnormalities requiring therapy. If needed, the following blood products should only be administered following CPB.

   a. Platelets should be available if indicated (thrombocytopenia, aspirin use, chronic renal failure, reoperations, and so on).

   b. Fresh frozen plasma or cryoprecipitate should be available for treatment of factor deficiencies or other coagulopathies.

   c. Desmopressin acetate (DDAVP) can be used to increase platelet aggregation in patients with chronic renal failure, von Willibrand's disease, or other platelet abnormalities. DDAVP may decrease chest tube bleeding when given to patients without known platelet abnormalities in the post-CPB period [9].

d. Additional blood products should be ordered from the blood bank as needed.

e. These blood products and DDAVP should not be given until heparin has been reversed. Blood products should not be administered unless a bleeding problem is clinically evident.

7. Ventilation

a. Adequate oxygenation and ventilation while the patient is on CPB must be ensured by checking arterial and venous blood gas measurements at routine intervals. pH should be kept within the normal range.

b. The lungs should be reexpanded with two to three breaths to a peak pressure of 30–40 cm H_2O with visual confirmation of bilateral lung expansion and resolution of atelectasis. An estimate of lung compliance can be made at this time.

c. Inspired oxygen fraction (FIO_2) should be 1.0. If air was used during CPB to prevent atelectasis it should be discontinued. Nitrous oxide should never be used on or after CPB to avoid increasing the size of air emboli.

d. The pulse oximeter should be turned on; if pulsatile flow exists it should be functional.

e. All airway monitors should be on line (apnea, FIO_2, end-tidal carbon dioxide, and so on).

f. Mechanical ventilation must be started prior to an attempt to terminate CPB. Terminating CPB without lung ventilation could have disastrous consequences. The timing of commencement of mechanical ventilation while the patient is still on CPB is controversial. Some practitioners believe that ventilation should begin when pulmonary blood flow is documented on CPB to avoid hypoxemia. However, this may not be necessary in normothermic, full-flow bypass [6] and may cause severe respiratory alkalosis of pulmonary blood. The pulse oximeter should be used to assess the need for ventilation during partial CPB.

g. Auscultation of breath sounds will confirm air movement and may reveal wheezing, rales, or rhonchi.

8. Vaporizer. Inhalation agents used during CPB for blood pressure control **should** be turned off at least 15–30 minutes prior to terminating CPB. These agents will decrease contractility and may take as long as 15 minutes to clear from the circuit [7] when a bubble oxygenator is used and may require a longer duration if a membrane oxygenator is used.

9. Volume expanders. Albumin or hetastarch should be available to increase preload if blood products are not indicated.

10. Visualization of the heart is important prior to terminating CPB. Primarily the right ventricle is available for visual inspection. It is possible to evaluate

a. Contractility: The heart will beat vigorously and "snap" with each beat in a normal contractile pattern.

b. Distention of the chambers.

c. Areas of infarct and wall motion abnormalities.

d. Conduction: Direct visual diagnosis of normal sinus rhythm or atrial dysrhythmias can be easier than using the electrocardiogram (ECG).

11. Protamine. The protamine dose should be calculated and drawn up in a syringe or ready as an infusion. The premature use of protamine is a catastrophe. Therefore, protamine should be prominently labeled and should not be placed where routine medications are stored to avoid accidental use. The surgeon, anesthesiologist, and the perfusionst should coordinate the use of this medication.

12. **Pressure.** Check the calibration of all transducers prior to terminating CPB. This will increase the accuracy of the information received from the monitoring lines.

13. **Pressors**
    a. Medications that are likely to be used should be ready to infuse at the appropriate initial rate with less than a 15-second delay. These medications include a vasodilator (nitroglycerin, nitroprusside, trimethaphan) as well as inotropic agents (dopamine, dobutamine, epinephrine, and so on).
    b. Nitroglycerin, sodium nitroprusside, and an inotropic agent should always be ready to infuse after CPB even if their use is not expected. Nitroglycerin can be used as a venodilator to allow additional volume to be infused in all patients after CPB.
    c. Volumetric infusion pumps **must** be used to deliver vasoactive substances accurately.

14. **Pacer.** An external pacemaker controller should be in the room, checked and set to the initial settings by the anesthesiologist. A pacemaker is often needed for treatment of bradycardia and asystole. In patients with heart block, an atrioventricular sequential pacemaker should be used.

15. **Potassium.** Blood chemistries should be checked prior to terminating CPB.
    a. **Hyperkalemia** may induce conduction difficulties and decreases in contractility. It is more common after long pump runs when large amounts of cardioplegic solution are used and absorbed, especially in patients with renal dysfunction.
    b. **Hypokalemia** can cause dysrhythmias.
    c. Other electrolytes and glucose should be evaluated as needed.

16. **Predictors**
    a. Assess the patient's risk for difficult weaning from CPB. Risk factors that can be identified **prior** to terminating CPB include:
       (1) Preoperative ejection fraction of less than 0.45 or dyssynergy [4]
       (2) Ongoing ischemia or evolving infarct in the pre-CPB period
       (3) Prolonged CPB duration (> 2–3 hours)
       (4) Inadequate surgical repair
           (a) Incomplete coronary revascularization
               (i) Small vessels (not graftable)
               (ii) Distal disease (diabetic patients)
           (b) Valvular disease
               (i) Valve replacement with very small valve (high transvalvular pressure gradient post-CPB)
               (ii) Suboptimal valve **repair** (residual regurgitation or stenosis)
       (5) Incomplete myocardial preservation during cross-clamping
           (a) ECG not asystolic (diastolic arrest incomplete)
           (b) Prolonged ventricular fibrillation prior to cross-clamping
           (c) Warm myocardium
               (i) Left ventricular (LV) hypertrophy (incomplete cardioplegia)
               (ii) High-grade coronary stenoses (no cardioplegia to that area of heart)
               (iii) Choice of grafting order (in an area of the heart served by a high-grade lesion without retrograde flow that

graft should be performed first so that cardioplegia may be infused early through the graft)

   (iv) Noncoronary collateral flow washing out cardioplegia

   (v) Poor LV venting

b. Additional preparations for high-risk patients

   (1) Prepare an **epinephrine** infusion (adults: 8–12 μg/ml) and fill a syringe (3-ml) with this dilute solution to facilitate administration of 2- to 8-μg bolus doses to promote rapid immediate effect prior to starting the infusion.

   (2) Discuss the need for additional **invasive monitoring** with the surgeon (i.e., left atrial or aortic pressure monitoring catheter).

   (3) Check for immediate availability of other **inotropic** drugs: amrinone, norepinephrine, prostaglandin E_1, and so on.

   (4) Check for immediate availability of **intraaortic balloon pump** and consider placement of a femoral arterial line for immediately available balloon access and improved BP monitoring.

   (5) Consider starting an inotropic infusion prior to terminating CPB in patients with exceptionally poor contractility. It must be remembered, however, that the Frank-Starling law implies that an empty heart will not beat very forcefully. Often a sluggishly contracting heart will start to "snap" once it is filled.

II. Sequence of events immediately prior to terminating CPB. Weaning from bypass describes the transition from an initial condition in which the bypass pump supplies 100% of the mechanical work needed to pump the blood to a final condition in which the heart provides 100% of this work. The transition should be gradual, recognizing that cardiac function post-CPB is not usually normal. (At times, though, cardiac function may be **improved** after bypass if ischemia is relieved or valvular dysfunction repaired.)

A. Final checklist prior to terminating CPB

   1. Confirm

      a. Ventilation

         (1) Lungs are ventilated with 100% oxygen, a visual confirmation.

         (2) Ventilatory alarms are enabled.

         (3) Esophageal stethoscope is reconnected to the ear.

         (4) Breath sounds and heart tones are heard.

         (5) All vaporizers are off.

      b. The patient is sufficiently rewarmed.

      c. The patient's heart, great vessels, and grafts have been properly de-aired.

      d. The patient is in optimal metabolic condition.

      e. All equipment and drugs are ready.

   2. Do not proceed until these criteria have been met.

   3. The time of weaning from CPB requires the utmost concentration and vigilance by the anesthesiologist, and all distractions should be eliminated.

B. What to look at during weaning. The greatest information is obtained from three sources: the invasive pressure display, the heart itself, and the ECG.

   1. Invasive pressure display

      a. Pressure waveforms (arterial, central venous pressure [CVP], and pulmonary artery [PA] or left atrial [LA], if used) are best displayed using a **common zero** (overlapping traces) with an **identical scale.**

      (1) Coronary perfusion pressure will be graphically depicted as the vertical height between the arterial pressure and the filling pressure during diastole.

      (2) The slope of the rise in **central aortic pressure** during systole may give some indication of LV contractility.

      (3) Valvular abnormalities can be diagnosed by examining CVP, pulmonary capillary wedge pressure (PCWP), or LA waveforms (e.g., mitral regurgitation may produce V waves in LA and PCWP tracings).

   b. Digital arterial pressure. The systolic and mean systemic arterial pressures should be continuously checked.

      (1) The **systolic** pressure describes the pressure generated by the heart's own contraction.

      (2) The **mean** pressure describes the work performed by the bypass pump and the vascular tone.

      (3) The **systolic-mean pressure difference** reflects the mechanical work done by the heart. As the heart assumes more of the circulatory work, this pressure difference increases. LV failure may be diagnosed by a decreased pressure difference.

      (4) Difficulty in weaning may be reflected by a small systolic-mean pressure difference in the presence of high atrial filling pressures when the venous return line is partially occluded.

      (5) It is important to remember that a radial artery line may not be accurate following CPB. During the first 30 minutes after CPB, a radial artery line tends to underestimate both the systolic and mean central aortic pressures [5]. Clinically significant hypotension measured by a radial artery line should be confirmed by a noninvasive blood pressure reading or a femoral artery line prior to treatment or resumption of CPB. Alternatively, an approximate pressure measurement from the aortic cannula still in the aorta can be obtained by the perfusionist monitoring the line pressure. A needle placed in the aortic root can also temporarily give a central aortic pressure measurement.

   c. CVP. Index of right heart filling before and during weaning.

   d. CVP-PA mean pressure step-up. The amount of mechanical work performed by the right ventricle is related to the difference between the CVP and the PA mean pressure. If the normal CVP to PA mean step-up in pressure is absent, the right ventricle (RV) is acting as a passive flow-through chamber, and severe RV failure is present.

 2. Visual inspection of the heart provides valuable information about contractility, conduction, and preload, although only the RV is usually visible. Poor contractility on inspection may predict difficulty in weaning from CPB.

 3. ECG changes such as heart block, dysrhythmias, or ischemia occur frequently and must be treated immediately, mandating frequent examination.

 4. Ventilation and oxygenation. While concentrating on the heart it is easy to overlook routine airway management issues as well as problems in the other major organ systems. The partial pressure of cabon dioxide ($PaCO_2$) should be kept at or below 40 mm Hg in the post-CPB period. Minor elevations in $PaCO_2$ can increase pulmonary vascular resistance (PVR) significantly [8].

III. Sequence of events during weaning from CPB

 A. Step 1: Retarding venous return to the pump

   1. Consequences of partial venous occlusion. Slowly the venous line is partially occluded (by the surgeon or perfusionist). This increase in venous line resistance causes right atrial pressure to rise and causes some blood to flow through the tricuspid valve into the RV instead of all draining to the pump. According to the Frank-Starling law, cardiac output increases as preload rises; therefore, the heart begins to eject blood more forcefully as the heart fills and enlarges.

2. **Preload.** The amount of venous line occlusion is carefully adjusted to attain and maintain a certain "optimal" preload or LV end-diastolic **volume** (LVEDV).

    a. **Estimating preload.** Unless an esophageal echocardiograph is in use, LV filling **volumes** cannot be measured directly. Instead, LVEDV is estimated from a filling **pressure** (PA diastolic, PCWP, or LA pressure [LAP]). The relationship of LVEDV to left atrial pressure and PCWP can be quite variable after bypass secondary to changes in diastolic compliance. Decreased compliance may be secondary to myocardial edema and ischemia. Therefore, the pulmonary wedge pressure is a relatively poor indicator of LVEDV in the post-CPB period [2], but this is usually the best available indicator.

    b. **Optimal preload** is the **lowest** filling pressure that provides an adequate cardiac output. Preload greater than the "optimal" value may cause:

        (1) Ventricular distention and increased wall tension (increased myocardial oxygen consumption [$M\dot{V}O_2$])

        (2) Decreased coronary perfusion pressure

        (3) Excessive or decreased cardiac output

        (4) Pulmonary edema

    c. **Typical weaning filling pressures.** For patients with good LV function preoperatively, a PCWP of 8–12 mm Hg often suffices. Abnormal contractility or diastolic stiffness may necessitate much higher filling pressures to achieve adequate filling volumes (20 mm Hg or higher), but in such cases it is imperative to monitor the **left** heart filling by a PA or preferably an LA line.

    d. **CVP/LAP ratio.** Normally, the LAP (usually estimated by the pulmonary wedge pressure) is higher than the CVP (CVP/LAP ratio < 1). If the ratio is elevated (> 1), the intraventricular septum may be forced toward the left, limiting left ventricular filling and cardiac output. In this situation termination of CPB may be impossible until the ratio is normalized [3] by improving RV function.

B. Step 2: Lowering pump flow into the aorta

1. **Attaining partial bypass.** The rise in preload causes the heart to begin to contribute to the cardiac output. This condition is termed **partial bypass** because the venous blood draining into the RA divides into two paths: Some goes to the pump, and some passes through the RV and lungs and is ejected into the aorta by the LV.

    a. Some institutions advocate keeping the patient on partial CPB for several minutes to wash vasoactive substances from the lungs before terminating CPB.

2. **Reduced pump outflow requirement.** Because two sources of blood are now supplying the aorta, the amount of arterial blood returned from the pump to the patient can be reduced as native cardiac output increases to maintain total aortic blood flow. Therefore, the perfusionist lowers the pump flow rate in 0.5–1.0 liter/min increments. This step is repeated, allowing gradual reductions in pump flow rate while cardiac function and hemodynamics are carefully monitored.

3. Readjusting venous line resistance. Some adjustment in the **venous** line resistance may be needed to maintain a constant filling pressure as the heart is given more work to perform. Also, as arterial pump outflow is reduced, less venous inflow is needed to keep the venous reservoir from being pumped dry. Therefore, the venous line clamp can be tightened further to achieve the desired increase in preload.

C. Step 3: Terminating bypass. If the heart is generating an adequate systolic pressure (typically 90–100 mm Hg for an adult) at an acceptable preload with pump flows of 1 liter/min or less, the patient is ready for a trial without CPB, and bypass is terminated. This means that the pump is stopped, and both arterial and venous pump cannulae are clamped shut. If these criteria are not met, CPB is reinstituted, and management of cardiovascular decompensation is begun (see sec. **V.D.** below).

1. Variant techniques. At some institutions, weaning is accomplished by abruptly clamping the venous line shut, then lowering pump flow as the heart rapidly begins to eject blood in response to the precipitous filling. Although this technique may be satisfactory for patients with good heart function, it requires that pump flows be quickly decreased because the venous reservoir would otherwise be pumped dry in the absence of venous return. It is not recommended for patients with compromised cardiovascular function.

IV. Sequence of events immediately after terminating CPB

A. Preload: infusing blood from the pump. If cardiac performance is inadequate, small increases in preload may be beneficial. For adult patients, volume is transferred in 50- to 100-ml increments from the venous pump reservoir to the patient through the aortic cannula. Before volume infusion, the aortic cannula should be inspected for air bubbles within its lumen. Ten to 50-ml increments are used in pediatric patients. During volume infusions from the pump, the blood pressure, filling pressure, and heart should be watched closely. **Continuous** infusion is contraindicated because overdistention of the heart may occur and the oxygenator reservoir may be emptied, embolizing air to the patient.

1. If BP and cardiac output do not change with increased preload, the patient is probably at the top (flat part) of the Starling curve, and further volume infusion is unlikely to be of benefit.

2. If BP does rise, the rise is probably due to a rise in cardiac output (CO), and further volume administration may be beneficial. In this manner, the optimal preload can be titrated after CPB.

3. Three factors often contribute to a need to give volume after CPB:

a. Continued rewarming of peripheral vascular beds results in vasodilation.

b. Changes in LV diastolic compliance alter "optimal" filling pressure.

c. Continued bleeding in the chest occurs from a higher mean arterial pressure (MAP) prior to heparin reversal.

B. Measuring cardiac function

1. Before taking the **relatively** irrevocable steps of removing the aortic cannula or administering protamine, cardiac function should be assessed. Particularly in adults, this is important because an adequate blood pressure may be the result of a low CO and a high systemic vascular resistance. Cardiac output may be measured using thermodilution or indocyanine ("green") dye dilution, depending on whether a PA catheter is in use. The derived **cardiac index** (cardiac output/body surface area) should be calculated. Generally a cardiac index of more than 2.0 liters $\cdot$ min^{-1} $\cdot$ m^{-2} should be present to consider permanent termination of CPB, although an index of greater than 2.3 is usually considered "normal." If heart rate is high, a normal CO can exist in spite of a low stroke volume. Therefore, a calculation of the **stroke volume index** (CI/HR) can be useful (normal = > 40 ml $\cdot$ beat$^{-1} \cdot$ m^{-2}).

2. **Measuring patient perfusion.** Signs of adequate **tissue** perfusion after CPB should be sought. Within the first 5–10 minutes after terminating CPB, arterial blood gases and pH should be measured, looking for signs of lactic acidosis as well as gas exchange abnormalities. Urine output normally rises after CPB, and lack of such a rise should be evaluated and treated immediately. The ideal perfusion pressure for adequate tissue oxygenation depends on the physiologic state of the other vital organ systems. Patients with renal insufficiency, cerebrovascular disease, or hypertension may require higher perfusion pressures than those necessary for patients without these abnormalities.

3. **Afterload and aortic impedance.** In the presence of good LV function (and absence of myocardial ischemia), the anesthesiologist avoids an elevated afterload to prevent excessive stress on the aortic suture lines and to reduce surgical bleeding. In adults, the usual desired range for systolic BP is 100–140 mm Hg.

   With impaired LV function or valvular regurgitation, systemic vascular resistance (SVR) should be reduced to the lowest level possible while maintaining adequate blood pressure for organ perfusion. Reducing the aortic impedance improves LV ejection and lowers systolic LV wall stress and myocardial oxygen demand. Impedance is related to blood pressure and SVR, and lowering SVR can result in increased CO with no change in BP.

4. **Heart rate and rhythm.** The optimal HR is usually 70–100 bpm.
   a. **Bradycardia** (HR < 60 bpm). **Low heart rates** can substantially reduce CO because the abnormal LV stiffness that is often present after CPB prevents the normal rise in stroke volume as HR falls. Pacing is the ideal means for increasing HR, especially atrial or atrioventricular sequential pacing, because of its controllability.
   b. **Tachycardia** (> 120 **bpm**) can be detrimental to LV filling and will increase MVO$_2$ and should be treated promptly.
   c. **Dysrhythmias** require appropriate and timely treatment as needed.

C. **Removing the venous cannula(e).** The presence of a large cannula(e) in the right atrium or in the vena cava will retard venous return to the heart, and if cardiac function is reasonable, the venous cannula is removed as soon as practical.

D. **Cardiovascular decompensation**
   1. The management of systemic hypotension during weaning from CPB is outlined in Fig. 8-1.
   2. Failure of the left or right ventricle, both of which are recovering from the ischemic insult of CPB, is the most common cause of cardiovascular insufficiency during the weaning process.
      a. **Left ventricular failure**
         (1) Differential diagnosis of LV failure after CPB is listed in Table 8-1.
         (2) Treatment of LV failure during weaning from CPB is as follows:
            (a) Initiate administration of inotropic agents (Fig. 8-1).
               (i) Most commonly dopamine or dobutamine is chosen as the first-line agent, although some institutions advocate the use of epinephrine initially. Regardless of choice, often a 4- to 8-μg bolus of epinephrine (adults) is utilized while commencing an inotrope infusion.

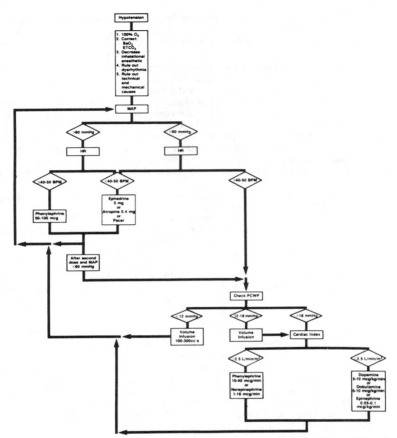

Fig. 8-1. The management of systemic hypotension during weaning from cardiopulmonary bypass. SaO_2 = arterial hemoglobin oxygen saturation; $ETCO_2$ = end-tidal carbon dioxide; HR = heart rate; PCWP = pulmonary capillary wedge pressure; SVR = systemic vascular resistance; IABP = intra-aortic balloon pump; CPB = cardiopulmonary bypass.

       ((a)) Dopamine may be more appropriate if HR is normal and SVR is low or normal.

       ((b)) Dobutamine or amrinone may be more appropriate if HR is elevated or SVR is increased.

    (b) Start nitroglycerin (NTG) if ischemia is present (consider use of calcium channel blockers)

b. Right ventricular failure

  (1) Diagnosis

    (a) The RV was once thought to be just a conduit to the pulmonary circulation. This is incorrect. Active pumping by the RV is mandatory for the optimal functioning of the cardiovascular system.

    (b) Patients most at risk include those with:

      (i) Pulmonary hypertension

        ((a)) Chronic mitral valve disease

        ((b)) Left-to-right shunts (atrial septal defect, ventricular septal defect, etc.)

Table 8-1. Differential diagnosis of left ventricular failure after CPB

I. Ischemia
  A. Graft failure
    1. Clot in graft
    2. Distal suture causing constriction
    3. Kinking of graft
    4. Air in graft
    5. Graft sewn in backwards (no flow through valves)
    6. Inadequate flow through internal mammary artery (IMA)
  B. Inadequate coronary blood flow
    1. Incomplete revascularization (secondary to distal disease or inoperable vessels)
    2. Inadequate coronary perfusion pressure
    3. Emboli in native coronary arteries—air or particulate matter (clot, atherosclerotic plaque)
    4. Coronary spasm
    5. Tachycardia (decreased diastolic filling time)
    6. Increased myocardial oxygen demand
    7. Surgical injury to native coronary artery
  C. Myocardial ischemia leading to myocardial damage
    1. Incomplete myocardial preservation during CPB
    2. Evolving myocardial infarction
II. Valve failure
  A. Prosthetic valve
    1. Sewn in backward
    2. Paravalvular leak
    3. Mechanical obstruction (immobile disc)
  B. Native valve—Acute mitral regurgitation (papillary muscle ischemia or rupture)
III. Gas exchange problems
  A. Hypoxemia
    1. Inadequate F_{IO_2}
    2. Mechanical ventilator failure
    3. Airway disconnected
    4. Severe bronchospasm
    5. Pulmonary edema ("pump lung" adult respiratory distress syndrome)
  B. Hypoventilation
IV. Inadequate preload
V. Excessive preload (can lead to distention of cardiac structures)
VI. Reperfusion injury
VII. Ventricular septal defect
VIII. Miscellaneous causes of decreased contractility
  A. Medications
    1. Beta blockade
    2. Calcium channel blockers
    3. Inhalational agents
  B. Acidemia
  C. Electrolyte abnormalities
    1. Hyperkalemia
    2. Hypocalcemia
  D. Preexisting LV failure

((c)) Massive pulmonary embolism
((d)) Primary pulmonary hypertension
((e)) Acute mitral regurgitation
((1)) Valvular dysfunction
((2)) Papillary muscle rupture
((f)) Air embolism
(ii) RV ischemia or infarct
(c) Physiologic findings include
(i) Depressed cardiac output
(ii) Inappropriate elevation in CVP compared to PCWP (unless biventricular failure exists)
(iii) Increase in PVR of more than 2.5 Wood units (> 200 dynes·sec·cm^{-5})
(iv) Pulmonary hypertension
(v) Absence of the CVP-mean PA pressure step-up (see sec. **III.B.1.d.**)
(2) Treatment
(a) Treat signs of ischemia by
(i) Giving NTG infusion
(ii) Increasing coronary perfusion pressure
(b) Increase preload
(c) Increase inotropic support
(i) Isoproterenol is the agent of choice because it will increase contractility of the RV and will also decrease PVR
(d) Use adjuncts to decrease PVR
(i) Hyperventilation will induce hypocapnia. This should be accomplished by means of a high respiratory rate because an increase in tidal volume may increase PVR.
(ii) Avoidance of hypoxia
(iii) Avoidance of acidemia
(iv) Maintenance of normal core temperature
(v) Use of vasodilators
(e) Administer prostaglandin E_1 (PGE$_1$). PGE$_1$ infusion through an RA line will induce pulmonary vasodilation (this requires concomitant norepinephrine infusion into the systemic circulation through an LA line to avoid marked SVR reduction)[1].
(f) Use an RV assist pump (experimental)
(g) Use pulmonary artery balloon counterpulsation (experimental)

E. Resumption of CPB

1. The decision to resume CPB after a trial of native circulation must not be made prematurely because there are dangers to resuming CPB (inadequate heparinization, hemolysis, etc.), but CPB must be restarted before permanent ischemic damage is sustained by the heart, brain, and kidneys. If diagnosis and treatment of cardiovascular derangements mentioned above cannot be made within 3–5 minutes, reinstitution of CPB is indicated. While the patient is on CPB, diagnosis and treatment should continue but may proceed without markedly increasing the risk of organ failure.
2. Heparin should be given as needed based on the last ACT measurement made while the patient was on CPB. (If any protamine was given, a **full dose** of heparin, 300 units/kg, is needed prior to resuming CPB.)
3. Any mechanical factors that could compromise cardiac performance must be looked for and surgically corrected.

4. Unsuccessful "weaning" will necessitate the addition of more aggressive inotropic support. These are added to the first-line regimen.
  a. Second-line agents include the following.
    (1) Epinephrine will cause increased contractility and a slight decrease in SVR at low to moderate dosages and increased SVR at high dosages.
    (2) Norepinephrine will cause markedly increased SVR and an increase in contractility.
    (3) Amrinone will cause increased contractility and a moderate decrease in SVR.
5. Increase monitoring. Left atrial pressure is a better estimate of LVEDP than pulmonary artery pressures. Aortic or femoral arterial pressures may be more accurate than radial pressures. Increasing the accuracy of information by the insertion of these monitoring lines may facilitate weaning.
6. If the second attempt to wean is unsuccessful, continue to optimize preload and afterload with vasodilators or volume infusion as needed.
  a. An intraaortic balloon pump that will augment diastolic blood pressure, increase coronary perfusion, and decrease afterload should be considered.
  b. If available, ventricular assist devices can be life-saving after multiple failed attempts to separate the patient from CPB. These are usually used either for 24–96 hours to rest the "stunned myocardium" or as a bridge to heart transplantation (see Chapter 22).

REFERENCES

1. D'Ambra, M. N., LaRaia, P. J., and Philbin, D. M. Prostaglandin E$_1$. A new therapy for refractory right heart failure and pulmonary hypertension after mitral valve replacement. *J. Thorac. Cardiovasc. Surg.* 89:567–71, 1985.
2. Hansen, R. M., Viquerat, C. E., Matthay, M. A., et al. Poor correlation between pulmonary arterial wedge pressure and left ventricular end-diastolic volume after coronary artery bypass graft surgery. *Anesthesiology* 64:764–770, 1986.
3. Kopman, E. A., and Ferguson, T. B. Interaction of right and left ventricular filling pressures at the termination of cardiopulmonary bypass. *J. Thorac. Cardiovasc. Surg.* 89:706–708, 1985.
4. Mangano, D. T. Biventricular function after myocardial revascularization in humans: Deterioration and recovery patterns during the first 24 hours. *Anesthesiology* 62:571–577, 1985.
5. Mohr, R., Lavee, J., and Goor, D. A. Inaccuracy of radial artery pressure measurement after cardiac operations. *J. Thorac. Cardiovasc. Surg.* 94:286–290, 1987.
6. Moore, R. A., Gallagher, J. D., Kingsley, B. P., et al. The effect of ventilation on systemic blood gases in the presence of left ventricular ejection during cardiopulmonary bypass. *J. Thorac. Cardiovasc. Surg.* 90:287–290, 1985.
7. Nussmeier, N. A., Moskowitz, G. J., Weiskopf, R. B., et al. In vitro anesthetic washin and washout via bubble oxygenators: influence of anesthetic solubility and rates of carrier gas inflow and pump blood flow. *Anesth. Analg.* 67:982–987, 1988.
8. Salmenpera, M., and Heinonen, J. Pulmonary vascular responses to moderate changes in PaCO$_2$ after cardiopulmonary bypass. *Anesthesiology* 64:311–315, 1986.
9. Salzman, E. W., Weinstein, M. J., Weintraub, R. M., et al. Treatment with desmopressin acetate to reduce blood loss after cardiac surgery. *N. Engl. J. Med.* 314:1402–1406, 1986.

SUGGESTED READING

Kaplan, J. A. *Cardiac Anesthesia* (vol. 2). Orlando: Grune & Stratton, Inc., 1987.

Lappas, D. G., Powell, W. M. J., and Daggett, W. M. Cardiac dysfunction in the perioperative period: Pathophysiology, diagnosis and treatment. *Anesthesiology* 47:117–137, 1977.

Lazar, H. L., and Roberts, A. J. Recent advances in cardiopulmonary bypass and the clinical application of myocardial protection. *Surg. Clin. North Am.* 65 (June):455–476, 1985.

Ream, A. K. Cardiopulmonary Bypass. In A. K. Ream (ed.), *Acute Cardiovascular Management—Anesthesia and Intensive Care*. Philadelphia: Lippincott, 1982. Pp. 420–455.

Tinker, J. H. Management of Cardiopulmonary Bypass. International Anesthesia Research Society, Review Course Lecture. April Supplement, 1989. Pp. 47–54.

The Postcardiopulmonary Bypass Period: A Systems Approach

Scott K. Clark and Jerrold H. Levy

The postcardiopulmonary bypass period is characterized by recovery from the major physiologic insults of cardiopulmonary bypass (CPB). The rate and extent of recovery and the need for multisystemic support depend on (1) preexisting disease, (2) particular organ system dysfunction, (3) the adequacy of the surgical repair, and (4) the nature of ongoing physiologic derangements in the postbypass period.

I. **Cardiovascular system.** Both bypass and postbypass risk factors influence management during this time period:

Physiologic stress related to the CPB period
Length of the bypass period
Adequacy of surgical repair
Adequacy of myocardial protection
Reperfusion injury

Physiologic stress in the postbypass period
Mechanical manipulation of the heart
Decannulation
Protamine administration
Surgical bleeding and coagulation abnormalities
Chest closure and mechanical ventilation
Coronary spasm

A. **Physiologic Stress related to the CPB period**
1. **Length of bypass period.** In an adequately protected myocardium, an aortic cross-clamp time of less than 120 minutes should not be associated with significant myocardial damage. Cross-clamp times of greater than 120 minutes and inadequate protection will lead to myocardial damage and subsequently, impaired myocardial performance. The duration of cardiopulmonary bypass also correlates with the degree of complement activation and potential organ dysfunction[6].
2. **Incomplete repair**
   a. **Congenital disease.** Hemodynamic instability after congenital heart surgery often is due to an inadequate repair. If the dysfunction is moderate to severe, the surgeon should reevaluate the patient for potential anatomic or mechanical problems and consider immediate reoperation. Epicardial two-dimensional (2-D) echocardiography can help delineate problems in this situation. For instance, after repair of an atrioventricular canal defect, the presence of residual mitral regurgitation will prevent adequate forward flow and lead to hemodynamic impairment. However, reoperation may not solve every hemodynamic derangement post bypass, especially when palliative procedures are performed.
   b. **Malfunctioning prosthetic valve.** When the heart appears to be contracting with sufficient vigor but is not ejecting, one should suspect a mechanical difficulty with the newly implanted prosthetic valve. One of the valve leaflets could be stuck, or the valve may be sewn in a direction opposite to that intended. The patient may also have dysfunction of one of the remaining native valves. For example, after mitral valve replacement the patient may have residual tricuspid regurgitation.
   c. **Diffuse or distal coronary vascular disease.** Most often seen in diabetic and elderly patients, the distribution and degree of distal vascular disease will offset any increased proximal flow from a coronary graft. Reversal of anticoagulation by protamine in an area of poor distal flow may lead to occlusion of the graft.
   d. **Technically unsatisfactory anastomosis.** The quality of the vessel (both vein and internal mammary artery) and the quality

of the anastomosis will affect postbypass myocardial blood flow and hence myocardial performance.

3. Inadequate myocardial protection (see Chapter 21)

a. Left ventricular distention during bypass. Left ventricular distention during bypass increases wall tension and thus increases myocardial oxygen demand.

b. Inadequate myocardial cooling. Myocardial warming will increase oxygen demand. Causes of myocardial warming include heat from surrounding tissues and operating room lights, bronchial and thebesian venous return, inadequate surface cooling of the myocardium, inadequate cardioplegia volume, and administration of cardioplegia with a temperature of greater than 4–8°C for crystalloid cardioplegic solutions. Less than total drainage of the patient's venous return into the venous cannula will allow the venous blood which has a relatively higher temperature, to come into contact with and warm the right ventricle and the septum.

c. Inadequate cardioplegic protection. Cardioplegia must be distributed throughout the myocardium to provide electrical and mechanical quiescence and adequate cooling. Left ventricular hypertrophy, aortic valvular insufficiency, and distal coronary artery disease may make this difficult. The longer inadequate protection goes unrecognized, the greater the myocardial damage that results.

d. Ventriculotomy. Ventriculotomy will increase the incidence of air and debris embolization to the coronary circulation. Ventriculotomy will also cause significant trauma to the ventricular muscle with formation of edema in the ventricular wall. This may lead to ventricular dysfunction in the postbypass period.

e. Prolonged ventricular fibrillation. Prolonged ventricular fibrillation, especially at normothermia, will decrease subendocardial blood flow and increase myocardial oxygen demand.

f. Air or debris in coronary arteries. Air or debris may enter the coronary circulation after removal of the aortic cross-clamp or the side-biting aortic clamp. This may produce regional or global myocardial ischemia with deterioration of myocardial performance. The surgeon should aspirate any visible air out of the coronary arteries with a fine needle (27-gauge). If myocardial function does not improve, increasing coronary perfusion pressure with vasoconstrictors to increase coronary perfusion pressure may improve ventricular performance. Resolution of myocardial dysfunction from intracoronary air emboli may require reinstitution of bypass to "rest" the heart and allow resorption of the air.

g. Surgical trauma to the native coronary arteries. Surgical trauma may occur during aortotomy (during aortic valve replacement), during mitral valve replacement (left circumflex coronary artery), or by direct cannulation or incision of an aberrant coronary artery during any type of cardiac surgical procedure.

4. Reperfusion injury. When less than optimal myocardial preservation occurs during bypass, removal of the aortic cross-clamp may cause further myocardial damage in areas of ischemia, producing cellular edema, membrane dysfunction, and mitochondrial dysfunction. Paradoxically, oxygen may play a role in this cellular damage through free radical formation. Free radical scavengers, osmotic agents, coronary vasodilators, and drugs that inhibit platelet aggregation have been used to treat reperfusion injury. Because initial use of high pressure (> 100 mm Hg) and high flow (> 150 ml $\cdot$ kg^{-1} $\cdot$ min^{-1}) may also exacerbate reperfusion injury, some surgeons advocate the use of controlled reperfusion of the coronary arteries prior to aortic cross-clamp removal while the coronary arteries are still isolated (see Chap. 21).

B. Physiologic stress in the postbypass period

1. **Manipulation of the heart.** Early in the postbypass period the surgeon will often manipulate the heart to examine anastomotic sites, examine the position in which the vein grafts lie, and search for areas of bleeding. This manipulation often causes hypotension due to dysrhythmias, decreased venous return, air or particulate emboli, and impedance of arterial outflow. If the surgeon lifts or compresses the heart for a prolonged period and the mean arterial pressure remains below 70 mm Hg or continues to fall, the anesthesiologist should communicate this abnormality to the surgeon and suggest that he allow the heart to recover. Since this hypotension is mechanical, pharmacologic intervention should not be necessary unless the heart becomes ischemic and recovers very slowly.

2. **Decannulation** may occur prior to the administration of protamine or after administering approximately half of the protamine. The timing of decannulation varies from institution to institution. Generally, cannula removal occurs uneventfully. However, rapid blood loss and dysrhythmias may occur during decannulation. Allowing the aortic cannula to remain in place during at least the initial portion of protamine administration will still allow infusion of fluid from the bypass machine through the aortic cannula, rapidly if necessary, in the event of bleeding during venous cannula(e) removal or hypotension due to protamine administration. The main disadvantage of allowing the cannulae to remain in place is thrombus formation on the cannula and subsequent embolization of this thrombus. Regardless of the timing of decannulation, many surgeons keep the cannulae and bypass pump tubing on the surgical field until the end of the procedure in the event of rapid deterioration of the patient's condition requiring reinstitution of bypass.

3. **Protamine administration.**

   a. **Rate.** Protamine should be administered intravenously in a dilute solution (protamine 10 mg/ml mixed with an equal volume of 5% D/W) and infused no faster than 50 mg/min. A Buretrol or similar device can be used for dilution and administration of the protamine. Slow administration of a dilute solution of protamine should prevent any adverse hemodynamic events directly attributable to protamine. Morel has shown that rapid protamine administration may produce transient white cell sequestration in the pulmonary vasculature, which may explain some of its nonimmunologic adverse acute hemodynamic effects[9].

   b. **Route.** There is no convincing evidence to suggest that the particular route of protamine administration (left heart versus right heart) can prevent adverse hemodynamic effects. Therefore, the patient should be carefully monitored for adverse cardiopulmonary effects regardless of the route chosen.

   c. **Direct cardiovascular effects.** Protamine, if administered slowly, produces minimal hemodynamic effects in most patients. According to most animal and human studies, protamine probably does not directly decrease myocardial contractility. Hypotension is due to a decrease in preload and systemic vascular resistance and is probably related to the speed of administration. Hypotension may therefore be exaggerated in the hypovolemic patient. If hypotension occurs despite the slow administration of protamine, volume should be administered as well as 50–100 μg doses of phenylephrine. If these corrective measures do not result in normotension, protamine administration must be temporarily discontinued to allow volume administration and return of an adequate blood pressure.

d. Idiosyncratic protamine reactions. A spectrum of reactions to protamine has been described, some as serious as life-threatening cardiopulmonary dysfunction. (Table 9-1). Three different mechanisms may be responsible.

(1) **Anaphylactic reactions.** True allergic reactions of an immediate hypersensitive nature (anaphylaxis) are due to IgE or IgG antibodies. These reactions may be immediate or delayed up to 20 minutes following initial protamine administration. However, when administering protamine and blood products together, it may be unclear which agent is responsible for the anaphylactic reaction. For these reasons, it is best to administer protamine and wait 20 minutes prior to transfusing any blood products. Management of an anaphylactic reaction to protamine is described in Table 9-2. Management of anaphylactoid reactions and the initial management of catastrophic pulmonary vasoconstriction reactions are similar.

(2) **Anaphylactoid reactions.** These reactions are nonimmunologic and do not involve antibodies. The heparin-protamine complex can activate the classic complement pathway, liberating complement fragments that degranulate mast cells or basophils and release vasoactive substances into the circulation[7]. Nonimmunologic complement activation may also be responsible for some reactions that produce pulmonary hypertension.

(3) **Catastrophic pulmonary vasoconstriction reactions** (see Chap. 18). Catastrophic pulmonary hypertension and bronchoconstriction, mediated by thromboxane A_2 (generated through immunologic (IgG) or nonimmunologic complement activation), is part of the spectrum of protamine reactions. Persistent pulmonary hypertension refractory to nitroglycerin or isoproterenol may require infusion of prostaglandin E_1 into the right atrium along with left atrial administration of norepinephrine to support systemic blood pressure.

4. Surgical bleeding and coagulation disorders. The potential exists for greater postbypass blood loss during reoperation and in patients with pericarditis due to bleeding from virtually every tissue surface subjected to lysis of pericardial adhesions. Therefore, platelets should be available preoperatively in all such patients. After bypass, if continuous nonsurgical bleeding occurs despite documentation of adequate heparin reversal, platelets (0.1 units/kg) should be given empirically (see Fig. 18-6).

5. Chest closure. Patients with **good ventricular function** who have an adequate preload usually tolerate chest closure without difficulty. However, patients with **inadequate preload** or **poor ventricular function** may become acutely hypotensive. Chest closure is analogous to mechanical tamponade, in which venous return decreases due to the increased intrathoracic pressure from chest closure. Patients who are hypovolemic usually respond to volume administration and perhaps adjustment of their ventilatory pattern (decrease in tidal volume or peak inspiratory pressure) and an increase in heart rate (usually by pacing). In patients with poor ventricular function, catecholamine therapy may also improve ventricular function. If these manipulations are not effective the surgeon may need to reopen the chest and reevaluate and remedy the patient's hemodynamic situation. Occasionally, during chest closure, one of the vein grafts may become trapped or kinked causing regional myocardial ischemia, dysfunction, dysrhythmias, and hypotension. The surgeon will need to repair any mechanical problems involving the vein grafts.

Table 9-1. Idiosyncratic protamine reactions

Type of reaction	Antibody responsible	Humoral mediator	Systemic effect	Treatment
Anaphylactic	IgE, IgG$_4$	Histamine and other vasoactive mediators	Edema, hives, bronchospasm, low BP, CVP, PAP	See Table 9-2
Anaphylactoid	None	Complement, histamine, and other vasoactive mediators	Decreased SVR	See Table 9-2
Catastrophic pulmonary vasoconstriction	?IgG	Complement, thromboxane A$_2$, polymorphonuclear leukocytes	Bronchospasm; low LAP, BP; high PAP, CVP	See Table 9-2

SVR = systemic vascular resistance, BP = systemic blood pressure, CVP = central venous pressure, PAP = pulmonary artery pressure, LAP = left atrial pressure, PGE$_1$ = prostaglandin E$_1$.

Table 9-2. Therapy for idiosyncratic protamine reactions

Initial therapy

1. Stop administration of protamine.
2. Maintain airway with 100% oxygen.
3. Discontinue all anesthetic agents.
4. Start intravascular volume expansion (2–4 liters of crystalloid with hypotension).
5. Give epinephrine (4–8 µg IV bolus with hypotension, titrate as needed; 0.1–1.0 mg IV with cardiovascular collapse).
6. Reinstitute cardiopulmonary bypass for severe reactions to allow time for drug therapy to take effect.

Secondary treatment

1. Antihistamines (0.5–1 mg/kg diphenhydramine, 300 mg cimetidine, 20 mg famotidine, or 50 mg ranitidine)
2. Catecholamine infusions (starting doses: epinephrine 2–4 µg/min, norepinephrine 2–4 µg/min, *or* isoproterenol 0.5–1.0 µg/min as a drip, titrated to desired effects)
3. Aminophylline (5–6 mg/kg over 20 min with persistent bronchospasm) followed by infusion
4. Corticosteroids (0.25–1.00 g hydrocortisone; alternatively, 1–2 g methylprednisolone)*
5. Sodium bicarbonate (0.5–1.0 mEq/kg with persistent hypotension or acidosis)
6. Airway evaluation (prior to extubation)

Specific treatment for catastrophic pulmonary vasoconstriction

Therapy as above; once diagnosed, treatment of pulmonary hypertension, right heart failure, and bronchoconstriction should include immediate hyperventilation and one or more of the following treatments: Nitroglycerin; isoproterenol; aminophylline; prostaglandin E_1; amrinone.

*Methylprednisolone may be the drug of choice if the reaction is suspected to be mediated by complement.
Source: Modified from J. H. Levy. *Anaphylactic Reactions in Anesthesia and Intensive Care.* Boston: Butterworths, 1986. Pp. 104. With permission.

Failing these maneuvers, the skin and fascia of the chest may be closed with retention sutures, leaving the sternum unapproximated for closure at a later time. This maneuver should prevent large increases in intrathoracic pressure and tamponade, therefore improving venous return and ventricular performance.

6. **Coronary spasm.** Although inadequate myocardial preservation and inadequate revascularization are the most common reasons for poor myocardial performance after bypass, coronary spasm represents another important cause. Spasm may occur at any time in the postbypass period, including the postoperative period in the intensive care unit and also may occur in patients undergoing cardiac procedures other than coronary revascularization. Coronary spasm often presents with ST-segment elevation (although ST-segment depression may also occur, especially with nontransmural ischemia) in the absence of hemodynamic compromise. The patient may then progress to dysrhythmias (often refractory to the usual measures), atrioventricular block, hypotension, decreased cardiac output, and possibly even sudden cardiac arrest. The diagnosis of coronary artery spasm is often one of exclusion. Established coronary spasm can be difficult to treat and may not respond to intravenous nitroglycerin. **Intracoronary** nitroglycerin and sublingual nifedipine represent addi-

tional current therapeutic modalities. Treatment of coronary spasm with either of the above drugs may take several minutes to become effective, and ventricular function may not recover completely for several hours.

C. **Postbypass hemodynamic management. Cardiovascular deterioration** in the postbypass period may occur gradually or rapidly, depending on the cause. Etiologic factors and their treatment are listed in Table 9-3. During an uneventful case, **the patient's hemodynamic status should continually improve during the first 30–60 minutes after weaning from CPB.** Unfortunately, some patients may initially improve hemodynamically and later deteriorate owing to the physiologic stresses of the CPB and the post-CPB periods. Evaluation and treatment of the patient's postbypass hemodynamic status requires an organized and methodical plan (Fig. 9-1).

1. **First, optimize the heart rhythm and rate.** In the postbypass period a heart rate of 80–90 bpm in adults will optimize cardiac output and prevent ventricular distention. Patients with coronary artery disease or stenotic valvular lesions who have **an adequate repair** will no longer need the slow heart rate they required prebypass. Most often, increasing the heart rate can be accomplished with epicardial pacing. Because synchronous atrial contraction may supply up to 40% of ventricular filling in patients with noncompliant ventricles, one should initiate atrial pacing in patients with a low heart rate and normal atrioventricular conduction time. With advanced atrioventricular block and a low heart rate, pacing may be accomplished using an atrioventricular sequential pacemaker, with the atrial rate set at 80–90 bpm and an atrioventricular interval that optimizes cardiac output, generally about 120–150 msec in adults. It is also desirable to initiate a rhythm that maximizes cardiac output, usually sinus rhythm. While the chest is open, rhythms such as supraventricular tachycardia (SVT) and atrial fibrillation are best treated by cardioversion. Atrial fibrillation refractory to cardioversion may require ventricular pacing to optimize cardiac output. Bradydysrhythmias are treated with atrial or atrioventricular sequential pacing as described above. Pharmacologic manipulation of rhythm may eventually be necessary to maintain a stable rhythm (see Chapter 3).

2. **Second, optimize the patient's preload.** Several methods exist to determine the patient's preload.
   a. **Pulmonary capillary wedge pressure (PCWP).** This value should be comparable to the prebypass value but must be established individually for each patient. Often, in the early postbypass period, the PCWP may need to be maintained higher than the prebypass value by 3–5 mm Hg to generate the same forward stroke volume because myocardial compliance is decreased. This decrease in myocardial compliance may result from cardioplegic arrest and subsequent myocardial edema. Patients with some types of valvular heart disease may require a lower PCWP in the postbypass period.
   b. **Examination of the heart.** Examine the heart to determine its volume because the PCWP may be less reliable in the early postbypass period (decreased myocardial compliance).
   c. **Two-dimensional transesophageal echocardiography** (2D-TEE). Examine the cross-sectional area of the left ventricular cavity at the level of the papillary muscle with 2D-TEE.

3. **Third, assess myocardial contractility and cardiac output,** both by looking at the heart for global and regional defects in contractility and by determining thermodilution cardiac outputs. Remember that

Table 9-3. Etiologies of postbypass cardiovascular deterioration

Condition	Causes	Treatment
Inadequate HR or rhythm	Low HR	Atrial, ventricular pacing
	A-V block	A-V sequential pacing
	Ventricular or atrial dysrythmias	Appropriate antidysrhythmics, overdrive pacing
	High HR, SVT	Cardioversion volume, verapamil, beta-blockers
Inadequate preload		
Absolute	Inadequate intravascular volume	Volume replacement
	*Excessive urine output	
	*Obvious bleeding	
	*Occult bleeding (intraabdominal, groin)	
Relative vasodilation	Drugs (NTG, SNP, protamine); transfusion reaction (if anaphylaxis is present, see Table 9-2)	Decrease or stop drug infusion; Stop blood transfusion, repeat cross match
Mechanical	Chest closure	Volume replacement, adjust tidal volume, increase HR
	Surgical manipulation of the heart and great vessels	Notify surgeon

Table 9-3 (continued)

Condition	Causes	Treatment
Inadequate contractility	Residual cardioplegia and effect of ischemic cardioplegic arrest; reperfusion injury; ischemia	CaCl₂
	Vasospasm	NTG, nifedipine
	Fixed lesion	NTG, nifedipine
	Mechanical problem with graft	Fix mechanical problem with graft
	Air in coronaries	Remove air, give phenylephrine to increase coronary perfusion pressure, NTG
		Catecholamines, vasoconstrictors
	Hemodynamic abnormalities leading to decreased coronary flow	Inotropes
	Intrinsic cardiomyopathy	Decrease or stop drug
	Other drugs including anesthetics	
Altered afterload	Low	
	Drug reaction or side effect (including protamine)	Decrease or stop drug
	Transfusion reaction	See above
	Increasing core temperature	Vasoconstrictors
	High	
	"Light" anesthesia	Increase depth of anesthesia
	Intrinsic vascular disease	Vasodilators (SNP, hydralazine, amrinone)
	Aortic dissection	Surgical repair
	Iatrogenic	Discontinue vasoconstrictors

HR = heart rate, SVT = supraventricular tachycardia, A-V = atrioventricular, NTG = nitroglycerin, SNP = sodium nitroprusside, CaCl₂ = calcium chloride.

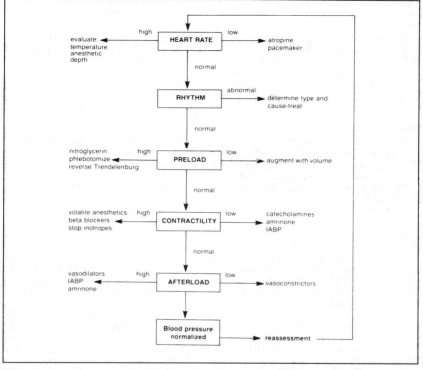

Fig. 9-1. Management scheme for cardiovascular deterioration in the postbypass period. IABP = intra-aortic balloon pump.

the right ventricle comprises most of the heart visible through a median sternotomy. The use of 2D-TEE may also help by providing a qualitative assessment of contractility. Diminished myocardial contractility may be due to regional or global ischemia.

It is important to establish an adequate coronary perfusion pressure to maintain myocardial oxygen supply and hence myocardial performance. Subendocardial coronary perfusion pressure equals the diastolic arterial pressure minus left ventricular end-diastolic pressure (PCWP may be used to estimate left ventricular end-diastolic pressure).

Refer to Chapters 3 and 8 for a discussion of specific options for inotropic augmentation.

4. **Fourth, evaluate the afterload.** Afterload is the impedance against which the ventricle must contract to eject the stroke volume. The systemic vascular resistance (SVR) comprises the majority of the afterload on the left ventricle and should almost always be the last hemodynamic parameter manipulated. With normal or high blood pressure, afterload reduction may be accomplished pharmacologically with vasodilators. With low blood pressure, reduction of the afterload may be accomplished with the use of an intraaortic balloon pump, effectively decreasing the impedance to ejection for the heart. Patients with a low cardiac output, low systemic arterial pressure,

Table 9-4. Summary of mechanisms and etiologies of hypoxia and hypercarbia

Hypoxia

Hypoventilation: Airway mishap, ventilator mishap, insufficient O_2 supply
$\dot{V}/\dot{Q}$ mismatch: Pulmonary edema, bronchospasm, pulmonary emboli, aspiration
   of foreign material or blood, pneumothorax, atelectasis
Intrapulmonary shunt: Mainstem bronchial intubation, tension pneumothorax,
   vasodilators (release of hypoxic pulmonary vasoconstriction)
Intracardiac shunt: Congenital or acquired
Diffusion abnormality: Preexisting lung disease, pulmonary edema

Hypercarbia

Decreased CO_2 elimination: Chronic obstructive pulmonary disease, restrictive
   disease (leading to increased dead space), hypoventilation, exhausted soda
   lime, inadequate fresh gas flows (in systems without CO_2 absorbers),
   decreased pulmonary blood flow
Increased CO_2 production: Shivering, "light" anesthesia, excess $NaHCO_3$
   administration

---

high SVR, and already on maximal pharmacologic inotropic support
will require an intraaortic balloon pump to reduce left ventricular
afterload and increase cardiac output. Pharmacologic manipulation
of the afterload first would almost always produce disastrous
hypotension.

In patients with low SVR the heart rate, preload, and contractility should be optimal before an attempt is made to increase
the SVR. Simply raising the SVR to raise a low systemic blood pressure may have deleterious effects on cardiac output and subsequently
on organ blood flow. However, if the patient has a sinus rhythm of
80–90 beats/min, the preload is optimal, and the cardiac output is
adequate (or high) for satisfactory organ perfusion, the use of a pharmacologic agent to increase SVR and normalize blood pressure is
appropriate.

5. **Finally,** one must continually return through each of these steps in
   sequence to maintain the patient's hemodynamic status.

II. **Respiratory System.** The usual causes of hypoxia and hypercarbia that
can occur during any anesthetic may also occur during the postbypass
period (Table 9-4). Some causes of hypoxia and hypercarbia especially
important to the postbypass patient include:

Pulmonary edema
   "Pump lung"
   Left ventricular dysfunction
   Residual pulmonary edema
   Drug or transfusion reaction
Mechanical difficulties
   Pneumothorax or hemothorax
   Endotracheal tube movement during CPB
Airway bleeding during heparinization
Protamine reactions
Intracardiac shunts
Pulmonary shunts ($\dot{V}/\dot{Q}$ mismatching)

A. **Causes of hypoxia and hypercarbia unique to the postbypass
   patient**

1. **Pulmonary edema**
   a. **"Pump lung"** (also called postperfusion lung) is a form of adult respiratory distress syndrome (ARDS). Although this syndrome usually develops in the postoperative period, it may become manifest during the postbypass period and can be quite severe. This entity usually presents with a gradually widening alveolar-to-arterial oxygen gradient, increasing physiologic shunt, decreasing pulmonary compliance, and progressive arterial hypoxemia. The risk factors for developing pump lung include preexisting pulmonary disease or pulmonary edema, high bypass flow rates, high pulmonary hydrostatic pressures (due to inadequate venting or increased bronchial blood flow) during bypass, and prolonged bypass duration[4]. Release of lysosomal granules and vasoactive substances from embolized platelet and leukocyte aggregates have been implicated as the cause of the increase in capillary permeability seen with pump lung. Other proposed causes include surfactant depletion, ischemic lung damage, and the use of bubble oxygenators. Pump lung rarely occurs with today's perfusion technology, especially in patients with no underlying lung disease. However, as we treat a "sicker" patient population and attempt surgical procedures of greater difficulty, pump lung should always be kept in the list of differential diagnoses for postbypass hypoxemia.
   b. **Left ventricular dysfunction.** Increase in pulmonary artery and capillary hydrostatic pressures may cause pulmonary edema.
   c. **Residual pulmonary edema.** Preexisting pulmonary edema may persist in patients with such diseases as ischemic and other cardiomyopathies, valvular heart disease (especially mitral stenosis), and some types of congenital heart disease.
   d. **Drug or transfusion reaction.** A reaction to a drug or blood product may cause either an increase in capillary hydrostatic pressure or an increase in capillary permeability, due to allergic mechanisms.
2. **Mechanical difficulties**
   a. **Pneumothorax.** Pneumothorax may occur spontaneously or may arise from excessive ventilatory pressures or inadvertent opening of the pleura and may only be recognized or become more significant after chest closure.
   b. **Hemothorax.** Blood may collect in the pleural space either after dissection of an internal mammary artery or from overflow of blood in the pericardial sling. The surgeon should routinely suction accumulated blood and fluid from the open pleural spaces prior to termination of bypass.
   c. **Movement of the endotracheal tube.** Because of the draping necessary to expose the field for cardiac surgery, the patient's head is often out of the anesthesiologist's direct vision. This arrangement may allow displacement of the endotracheal tube (either into a mainstem bronchus or out of the trachea), which may go unnoticed during bypass. This underscores the importance of listening for breath sounds and observing both lungs expand in the surgical field early in the process of weaning from bypass. Many anesthesiologists avoid the use of angulated connections between the breathing circuit and the endotracheal tube to prevent its migration if the surgeon leans on the tube or breathing circuit.
3. **Airway bleeding.** Full systemic heparinization makes bleeding from even the mildest trauma or unsuspected vascular lesion much more likely. Although systemic heparinization is the culprit, some of the more common sites of airway bleeding include the following:

a. **Traumatic lesions.** Heparinization will increase the quantity of extravascular blood in the respiratory system when trauma to the airway occurs. Blood will inactivate lung surfactant, causing atelectasis and ventilation-perfusion ($\dot{V}/\dot{Q}$) mismatching.

b. **Bronchial lesions.** Bronchial bleeding may occur with excessive lung manipulation, trauma from the endotracheal tube, or an unsuspected vascular tumor in the fully heparinized patient.

c. **Pulmonary artery perforation.** The pulmonary artery catheter may migrate into the "wedge" position with manipulation of the heart, and subsequent balloon inflation could perforate the pulmonary artery. During the hypothermic period, the catheter will become stiff, which will make pulmonary artery perforation more likely in these patients than in the general population. Other patients at increased risk for catheter-induced pulmonary artery perforation include women, anticoagulated patients, and possibly patients with pulmonary hypertension[5].

4. **Protamine reactions.** See discussion of protamine administration in sec. **I.B.3.**

5. **Intracardiac shunts.** If hypoxia persists despite evaluating and excluding the above abnormalities, one should entertain the diagnosis of a residual right-to-left intracardiac shunt. This diagnosis should also be suspected if positive end-expiratory pressure (PEEP) exaggerates hypoxia. One may confirm the diagnosis by using an indocyanine green dye measurement of cardiac output (see Chap. 13). Obtaining a left atrial blood gas saturation measurement may be helpful if the shunt is known or suspected to be at the ventricular level. If the left atrial blood is 100% saturated, then the cause of hypoxia is not pulmonary.

6. **Intrapulmonary shunts.** Large doses of vasodilators used to treat hypertension may reverse hypoxic pulmonary vasoconstriction and produce $\dot{V}/\dot{Q}$ mismatching. Hypoxemia may result from severe $\dot{V}/\dot{Q}$ mismatching.

7. **Summary.** Table 9-4 summarizes the mechanisms and etiologies that lead to hypoxia and hypercarbia.

B. **Postbypass respiratory management**

1. **Ensure adequate fresh gas flow.** One may forget to turn on the oxygen after bypass with the other duties that distract the anesthesiologist during this busy time.

2. **Check lung expansion.** Observe the field and listen to the lungs for wheezing or secretions.

3. **Ensure that the ventilator is on and securely connected to the patient.** Again, one may become distracted with the patient's hemodynamic management and forget to turn on the ventilator or not notice that the circuit has become disconnected during or after bypass. Therefore, one must take the time to check the breathing circuit specifically prior to terminating bypass.

4. **Check airway (including endotracheal tube) for obstruction.** One should always check the endotracheal tube for kinking or accumulation of secretions or blood and for tube migration.

5. **Check noninvasive monitors.** One should check these monitors immediately after separating from bypass. The pulse oximeter may not track the pulse if the patient is vasoconstricted, owing to either low peripheral temperature or administration of vasoconstrictors. The arterial-to-end-tidal carbon dioxide gradient may exceed 10–25 mm Hg on the basis of low cardiac output or pulmonary dysfunction. Bermudez[1] has suggested that the arterial-to-end-tidal carbon diox-

ide gradient results from closure of some pulmonary capillaries during bypass, causing an increase in total dead space. These capillaries reopen very slowly in the postbypass period. This phenomenon occurs regardless of whether patients are smokers or receive blood products. Also, examine the capnograph for an obstructive pattern.

6. **Arterial blood gas.** Despite the utilization of noninvasive monitoring of SaO_2 (by pulse oximetry) and carbon dioxide (by capnometry), one should always obtain an arterial blood gas measurement to ensure adequate minute ventilation and oxygenation and to assess acid-base status.

7. **Treatment of intrinsic pulmonary problems.** The treatment of pump lung and pulmonary edema may require high inspired concentrations of oxygen, PEEP, bronchodilators, diuretics, and circulatory support.

III. Hematologic considerations; coagulation

Coagulation in the postbypass period
Protamine reversal
Evaluation of postbypass bleeding
Blood conservation in the perioperative period

A. Protamine reversal
1. **Mechanism of action.** Protamine antagonizes heparin by a nonspecific polyanionic-polycationic interaction that displaces heparin from antithrombin III on an equal weight basis (i.e., 1 mg of protamine reverses 1 mg of heparin). For further discussion of protamine reversal, see Chapter 18.

2. **Determining the dose.** The protamine dose required for reversing the anticoagulant effect of heparin can be determined while rewarming is proceeding or just prior to separating from cardiopulmonary bypass by one of the following methods.

    a. **A heparin-protamine titration (HPT) test** to determine the circulating heparin concentration. The required dose of protamine needed is automatically calculated (Fig. 9-2). This technique is the most clinically precise method and reduces the protamine dose compared to a fixed protamine–total heparin dose ratio. See Chapter 18 for a detailed description of this technique.

    b. **Estimation** from a dose-response curve using the postrewarming activated clotting time (ACT) to calculate circulating heparin activity (method of Bull, see Chapter 18). However, this assumes a linearity between the ACT and heparin dose that will tend to overestimate protamine reversal requirements when hemodilution, hypothermia, or an ACT of greater than 600 seconds is present[2,3].

    c. **Empiric administration of 1.0–1.5 mg protamine/100 units of heparin given.** This method assumes that no heparin dilution or metabolism has occurred and therefore overestimates the required protamine dose.

    d. **Theoretically, excess protamine administration should be avoided** to prevent excess postoperative blood loss, although some authorities believe that anticoagulation from excess circulating protamine is not clinically significant.

3. **Monitoring the effectiveness of protamine**

    a. **One should observe the surgical field** for the amount of bleeding present and whether it is localized or generalized. Localized bleeding suggests a surgical cause, whereas generalized bleeding may indicate unneutralized heparin or another coagulation abnormality.

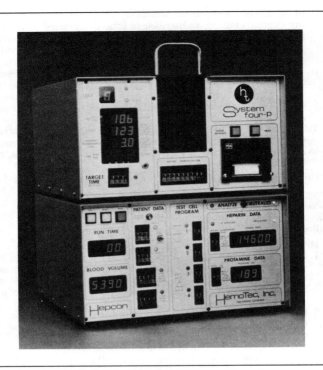

Fig. 9-2. Automated heparin-protamine titration system.

    b. Ten minutes after the initial protamine dose is administered, an ACT as well as a low-range HPT can be performed. If the results of the tests indicate the presence of circulating heparin, additional protamine may be required. Additional protamine (about 25–50 mg/500 ml of blood) may be required for blood scavenged from the chest or other blood that is administered from the cardiopulmonary bypass circuit. After administration of the additional protamine, the ACT should be repeated. If the results of the ACT are at or near the precardiopulmonary bypass baseline, it can be assumed that the patient has returned to normal hemostasis. If additional bleeding occurs, the probability is that a mechanical bleeding site is present. However, if the patient is still bleeding and no "rebound" heparin can be found using a heparin-protamine titration test, the ACT is normal or abnormal and the surgeon cannot find a surgical cause for the bleeding, a more comprehensive coagulation workup and platelet transfusions may be indicated.

B. Postbypass bleeding. Inadequate surgical hemostasis and unneutralized heparin are the most common causes of postbypass bleeding. However, one should bear in mind that postbypass bleeding may have multiple causes and keep a high index of suspicion for less common abnormalities such as deficiency or decreased adhesiveness of platelets, fibrinolysis, specific factor deficiency, transfusion reaction, and disseminated intravascular coagulation (DIC) (see Chapter 18).

C. **Blood conservation.** With increasing concern about the transmission of infectious agents, especially HIV, through blood transfusions, many clinicians allow lower intraoperative hemoglobin values. Methods for the conservation of blood during surgery have been developed.

1. **Use of bypass suction.** After administration of heparin and attainment of an adequate ACT, the bypass suction (also called cardiotomy suction) may be used. However, a significant amount of blood may be lost both before heparin administration and after its reversal, and greater hemolysis may occur with cardiotomy suction.

2. **Cell salvage.** Many centers now use cell salvage for the periods before and after bypass. A study done at the Mayo Clinic[8] showed a significant decrease in the use of banked red blood cells, fresh frozen plasma, and platelets when intraoperative cell salvage was performed.

3. **Reinfusion of shed mediastinal blood.** Another method of cell salvage includes the use of blood shed from the chest and mediastinum during the postoperative period.

4. **Removal of 500–1000 ml of autologous blood prior to bypass.** See Chapter 6.

5. **Acceptable postbypass hematocrits and fluid management** remain areas of controversy. Because many patients will still have a low hematocrit in the postbypass period owing to hemodilution, administration of blood would seem to be the logical choice. However, the administration of banked blood carries a small but definite risk, both from the standpoint of infectious disease and that of transfusion reaction. In patients with good ventricular function, a hematocrit of 21–25% or greater will usually suffice. Many patients, especially those with poor ventricular function, older patients, diabetics, and patients with inadequate revascularization will require the increased oxygen-carrying capacity afforded by an increased hematocrit. This group of patients will generally require a hematocrit of approximately 30%, or perhaps even greater, if clinical circumstances demonstrate a need for a higher oxygen-carrying capacity. Infusion of salvaged or autologous blood will optimize both the preload and oxygen-carrying capacity with an extremely low risk. These patients will require banked blood if an insufficient supply of autologous blood exists.

    For patients in whom the administration of banked blood is not justified based on the hematocrit and autologous blood is not available, the question arises whether to give colloid or crystalloid when the patient's preload requires augmentation. Colloid solutions may remain in the vascular space for a longer period of time, and therefore less total volume may be needed to achieve the desired effect on preload. The sustained effect of colloids in the postbypass period is probably their best recommendation. Both albumin and hetastarch are eliminated by the kidneys, both lasting up to 24 hours. One should limit hetastarch administration, including pump prime, to 20 ml/kg to prevent possible adverse effects on blood coagulation and blood typing associated with the administration of larger volumes. Most studies demonstrate similar hemodynamic profiles and volume requirements when either albumin or hetastarch is used for volume replacement.

IV. **Renal and metabolic systems**

Bypass insults
  Low blood pressure
  Low flow
  Deep hypothermic circulatory arrest
  Free hemoglobin

Table 9-5. Treatment of hyperkalemia

1. Diuresis
2. Sodium bicarbonate, 1–2 mEq/kg in children and one amp (44.6 mEq) in adults
3. Infusion of dextrose and insulin, 1–2 g glucose/kg with 0.3 units regular insulin/g of glucose in children; 25 g (1 amp of D_{50}) of glucose and 10 units of regular insulin in adults
4. Calcium, 20 mg/kg of calcium gluconate over a 5-min period for children and 500–1000 mg of calcium chloride for adults

> **Postbypass insults**
> Vasopressors
> Transfusion reaction
> Hypotension
> Low cardiac output
> Nephrotoxic drugs

A. **Postbypass renal dysfunction.** Many factors related to the bypass period have been implicated in postbypass renal dysfunction. Studies have shown that this dysfunction is not related **solely** to the pressure or flow technique used during bypass but rather to low cardiac output after bypass. Other factors such as nonpulsatile flow, preexisting renal dysfunction, the duration of bypass, circulatory arrest, free hemoglobin levels, and drugs such as gentamicin may also contribute to renal dysfunction.

   One should attempt to prevent or convert oliguric renal failure to nonoliguric renal failure because the former has a higher associated mortality. Treatments include dopamine 2–3 $\mu g \cdot kg^{-1} \cdot min^{-1}$; mannitol up to 1 g/kg if the patient has normal or low filling pressures (mannitol will increase filling pressures at least transiently); and loop diuretics such as furosemide, starting with low doses (5–10 mg) and gradually increasing the dose.

B. **Electrolyte abnormalities**

   1. **Hypokalemia** commonly occurs in the postbypass period.
      a. **The causes of postbypass hypokalemia include** urinary losses, intracellular sequestration, and hemodilution. The plasma potassium, however, will belie the total body potassium deficit, because most of the body's potassium is contained intracellularly (98%).
      b. **The treatment of hypokalemia is potassium replacement,** about 0.15–0.3 mEq $\cdot kg^{-1} \cdot hr^{-1}$, with potassium chloride. However, in children replacement is usually avoided unless severe dysrhythmias occur.

   2. **Hyperkalemia** generally does not occur after bypass.
      a. **If the patient receives a large cardioplegia dose** and has renal dysfunction, the serum potassium level may rise.
      b. **Patients with normal renal function** and mild hyperkalemia ($K^+ < 6.0$) generally need no treatment and may be observed by obtaining repeated determinations of the serum potassium concentration. Moderate hyperkalemia (K^+ between 6.0 and 7.0), often discovered by routine laboratory tests, generally resolves with time but may require some combination of the therapies listed in Table 9-5. With severe hyperkalemia ($K^+ > 7.0$ mEq/liter), especially with electrocardiographic (ECG) manifestations, virtually all patients will require therapy.

   3. **Hypocalcemia.** Some investigators believe that normal serum ionized calcium, although required to initiate excitation and contraction, has little influence on the amount of calcium that reacts with

troponin and hence little influence on contractility. They further assert that high extracellular calcium levels may inhibit diastolic relaxation and actually decrease contractility in some settings. They also believe that administration of exogenous calcium may precipitate coronary artery spasm and, in some patients, cellular death. Other investigators believe that the amount of sarcolemmal calcium depends greatly on the amount of ionized calcium in the extracellular fluid and, in turn, on the ionized calcium level in the blood[10].

    a. Hypocalcemia (total or ionized) may be caused by acute dilution, a large citrate load, an increase in pH, or elevation of parathyroid hormone. It often is manifest as myocardial depression and a prolonged QT interval.

    b. Although routine calcium administration post-CPB remains controversial, less controversial indications include hypotension associated with a low serum ionized calcium level or rapid blood administration (especially in children) and also severe hyperkalemia.

    c. The treatment is calcium, either the chloride or gluconate salt. Ten milliliters of 10% calcium gluconate contains 4.65 mEq of calcium. Ten milliliters of 10% calcium chloride contains 14 mEq of calcium. Most often the chloride salt is used because an equal molar amount of calcium may be administered with a smaller volume, and this salt produces a higher serum ionized calcium level than calcium gluconate.

4. Hypomagnesemia. Most of the body's magnesium is intracellular, and large losses may occur before the serum level falls. Normal serum magnesium ranges from 1.5–2.9 mg/dl. In patients with prolonged critical illness, hypomagnesemia may occur and may be manifest in the postbypass period. Hypomagnesemia may also result from dilution with a magnesium-free pump prime or may be due to intracellular sequestration during bypass.

    a. Hypomagnesemia causes prolonged PR and QT intervals and widened QRS complexes as well as myocardial depression.

    b. It is better to prevent hypomagnesemia than treat it, usually by supplying magnesium in the pump prime in a concentration of 2–5 mEq/liter. If supplementation is required in adults, 2–4 g is administered over 30–45 min. An infusion of 1 g/hr is begun and magnesium levels measured.

V. Central nervous system

  A. Surgical stimulation/anesthetic depth. Surgical stimulation in the postbypass period may vary. However, depending on the anesthetic technique chosen for the prebypass and the bypass periods and the current hemodynamic state, many patients may require an increase in depth of anesthesia and degree of neuromuscular blockade. The most stimulating portions of the postbypass period include electrocautery of the pericardium and pleura, manipulation of the pericardium and great vessels, and placement of the sternal wires and chest tubes.

    1. With a high-dose narcotic technique, patients may require small increments of narcotic (100–200 μg of fentanyl or 25–50 μg of sufentanil) unless they have very poor ventricular function and require aggressive catecholamine support. Patients with good ventricular function, especially those with hypertension, may require the addition of a volatile agent as well.

    2. The use of nitrous oxide in the postbypass period has the undesirable feature of enlarging any inadvertent intravascular air emboli and therefore is contraindicated in the postbypass period. Nitrous oxide also may increase pulmonary artery pressure in adults with preexisting pulmonary hypertension. Patients may also require high inspired concentrations of oxygen during this period (for pulmonary reasons or to increase the myocardial oxygen supply), and the use of nitrous oxide would limit the ability to deliver higher oxygen concentrations.

3. All anesthetic agents (including narcotics) should be titrated carefully in the postbypass period because the patient's hemodynamic status may change rather rapidly. Also, many patients depend heavily on endogenous sympathetic tone for circulatory homeostasis. Even small doses of opioids may diminish or abolish this response, with obvious adverse hemodynamic consequences.

4. Regardless of the patient's hemodynamic status, awareness may still occur, and one should consider administration of some amnestic agent such as scopolamine or additional sedative/hypnotics to reduce the incidence of awareness during periods of lighter anesthetic depth. However, sedative/hypnotics may decrease the systemic blood pressure.

B. **Neuromuscular blockade requirements.** Patients should receive adequate neuromuscular blockade at this point in the operation to prevent shivering, including microscopic shivering, which may increase total body oxygen consumption by 300–400%. The specific neuromuscular blocking agent should be chosen for its hemodynamic properties and duration of action.

C. **Postbypass temperature regulation.** The phenomenon of "afterdrop," or decrease in core body temperature after rewarming on bypass, occurs in virtually all patients who undergo hypothermic cardiopulmonary bypass. Several investigators have found that although the SVR decreases in the core circulation during rewarming, several vascular beds (e.g., muscle) are still severely vasoconstricted. These areas then become vasodilated during the 45–90 minutes following the termination of bypass, causing a decrease in core temperature. Afterdrop occurs as the lower temperature of the "shell" equilibrates with the core temperature. Afterdrop may cause an increase in oxygen demand (if shivering occurs) and may also alter coagulability of the blood. Several methods are used to attenuate afterdrop, including using warm irrigation fluids in the chest cavity, warmed inspired gases, warming blankets, warm ambient temperature, using vasodilators along with increased bypass flows during the warming period, lengthening the period of rewarming to increase the rectal temperature to about 33°C, and minimizing the length of time that the chest is open postbypass. The effectiveness of each of these methods is a subject of some debate because each has studies proving as well as disproving their efficacy. Despite the use of all the above measures, patients commonly arrive in the ICU with rectal temperatures in the 34–36°C range. In most patients the core temperature returns to normal during the next few hours, the greatest increase in temperature occurring 2–4 hours postoperatively, with a slight overshoot before stabilizing. One should carefully watch and correct the patient's pH and PCO_2 to prevent acute respiratory acidosis from developing during this postoperative warming period.

VI. **Conclusion.** The postbypass period is a time when some clinicians may allow their vigilance to wane as the end of the case approaches. This chapter underscores the need for **increased** vigilance during this busy period when the high technology aspects of the case distract the anesthesiologist from the basics of anesthetic management.

REFERENCES

1. Bermudez, J., and Lichtiger, M. Increases in arterial to end-tidal CO_2 tension differences after cardiopulmonary bypass. *Anesth. Analg.* 66:690–692, 1987.

2. Bull, B. S., Korpman, R. A., Huse, W. M., et al. Heparin therapy during extracorporeal circulation—I. Problems inherent in existing heparin protocols. *J. Thorac. Cardiovasc. Surg.* 69:674–684, 1975.

3. Bull, B. S., Huse, W. M., Braver, F. S., et al. Heparin therapy during extracorporeal circulation—II. The use of a dose-response curve to individualize heparin and protamine dosage. *J. Thorac. Cardiovasc. Surg.* 69:685–689, 1975.

4. Edmunds, L. H., and Alexander, J. A. Effect of Cardiopulmonary Bypass on the Lungs. In A. P. Fishman (ed.), *Pulmonary Diseases and Disorders* (1st ed.). New York: McGraw-Hill, 1980. Pp. 1728–1734.

5. Fletcher, E. C., Mihalick, M. J., and Siegel, C. O. Pulmonary artery rupture during introduction of the Swan-Ganz catheter: Mechanism and prevention of injury. *J. Crit. Care* 3:116–121, 1988.

6. Kirklin, J. W., and Barratt-Boyes, B. G. Hypothermia, Cardiac Arrest, and Cardiopulmonary Bypass. In J. W. Kirklin and B. G. Barratt-Boyes (eds.), *Cardiac Surgery.* New York: Wiley, 1986. Pp. 29–82.

7. Levy, J. H. Common Anaphylactic and Anaphylactoid Reactions the Anesthesiologist Sees. In J. H. Levy (ed.), *Anaphylactic Reactions in Anesthesia and Intensive Care.* Boston: Butterworth, 1986. Pp. 53–74.

8. McCarthy, P. M., Popovsky, M. A., Schaff, H. V., et al. Effect of blood conservation efforts in cardiac operations at the Mayo Clinic. *Mayo Clin. Proc.* 63:225–229, 1988.

9. Morel, D. R., Zapol, W. M., Thomas, S. J., et al. C5a and thromboxane generation associated with pulmonary vaso- and broncho-constriction during protamine reversal of heparin. *Anesthesiology* 66:597–604, 1987.

10. Vitez, T. S., and Koski, G. Calcium salts are contraindicated in the weaning of patients from cardiopulmonary bypass. *J. Cardiothorac. Anesth.* 2:567–575, 1988.

Care of the Cardiac Surgical Patient: The First 24 Hours Postoperatively

Garfield B. Russell, John L. Myers, and W. Andrew Kofke

The postoperative transition from termination of anesthesia and surgery to reestablishment of independence from ventilatory and hemodynamic support can be a precarious one for the cardiac surgical patient. This chapter will deal with methods of evaluation, diagnosis, and treatment during the early postoperative period and complications that arise during this period in cardiac surgical patients. Because many of these topics will be applicable to adults only, a separate section of the chapter deals with postoperative care in pediatric patients. The pediatric patient often requires a different approach to both clinical evaluation and therapy.

I. Transportation from the operating room to the intensive care unit (ICU)

A. General principles. The postoperative cardiac surgery patient must be viewed as capable of immediate and catastrophic decompensation at any time during transport. The transportation process must be viewed as a continuation of intraoperative care. At the conclusion of the surgical procedure, both surgical and anesthesiology teams must assess both surgical and cardiorespiratory stability. A simple maneuver, such as lifting the patient off the operating table, can cause dysrhythmias and marked blood pressure variations in the volume-depleted or incompletely anesthetized patient.

B. The moving process (Table 10-1)

1. Transition to transport monitors. At no time should the patient be without electrocardiographic and hemodynamic monitoring. When changing to transport monitors, disconnect a single monitor at a time. Zero and calibrate each unit individually. All monitoring catheters, including the pulmonary artery catheter, urinary catheter, arterial lines, and chest tubes should be secured.

2. Ventilation during transport. Until all preparations have been made for the patient to leave the operating room, continue ventilation with the anesthesia machine ventilator. During transport, vigorous manual ventilation of patients with a self-inflating bag and 100% oxygen is required to maintain normocarbia and thus avoid the increased incidence of dysrhythmias and pulmonary artery pressure changes associated with hypercarbia. Endotracheal tube position should be checked with each change in patient position, and breath sounds should be continuously auscultated during transport.

3. Drug infusions. All drug infusions received by the patient should be continued on battery-powered infusion pumps. Transport personnel should ideally include aides whose only duty is patient transport. Members of the anesthesiology and surgical team should be present to oversee the transport and recognize and treat any medical problems that arise.

C. Delivery of the patient to ICU personnel. On arrival in the ICU, coordination of personnel and meticulous attention to detail is required. It is at this time that loss of continuity of care and inadequate transfer of information is most likely. The operating room (OR) team must give a full, complete report to the receiving physician and the nursing staff who will be taking part in postoperative care. During this period, the ICU staff must evaluate the patient for changes in medical status occurring during transport, institute mechanical ventilation, take blood samples for arterial blood gas analysis and blood chemistry measurements, and form a management plan.

1. The initial postoperative report on arrival in the ICU

a. General data required. The patient's name, age, and other specific relevant data should be included.

b. Preanesthetic status

Table 10-1. Requirements during transport of postoperative cardiac patients to the intensive care unit

Monitoring
1. Minimum of a two-channel oscilloscope to visualize ECG and systemic blood pressure
2. Ability to monitor PA pressures, particularly if refractory pulmonary hypertension is present
3. Precordial or esophageal stethoscope
4. Pulse oximeter

Respiratory support equipment
1. E-tanks of oxygen with yoke, regulator, and key
2. Tubing connecting the oxygen supply to a 3-liter, self-inflating reservoir bag
3. Portable suction; Yankauer and catheter suction tubes
4. Laryngoscope and appropriate endotracheal tubes
5. PEEP valve (5 cm H_2O) for attachment to expiratory limb of the self-inflating bag to maintain intraoperative PEEP (if indicated)

Circulatory support
1. All drugs infusing prior to transport
2. Vasopressors (i.e., phenylephrine, epinephrine)
3. Antihypertensives (i.e., nitroglycerin, nitroprusside, trimethaphan)
4. Inotropes (i.e., calcium chloride, dopamine)
5. Sedatives or anesthetics (i.e., midazolam, opiates such as fentanyl or sufentanil)
6. Muscle relaxants
7. Intraaortic balloon pump or other assist device if needed

---

      (1) Preoperative status should include a description of the cardiac lesions, cardiac catheterization report, pulmonary history and report of abnormal pulmonary function tests, allergies, medications, laboratory studies, and any other pertinent medical information.
      (2) Patient response to preanesthetic medications and monitoring line insertion should be included as well.
   c. The anesthetic itself
      (1) The report on the intraoperative course should include the anesthetic technique (including drugs and doses used), any problems encountered (i.e., a difficult intubation, the need for vasopressors or inotropes on discontinuing cardiopulmonary bypass), medications and dosages presently infusing, blood products given, and the most recent results of intraoperative laboratory studies.
      (2) Any problems anticipated based on the intraoperative course should be elucidated, including any evidence of postbypass pulmonary dysfunction.
   d. Aspects of the surgical procedure
      (1) Describe the procedure performed and any technical problems encountered.
      (2) Are there anticipated problems (i.e., hemostasis)?
II. Initial patient evaluation in the ICU
  A. Review of systems
    1. Initial overview
      a. Base the initial evaluation on the ABCs of cardiopulmonary resuscitation. Ensure airway patency, adequate ventilation, and circulatory stability.

b. Make sure that all monitoring lines, IVs, chest tubes, and urinary catheters are patent and functioning.

c. Ensure that all ICU monitors are calibrated and connected by a monitor technician whose only duty is the operation of required monitors.

2. **Respiratory system**

a. Ensure that a respiratory therapist is present for immediate ventilator connection and adjustment.

b. Check endotracheal tube position and cuff volume.

c. Auscultate the lung fields for breath sound quality and air distribution during hand-bagging prior to mechanical ventilation.

d. Ensure that the chest tubes are patent and draining.

e. When mechanical ventilation is instituted in the ICU, start with an FIO_2 of 70–100% and the other ventilator settings utilized in the operating room until the initial ABG and chest x-ray (CXR) are evaluated. This ensures optimal oxygenation until the first results of arterial blood gas measurements are obtained.

f. If end-tidal carbon dioxide ($ETCO_2$) monitoring is present observe the waveform to ensure that the endotracheal tube is in position and there is no significant gas flow obstruction.

g. Transcutaneous pulse oximetry provides immediate evaluation of arterial oxygenation.

3. **Circulatory system**

a. Check the heart rate and rhythm

(1) Observe the monitor screen (a lateral chest lead, preferably lead V_5 for ischemia and lead II or MCL_1 for rhythm).

(2) Note function of artificial pacemaker when present.

b. Assess systemic perfusion

(1) Compare the arterial line blood pressure (BP) to a BP reading taken by sphygmomanometer.

(2) Assess peripheral pulses, skin color, temperature, and urine output.

(3) Determine the pulmonary artery (PA) pressures, pulmonary capillary wedge pressure (PCWP), central venous pressure, and the left atrial pressure (if a left atrial line is present).

(4) Measure a thermodilution cardiac output, and calculate cardiac index and systemic and pulmonary vascular resistance.

c. Assess postoperative bleeding. Note any active bleeding from the chest and leg incisions (if a saphenous vein graft has been harvested) as well as the volume of blood in the chest tube collection reservoir.

4. **Central nervous system (CNS).** Note the level of consciousness present. Since the patient is usually anesthetized and paralyzed from muscle relaxants, complete CNS assessment cannot be performed.

5. **Renal system**

a. Assess urine output during the surgery and the initial period in the ICU.

b. Assess the character of the urine (i.e., concentration, presence of hemoglobinuria or hematuria).

6. **Gastrointestinal system.** Check patency and placement of the nasogastric tube. Look for blood in the gastric drainage.

7. **Integument.** Look for signs of skin damage at pressure points.

8. **Temperature**

a. Note both the core and peripheral temperatures.

b. Use both warming lights and heating blankets to treat rectal temperatures of 35°C or lower.

c. Note and treat any shivering (see sec. **V.B.**).

B. Recommended postoperative tests

1. **Evaluate the cardiorespiratory system with**
   a. Arterial blood gases for oxygenation, ventilation and acid-base status, creatinine phosphokinase (including Mb fraction).
   b. A chest x ray for correct endotracheal tube and Swan-Ganz catheter position, cardiac and mediastinal widening, pulmonary edema, atelectasis, pleural effusions, and pneumothoraces.
   c. An electrocardiogram (ECG) for evidence of new ischemia, infarction, conduction defects, and arrhythmias.
2. **Metabolic and hematologic evaluation can be performed by clinical and blood chemistry analysis**
   a. Arterial blood gas determination allows assessment of acid-base balance with evaluation of the base excess, bicarbonate, and pH.
   b. Electrolytes (particularly potassium) can affect rhythm and contractility. Measured levels can be affected by the systemic pH.
   c. Urea nitrogen and creatinine levels reflect baseline renal functions and intravascular fluid status. Values obtained 24 hours after surgery should be compared with those obtained preoperatively.
   d. Glucose levels can be affected by surgical stress. If the patient is diabetic, abnormal glucose levels can make acid-base status more difficult to control.
   e. Hemoglobin and hematocrit levels help determine oxygen delivery, need for transfusion, and the presence of continued surgical bleeding.
3. **Evaluate hemostasis if bleeding from the chest tubes or incisions is excessive.** Included in this evaluation should be an activated coagulation time (ACT), prothrombin time (PT), activated partial thromboplastin time (PTT), platelet count, and fibrinogen determination. (see Chap. 18).

III. **Respiratory support following cardiac surgery.** Most adult and pediatric patients require postoperative mechanical ventilation. Slow emergence and gradual withdrawal of ventilatory support provide stability during this potentially unstable period.

After cardiac surgery, management of mechanical ventilation involves consideration of the patient's basic disease process and physiologic changes that occur with the sternotomy or thoracotomy incisions, general anesthesia, cardiopulmonary bypass, and the medications administered. These changes affect both the pulmonary circulation and alveolar ventilation. **Pulmonary dysfunction is usually maximal approximately 24 hours postoperatively and improves during the following week.**

A. **Pulmonary changes after cardiac surgery**
1. **Pulmonary mechanical effects**
   a. It takes about 2 weeks for vital capacity to return to preoperative values. On the third postoperative day it may still be only 50% of the preoperative value.
   b. There is decreased total lung capacity, inspiratory capacity, and functional residual capacity. Following sternotomy almost all patients have some degree of atelectasis. Left lower lobe atelectasis occurs in more than 50% of patients with myocardial revascularization.
   c. Postoperatively, total lung compliance decreases to 75% of baseline and is associated with increased dead space (V_D/V_T).
   d. Increased intrapulmonary shunting is often present owing to decreased functional residual capacity and lung compliance. Following cardiopulmonary bypass, the alveolar-arterial oxygen gradient ($A-aDO_2$) is increased, and the measured shunt is increased a mean of 13% from a preoperative normal shunt value of 5% or less.

Table 10-2. Initial ventilator settings for routine postoperative cardiac patients*

1. FIO_2: 0.7–1.0
2. Tidal volume: 12–15 ml/kg
3. Respiratory rate: 8–12 breaths/min
4. PEEP: 5 cm H_2O
5. Inspiratory/expiratory ratio: 1:2
6. Inspiratory flow rate: at least 30 liters/min

*Patients with internal mammary artery grafts or preexisting pulmonary disease may require different settings.

    e. The increased extravascular lung water present contributes to atelectasis and decreased compliance.

    f. An increased $A–aDO_2$ (often with associated hypoxemia and a PaO_2 of 70 mm Hg or less on room air) is found in more than 50% of patients during the first three postoperative days.

    g. Increased work of breathing (about 20%) is associated with decreased vital capacity and lung compliance during spontaneous respiration. Work of breathing increases in direct proportion to the decrease in vital capacity.

2. Pharmacologic effects

    a. Intraoperative narcotics and sedatives depress ventilation and blunt the respiratory response to hypercapnia and hypoxemia.

    b. Anticholinergics (scopolamine or atropine) dilate the airways, which may increase VD/VT by 25%. This may occur even when anticholinergics are given only as part of the premedication.

    c. Dopamine may have a central depressant effect on ventilation.

    d. After cardiopulmonary bypass (CPB) pulmonary vascular resistance (PVR) increases and remains above control values for the first 1–2 hours. PVR may also be increased by hypercapnia or hypoxemia or any catecholamine or vasoconstrictor with alpha activity.

    e. Inhibition of hypoxic pulmonary vasoconstriction (HPV) results from several agents.

        (1) Beta agonists, such as isoproterenol, decrease HPV, resulting in an increased $A–aDO_2$ and an increased shunt fraction. Clinically, this is important only when underlying lung disease is present.

        (2) HPV is also reduced by vasodilators, including nitroglycerin (NTG) and nitroprusside (NP).

B. Ventilator settings on arrival in the ICU (Table 10-2)

    1. FIO_2. Start ventilation with 100% oxygen if any question exists about cardiorespiratory stability. If intraoperative oxygenation has been adequate, then 70–80% oxygen may be used.

    2. A tidal volume of 12–15 ml/kg helps prevent atelectasis. In some patients who have had internal mammary artery (IMA) grafts, large tidal volumes may place tension on the IMA from its origin to the coronary anastomosis on the heart. In these patients, higher respiratory rates and smaller tidal volumes (6–10 ml/kg) are recommended so that adequate minute ventilation (100 ml/kg/min) is maintained.

    3. A respiratory rate of 8–12 breaths/minute should maintain a normal $PaCO_2$ (35–45 mm Hg). In patients with anticipated higher metabolic requirements or increased carbon dioxide production (i.e., patients who are initially hypothermic who shiver during rapid rewarming or those who are febrile), the initial rate may be set slightly higher even when a low normal $PaCO_2$ is present at the time. This maneuver usually prevents a respiratory acidosis from developing.

Patients with pulmonary artery hypertension (PAH) are hyperventilated, and a $PaCO_2$ of 25–28 mm Hg is maintained. This promotes pulmonary vasodilation and helps decrease PA pressure.

4. As a rule, 5 cm H_2O of **positive end-expiratory pressure** (PEEP) should be added to help prevent atelectasis and perhaps reverse the atelectasis that has developed intraoperatively. In patients with hypotension or poor cardiac output, PEEP may interfere with systemic venous blood return to the right side of the heart, decreasing cardiac output (CO). Higher PEEP may also increase pulmonary vascular resistance. In this situation, no PEEP (ZEEP or zero end-expiratory pressure) is used until the patient's condition is stabilized. When there is increased mediastinal bleeding postoperatively and no hemodynamic contraindication, PEEP is often increased to 10 cm H_2O. Higher levels of PEEP may help tamponade bleeding sites on the chest wall.

5. **The initial inspiratory/expiratory (I:E) ratio** setting is usually 1 : 2. A shorter inspiratory time leads to higher peak inflation pressures (PIP) and increased ventilation-perfusion mismatching. In the average adult, PIP is usually equal to or less than 30 cm H_2O and ideally should not be equal to or more than 35 cm H_2O.

6. **Inspiratory gas flow rates** must be able to maintain an even distribution of ventilation and constant gas flow during all phases of the respiratory cycle. Each patient's tidal volume, respiratory rate, and I:E ratio must be considered. Limits on the gas flow rate can vary between ventilators. The usual inspiratory flow rate is 30 liters/minute.

7. **The mode of mechanical ventilation** must also be decided. Most adults are ventilated with a volume ventilator. Initially, ventilation can be controlled (CMV), but as the patient recovers from anesthesia and spontaneous respirations resume, synchronous intermittent mandatory ventilation (SIMV) or extended mandatory minute ventilation (EMMV) may be used to facilitate weaning. During weaning a pressure support (PS) or pressure assist (PA) mode is often chosen. The available modes of mechanical ventilation include:

   a. **Controlled ventilation.** Controlled ventilation may be volume (usual for adults) or pressure limited. A preset rate and tidal volume or a preset peak pressure and rate is delivered regardless of spontaneous ventilatory efforts.

   b. **Assist control.** With volume-limited ventilation a negative inspiratory effort results in the ventilator delivering a preset tidal volume at the patient-generated rate.

   c. **Synchronized intermittent mandatory ventilation.** The patient's own inspiratory effort triggers the ventilator. The breaths given independent of effort are synchronized so that patient- and machine-initiated breaths do not occur simultaneously. The IMV mode does not have this synchronization.

   d. **Pressure support ventilation.** A preset maximum pressure is delivered at a patient-initiated rate. Because the patient can control the rate and tidal volume, there is often a greater sense of control and comfort in awake patients during weaning.

   e. **Extended mandatory minute ventilation.** The desired minute volume is set. If the patient attains this level spontaneously the ventilator does not give additional breaths. If not, breaths at a preset tidal volume attain the predetermined minute ventilation.

Table 10-3. The hemodynamic effects of mechanical ventilation

Effect	Mechanism
Decreased cardiac output	1. Increased intrathoracic pressure increases right atrial pressure, decreasing venous return and right ventricular end-diastolic volume, thus decreasing right ventricular stroke volume.
	2. Leftward shift of the interventricular septum decreases left ventricular diastolic compliance, decreasing left ventricular end-diastolic volume and stroke volume.
Increased pulmonary vascular resistance	A tidal volume of 5–10 ml/kg increases PVR by about 12% at end inspiration. Blood vessel compression and air space dilation are responsible.
Inaccurate PCWP measurements	Hyperinflation with high tidal volumes and PEEP of > 12 cm H_2O decrease the accuracy of PA catheter wedge pressure determinations.
Decreased required oxygen delivery	Breathing normally utilizes 5% of the total oxygen consumption. In respiratory failure prior to mechanical ventilation respiratory muscle O_2 consumption may increase to 50% of total O_2 consumption. The cardiorespiratory requirements for this increased oxygen delivery are relieved with mechanical ventilation.
Negative inotropy	A reflex vasodilation, bradycardia, and negative inotropic effect **may** occur with lung hyperinflation and is directly proportional to tidal volume.

C. **Hemodynamic effect of mechanical ventilation.** The hemodynamic effect of mechanical ventilation and PEEP are described in Table 10-3.

D. **Alternate modes of ventilating**

1. **Rapid rates and smaller tidal volumes.** High-frequency ventilation may be performed simply by decreasing the tidal volume (TV) to 6–8 ml/kg and increasing respiratory rates to 18–20 breaths/minute with a ventilator such as the Siemans 900 C. Other methods utilize high-frequency jet or oscillatory movement of the tidal volume. Often tidal volumes are decreased and respiratory rates increased (although usually quite conservatively) for prevention of stretch of a mammary artery graft or to decrease the peak inspiratory pressure and prevent potential barotrauma in a patient with postoperative pulmonary compromise (i.e., capillary leak syndrome). There is seldom a need for high-frequency jet ventilation (HFJV) or high-frequency oscillation in the postoperative cardiac patient.

2. **High positive end-expiratory pressure.** The usual PEEP level utilized is 5 cm H_2O, or 10 cm H_2O to help control increased chest wall bleeding. However, higher levels may be required. With a severe pulmonary insult, such as that seen with "pump lung," a severe capillary leak syndrome with an adult respiratory distress syndrome (ARDS)-like picture after cardiopulmonary bypass (Chap. 9), PEEP levels as high as 20–30 cm H_2O may be required to maintain an adequate PaO_2.

3. **Reverse I:E ratios.** Prolonging the inspiratory phase may allow ventilation with lower peak inspiratory pressures because the same

tidal volume can be forced through the airway in a longer time interval. In patients with postoperative pulmonary dysfunction (i.e., adult respiratory distress syndrome) and high inflation pressures with increased risk of barotrauma, inverse ratio ventilation (with a longer inspiratory than expiratory phase) may be beneficial and may result in lower PIP and less interference with cardiac output. This can improve PaO_2 as well. Conversely, the expiratory phase may need to be more prolonged, particularly in patients with obstructive pulmonary disease, to allow adequate exhalation and prevent stacking of lung volumes.

4. **Inspiratory hold.** A pause at the end of inspiration before expiration may improve oxygenation because it encourages alveolar recruitment and helps to prevent further atelectasis.

E. **Ventilators.** Ventilators are either negative-pressure or positive-pressure devices. The classic negative-pressure ventilators is the *"iron lung"* used during the polio epidemic of the fifties. Another is the cuirass ventilator, which consists of a lightweight plastic thoracic shell with an airtight bag that encloses the thorax. It is still occasionally used for the treatment of neuromuscular respiratory failure and occasionally after correction of some congenital heart defects. Positive-pressure ventilators are much more common and require the presence of an endotracheal tube. Positive-pressure ventilators inflate the lungs with ventilating gas under a positive pressure that is either volume (most common) or pressure limited. Table 10-4 describes some characteristics of commonly used volume ventilators.

1. **Volume ventilators commonly used in postoperative cardiac patients.** Different ventilators offer different advantages under varied clinical conditions.

a. Use of the Engstrom Erica has a number of advantages. It has an easy to read front face with set dials, and LED readings and toggle switches allow direct visualization of settings and variables such as compliance, exhaled tidal volume, and minute volume. The extended mandatory minute ventilation (EMMV) mode is a major advantage. Its major disadvantage lies in the increased work of breathing that is necessary during spontaneous ventilation through its valved gas flow pathway. Its true maximal minute volume can also be suboptimal for those with high ventilatory requirements.

b. The Siemans Servo 900 C ventilator has capabilities for high gas flows, high effective respiratory rates (to 120/minute), and low delivered tidal volumes that make ventilation of adults, children, infants, and neonates at slow rates or at rates classified as high-frequency positive-pressure ventilation (HFPPV) easily attainable. The servo mechanisms on both the inspiratory and expiratory limbs allows accurate delivery of set volumes. The machine is often modified with a continuous flow circuit when ventilating infants following cardiac surgery.

c. The Bennett MA Series and Bear ventilators are widely used. The Bennett MA Series at University Hospital, The Pennsylvania State University are modified to provide a high constant gas flow without as much resistance as the Engstrom Erica valve system. It is a good machine for patients for whom weaning is difficult and for patients requiring higher than normal minute volumes. The Bear ventilators are available for adults, and the Bear Cub infant ventilator, which is pressure controlled, is used in infants.

Many other ventilators are available. Choice of ventilator should depend on individual patient circumstances and the particular ventilating requirements desired by the attending physician.

Table 10-4. Commonly used volume-limited ventilators

Ventilator	Tidal volume delivery system	Modes of function	Respiratory rate limits (breaths/min)	PEEP range (cm H_2O)
Emerson IMV and 3PV	Piston driven	IMV, CMV, CPAP	0.2–25.0 (IMV) 0.2–50.0 (3PV)	0–25
Bournes Bear-2	Pneumatic flow generator	SIMV, CPAP, CMV, A/C	0.5–60	0–50
Bennett MA-1	Compressor-powered bellows	CMV, A/C, IMV, CPAP with modification	1–60*	0–15
Puritan Bennett 7200	Pneumatic flow generator (microprocessor-controlled)	SIMV, CMV, A/C, CPAP, PS	0.5–70	0–45
Engstrom Erica	Pneumatic flow generator (microprocessor-controlled)	SIMV, CMV, A/C, EMMV, CPAP	0.4–40*	0–30
Siemans 900 C	Pneumatic flow generator (microprocessor-controlled)	SIMV, A/C, CPAP, PS, and PC	0.5–120	0–50

*Rates may be higher but tidal volume may be inaccurate.

A/C = assist/control, CPAP = continuous positive airway pressure, CMV = continuous mandatory ventilation, EMMV = extended mandatory minute ventilation, IMV = intermittent mandatory ventilation, PC = pressure control, PS = pressure support, SIMV = synchronized intermittent mandatory ventilation.

Source: Modified from W. A. Kofke. Postoperative Respiratory Care Techniques. In W. A. Kofke and J.H. Levy (eds.), *Postoperative Critical Care Procedures of the Massachusetts General Hospital.* Boston: Little, Brown, 1986. P. 64. With permission.

F. **Monitoring postoperative cardiac patients during mechanical ventilation**

1. **Arterial blood gases.** The initial ABG measurement taken after ICU admission is vital to the assessment of the physiologic changes that have occurred during transport, the adequacy of ventilator settings, and acid-base status. When ABGs are the only objective means of ventilation and oxygenation assessment they should usually be measured at regular intervals, depending on the individual patient during the initial postoperative period, and 15–30 minutes after each change in ventilator setting. Even if no changes are made in ventilating parameters, increased carbon dioxide production associated with rewarming can result in significant respiratory acidosis.

2. **ETCO$_2$.** Monitoring of breath by breath ETCO$_2$ by mass spectrometry or infrared capnometry can provide constant and vital information, especially (1) during rewarming when the patient is hypothermic on admission, (2) in the patient with pulmonary hypertension in whom hyperventilation and relative hypocarbia is indicated in the initial postoperative period, and (3) during the weaning of ventilatory support. Continuous capnometry may result in fewer ABG determinations and maintenance of a narrower range of acid-base changes.

3. **Pulse oximetry.** A constant noninvasive measure of oxygen saturation has become a standard of care in the monitoring of mechanically ventilated patients. It is especially important in patients who are being rapidly weaned or recently extubated or who have borderline oxygenation. After a change in ventilator settings (i.e., increased PEEP), the effects on oxygenation can be observed immediately and continuously, not just with intermittent ABGs. In a patient with good myocardial and pulmonary function, a combination of ETCO$_2$ and pulse oximetry monitoring may allow fewer ABGs to be measured.

4. **Mixed venous oxygen saturation ($S\bar{v}O_2$).** Fiberoptic pulmonary artery catheters can continuously measure $S\bar{v}O_2$. $S\bar{v}O_2$ reflects arterial oxygen content, oxygen utilization, and cardiac output. With both a constant display of saturation and a graph of $S\bar{v}O_2$ trends over a period of time, reduction of cardiac output by PEEP or changes in oxygen utilization by an inappropriately rapid rate of ventilator weaning can be detected.

G. **Withdrawing ventilatory support.** Most patients are weaned from mechanical ventilation and extubated within 12–24 hours of cardiac surgery. The weaning plan begins when the patient returns from the operating room and the anesthesia and surgical procedures and any associated problems are assessed. Patients with valve replacements or poor ventricular function are often electively ventilated for the initial 24 postoperative hours, especially if PA pressures are elevated or increase significantly in response to a rise in PaCO$_2$. However, after a routine coronary artery bypass graft (CABG) procedure in an otherwise healthy patient who has had a low-dose narcotic anesthetic supplemented by a volatile agent, extubation may be performed within 4–8 hours of surgery.

1. **Criteria to be filled prior to consideration for weaning and extubation.** Prior to weaning, the patient should demonstrate the following characteristics:

   a. **Hemodynamic stability.** Cardiac rhythm and measured hemodynamic variables (i.e., PCWP, BP, and CO) should be stable. Inotropic agents, vasopressors, and vasodilators should be weaned to low-range doses with a view to discontinuation. If an intraaortic balloon pump (IABP) is in use, it should be weaned to a low rate

Table 10-5. Respiratory criteria for weaning from mechanical ventilation

1. $PaO_2 \geq 100$ mm Hg with an FIO_2 of 0.5
2. $PaCO_2 \leq 50$ mm Hg
3. Arterial pH of ≥ 7.32, unless cause clearly known and improvement expected
4. PEEP ≤ 5 cm H_2O
5. Stable chest x ray
6. Awake without residual neuromuscular blockade

Respiratory criteria for extubation
1. Negative inspiratory force of at least -20 (preferably -30) cm H_2O
2. Vital capacity of at least 10 ml/kg (2–3 times the tidal volume)
3. Resting minute ventilation of ≤ 10 liters
4. Maximum voluntary ventilation ≥ 2 times resting level
5. Patient is comfortable breathing spontaneously with CPAP of ≤ 5 cm H_2O with respiratory rate < 30

PEEP = positive end-expiratory pressure, CPAP = continuous positive airway pressure.

of support (i.e., 1 : 4), or a distinct plan of long-term support should be established by the patient care team.
  b. Surgical hemostasis. Hemostasis should be present and chest tube drainage should be equal to or less than 1–2 ml/kg/hr or equal to or less than 100 ml/hr.
  c. Adequate neurologic function. The patient is awake, has a gag reflex, and is cooperative.
  d. No planned intervention that would require further sedation or analgesia.
  e. Normothermia. Increased carbon dioxide production occurs with rewarming as well as with a fever.
  f. No acute changes shown on CXR that would compromise the patient.
  g. Satisfaction of the respiratory criteria shown in Table 10-5.
2. **The weaning process.** It is important to observe patients closely during weaning from mechanical ventilation to evaluate changes in hemodynamics that might occur. The following steps should be followed to implement weaning from mechanical ventilation safely.
  a. Withhold narcotics that may depress respiration. An agitated patient who is not in pain may be sedated without depressing ventilation by a small dose of haloperidol (1 mg IV or 1–5 mg SQ).
  b. Decrease the respiratory rate 2–4 breaths/minute at regular intervals, noting the response to each change. Usually **ABG** measurements are made after each change in ventilator settings. With an $ETCO_2$ monitor and a pulse oximeter this is not always necessary.
  c. Clinical and ABG assessment is made at respiratory rate of 4. In patients without underlying oxygenation problems who cannot be weaned, hypoxemia usually does not develop until the respiratory rate is decreased to 4 breaths/minute. If the patient is progressing well, discontinue mechanical ventilation and substitute a continuous positive airway pressure (CPAP) of 5 cm H_2O.
  d. Maintain the patient on CPAP for 45–60 minutes with a clinical and ABG assessment. Extubation criteria in Table 10-5 should be satisfied.
  e. There will obviously be vigorous patients in whom weaning can progress directly from full ventilation to CPAP as well as those for whom even a conservative, graded approach is too rapid.

Table 10-6. Methods of oxygen delivery to the extubated patient

Method	O$_2$ flow (liters/min)	Percent O$_2$ delivered
Nasal cannula	1–6	25–45
Face tent	15	30–45
Face masks		
Simple	6–15	35–65
Aerosol	6–15	40–70
Partial rebreathing	Enough to keep the reservoir bag	60–80
Nonrebreathing	from collapsing	85–95

3. **The extubation process.** At the time of extubation, all preparations should be made for immediate emergency airway support and reintubation. All equipment should be nearby, checked, and ready. An anesthetic plan for intubation should be formulated.

   a. **Position the patient** in a semiupright position, preferably 30–45 degrees, if there are no contraindications.

   b. **Suction** the endotracheal tube and then the mouth and pharynx. This should be done 2–3 minutes before extubation so that any airway irritation or hypoxemia caused by too vigorous suctioning is corrected.

   c. Have the postextubation **oxygen delivery system** ready.

   d. Have a **selfinflating 3-liter resuscitation bag** available to connect to the endotracheal tube (ETT).

   e. Deflate the endotracheal tube cuff and **remove the tube** with positive pressure on the breathing bag, allowing forced expiration to clear residual secretions.

   f. Clear any **oral secretions.**

   g. Apply **face mask** oxygen.

   h. Follow the **oxygen saturation** by pulse oximetry and obtain an ABG measurement in 20 minutes, or sooner if indicated.

   i. The patient must be carefully **observed** for **10–15 minutes after extubation** to ensure continued adequate spontaneous ventilation.

   j. **Maintain an NPO status** for at least 6 hours postextubation. There is often residual vocal cord dysfunction that temporarily decreases the patient's ability to protect the airway.

H. **Postextubation respiratory support.** In most cases after extubation there is a rapid transition first to oxygen by high-humidity face mask, then to oxygen by nasal cannula, and finally to room air breathing (Table 10-6). However, some patients do not go through this period without requiring additional respiratory intervention ranging from the use of a bronchodilating drug to oxygen delivery to combined nasal cannula and face mask, to reintubation and reintroduction of mechanical ventilation.

I. **Management of postoperative respiratory complications**

   1. **Causes of postoperative respiratory failure.** Many pulmonary and systemic factors can contribute to postoperative hypoxemia and hypercapnia (Table 10-7). Several of these factors uniquely related to cardiac surgery require specific mention:

      a. **Phrenic nerve palsy.** The iced slush solution used to produce topical myocardial hypothermia and supplement myocardial protection from cardioplegic arrest can damage one or both phrenic nerves. The phrenic nerve is also at risk of surgical injury during internal mammary artery dissection. Often the clinical signifi-

Table 10-7. Physiologic mechanisms of hypoxemia and hypercapnia

Hypoxemia	Hypercapnia

Decreased alveolar oxygen concentration ($P_{A}O_2$)
   Hypoventilation (residual anesthesia, sedation)
   Hypoxic gas mixture
	Hypoventilation
	   Decreased minute ventilation
	   Increased respiratory dead space

Increased right-to-left shunt (cardiac, pulmonary)
   Atelectasis
   Lobar collapse
   Pneumonia
	Increased carbon dioxide production
	   Hypermetabolic states (i.e., sepsis)
	   Hyperalimentation
	   Hypothermia with shivering

Decreased oxygen in mixed venous blood
   Increased oxygen consumption (hypermetabolic states such as sepsis and shivering)
   Decreased cardiac output
   Decreased oxygen content in arterial blood	

Decreased alveolar-capillary diffusion	

cance of this damage is not apparent until weaning is attempted or extubation is completed. Many patients can be weaned without difficulty when the deficit is unilateral. The patient often does not manifest the classic paradoxical respiratory pattern but exhibits a vital capacity and negative inspiratory force that, although not normal, fulfill extubation criteria. Then within several hours after extubation, respiratory failure develops, and reintubation becomes necessary. Evaluation of diaphragmatic movement by fluoroscopy or ultrasound is usually diagnostic. Continued ventilatory support when necessary and the passage of time usually result in eventual recovery of phrenic nerve function.

b. Hypoventilation. In the postoperative period during weaning, some patients are adequately oxygenated but hypoventilate and become hypercapneic. This situation is often related to the total dose of perioperative narcotics or to additional sedation given in the ICU. A long plasma half-life of narcotics can be expected in some patients, for example the $t_{1/2}$ of fentanyl can be prolonged from about 220 minutes up to 18 hours in patients with congestive heart failure and associated decreased liver perfusion.

Less common causes of hypoventilation include underlying neuromuscular disease and chronic obstructive lung disease in patients who rely on a hypoxic ventilatory drive.

Some older patients (usually >65 years) exhibit a sedated and confused behavior from scopolamine, which is often used as part of the anesthetic premedication. This is reversible with titration of low-dose physostigmine (Antilirium). Often less than a total dose of 1 mg is required. In the narcotized patient, it may be tempting to give a narcotic antagonist (i.e., naloxone). However, the potential for marked increases in blood pressure and even pulmonary edema following reversal of analgesia usually makes waiting for spontaneous reversal the preferred choice.

   c. **Venous admixture.** Vasodilators such as nitroglycerin and nitroprusside counteract hypoxic pulmonary vasoconstriction and
   may open some previously closed arteriovenous connections. This
   causes increased right-to-left shunting of blood and lowers the
   PaO_2. The effect varies with the individual patient and overall
   clinical situation. It is impossible to predict the effect of any particular drug infusion on blood shunting.
2. **Treatment of hypoxemia or hypercarbia.** Increased pulmonary
   secretions, atelectasis, preexisting lung disease, and bronchospasm
   may result in pulmonary compromise in postoperative cardiac surgical patients.
   a. **Management of atelectasis and increased secretions.**
      (1) **Pulmonary physiotherapy.** Postural drainage, percussion,
          vibration, coughing, and suctioning are intended to encourage
          thoracic expansion and improve clearance of secretions. Early
          ambulation is beneficial.
      (2) **Humidification.** Moist secretions are more easily mobilized.
          Inspired gas bypassing the nose and upper airway through the
          ETT and perioperative use of anticholinergics can have a marked
          drying effect. Keeping inspired gas at or more than 80% humid-
          ified and normothermic is very helpful. Monitoring inspired
          gas temperatures is essential. At times, aerosol treatments are
          also needed, but overhydration and bronchospasm can result
          from this treatment.
      (3) **Flexible bronchoscopy.** Diagnostic visualization of pulmo-
          nary segments and recovery of sputum samples for bacterio-
          logic assessment can be valuable for diagnosis and treatment.
          Directed suctioning and saline lavage as well as visualization
          of the effects of chest physiotherapy on secretion mobilization
          allow assessment of the effects of physiotherapy maneuvers.
      (4) **Pharmaceutical assistance.** Several drugs can improve mo-
          bilization of secretions.
          (a) **Acetylcysteine.** This agent acts as a mucolytic that lyses
              mucus disulfide bonds with its free sulfhydryl group. Mucus
              viscosity is thus decreased. When given by inhalation via
              jet nebulizer (2–5 ml of a 5–20% solution q4–8h) it liquifies
              secretions within 1 minute, and its effects peak within 10
              minutes. Alternatively, 1–2 ml of a 10–20% solution can be
              instilled through an ETT or, perhaps with fewer side effects,
              in a locally directed manner through a flexible broncho-
              scope. The known side effects include bronchospasm, nausea
              and vomiting, and irritation of the bronchial mucosa.
          (b) **Racemic epinephrine.** This agent produces bronchodila-
              tion and decreased airway edema, aiding clearance of air-
              way secretions. Up to 0.5 ml of a 2.25% solution is given
              by nebulizer. Because of the high potential for beta-1 car-
              diac stimulation, treatments should be carefully ordered
              and monitored.
          (c) **Beta-adrenergic agonists.** Nebulized beta-adrenergic ag-
              onists promote mucociliary clearance of airway secretions
              (Table 10-8). Their bronchodilating effect is comparable to
              and can be superior to that of parenterally administered
              aminophylline. Given by nebulizer they are relatively beta-
              2-specific compared with isoproterenol. However, when given
              parenterally, (i.e., terbutaline 0.25–0.50 mg), the specificity
              is lost, and the resulting tachycardia can be as marked as
              that seen with epinephrine.

Table 10-8 Commonly used beta-adrenergic agonists

Name	Route	Usual dose	Potential advantages	Disadvantages
Albuterol Ventolin Proventil	Oral Inhaled	10–20 mg q6–8h 0.5 ml (0.5%) in 2.5 ml saline q4–6h	Perhaps fewer beta-1 effects	Has been used for a shorter time in the United States than others
Metaproterenol Alupent Metaprel	Oral Inhaled	2–4 mg q6–8h 0.3 ml (5%) in 2.5 ml of normal saline q4–6h	Minimal beta-1 effects when inhaled	Tolerance may develop
Terbutaline Brethine Bricanyl	Oral Inhaled SQ	5 mg q6h 2 sprays q4–6h 0.25 mg (may be repeated in 15–30 min once)	As effective as epinephrine when given parenterally	Beta-1 stimulation marked SQ; nervousness and tremors are common
Isoetharine Bronkosol	Inhaled	0.5 ml (1%) in 3 ml normal saline q4–6h	Has been available and in use longer than others	Less beta-2 selective

(5) Improving chest expansion. The decreases in vital capacity, functional residual capacity, and inspiratory and expiratory reserve volumes that are present after surgery increase the risk of postoperative pulmonary complications. Incentive spirometry, intermittent positive-pressure breathing (IPPB), and CPAP are used to help expand the lungs and prevent further development of atelectasis.

   (a) Incentive spirometry involves a variety of methods that encourage deeper, more forceful inspirations and provide a measure of inspiratory effort. The positive reinforcement of these visual measurements allows the patient to see the extent of each inspiratory effort and the improvement that occurs with repetition.

   (b) IPPB has been used to help pulmonary expansion. A pressure-limited ventilator with an attached mouthpiece is used for about 15 minutes every 2–6 hours to produce passive lung expansion. Benefits are maximal in patients who have a poor vital capacity or chest wall deformities that prevent maximal voluntary lung expansion. Overall, use of this technique has decreased because of controversy about its efficacy.

   (c) CPAP is often used instead of IPPB. In the extubated patient, CPAP can be given either by a tight-fitting mask covering the mouth and nose or a specially devised nasal mask. Besides preventing and reversing airway collapse, it may also promote air movement between adjacent lung segments. Nasal CPAP is associated with less risk of aspiration than CPAP with a mask covering the face. Gastric insufflation is cited as a complication, but its extent and the level of CPAP causing it are poorly documented.

b. Bronchospasm. Aside from the aerosolized beta-adrenergic agonists (Table 10-8), theophylline derivatives are utilized to promote bronchodilation.

   (1) Theophylline. The theophyllines are available both as oral and parenteral agents. In the ICU, intravenous administration of aminophylline is most common. The degree of bronchodilation and the side effects are directly related to the serum level attained. The dosage should vary with the patient's physical status, liver perfusion (metabolism is primarily hepatic), and coadministration of medications (i.e., cimetidine) that can increase serum levels. The initial loading dose is 3–9 mg/kg followed by an infusion rate of 0.4–1.0 mg/kg/hr. Higher rates of infusion are required most often in adult smokers. The overall effects of aminophylline include bronchodilation, central stimulation of respiration, increased diaphragmatic contractility, and increased cardiac output. Significant tachyarrhythmias can occur. With the availability and effectiveness of beta-2 agents, aminophylline is used less frequently.

   (2) Anticholinergics. Although these are drying agents, they also produce bronchodilation by reducing the basal vagal tone of the airway musculature. When given by inhalation, the drying effect is less and the bronchodilation achieved is as pronounced as when given parenterally. Ipratropium (1–2 puffs q4–6h) and, less frequently, atropine (1.2 mg in 5 ml saline) or glycopyrrolate (0.6 mg in 5 ml saline) are more effective for maintaining bronchodilation than for the initial treatment of acute bronchospasm.

Table 10-9 Respiratory indications for endotracheal intubation and ventilatory support

1. PaO_2 < 50 mm Hg
2. $PaCO_2$ > 55 mm Hg
3. Shunt fraction > 20%
4. Dead space > 60% of tidal volume
5. Vital capacity < 10 ml/kg

(3) **Corticosteroids.** Unless the patient is steroid dependent, steroids are rarely used in the immediate postoperative period. Generally, it takes 4–6 hours for steroids to affect bronchospasm. Postoperatively, consideration must also be given to the potentially increased risk of infection and the delayed wound healing that are associated with these agents.

3. **Failed extubation.** Periodically, patients go into respiratory failure after extubation and require reintubation. When determining the need for reintubation, the total patient must be evaluated. Emergency intubations are required for hemodynamic collapse (cardiac arrest) or respiratory arrest. Urgent intubation may be required for impending respiratory failure, acute left ventricular failure, or sudden deterioration in the level of consciousness with loss of airway protective reflexes such as may occur with a cerebrovascular accident. Table 10-9 outlines the respiratory indications for intubation.

J. **Anesthetic technique for intubation of postoperative cardiac surgery patients.** When patients who have recently undergone cardiac surgery need intubation, the anesthetic technique used must be carefully chosen. Whether intubation is performed with the patient awake or under a general anesthetic is determined by the physical condition of the patient, the speed with which intubation is required, the patient's desires, and the experience of the physician performing the intubation.

Endotracheal intubation often results in hypertension, tachycardia, increased myocardial oxygen demand, and an increased incidence of dysrhythmias. Heart rate and blood pressure peak within 1 minute and generally return to baseline levels within 5 minutes. These cardiovascular reflexes need to be blunted by anesthetic techniques that cause minimal depression of baseline cardiovascular function.

1. **Regional anesthesia for endotracheal intubation**

a. **Two percent lidocaine spray** may be used to provide topical anesthesia of the mouth, tongue, and hypopharynx. Topical anesthesia can also be provided with 4% Xylocaine ointment on a tongue depressor used as a lollipop. Obviously this requires a cooperative patient and nonemergent situation.

b. **The "triple block"** (Fig. 10-1). Endoscopy and intubation of conscious patients can be performed by producing anesthesia in the sensory distribution of the glossopharyngeal and vagus nerves supplying the pharynx and larynx. This block involves an anesthetic spray (usually 2% or 4% lidocaine) to the mouth and tongue, bilateral superior laryngeal nerve blocks, and transtracheal injection of local anesthetic. For superior laryngeal nerve block, local anesthetic is injected near the nerves on each side of the neck. A 2.5-cm, 25-gauge needle is inserted at the cornu of the thyroid cartilage. Up to 5 ml of 1% lidocaine is infiltrated superficially and also deep to the thyrohyoid membrane. Anesthesia resulting from this latter block extends from the inferior epiglottis down to the vocal cords. For the transtracheal injection, a 20- or 22-gauge needle is inserted in the midline through the cricothyroid mem-

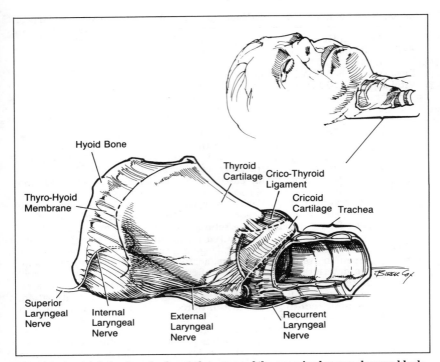

Fig. 10-1. Anatomic landmarks for performance of the superior laryngeal nerve block. Regional anesthesia blunts the laryngeal reflexes, allowing endotracheal intubation. Oropharyngeal local anesthetic spray, superior laryngeal nerve block (from perineural infiltration), and recurrent laryngeal nerve block (from transtracheal local anesthetic injection through the cricothyroid membrane) achieve this goal.

brane. Air is aspirated, and 3–5 ml of 2% lidocaine is injected, resulting in coughing and spread of anesthesia up and down the trachea. Laryngeal reflexes are blunted, and the patient is susceptible to aspiration. Therefore, either the superior laryngeal nerve block or the transtracheal injection is often not performed when the risk of aspiration is high.

2. **General anesthesia.** The choice of induction agent for general anesthesia is vital and needs to be considered on an individual patient basis. No anesthetics are innocuous, and all can have exaggerated effects in patients who are hemodynamically unstable. When general anesthesia is used, muscle relaxants are also usually required. For many patients, endotracheal intubation involves administration of an induction agent, a narcotic, and a relaxant. (See Chapter 5 for a more detailed discussion.)

   a. **Intravenous induction agents**

      (1) **Sodium thiopental (Pentothal Sodium) 1–4 mg/kg.** Although used periodically for intubation of critical care patients, this agent can be a potent myocardial depressant and should be used with extreme caution. If carefully administered in smaller than the usual doses and given very slowly, hemodynamic depressant effects can be minimized.

(2) **Etomidate (Amidate) 0.1–0.3 mg/kg.** This imidazole derivative results in greater hemodynamic stability than the barbiturates. In patients who already have a compromised
cardiovascular system, hemodynamic depression can be more
marked. Short-term adrenal cortex suppression (8 hours or less)
can result after this agent is given. Clinically, this suppression
is usually significant only if the agent is infused for long-term
sedation.

(3) **Ketamine (Ketalar) 1–2 mg/kg.** Ketamine is generally reserved for induction of general anesthesia in patients who have
acute decompensation secondary to cardiac tamponade. Ketamine is a myocardial depressant even though it has an indirect
sympathomimetic effect. Therefore, in patients with high preoperative sympathetic tone, ketamine may cause cardiovascular depression. Conversely, the sympathomimetic effect can
be potentially deleterious in patients who have cardiac ischemia or dysrhythmias or are receiving potentially dysrhythmogenic medications (i.e., aminophylline).

(4) **Midazolam (Versed) 0.15–0.30mg/kg.** This water-soluble
benzodiazepine has generally supplanted diazepam for anesthetic induction. It can lead to a decrease in systemic vascular
resistance and resultant hypotension. Respiratory depressant
effects from narcotics are potentiated. Older patients may exhibit agitation. It is more commonly used for sedation during
procedures on awake patients in small incremental doses of
(0.5–2.0 mg).

b. **Narcotics.** Fentanyl (Sublimaze), sufentanil (Sufenta), and alfentanil (Alfenta) are narcotics that classically are associated with
hemodynamic stability. However, in patients who are acutely de-
compensating from a significant cardiorespiratory insult, even reduction of the patient's "sympathetic drive" by a small narcotic
dose can result in rapid deterioration. In most ICU patients, use
of a small narcotic dose (i.e., fentanyl 1–2 µg/kg, sufentanil 0.1–
0.2 µg/kg, or alfentanil 5–10 µg/kg) helps blunt the sympathetic
response to intubation. In ICU patients, morphine (1–5 mg), although useful as a sedative during mechanical ventilation, is not
used as frequently for intubation. High-dose narcotic inductions
(i.e., fentanyl 50–75 µg/kg) are rare in the ICU unless the patient
is stable and surgery is imminent.

c. **Muscle relaxants.** Before deciding which muscle relaxant to use
for endotracheal intubation consider the speed of onset, duration
of action, desirable and undesirable physiologic changes, and
hemodynamic effects, both desired and undesired. In many situations, a rapid-acting agent may be necessary. Utilize each drug's
side effects to advantage when possible (see Chap. 5).

IV. **Postoperative management of the cardiovascular system**

A. **Low cardiac output** (see Chap. 3). Thermodilution cardiac output
measurements are done routinely, beginning on arrival in the ICU.
When cardiac output is inappropriately low (cardiac index < 2.0–2.5
liters $\cdot$ min$^{-1} \cdot$ m^{-2}), a thorough assessment of the patient is mandatory.

1. **Causes of low cardiac output** (Table 10-10)

a. **Perioperative myocardial infarction.** Some patients come to
coronary artery bypass grafting with a recent myocardial infarction. Myocardial infarction may also occur perioperatively in up
to 10% of cases. If enough myocardium is damaged, pumping ability can be impaired, and low output states may result.

b. **Myocardial ischemia.** Surgery is not always successful. Myocardial ischemia may persist postoperatively. Failure may result

Table 10-10 Etiologies and treatments of low cardiac output in the postoperative period

Causes	Treatments	Therapeutic considerations
Decreased preload	Volume augmentation: Whole blood for continuing bleeding Packed blood cells for low hematocrit Colloid (5% albumin) Crystalloid (normal saline, Ringer's lactate)	If deterioration has been acute, is there a surgical problem such as cardiac tamponade? Assess the whole patient.
Pump failure	Symptomatic treatment (i.e., diuretics, inotropes) Intraaortic balloon pump Left ventricular assist device Artificial heart Transplantation	Causes include idiopathic, valvular, congenital or ischemic disorders. Long-term prognosis is poor.
Myocardial ischemia or infarction	Nitroglycerin infusion Intra-aortic balloon pump Reoperation	Is there a surgically correctable cause, such as entrapment of a vein graft by the wound closure?
Increased intravascular volume (with left ventricular failure)	Diuresis Inotropic agents (i.e., dobutamine, amrinone) Ventilatory support with PEEP if necessary	Mechanical ventilation may allow a significant decrease in myocardial oxygen consumption.
Dysrhythmias	Defibrillation of ventricular fibrillation Cardioversion for hemodynamically disruptive ventricular tachycardia or supraventricular tachycardias Atropine, Isuprel, or cardiac pacing for symptomatic bradycardia Antidysrhythmic agents for stabilization (i.e., lidocaine, verapamil)	Both tachyarrhythmias and bradyarrhythmias can predispose to myocardial ischemia and cardiac failure.
Increased systemic vascular resistance	Fluids if increased SVR is secondary to hypovolemia Rewarming if hypothermia (<35°C) is present Nitroglycerin Nitroprusside Calcium channel blockers (nifedipine)	Correct abnormal physiologic responses of SVR to hypothermia or hypovolemia if present.
Mechanical disruptions	Emergent surgery	At times the urgency of the situation may make it necessary to perform sternotomy and immediate surgical repair in the ICU.

from incomplete revascularization of the heart due to small, diffusely diseased vessels, intramyocardial vessels that could not be found, lack of sufficient vein graft to bypass all diseased vessels, intracoronary air; or vein graft occlusion. Sometimes a bedside echocardiogram may allow determination of ventricular function, location of areas of hypokinesis indicative of ischemia or infarction, and an estimation of the ejection fraction. Myocardial ischemia may also be exacerbated by hypotension or systemic hypoxia.

c. **Fluid overload** may occur if overzealous volume replacement occurs intraoperatively or postoperatively. Increased pulmonary capillary wedge pressures result, increasing myocardial wall tension and work. Pulmonary edema may develop.

d. **Decreased preload** may occur if perioperative fluid and blood replacement has been inadequate or if blood loss is continuing without adequate replacement. As postoperative hypothermia resolves, the intravascular space expands, and relative hypovolemia can occur. Intrathoracic loss may be concealed within the thoracic cavity. Excessive diuresis may result from diuretics or the presence of glycosuria. Overzealous treatment of hypertension with vasodilators can also cause peripheral vascular pooling of blood and decreased venous return to the heart. Postoperative fluid loading with colloid (particularly 5% albumin) has been used to treat hypotension resulting from hypovolemia.

e. **Increased afterload.** Elevated systemic vascular resistance, particularly in patients with depressed ventricular function, can result in myocardial failure. Afterload reduction with vasodilator therapy can achieve marked improvement in cardiac output in these patients. Increased systemic vascular resistance occurs with hypothermia, vasopressor infusion, and hypovolemia and as a physiologic response to emergence from narcotic anesthesia.

f. **Dysrhythmias.** Bradycardia can significantly reduce cardiac output, even when stroke volume is maintained. Temporary atrial and ventricular pacing wires placed at the time of surgery can be used to treat bradycardia with atrial pacing alone or in combination with ventricular pacing when atrioventricular block is present.

Supraventricular tachycardias, in contrast, result in insufficient ventricular diastolic filling time. Atrial pacing wires can be connected to a standard ECG machine to obtain an atrial electrocardiogram, facilitating diagnosis of many dysrhythmias, including differentiation between atrial and ventricular rhythms. The leg leads are connected as for a routine electrocardiogram. However, the transthoracic atrial wires are connected to the ECG machine arm leads (often by metal alligator clips). Fig. 10-2 shows an example of atrial electrocardiogram used for the diagnosis of a rhythm disorder. Rapid, acute supraventricular dysrhythmias, ventricular fibrillation all require immediate countershock to restore a regular cardiac rhythm.

g. **Mechanical causes of myocardial failure.** In the postoperative period decreased cardiac output may be caused by problems related to the surgical procedure. Cardiac tamponade with decreased cardiac output, tachycardia, and hypotension may develop from accumulated blood in the pericardial sac. A tension pneumothorax may cause a mediastinal shift and decrease venous return to the heart. Graft closure, prosthetic valve dysfunction, or a disrupted intracardiac repair may also cause cardiac decompensation.

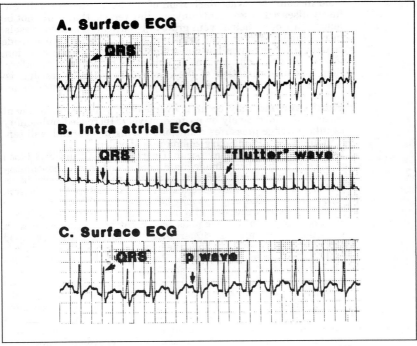

Fig. 10-2. Intra-atrial ECG used to diagnose a supraventricular tachyarrhythmia. *(A.)* Surface ECG showing rapid ventricular rate without obvious atrial activity. *(B.)* Intra-atrial ECG of same patient showing atrial flutter waves. *(C.)* Surface ECG showing normal sinus rhythm after successful cardioversion.

B. **Hypotension.** In the immediate postoperative period hypotension is most commonly due to decreased intravascular volume. Hypotension, by definition, must result from either low cardiac output or low systemic vascular resistance. The causes and treatment of low cardiac output are summarized above. In the immediate postoperative period, hypotension is most commonly due to decreased intravascular volume. Reduced systemic vascular resistance often results from:

1. Rewarming with vasodilation
2. Drug reactions (especially to protamine)
3. Hemolytic transfusion reactions
4. Overdose of vasodilators
5. Sepsis
6. Hyperthermia
7. Hyperthyroidism
8. Anemia

C. **Dysrhythmias in the postoperative period.** Dysrhythmias may be well tolerated or may result in rapid hemodynamic decompensation. Those that result in a decrease in cardiac output and hypotension need immediate therapy (Table 10-11). (See also Chap. 3.)

1. **Factors contributing to dysrhythmias**

Table 10-11. Dysrhythmias and their treatment (adults)

Common dysrhythmias	Acute treatments

Supraventricular tachycardia
  Atrial flutter
  Atrial fibrillation
	Digitalis (0.5–1.0 mg loading dose)
	Verapamil (5–10 mg bolus) given slowly
	Procainamide (100 mg q2–5min to effect, toxicity, or total of 12 mg/kg)
	Edrophonium (5–10 mg bolus)
	Quinidine (usually PO, rarely given IV)
	β blockers: propranolol (0.5–1.0 mg boluses to a total of 0.15 mg/kg), metoprolol, esmolol
	Cardioversion (synchronized, start at 10–20 joule). Because atrial fibrillation is often chronic, it may be more resistant to pharmacologic intervention. Cardioversion may require 80–200 joule.
	Overdrive pacing

Sinus bradycardia	Atropine (0.4–0.6 mg boluses to a total vagolytic dose of 2.0 mg if needed) Atrial pacing Isoproterenol (0.5–20 µg/min)
Nodal bradycardia	As for sinus bradycardia; pacing has a higher likelihood of being used
Ventricular tachycardia	Lidocaine if patient is stable (1.0 mg/kg/bolus, with a repeat bolus of 1.0 mg/kg and an infusion at 1–4 mg/min) Cardioversion (50–200 joule) Bretylium 5–10 mg/kg given over 10 min; repeat q15min to a maximum of 30 mg/kg; start infusion Procainamide (as above) Disopyramide (150–300 mg loading dose) Magnesium (if condition is refractory and lack of Mg^{2+} is the cause; 2 gm given over 30 min; then 10 gm in 500 ml 5% D/W given over 5 h
Ventricular fibrillation or pulseless ventricular tachycardia	Defibrillation (200–400 joule) first; if initial attempts fail, then epinephrine 0.5–1.0 mg. Other useful drugs include lidocaine, bretylium, procainamide in doses as above

    a. Myocardial ischemia. All patients who have undergone hypothermic cardiopulmonary bypass with cardioplegic arrest of the heart have had at least one recent ischemic episode.
    b. Myocardial hypertrophy may increase the likelihood of dysrhythmias. Atrial hypertrophy in the patient with mitral stenosis predisposes to atrial fibrillation.
    c. Electrolyte abnormalities commonly result from perioperative fluid shifts.
        (1) Hyperkalemia, if present, is usually due to overaggressive replacement or is secondary to an extracellular shift with respiratory or metabolic acidosis.
        (2) Hypokalemia is more common. Commonly, it is dilutional or secondary to intracellular ion shifts during hyperventilation and secondary to urinary losses. Diluted aliquots of potassium (generally 20 mEq/50ml) can be administered into a central

venous line to help correct the disorder rapidly in adults. Too rapid potassium infusion can also induce lethal dysrhythmias.

(3) **Hypocalcemia** may be related to rapid transfusion of large blood volumes. Treatment may involve 250–1000-mg doses (adults) of calcium chloride or gluconate given intravenously with careful attention to heart rhythms.

(4) **Hypomagnesemia** may be a contributing factor to cardiac rhythm disturbances. If required in adults, 2–4 g is administered over 30–45 min. An infusion of 1 g/hr is begun and magnesium levels measured. In refractory dysrhythmias (particularly ventricular dysrhythmias) a normal serum magnesium concentration may not reflect decreased total body stores, and there still may be a favorable response to magnesium therapy. Magnesium levels usually parallel changes in potassium.

d. Hypothermia. Low core body temperature increases myocardial irritability. In most cases, if this is the only abnormality present, supraventricular arrhythmias tend to occur at core temperatures of below 33°C and ventricular arrhythmias at core temperatures of below 28°C.

e. Acid-base disorder. Cell membranes and cellular function are affected by changes in pH. Serum levels of potassium ions are also affected. A pH decrease of 0.1 increases the measured extracellular potassium by approximately 0.6 mEq/liter.

f. Inadequate tissue oxygenation or perfusion may be related to decreased cardiac output, peripheral or pulmonary embolism, and high systemic vascular resistance. Lactic acidosis may develop.

g. Mechanical impairment of heart function. Cardiac tamponade and tension pneumothorax are two of the many problems causing rhythm disturbances.

h. Pharmacological agents causing rhythm disturbances

(1) **Digitalis toxicity** is still seen periodically. Dysrhythmias may range from paroxysmal atrial tachycardia with block to ventricular bigeminy.

(2) **Tricyclic antidepressants** result in increased susceptibility to tachyarrhythmias. Monoamine oxidase inhibitors, which have traditionally been associated with dysrhythmias, are still used occasionally.

(3) **Bronchodilators,** particularly intravenous aminophylline, may increase the incidence of supraventricular tachyarrhythmias. Cimetidine increases blood levels of aminophylline by decreasing its rate of hepatic metabolism. If a patient's rhythm is unstable, even nebulized beta-1-specific agents such as albuterol may increase the frequency of rhythm disturbances.

D. Pulmonary hypertension. Resistance to blood flow across the normal pulmonary circulation is about one-fifth of the resistance across the systemic vascular bed. Normal PVR is 144 ± 33 dynes · sec· cm^{-5}. The normal mean PA pressure is 12 ± 2 mm Hg with a pulmonary circulation to left atrial gradient of 6 ± 2 mm Hg. Pulmonary hypertension is present when mean pulmonary artery pressure exceeds 20 mm Hg. Primary pulmonary hypertension is rare. Pulmonary hypertension postoperatively usually occurs in patients who have had preoperative elevation of pulmonary artery pressures secondary to pulmonary disease or who have acquired or congenital cardiac valvular disease (Table 10–12). Classically, mitral stenosis is associated with high pulmonary artery pressures when it is severe or of long duration.

The clinical presentation of pulmonary hypertension includes signs and symptoms of right ventricular failure. Physical signs include right ventricular heave, a palpable pulmonary artery pulsation, loud

Table 10-12 Causes of pulmonary hypertension

Primary pulmonary hypertension
Disorders of ventilation
  High altitude
  Primary central hypoventilation
  Obstructive sleep apnea
  Cystic fibrosis
  Chronic obstructive pulmonary disease
  Kyphoscoliosis
Congenital heart disease
  Intracardiac defects with left-to-right shunting
  Palliative systemic-to-pulmonary artery shunt
  Persistent fetal circulation
Valvular heart disease, commonly mitral valve disease
Left ventricular failure
Pulmonary embolism

Table 10-13. Treatment of pulmonary hypertension

Treatment	Recommended utilization
Hyperventilation	Electively hyperventilate for the first 12–36 hr postoperatively. Maintain $PaCO_2$ at 25–28 mm Hg. Slowly wean patient from ventilator.
Isoproterenol (Isuprel)	Start IV infusion at 0.05 µg/kg/min Upper range for adults is ≤ 20 µg/kg/min
Nitroprusside (Nipride)	0.1–8.0 µg/kg/min
Nitroglycerin	0.1–7.0 µg/kg/min
Phentolamine (Regitine)	1.0–20.0 µg/kg/min
Tolazoline (Priscoline)	Initial dose 1–2 mg/kg; followed by infusion of 1–2 mg/kg/hr
Prostaglandin E_1	0.05–0.4 µg/kg/min

S_2 and S_4 heart sounds, distended jugular venous veins, hepatojugular reflux, and peripheral edema.

Because the pulmonary circulation is very sensitive to arterial carbon dioxide levels, patients with pulmonary hypertension are usually electively hyperventilated to a $PaCO_2$ of 25–28 mm Hg in the initial postoperative period. As $PaCO_2$ decreases, so does pulmonary vascular resistance. Hyperventilation is gradually withdrawn, and the response of PA pressures to weaning is closely followed. Vasodilators can also help decrease PA pressures. However, none of the vasodilators presently available are selective for the pulmonary circulation (Table 10-13). Prostaglandin E_1 is perhaps the most specific agent available at present. It is used primarily in pediatric patients. When pulmonary vasodilating properties are needed but systemic hemodynamic effects are marked, the vasodilator can be infused into the central venous line and a norepinephrine infusion given through the left atrial line to counteract the peripheral vasodilation and associated hypotension. It should be noted that since prostaglandin E_1 metabolism occurs pri-

marily in the lungs, metabolism may be decreased and systemic effects increased in patients with significant pulmonary disease.
  E. **Hypertension.** Hypertension in the postoperative patient increases myocardial oxygen consumption and increases the risk of perioperative ischemia, heart failure, and hemorrhage from vascular suture lines. Treatment varies with the specific cause.
    1. **Causes of postoperative hypertension**
      a. Surgical pain and the discomfort of an endotracheal tube
      b. Residual muscle paralysis
      c. Hypothermia with shivering
      d. Preoperative hypertension
      e. Iatrogenic hypertension
      f. Fluid overload
    2. **Treatment of postoperative hypertension (adults)**
      a. **Pain control.** Titrate analgesia to effect. Morphine sulfate in 1–4-mg increments are generally utilized.
      b. **Sedation.** Administer midazolam or diazepam (0.5–2-mg increments) if the narcotic alone is inadequate or if residual effects from preoperative scopolamine are present.
      c. **Rewarming** with blankets, heating lights, and warm intravenous fluids can help resolve shivering. If the patient is not extubated or is not ready for ventilator weaning, muscle relaxants can be given (along with sedatives) during the rewarming process to prevent shivering.
      d. Reinstitution of preoperative **antihypertensive medications** can begin only after oral intake resumes. Until then, parenteral medication must be used. The most commonly used intravenous vasodilators are nitroglycerin and nitroprusside.
      e. **β blockers.** Propranolol in 0.5-mg boluses (maximal dose 0.15 mg/kg), esmolol as a 50–200 μg/kg/min infusion, and labetalol boluses (5–20 mg q5min) can be utilized in patients with a hyperdynamic circulation). However, β blockers are usually avoided in the early postoperative period.
  V. **Postoperative management of the central nervous system**
    A. **Analgesia and sedation in the postoperative cardiac surgery patient (adults).** Postoperative cardiac patients require analgesia and sedation to control surgical pain and decrease the discomfort and agitation caused by the presence of an endotracheal tube and mechanical ventilation. Regional anesthesia techniques, such as thoracic epidural analgesia with local anesthetics, are not often used because of the systemic heparinization that present. Intravenous aliquots of narcotics, most frequently morphine sulfate (1–4-mg increments) and benzodiazepines (midazolam or diazepam 0.5–2.0-mg increments), are utilized. If prolonged ventilation is required, drug infusions may be utilized, such as fentanyl (3–10 μg/kg loading dose and generally 1–3 μg/kg/hr) or midazolam (0.1–0.2 mg/kg loading dose and 0.025–0.10 mg/kg/hr). Other benzodiazepines such as lorazepam (Ativan) or diazepam (Valium) can be given, but their longer half-life, active metabolic products, and lack of water solubility make intravenous administration less desirable in most situations.
    B. **Shivering.** Many patients are still hypothermic when they arrive in the ICU. A 300–600% increase in oxygen demand is imposed by shivering. The associated increase in carbon dioxide production can result in respiratory acidosis. Effective treatment must first involve rewarming and prevention of further temperature loss. Other therapies include (1) paralysis (with vecuronium 0.05 mg/kg), (2) meperidine (25–50 mg IV), and (3) sedation. Ventilatory requirements are increased.
  VI. **Postoperative management of metabolic factors**

A. Diabetes mellitus. Diabetes mellitus is frequently part of the disease profile in cardiac surgery patients. It has been well documented that hyperglycemia during cerebral ischemia results in more severe neurologic deficits. Careful control of the blood sugar level (preferably maintaining blood sugar at less than 200 mg/dl) with frequent monitoring of blood sugar concentration is indicated. Continuous infusion of regular insulin in a dextrose-containing solution (often starting at 0.1 units/kg/hr or less) with titration to effect can prevent hyperglycemia and such associated problems as lactic acidosis. (See Chap. 1.)

B. Acid-base disturbances. Respiratory acidosis is secondary to hypoventilation or increased carbon dioxide production. Monitoring of $ETCO_2$ during ventilation and postoperative weaning decreases the likelihood of respiratory acidosis and aids in following trends when hyperventilation is used as a partial compensation for metabolic acidosis.

Persistent metabolic alkalosis may be treated by administration of a carbonic anhydrase inhibitor (Diamox). However, since the alkalosis is usually due to volume contraction secondary to diuretics, chloride replacement with a saline solution may be all that is necessary.

VII. Surgical complications in the first 24 hours

A. Hemorrhage. Sudden hemorrhage from a suture line or cannulation site can cause profound hypotension due to hypovolemia or tamponade. Rapid volume infusion of blood, colloid, or crystalloid is necessary to maintain intravascular volume. If the patient can be quickly stabilized, immediate transfer to the operating room for sternotomy is necessary. Otherwise, emergency sternotomy in the ICU should be performed. For most adults, chest tube drainage greater than 500 ml in 1 hour, 400 ml in each of 2 successive hours, 300 ml in each of 3 successive hours, or 1000 ml in the first 4 hours is an indication for reexploration. Coagulation tests (PT, PTT, fibrinogen, platelet count) should be performed and appropriate component therapy instituted for abnormalities detected.

B. Cardiac tamponade. Excessive mediastinal bleeding with inadequate drainage (clotted chest tubes) or sudden massive bleeding can result in cardiac tamponade. The classic features of elevated central venous pressure and equalization of left and right atrial filling pressures may not occur when hypovolemia is present or when there is localized clot around one atrium or the other. Often the only signs are slowly deteriorating systemic perfusion with rising atrial pressures and an increase in the size of the cardiac silhouette on chest radiograph. A high index of suspicion is necessary. Tamponade can also occur in patients with left ventricular assist devices or artificial hearts in place when the inlet to the device itself becomes compressed.

C. Acute graft closure. After coronary artery bypass grafting acute graft closure can result in myocardial ischemia or infarction. If cardiac decompensation occurs and graft closure is the suspected cause, reexploration should be performed to evaluate graft patency. However, it is usually difficult to know preoperatively whether a graft has closed, and reexploration for this reason is uncommon. (See Chap. 17.)

D. Prosthetic valve failure. A rare cause of prosthetic valve failure in the early postoperative period may be empingement of the ends of sutures or chordal strands in the valve mechanism, causing it to stick in the closed or open position. This possibility should be suspected when sudden hemodynamic changes occur, particularly if the rhythm is unchanged and intermittent loss of the arterial waveform is noted on the monitor screen. Immediate surgical correction is necessary. Valve leaflet escape has been reported but rarely occurs in the immediate postoperative period. Likewise, valve dehiscence with a perivalvular leak is not usual in the early postoperative period.

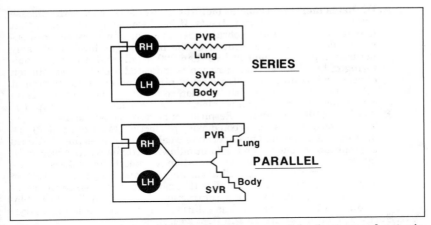

Fig. 10-3. Parallel circulations. This schematic shows parallel pulmonary and systemic blood flow, as compared to the normal series cardiac circulation. Mixing of systemic and pulmonary venous return in the heart (as shown in the parallel circulation) is exemplified by many congenital cardiac defects. These defects often result in the mixed ventricular blood being delivered into both the systemic and pulmonary circulations. RH = right heart, LH = left heart.

    E. Pneumothorax, hemothorax. A large pneumothorax, tension pneumothorax, or hemothorax impairs ventilation. Shift of mediastinal structures can cause mechanical obstruction of the vena cava or the heart itself and result in low cardiac output.

VIII. The pediatric cardiac surgery patient: The first 24 hours. Preoperative preparation, operative repair, and postoperative management of newborns, infants, and children with congenital heart disease requires strict attention to detail, continuous reassessment of the clinical course, and a thorough knowledge of the preoperative pathophysiology, operative repair, and expected postoperative physiology. Frequently "repairs" of congenital heart defects, such as the repair for hypoplastic left heart syndrome and the Fontan operation, are more palliative than truly corrective. In these cases the expected postoperative physiology is anything but "normal." A complete understanding of the cardiac anatomy, both before and after a repair, is necessary for personnel to provide optimal care for these patients. A thorough understanding is required of the parallel circulation, in which there is mixing of pulmonary and systemic venous return in the cardiac chambers, with the mixed ventricular blood delivered not only to the systemic circulation but also to the pulmonary circulation (Fig. 10–3). An example is a single ventricle with pulmonary atresia and a modified Blalock-Taussig (systemic-to-pulmonary artery) shunt. The effects of ventilatory manipulation on systemic and pulmonary vascular resistance (hyperventilation with hypocapnia lowers PVR) controls the systemic-to-pulmonary artery shunt flow (Table 10-14). This section will focus attention on those specific areas that are peculiar to patients with congenital heart disease.

    A. System by system evaluation and management

        1. Cardiovascular system

            a. Pediatric patients, especially newborns and infants, have a relatively fixed stroke volume. Cardiac output can be best improved by optimizing heart rate, rhythm, and contractility. Obviously, it is important to maintain adequate intravascular blood volume.

Table 10-14. Techniques used to control systemic-to-pulmonary shunt flow

Strategies to increase PBF
  Raise SVR: Vasopressors, catecholamines
  Lower PVR: O_2, hypocarbia, alkalosis
Strategies to decrease PBF
  Lower SVR: Vasodilators
  Raise PVR: FiO_2 = 0.21, hypercarbia, acidemia

PBF = pulmonary blood flow, SVR = systemic vascular resistance, PVR = pulmonary vascular resistance.

However, volume loading in a newborn or infant who already has adequate blood volume rarely increases the cardiac output to any significant degree. It usually results in the development of hepatomegaly, pleural effusions, and ascites. Afterload reduction using nitroprusside, nitroglycerin, or prostaglandin E_1 (particularly in patients with pulmonary artery hypertension) is used in nearly all pediatric patients. The decrease in systemic vascular resistance improves peripheral perfusion and hastens rewarming. Afterload reduction improves stroke volume in patients with ventricular dysfunction without increasing myocardial oxygen consumption. Patients with large left-to-right shunts and patients with signs of heart failure usually require chronic digoxin administration and often diuretic therapy as well.

b. With all the technologic advancements in monitoring, there is still nothing better than the clinician's physical examination. The presence of good skin color, brisk capillary refill, and strong pedal pulses is one of the best indicators of good circulation. When inotropic agents with vasoconstrictor properties and vasodilator agents are used, particularly in patients with systemic-to-pulmonary shunts and parallel circulation, it is important to consider carefully the effects on the ratio of pulmonary and systemic vascular resistances. These agents sometimes have beneficial but also sometimes quite adverse effects on systemic-to-pulmonary artery shunt flow, resulting in inadequate pulmonary blood flow (increased PVR/SVR ratio) or excessive pulmonary and inadequate systemic blood flow (decreased PVR/SVR ratio).

c. Drug infusions. In pediatric patients it is very easy to make errors in calculation of drug doses. A rigorous protocol for calculation of essential drug dosages before the patient enters the ICU is necessary. We have developed a computerized program that calculates pediatric drug doses for emergency bolus administration or continuous infusion. This program has been most helpful in maintaining a consistent approach to patient management for both the nursing and resident staff. All drug infusions are connected to a central venous catheter via a manifold arrangement by a low-volume (less than 0.5 ml) intravenous tubing. Infusion pumps with the capability of providing flow rate increments as low as 0.1 ml/hr are used.

d. Acid-base balance. Combining the results of the clinical examination with the acid-base balance derived from an arterial blood sample tells whether the circulation is meeting the metabolic demands of the patient. Metabolic acidosis in neonates should be treated with diluted solutions of sodium bicarbonate administered by slow infusion, often accompanied by measures to improve systemic blood flow.

Table 10-15. Monitoring devices used in children

Radial or umbilical (in newborns) artery catheter
Central venous catheter (percutaneous internal jugular vein)
Direct intracardiac left atrial, right atrial, and pulmonary artery catheters
Urinary catheter
Rectal and peripheral skin (foot) temperature probes
Multi-lead ECG
Transcutaneous pulse oximeter
End-tidal capnometer

e. **Urine output.** Because of high circulating levels of aldosterone and antidiuretic hormone, urine output frequently decreases to approximately 0.5 ml/kg/hr in the first 24–48 hours postoperatively in spite of optimal circulatory hemodynamics. There is often a poor response to diuretics used to treat oliguria during the first postoperative 24 hours after cardiopulmonary bypass in neonates and infants.

f. **Monitoring.** (Table 10-15). Proper monitoring of cardiac and other organ functions is paramount in interpreting the effectiveness of the operative repair and the results of interventions to optimize the patient's clinical condition. To obtain accurate pressure data all transducers must be properly calibrated and the zero level set to the midatrial level. In using these monitoring devices it is important to understand their limitations and always to evaluate the total clinical picture before making changes in therapy based on a single "number." Frequently, temporary atrial and ventricular pacing wires are placed to allow diagnostic atrial and ventricular electrocardiograms as well as therapeutic cardiac pacing.

2. **Respiratory system.** Postoperative management of the respiratory system in patients with congenital heart disease has a major impact on hemodynamics and patient survival. The importance of respiratory management is primarily related to the increased reactivity of the pulmonary vascular bed in general and the balance of pulmonary and systemic blood flow in patients with a parallel circulation. Most postoperative patients are placed on mechanical ventilation. The duration of mechanical support depends on the type of cardiac repair and the stability of the patient.

a. Endotracheal tubes must be carefully secured to ensure stability and positioned so that kinking cannot occur. This is especially important because the distance from the larynx to the carina is much shorter in infants and children. Leakage around the tube at pressures less than 30 cm H_2O usually allows adequate volume ventilation unless there is low pulmonary compliance.

b. **Mechanical ventilation.** The Siemans Servo 900C ventilator provides good flexibility. Because the maintenance of specific levels of $PaCO_2$ is required in many cases, a volume ventilator is best. The decreases in pulmonary compliance that occur postoperatively can result in major decreases in alveolar ventilation if a pressure-controlled ventilator is utilized. The tidal volume is set to maintain optimal chest expansion, and the respiratory rate is set to obtain the minute ventilation needed to maintain the desired arterial PCO_2. PEEP (2–3 cm H_2O) is frequently used to prevent atelectasis and to aid in postoperative alveolar recruitment. The FIO_2 used depends on the underlying anatomy and physiology. Patients with normal or completely corrected cardiac anatomy are started at

100% FiO_2 and the oxygen concentration is then reduced as indicated by arterial blood gas measurements. A PaO_2 of greater than 100 mm Hg is preferred in the immediate postoperative period. In patients with parallel circulation (Fig. 10-3), the FiO_2 can have a dramatic impact on the ratio of pulmonary to systemic flow. Oxygen tends to promote pulmonary artery vasodilation. Therefore, in patients with large left-to-right shunts the FiO_2 is decreased to a level that provides a PaO_2 of 35–45 mm Hg (SaO_2 about 85%). In patients with hypoxemia and diminished pulmonary blood flow, higher concentrations of oxygen are administered.

c. **Monitoring ventilation.** The pulse oximeter has become an important tool that allows continuous measurement of arterial oxygen saturation without repeat arterial blood gas measurements. Sudden changes in arterial oxygenation can be detected. The capnometer provides evidence of trends of end-tidal and instantaneous carbon dioxide levels in the expired gas. In patients with a parallel circulation the inequality between the pulmonary and systemic blood flows may cause a large difference in the end-tidal carbon dioxide and the arterial PCO_2. Specifically, when the ratio of pulmonary to systemic blood flow is reduced, the $ETCO_2$ may be quite low despite normal or elevated arterial PCO_2 levels. The capnograph is also a useful tool when one is observing spontaneous ventilation prior to extubation. The frequency and pattern of breathing are easily seen.

d. **Sedation and analgesia during mechanical ventilation.** Sedation is very important to maintain ease of ventilation and to prevent the patient from possibly dislodging the endotracheal tube and other monitoring catheters. In neonates with reactive pulmonary vasculature sedation helps prevent the precipitous increase in PVR that can occur with stimulation. We use intravenous morphine (0.05–0.10-mg/kg bolus) or low dose fentanyl infusions (1 μg/kg/hr). In addition, chloral hydrate given through a nasogastric tube is an excellent sedative and has little effect on hemodynamics or respiratory drive.

3. **Renal system**

a. A urinary catheter is inserted in all patients having cardiac surgery utilizing cardiopulmonary bypass and any other patient in whom a long operation is anticipated or precise hourly urine output assessment is required. The best management of oliguria in the early postoperative period is optimization of hemodynamics by volume challenges (10 ml/kg) which ensure an adequate circulating blood volume by improving contractility with inotropic agents and maintaining an optimal heart rate and rhythm.

b. **Diuretic therapy.** Indiscriminate use of diuretics to treat oliguria should be avoided. In volume-overloaded, edematous patients in whom cardiac function has already been maximized, aggressive diuretic therapy is necessary. We sometimes add chlorothiazide (IV or PO) 20–40 mg/kg/day when furosemide (1–2 mg/kg IV or PO initial dose) alone is ineffective. Aldactone (PO) 2–3 mg/kg/day can be added to help conserve potassium and block sodium reabsorption.

4. **Metabolism and fluid balance**

a. **Fluid and electrolytes**

(1) **Sodium.** Pediatric patients usually do not require much sodium in the first several days following cardiac surgery. Body reserves are **usually** sufficient. However, hyponatremia (Na <125 mEq/liter) is frequently treated by infusion of 3% sodium chloride in patients who are already fluid restricted and require

continued diuretic therapy. Close monitoring of serum sodium is essential.

(2) **Potassium.** In contrast to adults, potassium is not routinely given to neonates, infants, and small children until chronic diuretic therapy is started or until serum potassium is less than 2.5–3.0 mEq/liter with a normal acid-base balance. Postoperative pediatric patients rarely have dysrhythmias that are directly related to hypokalemia, particularly in the face of respiratory and metabolic alkalosis. Hyperkalemia, with its adverse effect on cardiac rhythm and function, can develop extremely rapidly in pediatric patients during sudden alterations in acid-base balance, and therefore it is safer for the patient to remain relatively hypokalemic (2.5–3.5 mEq/liter) in the immediate postoperative period. If needed, potassium can be administered in small incremental doses. Usually potassium requirements in newborns are 0.5–2.0 mEq/kg/day.

(3) **Maintenance fluids.** The intravenous maintenance fluids and solutions for drug infusions are usually made up in a 10% dextrose in water solution. Sometimes these are changed to 20% dextrose if low blood glucose levels are present. Radial and femoral arterial lines are usually flushed with one-half normal saline solution, which limits the acquired sodium load. Fluid requirements are usually 50 ml/kg/day with increments to 100 ml/kg/day during the first 3 postoperative days.

b. **Glucose.** It is important to avoid hypoglycemia by administration of adequate dextrose. Monitor blood glucose and maintain the blood sugar above 80 mg/dl in the sedated paralyzed patient. Nasogastric feedings of dilute formula (Isomil) are started on postoperative day one and advanced in caloric density and volume as tolerated.

c. **Calcium.** Low ionized calcium levels are frequently seen after cardiac surgery and the administration of blood products, resulting in the binding of calcium by citrate. Hypocalcemia may be a cause of seizures in the newborn and young infant and can depress ventricular function. Thus nearly all patients less than 2 years of age are placed on a continuous infusion of 10% calcium gluconate at 0.1 ml/kg/hr and are also given frequent boluses of calcium gluconate following administration of blood products.

d. **Routine metabolic status.** The most important metabolic parameters in newborns and infants include measurements of arterial blood gases, hematocrit, electrolytes, glucose, and ionized calcium. These should be measured every 2–4 hours in the first 24 hours postoperatively and more frequently in some cases.

5. **The central nervous system**

a. **Seizures.** Focal and localized seizures are sometimes seen postoperatively, most often in the newborn. The most common causes are the fluid and electrolyte shifts that occur during cardiopulmonary bypass, hypoglycemia, and hypocalcemia. Recurrent seizure activity (which is more common after deep hypothermia) is treated with phenobarbital. Unless structural pathology is found, the phenobarbital is usually discontinued after 3–4 days.

b. **Temperature control.** Neonates and infants have a large body surface area–to–body weight ratio, and thus their body temperature is very sensitive to changes in environmental temperature. This circumstance allows more rapid surface rewarming under radiant heat following deep hypothermic procedures as well as effective surface cooling during febrile episodes. Elevated core temperature and decreasing peripheral skin temperature is usually an indication of decreased cardiac output and increased systemic vascular resistance. The best treatment for this situation is vasodilator therapy (usually nitroprusside), which improves the peripheral circulation.

IX. **Summary.** Patients with congenital heart disease, and indeed all patients who have undergone cardiac surgery, may have limited physiologic reserves and have just suffered a major insult to virtually all body systems. These patients demand meticulous cardiovascular, respiratory, and metabolic support throughout the early postoperative period.

SUGGESTED READING

Ilabaca, P. A., Ochsner, J. L., and Mills, N. L. Positive end-expiratory pressure in the management of the patient with a postoperative bleeding heart. *Ann. Thorac. Surg.* 30:281–284, 1980.

Kane, P. B. Postoperative Management of the Cardiac Patient. In J. S. Israel, and T. J. DeKornfeld (eds.), *Recovery Room Care* (2nd ed.). Chicago: Year Book, 1987, Pp. 185–212.

Kirklin, J. K., and Kirklin, J. W. Management of the cardiovascular subsystem after cardiac surgery. *Ann. Thorac. Surg.* 32:311–319, 1981.

Kofke, W. A., and Levy, J. H. *Postoperative Critical Care Procedures of the Massachusetts General Hospital.* Boston: Little, Brown, 1986.

Lappas, D. G., Powell, W. M. J., and Daggett, W. M. Cardiac dysfunction in the perioperative period. *Anesthesiology* 47:117–137, 1977.

Morganroth, M. L., and Grum, C. M. Weaning from mechanical ventilation. *J. Intensive Care Med.* 3:109–120, 1988.

Stein, K L., Darby, J. M., and Grenvik, A. Intensive care of the cardiac transplant recipient. *J. Cardiothorac. Anesth.* 2(4):543–553, 1988.

Tarhan, S., White, R. D., and Moffitt, E. A. Anesthesia and postoperative care for cardiac operations. *Ann. Thorac. Surg.* 23:173–193, 1977,

Tobin, M. J., and Dantzker, D. R. Mechanical Ventilation and Weaning. In D. R. Dantzker (ed.), *Cardiopulmonary Critical Care.* Orlando: Grune & Stratton, 1986, Pp.203–262.

Vander Salm, T. J. Management of the Postoperative Cardiac Surgery Patient. In J. M. Rippe, R. S. Irwin, and J. S. Alpert, et al. (eds.), *Intensive Care Med.* Boston: Little, Brown, 1985. Pp. 996–1010.

Anesthetic Management for Specific Cardiovascular Disorders

Anesthetic Management for Myocardial Revascularization

Jan C. Horrow, Frederick A. Hensley, Jr.,
and Robert G. Merin

I. Introduction
A. **The patient with coronary artery disease.** The American Heart Association estimates that 1,500,000 Americans will sustain a myocardial infarction in 1989 and more than 500,000 die as a result. Coronary occlusive disease constitutes the leading threat to life in terms of its prevalence and mortality. Patients needing myocardial revascularization almost always have atherosclerotic cardiovascular disease, the notable exceptions being those with anomalous coronary anatomy or trauma to the coronary vascular bed. Patients with atherosclerotic coronary arteries often harbor arterial occlusive disease elsewhere. In particular, one may find obstructions in the carotid and cerebral arteries and the abdominal aorta as well as the renal, iliac, and femoral arteries. Diabetes mellitus, obesity, hypertension, and obstructive pulmonary disease from tobacco smoking increase the risk of atherosclerosis, explaining the high prevalence of these attendant disorders in patients for myocardial revascularization. Because survival of patients with chronic renal disease has improved, the number of dialysis-dependent patients requiring coronary artery surgery has increased as well.

B. **Symptoms and progression of coronary artery disease (CAD).** A complete description of angina pectoris and other symptoms related to coronary artery disease is included in Chapter 1. Unlike the usually predictable time course and progression of symptoms in patients with valvular heart disease, patients with CAD may have variable onset of symptoms as well as progression of disease characterized by discrete events such as angina or myocardial infarction. All aspects of preoperative evaluation of these patients (i.e., exercise stress testing and cardiac catheterization) are discussed in Chap. 1.

C. **Historical perspective of surgical intervention.** Early unsuccessful attempts at myocardial revascularization by inducing pericardial adhesions took place before the 1950s. In 1951 Vineburg implanted the internal mammary artery directly into the myocardium. Subsequent research showed that although myocardial blood flow did increase by this procedure, the additional blood flow was not enough to lead to symptomatic improvement of angina pectoris. In 1967 Favaloro and Effler at the Cleveland Clinic began performing reversed saphenous vein bypass grafting procedures as we know them today. In 1968 Green performed an anastomosis of the internal mammary artery directly to a coronary artery. A resurgence of interest in the internal mammary grafting procedure in the late 1970s and early 1980s occurred after a number of studies showed far greater graft patency rates for internal mammary grafts compared with saphenous vein grafts. In addition, better long-term survival was evident in patients receiving internal mammary grafts regardless of good or poor ventricular function.

Those factors associated with increased mortality after coronary artery surgery also predict a better long-term outcome with surgical management compared with medical management. For example, surgical patients with triple vessel disease associated with poor ventricular function and left main disease have increased survival compared with medically treated patients provided that surgical mortality is less than 6–7%. These statistics, combined with the facts that angioplasty is becoming a more common procedure and that medical management is further augmented by new drugs, make it likely that the patient population coming to the operating room in the future will be at even higher risk than that in the past and will be a further challenge to the skills of the cardiac anesthesiologist.

II. **Coronary artery anatomy.** One must have a thorough understanding of the coronary artery anatomy and distribution of blood flow to the myocardium to understand the surgical procedure as well as the extent and degree of myocardium at risk for ischemia and infarction during anesthesia and surgery.

A. **Right and left coronary arteries.** The blood supply to the myocardium comes from the aorta through two main coronary arteries (see Fig. 1-5). These are the left and right coronary arteries. The left main coronary artery extends for a short distance before dividing into the left anterior descending artery and the circumflex coronary artery.

   1. The **left anterior descending coronary artery** courses down the interventricular groove and gives rise to two types of branches, the diagonal and septal branches. The septal branches vary in number and size and course into the interventricular septum. One to three diagonal branches of variable size exist, and these branches distribute blood to the anterolateral aspect of the heart. The left anterior descending artery continues down the interventricular groove and usually passes all the way around the apex of the left ventricle.

   2. The **circumflex coronary artery** passes down the left atrioventricular groove. Its main vessels are the obtuse marginal branches. The obtuse marginal branches range from one to three in number. They supply the lateral free wall of the left ventricle.

   3. The **right coronary artery** passes down the right atrioventricular groove. It gives rise to acute marginal branches that supply the right anterior wall of the right ventricle. In approximately 85% of individuals the right coronary artery gives rise to the posterior descending artery to supply the posterior inferior aspect of the left ventricle. This blood supply pattern is classified as a right dominant system. Thus, in the majority of the population, the right coronary artery supplies a significant portion of blood flow to the left ventricle. In the other 15% of the population the posterior-inferior aspect of the left ventricle is supplied by either the circumflex coronary artery (left dominant system) or both right coronary and circumflex arteries (codominant system).

III. **Determinants of myocardial oxygen supply.** The myocardium maximally extracts oxygen from arterial blood at rest. With exertion or hemodynamic stress, the only way the oxygen supply can increase acutely to meet the myocardial energy demand is by increasing coronary blood flow. Ischemia occurs when coronary blood flow does not increase to a sufficient level to meet myocardial demand, and aerobic metabolism is impaired. The following approach achieves the clinical goal of ensuring that oxygen supply at least matches demand:

   1. Optimize the determinants of myocardial oxygen supply and demand.
   2. Select anesthetics and adjuvant agents and techniques according to their effects on oxygen supply and demand.
   3. Monitor for ischemia to detect its occurrence early and intervene rapidly.

The rest of this chapter elaborates on these segments of the clinical approach. One begins with an understanding of the determinants of myocardial oxygen supply and demand. First oxygen supply is discussed. The gross determinants of myocardial oxygen supply are arterial oxygen content and coronary blood flow.

A. **Arterial oxygen content.** Delivery of blood per se is not sufficient to supply oxygen: There must be adequate oxygen in that blood. Since oxygen content = [hemoglobin] $\times$ 1.34 $\times$ %saturation + 0.003 $\times$ PO_2, ensuring maximal oxygen content involves having a high hemoglobin level, highly saturated blood, and high PO_2. Warm temperature, nor-

Table 11-1. Control of coronary vascular resistance (CVR)

	Increase CVR	Decrease CVR
Metabolic	$\uparrow O_2$, $\downarrow CO_2$ $\downarrow H^+$	$\downarrow O_2$, $\uparrow CO_2$ $\uparrow H^+$ Lactate Adenosine
Autonomic nervous system	$\uparrow$ Alpha-adrenergic tone $\uparrow$ Cholinergic tone	$\uparrow$ Beta-adrenergic tone
Hormonal	$\uparrow$ Vasopressin (ADH) $\uparrow$ Angiotensin $\uparrow$ Thromboxane	$\uparrow$ Prostacyclin

mal pH, and high levels of 2,3 diphosphoglyceric acid (DPG) all favor release of oxygen at the tissues.

B. Coronary blood flow

1. **Determinants of blood flow in normal coronary arteries.** Coronary blood flow (CBF) varies directly with both the **pressure differential** across the coronary bed (coronary perfusion pressure [CPP]) and inversely with the resistance of the coronary vasculature (CVR) to give the relationship:

$$CBF = \frac{CPP}{CVR}$$

Metabolic, autonomic nervous system, hormonal, and anatomic parameters alter CVR, and hydraulic factors influence CPP. Coronary stenoses also increase CVR.

a. **Control of coronary vascular resistance.** Factors affecting coronary vascular resistance are outlined in Table 11-1.

(1) **Metabolic factors.** When increased coronary flow is required secondary to increased myocardial work load, metabolic control factors are primarily responsible. Hydrogen ion, carbon dioxide, and lactate may all play a role in metabolic regulation of coronary blood flow by inducing changes in CVR. However, adenosine is probably the most important metabolic blood flow regulator. When the oxygen supply of the myocardium is exceeded, adenosine from adenosine-triphosphate breakdown causes coronary vasodilation and increases blood flow with subsequent increased oxygen diffusion to the intracellular structures.

(2) **Autonomic nervous system.** The coronary arteries and arterioles are endowed with alpha and beta receptors. It has been hypothesized that an increased population of alpha receptors is responsible for episodes of coronary spasm in individuals with nonobstructed coronaries. Alpha-mediated neurogenic control of the coronary circulation may counter some of the metabolic vasodilation, especially in the resting basal state. However, under most circumstances such as increasing demands or ischemia, metabolic control factors will override alpha-mediated vasoconstriction [3].

(3) **Hormonal factors.** A number of hormones (blood-borne) may also affect the coronary arterioles. Two of the stress hormones, vasopressin (antidiuretic hormone [ADH]) and angiotensin, are known to be potent coronary vasoconstrictors. It is still unclear whether the blood levels of these hormones during major stress

are actually high enough to produce clinical coronary vasoconstriction.

The prostaglandin system also has major vascular effects, both constrictive and relaxing. Again, it is unclear what effect particular prostaglandins have. However, it has been postulated that thromboxane may participate in the thrombotic process and perhaps produce coronary vasospasm during myocardial infarction and perhaps that prostacyclin may be produced in an attempt to overcome the vasoconstricting effects of thromboxane.

(4) **Anatomic factors**

   (a) **Capillary/myocyte ratio** Almost a 1 : 1 ratio of capillaries to myocytes exists in the human myocardium. However, only three-fifths to four-fifths of these capillaries function during normal conditions. During exercise, episodes of hypoxia, or extreme myocardial oxygen demand, the additional unopened capillaries are recruited and increase blood flow, causing a decrease in CVR. This decreases the intercapillary distance and therefore the diffusion distance of oxygen to a given myocyte. This adaptation, along with coronary vasodilation, contributes to "coronary vascular reserve" [3].

   (b) **Coronary collaterals.** Coronary collateral channels exist in the human myocardium. Under most circumstances these are nonfunctional. However, in the presence of impeded coronary blood flow, these coronary channels may enlarge over time and become functional.

(5) **Other factors affecting CVR.** CVR varies linearly with blood viscosity. High hematocrit and hypothermia both increase viscosity dramatically, thus adversely increasing CVR. For these reasons, hemodilution is necessary when inducing hypothermia.

b. **Hydraulic factors and subendocardial blood flow**

   (1) **Left ventricular subendocardial blood flow.** Unlike coronary blood flow in the low-pressure right ventricular system, left ventricular subendocardial blood flow is intermittent and occurs only during the diastolic portion of the cardiac cycle. Because of the increased intracavitary pressure and excessive subendocardial myocyte shortening, subendocardial arterioles are essentially closed during systole. Of the total left ventricular coronary flow, 85% occurs during diastole and 15% occurs in systole (primarily in the epicardial region). Thus, the majority of blood flow to the epicardial and middle layers of the left ventricle and **all** the blood flow to the endocardium occur during diastole.

   (2) **Increased subendocardial myocyte shortening.** In addition to the intermittent decrease in subendocardial blood flow, the subendocardial region has higher rates of oxidative metabolism secondary to the increased myocyte shortening in this region. Little reserve for increased coronary vasodilation occurs in the subendocardium because most of these vessels are already maximally dilated. Because of the increased demand and intermittent limitations of blood flow in the subendocardial region, myocardial oxygen tension falls first here (Fig. 11-1). Thus, this region is more susceptible to an ischemic insult.

   (3) **Coronary perfusion pressure (CPP).** CPP equals the arterial driving pressure less the back pressure to flow across the coronary bed. For the left ventricle the driving pressure is the aortic blood pressure during diastole. The back pressure to flow

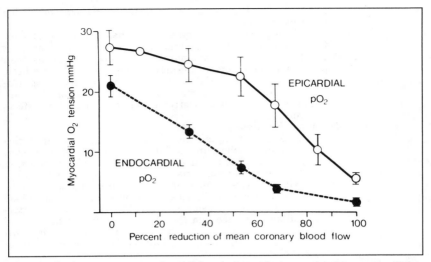

Fig. 11-1. Relationship of subendocardial oxygen supply (represented by myocardial O_2 tension) to reductions in coronary blood flow. Demonstrated is the increased vulnerability of the subendocardial zone compared to the epicardial zone. (Modified from M.M. Winbury, and B.B. Howe. Stenosis: Regional Myocardial Ischemia and Reserve. In M. M. Winbury, and Y. Abiko [eds.], *Ischemic Myocardium and Antianginal Drugs.* New York: Raven Press, 1979. P. 59. With permission.)

depends on the area of myocardium under consideration. Most blood returns via the coronary sinus, and the corresponding back pressure is that of the right atrium. However, for the endocardium, drainage occurs through thebesian veins directly into the ventricular cavities. Because the endocardium is the area most at risk, attention focuses on its flow. Thus, the calculation for subendocardial CPP utilizes left ventricular end-diastolic pressure (LVEDP) as the back pressure: CPP = diastolic blood pressure − LVEDP. Because diastole shortens relative to systole as heart rate increases, subendocardial blood flow is decreased at extremely rapid heart rates. Figure 11-2 demonstrates the total time per minute spent in diastole as a function of heart rate. Elevations in LVEDP (e.g., heart failure, ischemia) will also impede subendocardial blood flow. Thus, to optimize coronary perfusion pressure, one should aim for normal to high diastolic blood pressure, low LVEDP, and a low heart rate.

2. **Determinants of myocardial blood flow in stenotic coronaries.** In addition to the physiologic determinants of myocardial blood flow in normal coronary arteries, stenotic vessels add pathologic determinants of myocardial blood flow. Stenoses increase coronary vascular resistance and decrease coronary blood flow.

a. **Types of coronary stenoses**

(1) **Fixed or dynamic.** A fixed stenosis is composed of an atherosclerotic plaque. A dynamic stenosis can occur in a region of a normal coronary artery, such as occurs in Prinzmetal's variant angina or vasospastic angina. A combination of dynamic stenosis superimposed on an obstructive lesion may occur particularly in patients with unstable angina pectoris.

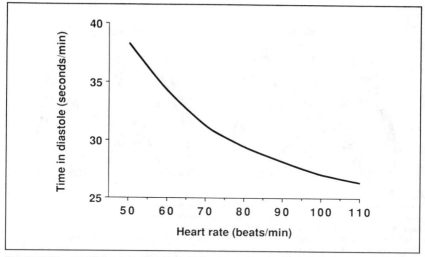

Fig. 11-2. The total time spent in diastole each minute is plotted as a function of heart rate in beats/minute. The reduction in diastolic interval leads to diminished left ventricular blood flow as heart rate increases.

(2) **Focal or segmental.** The length of a coronary artery lesion can be short (focal) or long (segmental). Given the same decrease in cross-sectional area, a longer segmental stenosis of a coronary artery increases CVR more, thus reducing coronary flow more than a short focal coronary stenosis (Poiseuille's law).

b. **Degree of stenosis.** Coronary blood flow is reduced in proportion to the fourth power of the vessel diameter. Angiographically, a 50% diameter decrease in lumen size corresponds to a 75% reduction in cross-sectional area, which is hemodynamically consistent with symptoms of angina on exertion. A 75% reduction in diameter at angiography corresponds to a 90% reduction in cross-sectional area, which correponds clinically to symptoms of angina at rest. Two discrete lesions in the same coronary artery will result in two tandem pressure drops, creating an impact on coronary flow in an additive fashion.

c. **Collateral channels.** If the stenotic coronary lesion develops slowly, then collateral channels will enlarge to provide additional blood supply to a jeopardized region of the myocardium. These channels directly connect one coronary artery to another or different segments of the same coronary artery without an intervening capillary bed. Often in the presence of a low-grade obstructive lesion these channels supply enough blood flow to prevent ischemia. However, as the degree of coronary stenosis increases, the collateral channels may not be adequate.

d. **Patterns of stenoses.** Certain patterns of stenoses have important clinical implications related to the amount of myocardium supplied and placed in jeopardy by the stenotic lesion(s). A left main coronary stenosis limits blood flow to a large amount of the left ventricular muscle mass. High-grade, very proximal stenotic lesions of both the circumflex and left anterior descending systems

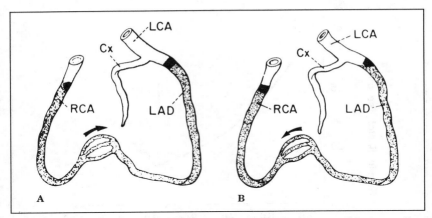

Fig. 11-3. Two examples of possible left main "equivalency." Two-vessel coronary disease with an occluded left anterior descending coronary artery (LAD) and myocardium jeopardized by a right coronary artery (RCA) stenosis *(A)* or an occluded RCA and myocardium jeopardized by a stenotic LAD *(B)*. LCA = left coronary artery; CX = circumflex coronary artery. (From A.M. Hutter, Jr. Is there a left main equivalent? *Circulation* 62:209, 1980. With permission.)

have the same **physiologic** implications as does a left main stenosis. **Prognostically,** however, a left main stenosis is more severe because only one vessel needs to become completely occluded to compromise a large amount of myocardial muscle. In addition, similar "left main equivalent" situations may exist when a severely stenosed coronary provides collateral blood flow to a region with a totally occluded vessel (Fig. 11-3).

  e. Diffuse distal coronary disease. In addition to discrete focal and segmental coronary lesions in graftable vessels, diffuse distal disease may be present in the small branches of the coronary vessels distal to where a graft could be placed. This diffuse disease reduces blood flow to the myocardium further and lessens the effectiveness of bypassing proximal coronary obstructions.

  f. Associated disease states

   (1) Diabetic patients. Diabetic patients have been shown to have abnormal microvasculatures consisting of thickened capillary basement membranes that limit the diffusion of oxygen to the myocytes.

   (2) Hypertensive patients. Hypertensive patients are at increased risk of subendocardial ischemia. Hypertension is associated with left ventricular hypertrophy (LVH). Because of increased wall thickness, the compressive forces on the coronary arteriole and oxygen demand in hypertensive patients are even greater in the subendocardium compared to normal individuals. A combination of LVH with severe coronary stenosis is an extremely risky scenario for the development of subendocardial ischemia.

IV. Determinants of myocardial oxygen demand. The three major determinants of myocardial oxygen demand are heart rate, contractility, and wall stress.

  A. Heart rate. If a relatively fixed amount of oxygen is consumed per heartbeat, one would expect the oxygen demand per minute to increase linearly with heart rate. Thus a doubling of heart rate would yield a doubling of oxygen demand. In fact, demand more than doubles with a twofold increase in heart rate. The source of this additional oxygen demand is the staircase phenomenon, in which increased heart rate causes a small increase in contractility, and increases in contractility mean more oxygen consumed (see sec. **B.** below).

B. **Contractility.** More oxygen is used by a highly contractile heart compared with a more relaxed heart. Contractility is extremely difficult to measure.

1. **Quantitative assessment.** Strictly defined, the contractile state of the heart is a dynamic intrinsic characteristic that is not influenced by preload or afterload. The rate of rise of LV pressure, dP/dt, had been used as a quantitative measure of contractility. Unfortunately, dP/dt depends on both preload and afterload. Currently, contractility is approximated in a load-insensitive fashion utilizing families of pressure-volume curves. These methods are not in routine clinical use.

2. **Qualitative measures.** One can easily observe the contractile state of the heart when the pericardium is open. Remember, though, that the right ventricle is more easily and most often viewed this way, whereas the left is more obscured. Clinically, we infer that contractility is good when there is a brisk rise in the arterial pressure tracing. Beware! The shape of the radial arterial tracing is heavily influenced by confounding factors (system resonant frequency, damping by air bubbles, compliance of the arterial tree, and reflections of pressure waves from arteriolar sites, to name a few). The presence of increased heart rate, blood pressure, and cardiac output more reliably predicts good contractility.

C. **Wall stress.** The stress in the ventricular wall depends on the pressure in the ventricle during contraction ("afterload"), the chamber size ("preload"), and the wall thickness. Calculated for a sphere (which we shall assume for the shape of the ventricle for the sake of simplicity)

$$\text{Wall stress} = \frac{\text{pressure} \times \text{radius}}{2 \ (\text{wall thickness})}$$

1. **Chamber pressure.** Oxygen demand increases with chamber pressure. Doubling the pressure doubles the oxygen demand. Systemic blood pressure usually reflects the chamber pressure; thus we equate systemic blood pressure with LV afterload. The heart's true afterload is more complex because there are elastic and inertial components affecting ejection. Mean systemic pressure, not peak systolic pressure, correlates with oxygen demand. In aortic stenosis, however, the left ventricle experiences very high chamber pressures despite more modest systemic pressures. The clinical goal is to keep afterload (and thus wall stress) low.

2. **Chamber size.** Doubling the ventricular volume increases the radius by only 26% (volume varies with the radius cubed). Thus, increased chamber size is associated with more modest increases in oxygen demand. Nevertheless, because preload determines ventricular size, we desire a low preload to keep wall stress (and thus oxygen demand) low. For example, much of the beneficial effect of nitroglycerin stems from venodilation and its attendant decrease in preload.

3. **Wall thickness.** A thicker wall means less stress over any part of the wall. Ventricular hypertrophy serves to decrease wall stress, although the additional tissue requires more oxygen overall. Hypertrophy occurs in response to the elevated afterload that occurs in chronic systemic hypertension or aortic stenosis. Although wall

Table 11-2. Regulation of oxygen supply and demand

Parameter	Demand	Supply	Oxygen balance
Low heart rate	↓	↑	Positive
Low RAP or PCWP	↓	↑ *	Positive
High heart rate	↑	↓	Negative
High RAP or PCWP	↑	↓	Negative
High temperature	↑	0	Negative
Low temperature	↑ ↓	↓	Variable
Low MAP	↓	↓	Variable
High MAP	↑	↑	Variable
Low hemoglobin	↓	↓ ↑	Variable
High hemoglobin	↑	↑ ↓	Variable

↑ = increased, ↓ = decreased, ↑ ↓ = may increase or decrease, 0 = unchanged, CBF = coronary blood flow, RAP = right atrial pressure, PCWP = pulmonary capillary wedge pressure, MAP = mean arterial pressure.
*However, a drastic decrease in filling pressure will decrease cardiac output.

thickness is essentially uncontrollable clinically, its effects should be considered.

   D. Summary. The factors increasing oxygen demand are increases in heart rate, chamber size, chamber pressure, and contractility. Table 11-2 summarizes the (sometimes) competing factors that contribute toward the goal of high myocardial oxygen supply and low oxygen demand. **The most deleterious physiologic perturbation is tachycardia,** which causes both a rise in oxygen demand and a fall in oxygen supply.

V. Anesthetic effects on myocardial oxygen supply and demand
   A. Intravenous nonopioid agents
      1. Thiopental and thiamylal. Induction doses of the ultra-short-acting barbiturates **decrease systemic vascular resistance and cardiac contractility and increase heart rate.** Oxygen demand is decreased by the first two effects and increased by the last. Oxygen supply is decreased by all three hemodynamic perturbations. The net effect on myocardial oxygen balance is not easily predicted. It depends on the initial conditions. For example, the hyperdynamic, hypertensive patient may benefit from restoration of more appropriate conditions of blood pressure and contractility, whereas a patient whose oxygen balance depends on a normal heart rate may respond to the resultant tachycardia with ischemia. One must remember that these data apply to induction only. Attempted intubation after thiobarbiturate administration alone will increase both heart rate and blood pressure.
      2. Ketamine. The hallmark of ketamine administration is an increase in sympathetic tone leading to **increases in systemic vascular resistance, filling pressures, contractility, and heart rate.** Myocardial oxygen demand is strongly increased whereas oxygen supply may be only slightly augmented, thus producing ischemia. The patient who is already maximally sympathetically stimulated may respond with decreased contractility and vasodilation. Ketamine is not recommended for routine use in patients with ischemic heart disease.
      3. Etomidate. Induction doses of etomidate **do not alter heart rate or cardiac output,** although mild peripheral vasodilation may lower

blood pressure slightly. As such, it is an ideal drug for rapid induction of anesthesia in patients with ischemic heart disease. Although this may be the case for induction, etomidate offers no protection from the increases in heart rate and blood pressure that accompany intubation. An induction dose will block adrenal steroidogenesis for 6–8 hours.

4. **Benzodiazepines.** Midazolam (0.2 mg/kg) or diazepam (0.5 mg/kg) may be used to induce anesthesia. Each drug produces **hemodynamic stability** in patients with ischemic heart disease, although blood pressure may decrease more with midazolam owing to more potent peripheral vasodilation. Negative inotropic effects are inconsequential. Blood pressure and filling pressures decrease with induction, whereas heart rate remains essentially unchanged. Addition of induction doses of a benzodiazepine to a moderate-dose narcotic technique, however, may result in profound peripheral vasodilation and hypotension.

5. **Propofol.** The cardiovascular effects of induction doses of propofol are similar to those of the thiobarbiturates: **systemic blood pressure, systemic vascular resistance, and cardiac contractility decrease.** Heart rate may increase less with propofol compared to thiopental.

B. **Volatile agents.** In general, **volatile anesthetics decrease both oxygen supply and demand.**

1. **Heart rate.** If heart rate is high, halothane decreases it; if low, halothane has little effect. Enflurane often increases heart rate. Isoflurane may also decrease heart rate if the decrease in systemic vascular resistance (SVR) is not profound, if the carotid baroreceptor function is impaired, or if the patient is fully beta-blocked. Junctional rhythms deprive the heart of an atrial kick and lead to decreased stroke volume, cardiac output, and CBF, which may offset the salubrious effects of low heart rate. Junctional rhythms are most often associated with enflurane but may occur with any volatile agent.

2. **Contractility.** All volatile anesthetics decrease contractility, which lowers oxygen demand. Reflex sympathetic activity in poorly beta-blocked patients receiving isoflurane may compensate for the negative inotropic effects, yielding little net effect on contractility. **Which volatile agent decreases contractility the most remains controversial** and is probably not clinical relevant.

3. **Afterload.** Decreases in cardiac output and systemic vascular resistance result in a decreased systemic blood pressure with volatile anesthesia. Venodilation and blunted contractility account for the decrease in cardiac output. Systemic vascular resistance decreases with isoflurane and perhaps enflurane but is essentially unchanged during halothane administration. The decrease in diastolic blood pressure (DBP) reduces myocardial oxygen supply, whereas the decreased afterload reduces oxygen demand.

4. **Preload.** Volatile agent anesthesia is characterized by maintenance of filling pressures; with halothane or enflurane, small increases in filling pressure are common. Coronary perfusion pressure (DBP − PCWP [pulmonary capillary wedge pressure]), as a result, decreases during volatile anesthesia.

C. **Nitrous oxide.** The mild negative inotropic effects of nitrous oxide yield a decrease in contractility, producing a reduction in both oxygen supply and demand. Adding nitrous oxide to a narcotic-oxygen anesthetic will decrease SVR owing to removal of the mild vasoconstrictive effects of 100% oxygen. Nitrous oxide has small negative inotropic effects on isolated cardiac tissue. Its sympathomimetic effects counterbalance any direct depression of contractility except in patients with poor LV function. Additional sympathetic tone in these patients is usually ineffective because the myocardium is already highly stimulated intrinsically.

If nitrous oxide is utilized in a technique that provides a "light" anesthetic that is inadequate to cover attendant stimulation, increases in SVR and afterload are likely. Controversy exists as to whether nitrous oxide per se induces ischemia in patients with coronary artery disease.

D. Opioids

1. **Heart rate.** All narcotics except meperidine decrease heart rate by a centrally mediated vagotonia (meperidine has an atropinelike effect). The dose of drug and speed of injection affect the degree of bradycardia. The result is less oxygen demand. By releasing histamine, morphine or meperidine may elicit a reflex tachycardia that decreases oxygen supply and increases oxygen demand.

2. **Contractility.** Aside from meperidine, which decreases contractility, the narcotics have little effect on contractility in clinical doses.

3. **Afterload.** With the onset of sleep from potent opioids, intrinsic sympathetic tone decreases. Compromised patients often depend on highly elevated sympathetic tone to maintain cardiac output and systemic resistance. This type of patient will experience a sudden drop in blood pressure, resulting in decreases in both oxygen supply and demand. Alfentanil may decrease SVR.

4. **Preload.** Despite a lack of histamine-releasing properties, fentanyl and sufentanil will reduce preload when administered in either moderate doses (25 µg/kg for fentanyl) or larger doses by decreasing intrinsic sympathetic tone. Oxygen demand is decreased.

5. **The hyperdynamic state.** Elevations of heart rate, blood pressure, and cardiac output with or without decreased filling pressures are common during pure narcotic-oxygen anesthetic techniques in patients with good ventricular function. This high-supply–high-demand state may be less preferable than the low-demand state achieved with volatile anesthesia. It is often difficult to treat the hypertension associated with hyperdynamic cardiovascular state with additional narcotic.

E. Muscle relaxants

1. **Succinylcholine.** This drug may cause a variety of **dysrhythmias,** (bradycardia, tachycardia, extrasystoles) that may have a negative impact on myocardial oxygen balance.

2. **Tubocurarine, metocurine iodide, and atracurium besylate.** These drugs **release histamine** at, respectively, 1, 2, and 3 times the ED_{95} for twitch blockade. None is the drug of choice for patients with ischemic heart disease. A combination of metocurine and pancuronium may be useful in this regard. One-fourth an intubating dose of each agent avoids the undesired side effects of each agent. With this combination a twofold synergism at the neuromuscular junction provides adequate relaxation.

3. **Pancuronium.** Prospective studies show that **heart rate elevations** of 18–22% result from pancuronium combined with a volatile anesthetic. With high-dose narcotic anesthesia, heart rate usually remains stable. An occasional patient will develop tachycardia and ischemia during induction or intubation [6]. Pancuronium is also known to increase systemic blood pressure, although the effects on oxygen balance in the heart are not predictable.

4. **Vecuronium.** The **flat cardiovascular profile** of vecuronium makes it the drug of choice with a low- or moderate-dose narcotic anesthetic and volatile agent technique. Extreme bradycardia may occur when vecuronium is given in conjunction with rapid injection of high doses

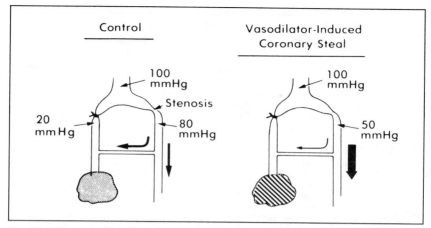

Fig. 11-4. Theoretical basis of coronary steal. The shaded, marginally ischemic area normally receives barely enough flow *(left)*. A potent vasodilator improves flow to the normal myocardium but does not affect the already maximally dilated area in jeopardy. This process decreases flow through the collateral from the nonischemic bed. This further impoverishment of the marginally ischemic area produces frank ischemia *(right)*. (Modified from L.C. Becker. Conditions for vasodilator-induced coronary steal in experimental myocardial ischemia. *Circulation* 57:1108, 1978. With permission.)

of the highly lipid-soluble narcotics; this technique is not recommended.

   F. **Regional myocardial blood flow.** Global measures of CBF may mask an intramyocardial "steal" phenomenon in which dilation of normal vascular beds diverts blood away from other beds that are ischemic and thus maximally dilated (Fig. 11-4). Nitroprusside, a potent systemic vasodilator, has been implicated in causing coronary steal by dilating coronary arteriolar resistance vessels. In contrast, nitroglycerin dilates the venous circulation, epicardial coronary vessels, and large collateral myocardial vessels and is not known to be associated with the steal phenomenon. Isoflurane-induced coronary steal is controversial. If systemic blood pressure is well maintained, steal has yet to be shown to occur with isoflurane.

   G. **Summary.** Volatile anesthesia provides a **low-supply–low-demand** environment. The narcotic-oxygen technique provides a **high-supply– high-demand** environment. Success with either technique depends on maintaining proper balance, with oxygen supply exceeding demand.

VI. **Associated cardiac pathology secondary to coronary artery disease.** Congestive heart failure, dysrhythmias, and mitral regurgitation are disease states that can develop secondary to coronary artery disease.

   A. **Congestive heart failure can be either acute or chronic.**
      1. **Acute congestive heart failure.** Onset of ischemia may lead to global diastolic dysfunction, with a decrease in left ventricular compliance leading to increased left atrial pressure and pulmonary congestion. This can occur in the presence of normal or relatively normal systolic ventricular function. This diastolic dysfunction may be the first and only sign of ischemia. In addition, ischemia of the papillary muscles may cause acute severe mitral regurgitation leading to pulmonary congestion.
      2. **Chronic congestive heart failure.** Multiple infarctions as a result of coronary disease or severe ischemia may compromise not only

diastolic function but also systolic function, and both can lead to the development of chronic congestive heart failure with a low forward output and pulmonary congestion.

B. **Dysrhythmias.** Whenever cardiac muscle is ischemic, dysrhythmogenic foci may develop. Ventricular ectopy is the most common dysrhythmia associated with coronary artery disease. Indeed, the severity of ventricular dysrhythmias correlates with the degree of coronary stenosis. Individuals with poor ventricular function and severe coronary disease have the highest incidence of ventricular ectopy. Ventricular dysrhythmias are especially common during myocardial infarction. In the anesthetized patient, new or unexplained dysrhythmias or bundle branch block may reflect ischemia or infarction.

C. **Mitral regurgitation.** Chronic congestive heart failure due to ischemia can lead to mitral valvular annular dilatation which in turn can lead to chronic mitral regurgitation. Acute ischemia of the papillary muscle also causes mitral regurgitation. Patients with coronary artery disease may have associated mitral valvular disease unrelated to their coronary artery disease, often of rheumatic origin.

VII. **Detection of myocardial ischemia.** Only half of intraoperative ischemic events can be related to a hemodynamic alteration (tachycardia, hypotension, or hypertension). Because patients who develop intraoperative ischemia are more likely to suffer a perioperative transmural myocardial infarction, we must monitor patients closely to detect and treat every ischemic episode. Angina is a symptom, not a sign, and requires an awake, communicative patient with an intact warning system. Ischemia is diagnosed with certainty by decreased lactate extraction of a regional myocardial circulatory bed. This technique is not feasible on a routine clinical basis, so we turn to picking up the clues that ischemia leaves in its wake: electrocardiographic (ECG) changes, pulmonary arterial pressure changes, and myocardial wall motion abnormalities. Chapter 4 provides additional information on monitoring.

A. **ECG changes.** The ST segment of the ECG changes with ischemia: Depression denotes endocardial ischemia and elevation denotes transmural ischemia. ST changes occur at least 60–120 seconds after the start of ischemia. The reference for the ST segment is usually taken as 80 msec after the J-point, which is the end of the QRS wave (Fig. 11-5). Significant changes are usually defined as 0.1 mV or 1 mm ST-segment elevation or depression at normal gain. Note the following details when interpreting ST-segment changes.

1. Differential diagnosis of ST-segment elevation includes the several causes of transmural ischemia (atherosclerotic disease, coronary vasospasm, intracoronary air), pericarditis, and ventricular aneurysm. One must also consider improper lead placement, particularly reversal of limb and leg leads, and improper selection of electronic filtering. **The diagnostic mode should always be chosen on machines equipped with a diagnostic-monitor mode selection switch.**

2. Modern monitoring systems now include automated real-time ST-segment analysis. Although this feature constitutes a definite advance in the "human engineering" aspects of ischemia monitoring, the machine is only as smart as the person interpreting its data. Beware of intraventricular conduction delays, bundle branch blocks, and ventricular pacing, all of which can render ST-segment analysis invalid. Check the machine's determination of where the ST segment occurs: 80 msec after the J-point is not always appropriate.

3. New T-wave alterations (flipped or flattened) may also indicate ischemia. These may not be detected by viewing the ST segment alone. Likewise, pseudonormalization of the ST segment or T wave (an

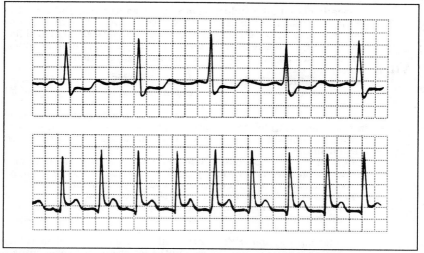

Fig. 11-5. The upper tracing shows ST-segment depression, an indicator of subendo-cardial ischemia. Transmural ischemia, one cause of ST-segment elevation, produces the pattern appearing in the lower tracing.

ischemic-looking tracing in a patient without ischemia reverting to a more normal-looking one) may indicate a new onset of ischemia and should be treated appropriately.

4. To increase detection of ischemia with the ECG, monitor more than one region of the heart. Simultaneous observation of an inferior lead (II, III, or aVF) and an anterior lead (V_5) provides detection superior to single lead monitoring. Modified chest leads may also be preferred.

B. **Pulmonary arterial pressure changes.** The absolute pulmonary artery (PA) pressure is not diagnostic of ischemia. Pulmonary hypertension, whether primary or secondary to valvular heart disease, is not uncommon. Elevations of PA pressure or PCWP may occur secondary to rapid volume infusion or light anesthesia in the absence of ischemia. The morphology of the waveform, however, is more predictive. Appearance of a new V wave in the PCWP waveform indicates functional mitral regurgitation, which is due to valvular pathology or papillary muscle dysfunction from ischemia (see Fig. 4-15). A new V wave suggestive of ischemia may occur before or in the absence of ECG changes. However, detection of changes in the pulmonary capillary wedge (PCW) waveform requires frequent wedging of the PA catheter, a questionable practice in heparinized patients owing to the possibility of PA rupture. Often the morphology of the PA pressure tracing will change when a new V wave appears in the wedge tracing. When the PA pressure wave changes shape, check the wedge for a new V wave.

C. **Ventricular wall motion abnormalities.** These may be the most sensitive indicator of ischemia available. Ultrasound permits real-time imaging of the ventricular wall. During cardiothoracic surgery, an anterior ultrasound probe is impractical, so the ventricle is viewed from its posterior aspect through a transesophageal probe. The equipment needed for transesophageal echocardiography (TEE) is bulky and expensive. The image must be continuously viewed; achieving and interpreting the image requires training and practice. Because the probe is usually placed after induction of anesthesia, the stressful induction period cannot be monitored with TEE. TEE is available with color-flow Doppler capability, showing the magnitude and direction of blood flow in the image. This feature is useful for diagnosing valvular abnormalities, such as ischemia-induced mitral regurgitation.

VII. Planning the case

A. Selection of anesthetic agents based on patient types.
The selection of premedication, induction, and maintenance anesthetic and adjuvant agents depends on the patient's condition. We consider three subgroups of patients, not mutually exclusive, undergoing revascularization: those with left main coronary artery disease or its equivalent; those with poor left ventricular function; and those with good left ventricular function.

1. **Left main or equivalent disease.** This type of patient depends heavily on adequate coronary perfusion pressure (oxygen supply). Avoid agents that could decrease blood pressure suddenly.

   a. **Premedication.** Choice of agent should be based on LV function: morphine (0.1 mg/kg IM) and scopolamine (6 µg/kg IM) suffice in all but highly anxious patients, for whom oral benzodiazepine should be added, and those with severely impaired LV function (ejection fraction [EF]<0.25). Half the usual doses of morphine and scopolamine may be used in the latter group. Scopolamine is the preferred adjuvant to morphine because it is an excellent amnestic and sedative. The dose should be reduced to 3 µg/kg in patients over age 70 and avoided in patients over age 80 owing to its dysphoric effects in the aged.

   b. **Induction.** Technique should provide high-supply–high-demand characteristics. Slow administration of a moderate (fentanyl 20–40 µg/kg) to high-dose (fentanyl 100 µg/kg) narcotic with pure oxygen is a good choice. A low-demand–low-supply technique, typically obtained with volatile agents, may compromise coronary perfusion pressure by decreasing diastolic BP and raising filling pressures.

   c. **Maintenance.** Maintenance doses should match the cardiovascular dynamics: Hyperdynamism should be controlled with low concentrations of volatile agents.

2. **Poor LV function (EF <0.40)**

   a. **Pre-medication.** The usual doses of morphine and scopolamine should be halved in patients with severely compromised LV function to prevent hypercarbia and hypotension from engendering preoperative cardiovascular deterioration.

   b. **Induction.** Since congestive heart failure is often present or easily incited, a volatile agent is best avoided. Slow administration of moderate doses of narcotic, such as 20–40 µg/kg fentanyl or 2–3 µg/kg of sufentanil over 5 minutes, achieves adequate protection against the stress of intubation in most patients.

   c. **Maintenance.** A repeat dose of narcotic prior to sternotomy will block the sympathetic response to that stimulus. If low dose volatile agents are added to control hypertension, cardiac output must be measured to ensure adequate flow and appropriate systemic vascular resistance. Volatile agents may also increase filling pressures, which compromise CPP and may increase oxygen demand.

3. **Good LV function**

   a. **Pre-medication.** Should be generous to avoid preoperative anxiety and its accompanying deleterious hyperdynamic state. Morphine, scopolamine, and oral benzodiazepine are appropriate.

   b. **Induction.** Volatile agents provide the low-demand–low-supply profile that characterizes a successful induction in these patients.

Table 11-3. Recommended choices of anesthetic agents for patient subgroups

Subgroup	Premedication	Induction	Maintenance
Left main or equivalent	Full-dose morphine/ scopolamine	High-dose opioid	Opioid ± volatile agent
Poor LV function	Full-dose or half-dose morphine/ scopolamine	High-dose opioid	Opioid ± volatile agent
Good LV function	Full-dose morphine/ scopolamine + oral benzodiazepine	Volatile agent with N_2O/O_2 and/or opioid	Opioid or volatile agent or both

With a narcotic-oxygen technique, breakthrough hypertension is common and is difficult to treat with additional narcotic; in such a case, adding a volatile agent is appropriate.

    c. **Maintenance.** A volatile agent is often required at some point to control heart rate and blood pressure responses to surgical stimulation.

        Table 11-3 summarizes the recommended choices of agents for each of the three patient subgroups mentioned. The choice between opioid and volatile anesthesia serves as an example only. Safe induction of anesthesia for myocardial revascularization may be provided with a variety of agents already discussed including etomidate, benzodiazepines, thiopental, and even ketamine.

B. Indications for a PA catheter for revascularization procedures. A PA catheter should be placed when the risks are outweighed by the benefits. If the catheter is placed, use it!

    1. Information. The PA catheter provides information on central venous pressure (CVP), PA pressure, and PCWP as well as core temperature, cardiac output, and in some cases, mixed venous oximetry.

    2. Other functions. The CVP port and other ports (side port of the introducing sheath as well as optional extra ports of various types) provide access to the central circulation for injection of medication and withdrawal of blood for analysis. Some catheters allow pacing of one or both chambers of the right heart, fiberoptic oximetry, or determination of right ventricular ejection fraction.

    3. Some specific indications for catheter placement

        a. Poor left ventricular function. In these patients there is little room for straying from optimal hemodynamics. Knowledge of filling pressures and cardiac output facilitates management. CVP alone is insufficient when there is a disparity of right-left ventricular function.

        b. The need to pace the heart. Catheters providing a port for placement of a pacing wire may be chosen when pacing is acutely needed and the chest is not open, although other therapies, such as external pacing or transvenous pacing wires, may also be appropriate. Occasionally, right bundle branch block (RBBB) will occur some time after PA catheter placement. This is possibly related to irritation of the right part of the interventricular septum, through which the conduction fibers pass. Patients who begin with a complete left bundle branch block (LBBB) may then develop complete heart block should RBBB occur. Thus, some clinicians prescribe

Table 11-4. Causes of perioperative ischemia in the myocardial revascularization patient

Prebypass	Bypass	Postbypass
Hemodynamic alterations[a]	Hemodynamic alterations[a]	Hemodynamic alterations[a]
Coronary spasm	Coronary spasm Cardioplegic arrest	Coronary spasm
Thrombus formation	Emboli (air, thrombus particulate matter)	Thrombus (native vessel/ graft)
High risk anesthetic-surgical events[b]	Ventricular fibrillation Ventricular distention	
	Surgical complications[b]	Surgical complications[b] Incomplete revascularization Excessive use of inotropes Distention of the lungs leading to occlusion of internal mammary graft flow

[a]Includes tachycardia, hypotension, hypertension, ventricular distention.
[b]See text for details.

a PA catheter with pacing capabilities for patients with preexisting LBBB. Additionally, a stand-by transcutaneous pacemaker during PA catheter placement in patients with LBBB is prudent should bradycardia or asystole occur.

c. **The desire to know cardiac output.** Although there are many indirect indices of cardiac output (blood pressure and urine output are two of them), we believe the risks of PA catheter placement are so small that every patient undergoing coronary revascularization deserves the benefit of measuring cardiac output by thermodilution. Claims that PA catheterization does not affect outcome[7] should be doubted until randomized studies provide validation.

d. **The desire to detect ischemia.** See sec. **VII. B.** above on detection of myocardial ischemia by PA pressure waveform configuration.

e. **The need to maintain preload.** A patient with coronary disease who has concomitant hypertrophic obstructive cardiomyopathy will benefit greatly from continual scrutiny and maintenance of preload.

IX. **Causes and treatment of perioperative myocardial ischemia.** Multiple factors may lead to development of ischemia in the perioperative period. Often several causes occur simultaneously. For purposes of discussion, causes of ischemia will be divided into those that are most common in the prebypass, bypass, and postbypass periods (Table 11-4). Factors leading to ischemia during one time period may enhance or worsen ischemia in subsequent time periods.

Any of the hemodynamic alterations (tachycardia, hypertension, hypotension, ventricular distention) outlined in the initial chapters on anesthetic management for cardiac surgery may be responsible for ischemia during any phase of the perioperative period. In addition, any factors that decrease oxygen content and delivery, such as poor oxygenation or anemia, may be additive to any ischemic event throughout the operative procedure.

A. Causes of ischemia in the prebypass period

1. **Ischemia associated with specific high risk anesthetic-surgical events.** Slogoff and Keats [4] identified specific events precipitating ischemia in the prebypass period in patients undergoing myocardial revascularization. These high-risk events were intubation, surgical stress (skin incision, sternal split), cannulation, and initiation of bypass. Many episodes of ischemia occurred during these high-risk events in the absence of hemodynamic changes.

2. **Ischemia associated with hemodynamic abnormalities.** The same study showed, however, that some episodes of ischemia during these high-risk periods were associated with hemodynamic abnormalities, (specifically, the authors looked at tachycardia, hypertension, and hypotension). There was a particularly high association of ischemia with tachycardia (>100 bpm). Every attempt should be made to minimize hemodynamic alterations to prevent myocardial ischemia because Slogoff and Keats also demonstrated a three-fold increase in myocardial infarctions in patients who developed ischemia in the prebypass period.

3. **Coronary spasm.** Coronary spasm in a normal coronary vessel or around an atherosclerotic lesion may cause myocardial ischemia in the prebypass period. Intense sympathetic stimulation or light levels of anesthesia could theoretically trigger coronary vasospasm. In addition, manipulation of the heart and coronary vessels by the surgeon may induce coronary spasm.

4. **Spontaneous thrombus formation.** Spontaneous thrombus formation at an atherosclerotic plaque leading to occlusion of a coronary vessel may be responsible for myocardial infarction. Although uncommon nothing precludes this scenario from occurring in the operating room in the pre-bypass period.

B. Causes of ischemia during bypass

1. **Bypass without aortic cross-clamp applied.** Hemodynamic alterations, mechanical factors during bypass, and ventricular fibrillation can influence the occurrence of ischemia (see Chap. 21) prior to application of the aortic cross-clamp and after removal of the aortic cross-clamp. In addition, particulate microemboli (thrombus, plastic, and other foreign material) is present in all bypass circuits and may lead to ischemia when the coronaries are perfused on bypass. Coronary air emboli can occur with imperfect de-airing of the vein grafts. Whenever the heart or aorta is opened, air embolism to the native coronary circulation is a potential problem.

2. **During aortic cross-clamping.** Once the aortic cross-clamp is applied, regardless of myocardial preservation techniques, ischemia is inevitable. As cross-clamp time increases, so does the potential for ischemic injury and subsequent infarction. Washout of cold cardioplegic solution owing to excessive noncoronary collateral flow (Chap. 21) may also be responsible for ischemia during this period. Unfortunately, once the aorta is cross-clamped and the cardioplegic solution is administered, the electrical and mechanical quiescence precludes monitoring for ischemia.

3. **Specific causes of ischemia after the aortic cross-clamp is removed**

   a. **Surgical and technical complications.** Surgical and technical complications still occur. However, they are a lesser problem than they were 10–15 years ago. Surgical complications include:

      (1) Inadvertent incision of the coronary back wall leading to coronary dissection

      (2) Improper handling of the vein graft with endothelial cell loss leading to graft thrombus formation

      (3) Twisting of vein grafts

      (4) Anastomosing the vein graft to the coronary vein

      (5) Suturing closed the artery while grafting or poor quality of anastomoses

      (6) Inadequate vein graft length leading to stretching of the vein when the heart is filled

      (7) Excess length of vein graft leading to vein kinking

  b. Etiology of ST-segment elevation after cross-clamp removal. After removal of the aortic cross-clamp, ST-segment elevation may occur. The length of cardioplegic arrest, residual electrophysiologic effects of cardioplegia, coronary air embolus, or coronary artery spasm may all contribute to the etiology of this ECG abnormality [5]. Often the ST-segment elevation is located in the inferior leads (i.e., right coronary distribution), implicating air embolus as the etiology (air seeks the high location of the right coronary ostium).

      Non-resolution and persistence of ST-segment changes after aortic cross-clamp removal may indicate ongoing ischemia secondary to coronary artery spasm or coronary air embolus and require appropriate therapy (see Table 9-3).

C. Causes of ischemia in the postbypass period

  1. Incomplete revascularization. It is important for the anesthesiologist to know whether or not the patient has been completely revascularized prior to the termination of cardiopulmonary bypass.

    a. Ungraftable vessels. Sometimes vessels are deemed ungraftable once the surgeon palpates and examines the caliber of the vessel. That region of the myocardium supplied by the unrevascularized stenotic vessel may have a greater chance of developing ischemia in the postbypass period than in the prebypass period because of the added insult of cardioplegic arrest.

    b. Diffuse distal disease and diabetes. Patients with diffuse distal disease and diabetic patients may be at risk for ischemia in the postbypass period. Severe distal disease is also a risk factor for early vein graft closure because the small distal vessels provide poor run-off for vein graft flow.

  2. Coronary spasm. Coronary spasm can occur in the postbypass period, most commonly in right coronary arteries that are undiseased. Surgical manipulation and exogenous as well as endogenous catecholamines may contribute to this problem.

  3. Mechanical factors. Mechanical factors such as vein graft kinking or stretching or occlusion of internal mammary flow secondary to overinflation of the lungs may cause ischemia in the postbypass period.

  4. Surgical and technical complications (see sec **B**).

  5. Thrombus formation. Thrombus formation in the native vessel or the bypass graft may occur postbypass, leading to severe ischemia and infarction. Coronary vasospasm or hypercoagulability arising from coagulation system manipulations or from patient disease may contribute to clot formation in vessels.

  6. Inotropes. Improper use of inotropes, including calcium, during weaning from bypass or in the postbypass period may also increase the risk of ischemia or potentiate ischemia during this period.

D. Treatment of myocardial ischemia. Table 11-5 lists conventional treatment of ischemia in the patient undergoing myocardial revascularization.

  1. Treatment of ischemia secondary to hemodynamic abnormalities

    a. Increasing or decreasing anesthetic depth

Table 11-5. Treatment of ischemia

Adequate oxygenation

Hemodynamic stability (e.g., adequate anesthetic depth)

Surgical correction

Specific pharmacologic treatment
  Nitroglycerin
  Calcium channel blockers
  β blockers (esmolol)

Inotropic support (ischemia secondary to a failing ventricle)

Mechanical support
  Intraaortic balloon pump
  Left ventricular assist device
  Right ventricular assist device

---

   b. Use of vasodilators or vasopressors when systemic vascular resistance is either high or low, respectively
   c. Use of a β-blocker, specifically esmolol, to treat tachycardia
   d. Use of atrioventricular sequential pacing. Specifically in the postbypass period this can be extremely beneficial to improve rate, rhythm, and hemodynamic stability
   e. Use of inotropes when failing ventricular function is diagnosed by decreased cardiac output and increased ventricular filling pressures. Pump failure leads to severe decreases in CPP because diastolic blood pressure is decreased and LVEDP is increased.
       Note: Indiscriminate use of inotropes may aggravate ischemia. Therefore, preload, heart rate rhythm, and afterload should all be maximized prior to the use of inotropes.
 2. Correction of surgical complications and mechanical problems
   a. Any surgical correctable factors leading to ischemia should be attended to in the postbypass period.
   b. Overinflation of the lungs when an internal mammary graft is present should be avoided.
 3. Treatment of coronary spasm. For a complete discussion of diagnosis and treatment of coronary spasm refer to Chapter 9.
 4. Specific pharmacologic treatment of ischemia. This treatment includes (1) nitroglycerin, (2) β blockers, (3) calcium channel blockers. Refer to Chapter 3 for these drugs' mechanisms of action and doses. Intravenous nitroglycerin is probably the most utilized pharmacologic treatment of ischemia in the operating room throughout the perioperative period. Specific prophylactic use includes the postbypass utilization of nitroglycerin in incompletely revascularized patients, patients with severe distal coronary disease, and diabetic patients.
 5. Mechanical support. Refer to Chapter 22 for a complete discussion of these devices.
   a. Intraaortic balloon pumps. Intraaortic balloon pumps have been utilized for many years as a treatment of ischemia by increasing coronary perfusion pressure, and decreasing afterload for left ventricular ejection. In patients with angina, insertion of a balloon pump often relieves symptoms in the presence of normal ventricular function. In patients with impaired ventricular function, elevation of coronary perfusion pressure and improved ventricular ejection may relieve ischemia and improve pump performance.
   b. Right and left ventricular assist devices. These devices may be useful for treating severe ischemia caused by myocardial failure

or ischemia that has led to myocardial failure. Data on their use as treatment for ischemia is still in question.

X. Unique anesthetic concerns for the patient undergoing myocardial revascularization reoperation. The indications for myocardial revascularization reoperation change with time.[1] In the early 1970s the indication for reoperation was incomplete revascularization at the primary operation or early graft closure, which was largely related to technical complications. Since the late 1970s the indications have been progressive coronary atherosclerosis in the native vessels as well as graft atherosclerosis or thrombosis.

An increased incidence of bleeding, perioperative ischemia, infarction, and pump failure are the main concerns that lead to increased morbidity and mortality in this subgroup of patients undergoing myocardial revascularization. Table 11–6 summarizes these special concerns as well as their causes and appropriate perioperative anesthetic management.

XI. Anesthesia for urgent revascularization. Urgent revascularization may arise in the setting of a failed attempt at balloon dilatation in the catheterization laboratory, following attempts at reperfusion using thrombolytic agents such as streptokinase or tissue plasminogen activator (tPA), or simply owing to acute ischemia refractory to maximal pharmacologic and mechanical (aortic balloon counterpulsation) therapy. These situations will be addressed individually and their special concerns summarized.

A. Anesthesia for balloon angioplasty. Most centers perform angioplasty without anesthesia. Small series from some institutions [2] show that anesthesia for angioplasty is safe and may be preferable to the awake state because it provides superior control of ventilation and hemodynamics. Because extubation at the end of the procedure is a goal, an oxygen-narcotic technique is not appropriate. Volatile anesthetics have been used successfully. Many patients for angioplasty with acute ischemia have full stomachs; rapid induction with etomidate may be helpful.

B. Revascularization after failed balloon dilatation angioplasty. There are four scenarios to consider:

1. **Angioplasty fails, no vascular damage.** The patient will be disappointed but in no immediate danger. Urgent revascularization, although popular in the past when angioplasty was a new procedure, is currently not in vogue. The interests of the patient are served best by a full evaluation and regularly scheduled surgical revascularization.

2. **Angioplasty fails, radiographs show arterial damage (usually dissection) despite absence of ischemia.** Some angiographers fear subsequent thrombus formation at the injured endothelium and argue for urgent revascularization. Evaluation, cannulation, and anesthetic induction should proceed in an unhurried fashion, and a full stomach should be given sufficient time to empty.

3. **Angioplasty fails, vascular damage and ischemia are present with hemodynamic stability.** The goal is to relieve the ischemia within 4–6 hours of its onset, before infarction occurs. Institution of aortic balloon counterpulsation often succeeds in ameliorating ischemia, following which revascularization should proceed in a prompt but unhurried fashion. With ongoing ischemia, time is limited. Induction should utilize vascular access (intravenous and arterial catheters) existing from catheterization. Attempts at appropriate central venous access may proceed in parallel with surgical preparation and draping.

4. **Angioplasty fails, vascular damage, ischemia, and hemodynamic instability are present.** Patients may arrive in the operating room alert with mild hypotension; others may be intubated and be

Table 11-6. Perioperative management of the myocardial revascularization reoperation patient

Perioperative problem	Cause	Management
Bleeding	Pericardial adhesions Preoperative antiplatelet or anticoagulant medication	Large-bore IV access Blood readily available and checked in the OR Careful dissection on reopening chest Femoral area exposed and ready for emergency cannulation Anticipated need for clotting factors and platelets in the postbypass period Availability of blood salvage equipment (cell saver, etc.)
Ischemia/ infarction	Increased incidence of unstable angina Long period before bypass instituted	Close monitoring of ischemia (ECG, PA catheter, two-dimensional TEE) Expeditious treatment of ischemia once detected
	Thrombus in vein grafts embolize to native vessels	Careful manipulation of vein grafts
	Interruption of vein graft flow (associated with 50–60% mortality)	Careful dissection around vein grafts
	Longer bypass and cross-clamp times	Minimal cross-clamp time
	Increased amount of noncoronary collateral flow	Mean perfusion pressure < 60 mm Hg when cross-clamp is applied to limit noncoronary flow
Pump failure post-bypass	Perioperative ischemia and infarction	Same as under perioperative ischemia Treat ischemia aggressively after bypass to improve myocardial function Anticipate need for intravenous inotropic and mechanical support

TEE = transesophageal echocardiography.

receiving chest compressions. Patients who are unresponsive with minimal blood pressure require paralysis, possibly supplemented with the amnestic scopolamine, and no anesthetic medication. In these patients, nothing should interfere with the goal of achieving cardiopulmonary bypass as quickly as possible.

C. **After fibrinolytic therapy.** Streptokinase and tPA are both available to break down thrombi in the coronary circulation. Streptokinase especially can alter the systemic coagulation cascade (see Chap. 18). Therefore, these patients arrive anticoagulated; special care should be exercised in placing monitoring catheters. Arterial catheters should be placed in vessels amenable to external pressure: The radial artery is preferred to the femoral artery. Central cannulation should be performed by experienced personnel, and venous placement verified prior to placement of a large-bore sheath. These patients tend to bleed more postoperatively. Administration of an anti-fibrinolytic drug, such as aminocaproic acid or tranexamic acid, is reasonable, but the effect is unproved. The fibrinolytic system is highlighted in Chap. 18 (see Fig. 18-5).

D. Acute ischemia refractory to therapy. This patient should be treated in a manner similar to that used for the failed angioplasty patient with ischemia.

E. Special considerations for urgent revascularization
   1. **Transport.** The unstable patient requires smooth, efficient transport with all necessary equipment readily available.
   2. **Operating room preparation.** One must avoid the hazard of a hastily prepared operating room. Preparation must proceed in parallel with patient transport to minimize ischemic time.
   3. **Full stomach.** An oxygen-narcotic induction with cricoid pressure is recommended, although etomidate has also been used successfully. Any rapid induction carries the risk of hypotension. Acute decreases in blood pressure often occur secondary to a loss of sympathetic tone, which can be quite high during myocardial ischemia and infarction. This hypotension may be transiently remedied with phenylephrine to restore preload and an inotrope if phenylephrine is unsuccessful alone or in patients with congestive heart failure, in whom phenylephrine should be avoided.
   4. **Anticoagulation.** Heparin is usually present. Some patients have received streptokinase or tPA. Cannulation precautions are warranted.
   5. **Dysrhythmia.** Since dysrhythmias are common, prophylactic antidysrhythmics have been recommended.
   6. **Inotropic support.** Patients who arrive in the operating room with ischemia more often require inotropic support to wean them from bypass. Inotropic support should be immediately available for these patients.

REFERENCES

1. Camann, W. R., Wojtowicz, S. R., and Mark, J. B. Reoperation for coronary artery bypass grafting: Anesthetic challenge. *J. Cardiothorac. Anesth.* 1:458–467, 1987.
2. Kates, R. A., Hill, R., and Reves, J. G. Reperfusion of the Acute Myocardial Infarction, Role of Anesthesia. In J. G. Reves (ed.), *Acute Revascularization of the Infarcted Heart.* Philadelphia: Grune & Stratton, 1987. Pp. 35–64.
3. Opie, L. H. Oxygen Supply: Coronary Flow. In L. H. Opie (ed.), *The Heart.* Philadelphia: Grune & Stratton, 1984. Pp. 154–165.
4. Slogoff, S., and Keats, A. S. Does perioperative myocardial ischemia lead to postoperative myocardial infarction? *Anesthesiology* 62:107–114, 1985.
5. Thomson, I. R., Rosenbloom, M., Cannon, J. E., et al. Electrocardiographic ST-segment elevation after myocardial reperfusion during coronary artery surgery. *Anesth. Analg.* 66(11):1183–1186, 1987.
6. Thomson, I. R., and Putnins, C. L. Adverse effects of pancuronium during high-dose fentanyl anesthesia for coronary artery bypass grafting. *Anesthesiology* 62:708–713, 1985.
7. Tuman, K. J., McCarthy, R. J., Spiess, B.D., et al. Effect of pulmonary artery catheterization on outcome in patients undergoing coronary artery surgery. *Anesthesiology* 70:199–206, 1989.

SUGGESTED READING

Lowenstein, E., and Reiz, S. Effects of Inhalation Anesthetics on Systemic Hemodynamics and the Coronary Circulation. In J. A. Kaplan (ed.), *Cardiac Anesthesia* (2nd ed.). Philadelphia: Grune & Stratton, 1987. Pp. 3–35.

Merin, R. Anesthesia and the Coronary Circulation. In R. K. Stoelting, P. G. Barash, and T. J. Gallagher (eds.), *Advances in Anesthesia,* Vol. 6. Chicago:Year Book, 1989. Pp. 195–218.

O'Connor, J. P., and Wynands, J. E. Anesthesia for Myocardial Revascularization. In J. A. Kaplan (ed.), *Cardiac Anesthesia* (2nd ed.). Philadelphia: Grune & Stratton, 1987. Pp. 551–588.

Reves, J. G. Myocardial ischemia and perioperative infarction. *Anesthesiol. Clin. North Am.* 6(3):461–654, 1988.

Ross, J. Jr., and Covell, J. W. Cardiovascular System. In J. B. West (ed.), *Physiological Basis of Medical Practice* (11th ed.). Baltimore: Williams & Wilkins, 1985. Pp. 236–262.

White, P. F. What's new in intravenous anesthetics? *Anesthesiol. Clin. North Am.* 6(2):297–318, 1988.

Anesthetic Management for the Treatment of Valvular Heart Disease

Roger A. Moore and Donald E. Martin

I. **Cardiac response to valvular heart disease.** The anesthetic management of patients undergoing valvular heart surgery requires a thorough understanding of:

1. The abnormal pressure and volume loads imposed by abnormal valves.
2. The structural and functional mechanisms by which the heart attempts to compensate.
3. The events that may signal the limits of compensation, such as arrhythmias, ischemia, and cardiac failure.
4. Secondary complications such as endocarditis or emboli.

A. **Ventricular function.** To anticipate the effect of valvular lesions on ventricular function, it is necessary to understand that ventricular function has two distinct components.
   1. **Systolic function** represents the ventricle's ability to contract and eject blood against an afterload. Systolic function allows the ventricle to respond to a pressure load and is best described by the ratio of the end-systolic pressure to end-systolic volume. As end-systolic pressure (afterload) increases, the ventricle cannot empty completely, and end-systolic volume increases. However, the ratio of end-systolic pressure to volume remains almost constant under most circumstances and is directly related to ventricular contractility.
   2. **Diastolic function** represents the ventricle's ability to relax and accept inflowing blood, or preload. Diastolic function is necessary for the ventricle to respond to a volume load and is best described by the relationship between end-diastolic pressure and end-diastolic volume, or ventricular **compliance. Both systolic and diastolic function require energy and can be compromised by ventricular ischemia.**
B. **Ventricular hypertrophy.** Chronic volume and pressure loads each evoke a characteristic ventricular response. Pressure loads usually result in a "concentric" ventricular hypertrophy, with an increase in ventricular wall thickness that allows the heart to maintain its normal concentric position within the chest cavity. Volume loading, on the other hand, leads to "eccentric" hypertrophy. The word *eccentric* in this context means that the heart dilates and, because of increased chamber size, assumes an eccentric position in the chest.
C. **Pressure-volume relationship.** Both systolic and diastolic components of ventricular function, along with the corresponding pressure and volume loads, can be represented graphically by a pressure-volume loop, which shows the pressure-volume relationship at each instant during a single cardiac cycle. Figure 12-1 shows a representative pressure-volume loop under normal conditions. Diastolic function is represented by a dashed line and includes phase 1, isovolumetric relaxation, and phase 2, ventricular filling. Systolic function is represented by a solid line and includes phase 3, isovolumetric contraction, and phase 4, ventricular ejection. The area inside the loop provides a rough index of the energy used to eject blood, or the stroke work. The shape of this loop changes with variations in ventricular load, ventricular compliance, and ventricular contractility. Each valvular lesion imposes its own unique set of variables on left and right ventricular function. These variations lead to specific hemodynamic profiles for each lesion that suggest the anesthetic and therapeutic priorities for patients with each type of valvular heart disease.

II. **Aortic stenosis**
   A. **Natural history**
      1. **Etiology.** Aortic stenosis is classified as valvular, subvalvular, or supravalvular based on the anatomic location of the stenotic lesion.

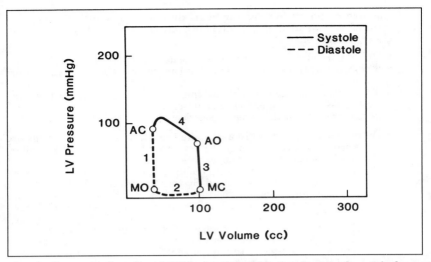

Fig. 12-1. Pressure-volume loop for the normal ventricle showing a peak ventricular systolic pressure equal to aortic systolic pressure of 105 mm Hg, aortic valve opening at a diastolic pressure of 80 mm Hg, left ventricular end-systolic volume of 30 ml and end-diastolic volume of 100 ml, and a low, almost constant left ventricular diastolic pressure of 5 mm Hg. AC = aortic valve closure, AO = aortic valve opening, MC = mitral valve closure, MO = mitral valve opening. Phase 1, isovolumetric relaxation; Phase 2, ventricular filling; Phase 3, isovolumetric contraction; Phase 4, ventricular ejection. (Modified from J.M. Jackson, S.J. Thomas, and E. Lowenstein. Anesthetic management of patients with valvular heart disease. *Semin. Anesth.* 1:240, 1982. With permission.)

Pure valvular aortic stenosis is the most common, accounting for more than 75% of patients. In the past, the primary cause of valvular aortic stenosis was **rheumatic** valvular degeneration. However, rheumatic carditis is becoming less common as streptococcal infections are more frequently recognized and treated. So, more recently, calcific degeneration of a **congenitally bicuspid aortic valve** has become the most common etiology. A congenitally bicuspid aortic valve occurs in approximately 1–2% of the general population, making it one of the most common congenital malformations. **Senile degeneration** of normal aortic valves can also occur. Thirty percent of patients over 85 years of age are found to have significant degenerative changes of the aortic valve on autopsy. A characteristic finding of senile valve degeneration is progression of the calcification from the base of the valve toward the edge, as opposed to rheumatic degeneration, in which calcification spreads from the edge toward the base.

2. **Symptomatology.** Patients with rheumatic aortic stenosis may be asymptomatic for 40 years or more. Patients with congenitally bicuspid aortic valves may develop symptomatic aortic stenosis anywhere between the ages of 15 and 65, but calcification of the valve more often occurs after age 30 and usually in the seventh or eighth decade of life. The onset of any one of a triad of symptoms is an ominous sign and indicates a life expectancy of less than 5 years:

a. **Angina pectoris.** Angina is the initial symptom in 50–70% of patients with severe aortic stenosis. It develops owing to either the presence of concurrent coronary artery disease or, more commonly, to an increasing disparity between myocardial oxygen supply and demand in a hypertrophied left ventricle. Patients with aortic stenosis are at high risk for subendocardial ischemia and the development of ventricular dysrhythmias. Angina secondary to aortic stenosis alone most commonly occurs with exertion. Angina at rest commonly indicates associated coronary artery disease.

b. Syncope. Syncope is the first symptom in 15–30% of patients. Once syncope appears, the average life expectancy is 3–4 years.

c. Congestive heart failure. Symptoms such as dyspnea, orthopnea, and paroxysmal nocturnal dyspnea herald the onset of congestive heart failure, which can rapidly progress to edema, hepatomegaly, and jugular venous distention. Once signs of left ventricular failure occur, the average life expectancy is only 1–2 years.

All patients with aortic stenosis are at increased risk for sudden death. Only 18% of patients are alive 5 years after stenosis has progressed to the point of a peak systolic pressure gradient of greater than 50 mm Hg or an effective aortic valve orifice size of less than 0.7 cm^2.

B. Pathophysiology

1. Natural progression

a. Stage 1: Mild aortic stenosis—asymptomatic with physiologic compensation. The normal adult aortic valve area is 2.6–3.5 cm^2, representing a normal aortic valve index of 2 cm^2/m^2. As stenosis progresses, the maintenance of normal stroke volume is associated with an increasing systolic pressure gradient between the left ventricle and the aorta. The left ventricular systolic pressure increases to as much as 300 mm Hg, while the aortic systolic pressure and stroke volume remain relatively normal. This higher gradient leads to increased myocardial pressure work and results in a compensatory **concentric left ventricular hypertrophy** (increased muscle mass in the left ventricular wall without dilation of the ventricular chamber). The resultant increase in left ventricular end-diastolic pressure is not a sign of left ventricular systolic dysfunction or failure but rather an indication of the decreased left ventricular diastolic function or reduced compliance.

b. Stage 2: Moderate aortic stenosis—symptomatic impairment. As stenosis progresses toward the critical orifice size of 0.7–0.9 cm^2, (aortic valve index of 0.5 cm^2/m^2) **dilation** as well as hypertrophy of the left ventricle may occur, leading to increases in both left ventricular end-diastolic volume and pressure. When this occurs, a decrease in ejection fraction may be noted, indicating compromise of left ventricular contractility. Ventricular contractility decreases more rapidly in some patients than in others but eventually is reduced in all untreated patients.

The increased left ventricular end-diastolic volume and pressure lead to increased myocardial work and oxygen demand. In this situation two of the primary determinants of myocardial oxygen demand (tension developed by the myocardium and duration of systole) are increased. At the same time, myocardial oxygen supply is impeded owing to an elevated left ventricular end-diastolic pressure, causing a decrease in coronary perfusion pressure. Finally, the Venturi effect of the jet of blood flowing through the aortic valve and past the coronary arteries may actually lower pressure in the coronary ostia enough to reverse systolic coronary blood flow. These factors produce a heart particularly

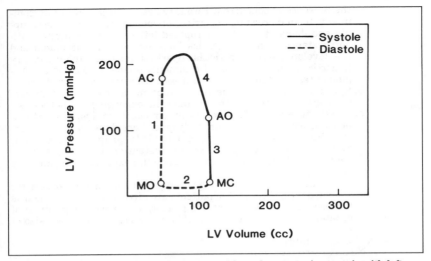

Fig. 12-2. Pressure-volume loop of a patient with moderate aortic stenosis with left ventricular compensation showing markedly elevated left ventricular systolic pressure, elevated end-systolic and end-diastolic volume, and increased diastolic pressure. AC = aortic valve closure, AO = aortic valve opening, MC = mitral valve closure, MO = mitral valve opening. Phase 1, isovolumetric relaxation; Phase 2, ventricular filling; Phase 3, isovolumetric contraction; Phase 4, ventricular ejection. (Modified from J.M. Jackson, S.J. Thomas, and E. Lowenstein. Anesthetic management of patients with valvular heart disease. *Semin. Anesth.* 1:241, 1982. With permission.)

at risk for ischemia and sudden death, even in the absence of concurrent atherosclerotic coronary disease.

The initial appearance of symptoms in patients with aortic stenosis is often associated with the development of atrial fibrillation. Normal patients depend on the atrial contraction for approximately 20% of the stroke volume. However, with the reduced ventricular compliance and increased left ventricular end-diastolic pressure (LVEDP) that is present in patients with aortic stenosis, passive ventricular filling is reduced, and the atrial contraction can supply as much as 40% of ventricular filling during diastole. Therefore, loss of sinus rhythm and atrial contribution to cardiac output can lead to rapid clinical deterioration.

c. **Stage 3: Critical aortic stenosis—terminal failure.** Continuation of the disease process with reduction of the aortic valve index to less than 0.5 cm²/m² leads to further decreases in ejection fraction and increases in LVEDP. Pressure builds up in the pulmonary venous circuit, leading to pulmonary edema when the left atrial pressure increases to more than 25–30 mm Hg. Normally, sudden death will intervene, but if the patient is able to survive, the increasing pulmonary arterial hypertension will eventually produce right ventricular failure.

2. **Pressure-volume relationship** (Fig. 12-2). As the pressure gradient across the aortic valve develops, stroke volume is preserved by an increase in left ventricular systolic pressure. During the early stages of left ventricular compensation, left ventricular end-diastolic pressure and volume are elevated, whereas the left ventricular end-systolic volume stays relatively normal. In the later stages of the

disease, compromise of left ventricular function can lead first to marked elevations of left ventricular end-diastolic pressure and end-diastolic volume and finally to elevation of left ventricular end-systolic volume and depression of stroke volume. Each of these changes, but especially elevated ventricular pressures, increase oxygen cost to an already compromised myocardium.

3. **Calculation of stenosis.** A determination of the aortic valve area is performed using the Gorlin modification of standard hydraulic formulas, as discussed in Chap. 1. The formula for calculating aortic valve area is summarized as follows:

Aortic valve area (cm²)

$$= \frac{\text{Cardiac output/(systolic ejection period} \times \text{HR)}}{1 \times 44.5 \times \sqrt{\text{Mean aortic pressure gradient}}}$$

where 1 = Aortic orifice constant

A simplified version of the Gorlin formula that is accurate enough to be clinically useful at normal heart rates is

$$\text{Aortic value area (cm}^2) = \frac{\text{Cardiac output (1/min)}}{\sqrt{\text{Mean pressure gradient}}}$$

This simplified version of the formula is valid only because the product of the heart rate, systolic ejection period, and the constant approximates unity.

There is a direct relationship between the aortic valve area and the flow across the aortic valve. A series of relationships can be derived between the rate of aortic valve blood flow and the mean systolic pressure gradient for any aortic valve area (Fig. 12-3). At a constant valve area, small changes in cardiac output can have major effects on the pressure gradient. Further, as valve area decreases, there is a corresponding decrease in flow across the aortic valve. Blood flow is not significantly impeded, however, until the aortic valve area falls below a critical level of 0.5–0.7 cm².

4. **Pressure wave disturbances**
   a. **Arterial pressure** (Fig. 12-4). The arterial pulse pressure is usually reduced to less than 50 mm Hg in severe aortic stenosis. The systolic pressure rise is delayed with a late peak and a prominent anacrotic notch. As stenosis increases in severity, the anacrotic notch occurs lower in the ascending arterial pressure trace. The dicrotic notch is relatively small or absent.
   b. **Pulmonary arterial wedge pressure.** Due to the elevated left ventricular end-diastolic pressure, which stretches the mitral valve annulus, a prominent V wave can be observed, but with progression of the disease and the development of left atrial hypertrophy, a prominent A wave becomes the dominant feature.

C. **Goals of perioperative management**
1. **Hemodynamic profile**

	LV pre-load	Heart rate	Contrac-tile state	Systemic vascular resistance	Pulmo-nary vascular resistance
Aortic stenosis	↑	↓ (sinus)	Maintain constant	↑	Maintain Constant

   a. **Left ventricular preload.** Due to the decreased left ventricular compliance as well as the increased left ventricular end-diastolic

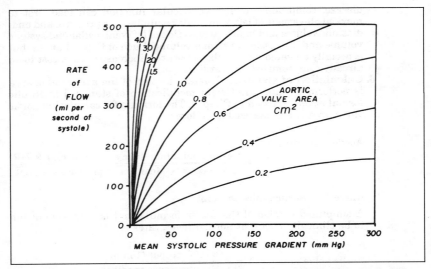

Fig. 12-3. Comparison between the rate of blood flow across the aortic valve and the mean systolic pressure gradient across the aortic valve in individuals with different aortic valve areas, as determined by the Gorlin formula. Below the critical aortic valve area of 0.5 cm², a major increase in the mean systolic pressure gradient across the valve produces a minimal increase in blood flow. (From R.C. Schlant. Altered Cardiovascular Function of Rheumatic Heart Disease and Other Acquired Valvular Disease. In J. W. Hurst, R. B. Logue, R. C. Schlant, et al. [eds.], *The Heart* [4th ed.]. New York: McGraw-Hill, 1978. P. 968. With permission.)

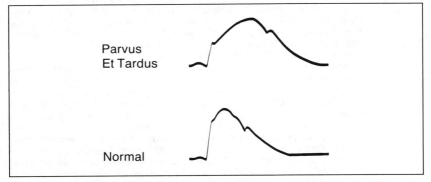

Fig. 12-4. A carotid arterial pressure trace frequently observed in patients with aortic stenosis is parvus et tardus. There is a delay in the upstroke and late peak of the pressure wave trace, as well as a prominent anacrotic notch. The dicrotic notch is relatively small. (Modified from J. W. Hurst, and R. C. Schlant. Examination of the Arteries and Their Pulsation. In J. W. Hurst, R. B. Logue, R. C. Schlant, et al. [eds.], *The Heart* [4th ed.]. New York: McGraw-Hill, 1978. P. 188. With permission.)

volume and pressure, preload augmentation is necessary to maintain a normal stroke volume, and the use of nitroglycerin may dangerously reduce cardiac output.

   b. **Heart rate.** Extremes of heart rate are not tolerated well. A high heart rate can lead to decreased coronary perfusion. A low heart rate can limit cardiac output in these patients with a fixed stroke volume. If a choice must be made, however, low heart rates (50–70 bpm) are preferred to rapid heart rates (over 90 bpm) to allow time for systolic ejection across a stenotic aortic valve. Supraventricular tachyarrhythmias should be aggressively treated because both the tachycardia and the loss of effective atrial contraction can lead to major physiologic deterioration. Ventricular irritability should also be treated aggressively, because cardioversion is frequently unsuccessful for patients whose heart rhythm deteriorates into ventricular fibrillation.

    c. **Contractility.** Stroke volume is maintained through preservation of a heightened contractile state. Beta blockade is not well tolerated and can lead to an increase in left ventricular end-diastolic volume and a decrease in cardiac output significant enough to induce clinical deterioration.

    d. **Systemic vascular resistance.** Most of the afterload to left ventricular ejection is caused by the stenotic aortic valve itself and thus is fixed. Systemic blood pressure reduction does little to decrease left ventricular afterload. However, the hypertrophied myocardium of the patient with aortic stenosis is at great risk for development of subendocardial ischemia. Coronary perfusion is dependent on maintenance of an adequate systemic diastolic perfusion pressure. Although blood pressure augmentation using alpha agents has little effect on total forward flow (the primary impedance to ventricular ejection occurs at the aortic valve), it can prevent falls in blood pressure which may be devastating for myocardial perfusion and lead to sudden death.

    e. **Pulmonary vascular resistance.** Except for end-stage aortic stenosis, pulmonary artery pressures remain relatively normal. Special intervention for stabilizing pulmonary vascular resistance is unnecessary.

2. Anesthetic techniques

    a. Light **premedication** is necessary to provide a calm patient without tachycardia. However, the use of a heavy premedicant with agents that markedly reduce either preload or afterload should be avoided. Either a combination of morphine 0.05–0.10 mg/kg IM and scopolamine 0.2–0.3 mg IM or lorazepam 1–2 mg PO alone can be used with little adverse hemodynamic effect.

    b. Thermodilution cardiac output **pulmonary artery catheters** are helpful in evaluating the cardiac output of patients prior to repair of the aortic valve. The pulmonary capillary wedge pressure, however, may underestimate the true end-diastolic pressure of a noncompliant left ventricle. There is also a small dysrhythmogenic risk during transventricular passage of a pulmonary artery catheter. If a patient does show dysrhythmias during advancement of a pulmonary artery catheter, the catheter tip should be left in a central venous position until repair of the aortic valve is completed.

    c. Any **anesthetic agent** leading to myocardial depression, blood pressure reduction, tachycardia, or other dysrhythmia should be used with caution. Each of these physiologic changes can lead to sudden and rapid deterioration. A narcotic-based anesthetic is usually chosen for this reason.

    d. During the induction and maintenance of anesthesia, a potent **alpha-adrenergic agent** such as phenylephrine should be handy for early and aggressive treatment of reductions in systemic systolic or diastolic pressures.

e. If the patient develops signs or symptoms of ischemia, **nitroglycerin** should be used with caution because its effect on preload or arterial pressure may actually make things worse.

f. Supraventricular **dysrhythmias** should be treated aggressively with **synchronized** DC shock. Ventricular ectopy should also be aggressively treated because patients whose rhythm deteriorates into ventricular fibrillation often cannot be successfully resuscitated.

g. **An experienced cardiac surgeon should be present, and perfusionists should be prepared before induction of anesthesia should rapid cardiovascular deterioration necessitate emergency use of cardiopulmonary bypass.**

h. In the presence of myocardial hypertrophy, adequate myocardial preservation with cold cardioplegic solution during bypass is essential to avoid myocardial "contracture" or "stone heart" caused by myocardial ischemia.

i. In the absence of preoperative ventricular dysfunction and associated coronary disease, inotropic support is often not required after cardiopulmonary bypass because valve replacement decreases ventricular afterload.

3. **Surgical intervention.** Due to the high risk of sudden death, symptomatic patients should all undergo surgery. Asymptomatic patients with a transvalvular gradient of greater than 50 mm Hg or a valve index of less than 0.5 cm^2/m^2 should have surgery. The initial surgical procedure is frequently a valvular commissurotomy performed under direct vision, which frequently leads to some residual aortic stenosis and aortic regurgitation. Eventually most patients require a prosthetic valve replacement. Surgical intervention should not be denied patients no matter how severe the symptomatology because irreparable left ventricular failure occurs only at the very end of the disease process. After aortic valve replacement, hospital mortality is 3–4%. Of the patients leaving the hospital 85% may expect to survive for at least 5 years.

4. **Postoperative care.** Following aortic commissurotomy or valve replacement, pulmonary capillary wedge and left ventricular end-diastolic pressures immediately decrease and stroke volume rises. Myocardial function improves rapidly, although the hypertrophied ventricle may still require an elevated preload to function normally. Over a period of several months, left ventricular hypertrophy regresses. It must be remembered that if a prosthetic valve has been used, a residual gradient of 7–19 mm Hg may be present, and if a commissurotomy has been performed, concurrent aortic regurgitation may also be present. Most patients do very well following surgery for aortic stenosis provided intraoperative myocardial preservation is adequate.

D. **Idiopathic hypertrophic subaortic stenosis (hypertrophic cardiomyopathy).** This disease process represents a **dynamic stenosis** of the aortic outflow tract, unlike valvular aortic stenosis, which is fixed. The response of the myocardium to this disease process is similar to that seen in valvular aortic stenosis; however, the increased muscle mass in the subaortic region eventually leads to total obstruction of left ventricular outflow. In this special situation, beta blockade or halothane anesthesia may have a beneficial effect on hemodynamic stability. These patients also benefit from preload augmentation for maintaining left ventricular volume, from afterload augmentation for increasing diastolic perfusion through the hypertrophied muscle mass, and from slow heart rates.

III. **Aortic regurgitation**

A. Natural history

1. **Etiology.** Aortic regurgitation may be caused by a wide variety of etiologic agents. **Rheumatic fever** and **syphilitic aortitis** were the primary causes in the past; however, with early identification and successful treatment of these diseases, these causes for aortic regurgitation are now seen infrequently. Increasingly, **bacterial endocarditis,** trauma, aortic dissections, and a variety of congenital diseases leading to abnormal collagen formation are becoming the primary etiologies.

2. **Symptomatology.** Patients with **chronic aortic regurgitation** may be asymptomatic for up to 20 years. The 10-year mortality for asymptomatic aortic regurgitation varies between 5% and 15%. However, once symptoms develop, patients progressively deteriorate and have an expected survival rate of 5 years. Early symptoms include dyspnea, fatigue, and palpitations. Angina pectoris is normally a late symptom and is an ominous sign. Patients with **acute aortic regurgitation,** on the other hand, may deteriorate rapidly, and the prognosis is guarded.

B. Pathophysiology

1. **Natural progression**

   a. **Acute aortic regurgitation.** The sudden occurrence of acute aortic regurgitation places a major volume load on the left ventricle. An immediate compensatory mechanism for the maintenance of adequate forward flow is increased sympathetic tone, producing tachycardia and an increased contractile state. Fluid retention leads to an augmentation of preload. The combination of increased left ventricular end-diastolic volume and increased total stroke volume and heart rate may not be sufficient to maintain a normal cardiac output. Rapid deterioration of left ventricular function can occur, necessitating emergency surgical intervention.

   b. **Chronic aortic regurgitation**

      (1) **Stage 1: Mild aortic regurgitation—asymptomatic with physiologic compensation.** The onset of aortic regurgitation leads to left ventricular systolic and diastolic volume overload. The increased volume load leads to eccentric hypertrophy of the left ventricle, with increases in both the thickness of the left ventricular wall and the size of the ventricular cavity. Because the left ventricular end-diastolic volume increases slowly, the left ventricular end-diastolic pressure remains relatively normal. Because volume work is less expensive metabolically than pressure work, no major increase in myocardial oxygen demand occurs in spite of an increased ejection fraction. Forward flow is aided by the presence of chronic peripheral vasodilation, which occurs along with a large stroke volume in patients with mild aortic regurgitation. Minimal symptomatology occurs as long as the regurgitant fraction remains less than 40% of the stroke volume.

      (2) **Stage 2: Moderate aortic regurgitation—symptomatic impairment.** As the amount of aortic regurgitation progresses to more than 60% of stroke volume, continued left ventricular dilation and hypertrophy occur, finally leading to irreversible left ventricular myocardial tissue damage. An early sign of these changes is an increase in left ventricular end-diastolic pressure, indicating left ventricular dysfunction. An LVEDP greater than 20 mm Hg suggests left ventricular dysfunction. Left ventricular dysfunction is followed by an increase in pulmonary arterial pressure with symptoms of dyspnea and congestive heart failure.

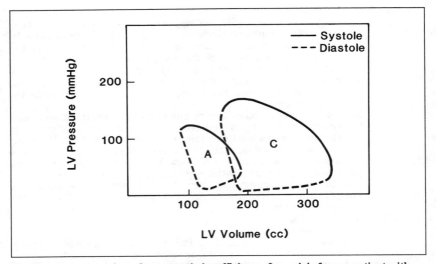

Fig. 12-5. Pressure-volume loops, aortic insufficiency. Loop A is from a patient with acute aortic insufficiency, showing moderately elevated left ventricular systolic and diastolic volumes as well as an increase in ventricular volume during ventricular relaxation due to regurgitant flow, and a high left ventricular end-diastolic pressure. Loop C represents a patient with chronic aortic insufficiency, showing markedly increased systolic and diastolic volumes but lower end-diastolic pressure. (Modified from J.M. Jackson, S.J. Thomas, and E. Lowenstein. Anesthetic management of patients with valvular heart disease. *Semin. Anesth.* 1:247, 1982. With permission.)

    (3) Stage 3: Severe aortic regurgitation—terminal failure. Following the onset of symptomatology, left ventricular dysfunction continues to progress and eventually becomes irreversible. Symptomatology is rapidly progressive, and surgical intervention at this point is not always successful. Angina pectoris may occur owing to the reduction in diastolic aortic pressure with decreased diastolic coronary perfusion, ventricular dilation with increased wall tension, and the presence of a hypertrophied left ventricle. As a compensatory mechanism for the poor cardiac output and poor coronary perfusion, sympathetic constriction of the periphery occurs, leading to further decreases in cardiac output.

  2. Pressure-volume relationship (Fig. 12-5). In acute aortic regurgitation, a sudden volume load is placed on a normally compliant left ventricle. This leads to increases in both left ventricular end-diastolic and end-systolic volumes. Because the left ventricle does not have time to compensate through eccentric hypertrophy, the result is a sudden increase in left ventricular end-diastolic pressure. The compensatory mechanism of sympathetic stimulation may not be sufficient to maintain an adequate stroke volume.

    In chronic aortic regurgitation eccentric hypertrophy occurs, leading to massive increases in left ventricular end-diastolic and end-systolic volumes. An increase in left ventricular compliance over time allows the left ventricular end-diastolic pressure to remain only mildly elevated. With this compensatory mechanism the stroke volume can be maintained initially.

  3. Determination of severity

a. Qualitative estimate. The amount of aortic regurgitation is usually estimated based on angiocardiographic clearance of injected dye into the aortic root.

+ 1   Slight reflux of dye into the left ventricle during left ventricular diastole with opacification limited to the left ventricular outflow tract; dye is completely cleared with next systole.

+ 2   Moderate reflux of dye into the left ventricle during diastole; dye is not completely cleared with the next systole.

+ 3   Complete opacification of the left ventricle for several systoles.

+ 4   Complete opacification of the left ventricle by the end of the first diastole with maintenance of opacification for several systoles. Density of the dye in the left ventricle is greater than that in the aorta.

b. Calculation of regurgitant fraction (see Chap. 1). A more quantitative estimate of the severity of aortic regurgitation may be obtained by comparing forward flow (thermodilution cardiac output) with total volume of blood ejected by the left ventricle (angiographic cardiac output). The regurgitant fraction, or fraction of each stroke volume flowing back into the left ventricle, can be calculated using the equation:

$$\text{Regurgitant fraction} = \frac{[(EDV - ESV) \times HR] - CO}{(EDV - ESV) \times HR}$$

where EDV = end-diastolic volume
ESV = end-systolic volume
HR = heart rate
CO = thermodilution cardiac output (forward flow)

4. Pressure wave disturbances

a. Arterial pressure. Patients with aortic regurgitation show a wide pulse pressure with a rapid rate of rise, a high systolic peak, and the presence of a low diastolic pressure. The pulse pressure may be as great as 80–100 mm Hg. The rapid upstroke is due to the large stroke volume, and the rapid downstroke is due to the rapid loss of blood volume from the aorta back into the ventricle and into the dilated peripheral vessels. The occurrence of a double peaked or bisferiens pulse trace is not unusual owing to the occurrence of a "tidal" or backwave (Fig. 12-6).

b. Pulmonary capillary wedge trace. Normally, stretching of the mitral valve annulus leads to functional mitral regurgitation, a prominent V wave, and a rapid Y descent. The V wave is more prominent in acute regurgitation and with the onset of left ventricular failure.

C. Goals of perioperative management

1. Hemodynamic management

	LV pre-load	Heart rate	Contrac-tile state	Systemic vascular resistance	Pulmo-nary vascular resistance
Aortic regurgitation	↑	↑	Maintain	↓	Maintain

a. Left ventricular preload. Due to the increased left ventricular volumes, maintenance of forward flow is dependent on preload augmentation. Pharmacologic intervention that produces venous

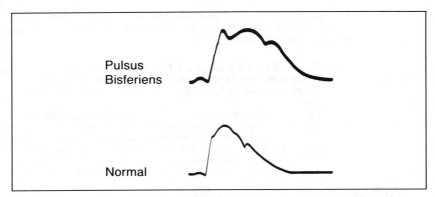

Fig. 12-6. A carotid arterial pressure trace frequently seen in patients with aortic regurgitation is pulsus bisferiens. The pulse pressure is wide, and the secondary peak results from a back pressure or "tidal" wave effect. (Modified from J.W. Hurst, and R.C. Schlant. Examination of the Arteries and Their Pulsations. In J. W. Hurst, R. B. Logue, R. C. Schlant, et al. [eds.], *The Heart* [4th ed.]. New York: McGraw-Hill, 1978. P. 189. With permission.)

dilation may significantly impair cardiac output in these patients by reducing preload.

b. **Heart rate.** Patients with aortic regurgitation show a significant increase in forward cardiac output with an increase in heart rate. The decreased time spent in diastole during tachycardia leads to a decreased regurgitant fraction. Actual improvement in subendocardial blood flow is observed with tachycardia owing to a higher systemic diastolic pressure and a lower left ventricular end-diastolic pressure. This explains why a patient who is symptomatic at rest may show an improvement in symptomatology with exercise. On other hand, bradycardia leads to a prolongation of the diastolic period and is associated with increased regurgitation per stroke volume. A heart rate of 90 bpm seems to be optimal, improving cardiac output while not inducing ischemia. Maintenance of sinus rhythm is not as important as it is in patients with stenotic lesions, and the presence of atrial fibrillation is common.

c. **Contractility.** Left ventricular contractility must be maintained. In patients with impaired left ventricular function, use of pure beta agents can increase stroke volume through a combination of peripheral dilatation and increased contractility.

d. **Systemic vascular resistance.** Normally, patients with chronic aortic insufficiency compensate initially for the limitation in cardiac output by dilatation of the peripheral arterioles. The forward cardiac index can be further improved with afterload reduction. Increases in afterload result in decreased stroke work and can significantly increase the left ventricular end-diastolic pressure. The patient in end-stage aortic regurgitation with left ventricular impairment benefits most from therapy with afterload-reducing agents.

e. **Pulmonary vascular resistance.** Pulmonary vascular pressure remains relatively normal except in patients in end-stage aortic regurgitation associated with severe left ventricular dysfunction.

2. **Anesthetic technique**
   a. **Premedication** that dilates the capacitance vessels should be avoided. A light premedication is recommended to maintain myo-

cardial contractility and heart rate because tachycardia can actually be helpful for these patients. Increases in systemic vascular resistance that may arise from anxiety, however, may be detrimental.

  b. The choice of agent for **induction** and maintenance of anesthesia should be directed at preserving the patient's preload, maintaining the peripheral arterial dilatation, improving normal contractility, and keeping the heart rate around 90 bpm. Use of isoflurane and pancuronium in combination with fluid augmentation is acceptable except in patients with end-stage disease with reduced ventricular function, in whom a synthetic narcotic in combination with pancuronium is better tolerated.

  c. In patients with acute aortic regurgitation associated with poor ventricular compliance, left ventricular pressure may increase fast enough to close the mitral valve before end diastole. In this situation the continued regurgitation of blood raises LVEDP above left atrial pressure, and the **pulmonary capillary wedge pressure** can significantly underestimate the true LVEDP.

  d. Intraaortic balloon pump is contraindicated in the presence of aortic regurgitation because augmentation of the diastolic pressure will increase the amount of regurgitation flow.

3. Surgical intervention. Surgical repair of aortic regurgitation can be performed with an annuloplasty or valvular plication but is most frequently provided through the use of valvular replacement with a prosthetic valve. Surgery is indicated if the patient is symptomatic, or preferably as soon as echocardiographic evidence of left ventricular dysfunction exists in the asymptomatic patient. It is important to intervene surgically before severe left ventricular dysfunction develops.

4. Postoperative care. Immediately following aortic valve replacement, the left ventricular end-diastolic pressure and volume decrease. However, the left ventricular hypertrophy and dilatation persist. In the immediate postbypass period, preload augmentation must be continued to maintain filling of the dilated left ventricle. In the early postoperative period a decline in left ventricular function may necessitate inotropic or intraaortic balloon pump support. If surgical intervention is delayed until major left ventricular dysfunction has occurred, the prognosis for long-term survival is not good. The 5-year survival rate for patients whose hearts do not return to a relatively normal size within 6 months following surgical repair is only 43%. If surgery is performed early enough, the heart will return to relatively normal dimensions, and a long-term survival rate of 85% after 6 years can be expected.

IV. Mitral stenosis

A. Natural history

1. Etiology. Mitral stenosis is almost always secondary to rheumatic heart disease, which leads to scarring and fibrosis of the free edges of the mitral valve leaflets. Fusion of the valvular commissures, progressive scarring of the leaflets, and contraction of the chorda tendineae lead to the development of a funnel-shaped mitral apparatus that can become secondarily calcified.

2. Symptomatology. Patients are normally asymptomatic for 20 years or more following an acute episode of rheumatic fever. However, as stenosis develops, symptoms appear, associated at first with exercise or high cardiac output states. Twenty percent of patients who are diagnosed with symptomatic mitral stenosis die within 1 year, and 50% die within 10 years following diagnosis, without surgical intervention. The natural history is a slow progressive downhill course with repeated episodes of **pulmonary edema, dyspnea, paroxys-mal nocturnal dyspnea, fatigue, chest pains, palpitations,** and **hemoptysis** as well as hoarseness due to compression of the left recurrent laryngeal nerve by a distended left atrium and enlarged pulmonary artery. Symptoms often become apparent with the onset of atrial fibrillation, and patients in atrial fibrillation are at an increased risk of forming left atrial thrombi and subsequent cerebral or systemic emboli. Medical management can be successful if it is initiated early in these patients' courses. Fortunately, due to the decreased incidence of rheumatic heart disease, the number of patients with mitral stenosis is decreasing.

B. Pathophysiology

  1. Natural progression

  a. Stage 1: Mild mitral stenosis—asymptomatic with physiologic compensation. Following an episode of rheumatic fever, stenosis slowly occurs over a 20–30 year period. The normal mitral valve area is 4–6 cm² (mitral valve index 4.0–4.5 cm²/m²). The patient can remain essentially symptom free during the period of slow progression of stenosis until a valve area of 1.5–2.5 cm² (or valve index of 1.0–2.0 cm²/m²) is reached. At this point moderate exercise may induce dyspnea. Exercise testing in the cardiac catheterization laboratory, by detecting increased filling pressures with exercise, can identify this stage of the disease. Further progression of mitral stenosis leads to increases in left atrial pressure and volume that are reflected back into the pulmonary circuit.

  b. Stage 2: Moderate mitral stenosis—symptomatic impairment. Between a valve area of 1.0 and 1.5 cm² increasing symptomatology appears with only mild to moderate exertion. Severe congestive failure can be induced either by the onset of atrial fibrillation or a variety of disease processes leading to high cardiac output states, such as thyrotoxicosis, pregnancy, anemia, or fever. In all these conditions the left atrial and pulmonary artery pressures suddenly rise as a result of the increased cardiac demand. The increase in pulmonary vascular resistance in response to a high left atrial pressure can eventually lead to right ventricular failure. Pulmonary arterial constriction, pulmonary intimal hyperplasia, and pulmonary medial hypertrophy eventually result in a picture of chronic pulmonary arterial hypertension associated with restrictive lung disease. Because atrial contraction contributes 30% of left ventricular filling in mitral stenosis, the onset of atrial fibrillation can lead to a significant impairment in cardiac output.

  c. Stage 3: Critical mitral stenosis—terminal failure. With a valve area below 1.0 cm² a patient is considered to have critical mitral stenosis, and symptoms are present even at rest. Not only are left atrial pressures on the border of producing congestive failure, but cardiac output may also be reduced. Chronic pulmonary hypertension eventually leads to right ventricular dilatation. The dilated right ventricle can cause a leftward shift of the intraventricular septum, thereby limiting the already reduced left ventricular size and further impairing left ventricular ejection. With further right ventricular dilatation tricuspid regurgitation results, leading to signs of peripheral congestion. A mitral valve area of 0.3–0.4 cm² is the smallest area compatible with life.

  2. Pressure-volume relationship (Fig. 12-7). Due to the restriction of flow from the left atrium to the ventricle, patients with significant mitral stenosis have a reduced left ventricular end-diastolic volume and pressure. Left ventricular end-systolic volume is also reduced,

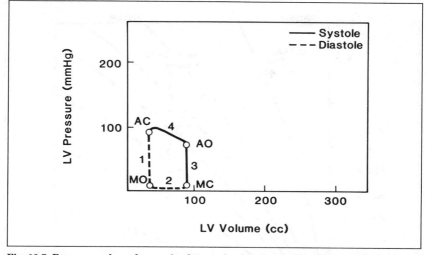

Fig. 12-7. Pressure-volume loop, mitral stenosis, showing decreased left ventricular systolic and diastolic volumes, reduced stroke volume, and decreased systolic and end-diastolic pressures. AC = aortic valve closure, AO = aortic valve opening, MC = mitral valve closure, MO = mitral valve opening. Phase 1, isovolumetric relaxation; Phase 2, ventricular filling; Phase 3, isovolumetric contraction; Phase 4, ventricular ejection. (Modified from J.M. Jackson, S.J. Thomas, and E. Lowenstein. Anesthetic management of patients with valvular heart disease. *Semin. Anesth.* 1:244, 1982. With permission.)

and stroke volume is reduced. The actual left ventricular performance is relatively normal. The limitation of stroke volume in these patients is entirely due to inadequate filling of the left ventricle.
3. **Calculation of mitral valve area.** Quantitative evaluation of mitral stenosis based only on the diastolic pressure gradient across the mitral valve is inaccurate, as with the aortic valve, because it does not take into consideration the important factor, **flow.** The Gorlin formula for the determination of the mitral valve area is:

$$\text{Mitral valve area (cm}^2\text{)} = \frac{\text{Mitral valve flow (ml/sec)}}{0.85 \times 44.5 \times \sqrt{\text{mean mitral gradient}}}$$

where 0.85   = mitral orifice constant

$$\frac{\text{mitral valve}}{\text{flow (ml/sec)}} = \frac{\text{Cardiac output (ml/min)}}{\text{diastolic filling period} \atop \text{(sec/beat)} \times \text{HR (beat/min)}}$$

Because tachycardia shortens the diastolic filling period, it compromises left ventricular filling and leads to clinical deterioration. Comparisons of the rate of blood flow and the mean diastolic pressure can be graphically represented (Fig. 12-8). It is apparent that, when the mitral valve area is 1.0 cm² or less, little additional flow can be obtained by increasing the pressure gradient across the valve.
4. **Pressure wave disturbances**
   a. **Pulmonary capillary wedge pressure.** Mitral stenosis produces a large A wave, and, if it is associated with an element of mitral

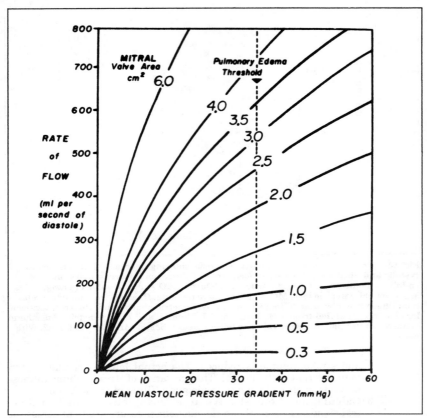

Fig. 12-8. Comparison between the rate of blood flow across the mitral valve and the mean diastolic pressure gradient across the mitral valve in individuals with different mitral valve areas, as determined by the Gorlin formula. Below a critical mitral valve area of 1.0 cm^2, a major increase in the mean diastolic pressure gradient across the mitral valve produces a minimal increase in blood flow. The point at which pulmonary capillary pressure exceeds plasma oncotic pressure leading to the transudation of fluid and the development of pulmonary edema is indicated on the graph. (From R.C. Schlant. Altered Cardiovascular Function of Rheumatic Heart Disease and Other Acquired Valvular Disease. In J. W. Hurst, R. B. Logue, R. C. Schlant, et al. [eds.], *The Heart* [4th ed.]. New York: McGraw-Hill, 1978. P. 972. With permission.)

regurgitation, a prominent V wave. In the presence of atrial fibrillation the A wave is absent. In addition, with increased impairment of left atrial contractility from severe mitral obstruction, the A wave may actually be small.

C. Goals of perioperative management

1. Hemodynamic management

Mitral stenosis	LV pre-load	Heart rate	Contrac-tile state	Systemic vascular resistance	Pulmo-nary vascular resistance
	↑	↓	Maintain	Maintain	↓

a. **Left ventricular preload.** Forward flow across the stenotic mitral valve is dependent on adequate preload. On the other hand, patients with mitral stenosis already have elevated left atrial pressures, so that overly aggressive use of fluids can easily send a patient who is in borderline congestive failure into florid pulmonary edema.

b. **Heart rate.** Blood flow across the mitral valve occurs during ventricular diastole. Tachycardia shortens the diastolic period so that at increased heart rates the flow across the stenotic mitral valve must be increased to maintain the same level of cardiac output. Based on Poiseuille's law, the atrial-ventricular pressure gradient is proportional to the fourth power of the instantaneous flow across the mitral valve, so any increase in instantaneous flow requires a large increase in left atrial pressure. At the same time, excessive bradycardia can be dangerous because stroke volume is relatively fixed.

   Atrial contraction in patients with mitral stenosis contributes approximately 30% of the left ventricular stroke volume. If atrioventricular pacing is initiated in these patients, a long PR interval of 0.15–0.20 msec is optimal to allow blood adequate time, after atrial contraction, to cross the stenotic mitral valve. Decreases in the PR interval will drop diastolic flow and result in a reduced cardiac output. In patients with atrial fibrillation, the contribution of atrial contraction is lost.

c. **Contractility.** Adequate forward flow is dependent on adequate right and left ventricular contractility. Chronic underfilling, however, leads to a cardiomyopathy with depressed ventricular contractility even in the face of restored filling. In end-stage mitral stenosis, depression of left ventricular contractility may lead to severe congestive heart failure. Depression of right ventricular contractility limits left atrial filling and eventually cardiac output. Therefore, many patients will require inotropic support before and especially after cardiopulmonary bypass.

d. **Systemic vascular resistance.** To maintain blood pressure in the presence of a limited cardiac output, patients with mitral stenosis normally develop an increased systemic vascular resistance. Afterload reduction is not helpful in improving forward flow because the limiting factor for cardiac output is the stenotic mitral valve. It is recommended that the afterload be kept in the normal range for that patient.

e. **Pulmonary vascular resistance.** These patients frequently have **elevated pulmonary vascular resistances** and are prone to exaggerated pulmonary vasoconstriction in the presence of hypoxia. Particular attention should be taken to avoid any increases in pulmonary artery pressure due to injudicious use of anesthetic agents, particularly nitrous oxide, or to inadvertent acidosis, hypercarbia, or hypoxemia.

2. **Anesthetic technique**

   a. **Premedication** should be light to avoid either an acute decrease in preload or the possibility of sedation with resultant hypoxemia and hypercarbia. In addition, use of scopolamine rather than atropine should be considered to avoid tachycardia.

   b. Continue **digitalis** for heart rate control right up to the morning of surgery.
   c. Avoid pharmacologic agents or conditions that produce tachycardia, increased pulmonary vascular resistance, decreased preload, or decreased contractility. In particular **tachycardia**, whether it is due to a sinus mechanism or atrial fibrillation, must be treated aggressively. An attempt should be made to maintain a sinus rhythm at all times with immediate use of cardioversion if new atrial fibrillation should occur. A narcotic anesthetic technique with high inspired oxygen concentration is usually chosen for these patients.
   d. **Pulmonary artery catheters** are almost always indicated for perioperative management. However, the catheters must often be inserted further than usual because of the dilated pulmonary arteries, and special care should be taken in the placement of the catheters due to the increased risk of pulmonary artery rupture. Further, the pressure data obtained from the catheters must be carefully interpreted. The pulmonary artery diastolic pressure often is not an accurate estimate of left atrial pressure because of significant pulmonary hypertension. Even a pulmonary capillary wedge pressure, which does reflect left atrial pressure, overestimates left ventricular filling pressure because of the stenotic mitral valve.
3. Surgical intervention. Surgical intervention should occur prior to the development of severe symptomatology because irreversible ventricular dysfunction may result if surgery is delayed too long. On the other hand, surgery is not recommended for the asymptomatic patient unless there is evidence of systemic embolization or progressive pulmonary hypertension. Mitral commissurotomy is the operation of choice, if the valve is not significantly calcified or severely fibrotic. Commissurotomy does not totally relieve the stenosis but rather makes it less severe. In addition, restenosis of the mitral valve will occur in as many as 30% of patients within 5 years after commissurotomy and in 60% after 9 years. Nevertheless, during this time the patient does not require anticoagulation and is at risk for less morbidity than with an indwelling prosthetic valve. If the valve is not amenable to commissurotomy, mitral valve replacement should be performed. After isolated mitral valve replacement, 95% of patients survive to leave the hospital, and, of these hospital survivors, 80% survive 5 years. More recently, a balloon-dilating technique used at catheterization can delay the necessity for open heart surgery by effectively relieving the mitral obstruction.
4. Postoperative care. Successful surgical intervention leads to a drop in pulmonary vascular resistance, pulmonary arterial pressure, and left atrial pressure while increasing cardiac output by the first postoperative day. However, immediately following bypass, even patients with seemingly normal preoperative left ventricular function may have major depression of myocardial contractility owing to their underlying cardiomyopathy combined with ischemic arrest. These patients frequently require inotropic support.
   Pulmonary vascular resistance in most patients will continue to decrease with time following surgery. Failure of the pulmonary artery pressure to decrease is usually indicative of irreversible pulmonary hypertension and probably irreversible left ventricular dysfunction. This places the patient in a prognostically poor group.
   Preload augmentation as well as afterload reduction should be undertaken in the immediate postbypass period to improve forward blood flow. Patients previously in chronic atrial fibrillation

may revert to a sinus rhythm following bypass, and overdrive atrial pacing at a rate of 110 bpm should be provided to maintain a sinus mechanism for as long as possible. It must be remembered that following prosthetic valve placement a residual 4–7 mm Hg gradient across the mitral valve will still be present.

One catastrophic complication that can occur within the first few days following valve replacement is atrioventricular disruption. One method suggested to help avoid this complication is to reduce LVEDP to as low a level as possible while maintaining adequate cardiac output. Atrioventricular disruption is a particular risk for the elderly patient with a relatively noncompliant left ventricle who experiences increased diastolic tension on the left ventricular wall following surgery. Thus, inotropes in the postbypass period can serve two functions by (1) increasing contractility, and (2) reducing left ventricular size and wall tension.

V. Mitral regurgitation
A. Natural history
1. **Etiology—chronic mitral regurgitation. Rheumatic** disease is an increasingly uncommon cause of mitral regurgitation. When rheumatic mitral regurgitation does occur, it is rarely pure. Usually it exists in combination with mitral stenosis. Rheumatic mitral regurgitation is a slow indolent process with an asymptomatic period that lasts 20–40 years. There is a gradual onset of fatigue and increasing dyspnea. Though mitral regurgitation can be tolerated for many years without ill effect, the onset of significant symptomatology (fatigue, dyspnea, or orthopnea) usually heralds a relatively rapid downhill course with death occurring within 5 years. A sequela such as bacterial endocarditis, atrial fibrillation, reactive pulmonary hypertension, or systemic embolization leads to rapid clinical deterioration. **Atrial fibrillation** occurs in about 75% of cases. Survival rates are better in patients when surgery is performed prior to the development of irreversible left ventricular dysfunction.

2. **Etiology—acute mitral regurgitation. Nonrheumatic** mitral regurgitation is being seen more frequently, especially mitral regurgitation on the basis of **papillary muscle dysfunction** due to myocardial ischemia. Papillary muscle dysfunction occurs in approximately 40% of patients who sustain a posterior septal myocardial infarction and in 20% of patients with an anterior septal infarction. **Bacterial endocarditis** is another frequent cause of nonrheumatic mitral regurgitation. Therefore, the spectrum of mitral regurgitation varies from acute forms, in which rapid deterioration of myocardial function can occur, to chronic forms that have slow indolent courses.

B. Pathophysiology
1. **Natural progression**
   a. **Acute.** Sudden development of mitral regurgitation leads to marked left atrial volume overload. Owing to the normal compliance of the left atrium the sudden volume overload leads to significant increases in left atrial pressure that are passed on to the pulmonary circuit. As immediate compensation for a decreased cardiac output, sympathetic stimulation increases contractility and produces tachycardia. In addition, the left ventricle functions on a higher portion of the Frank-Starling curve owing to increased left ventricular volumes. The acute increases in left atrial and pulmonary artery pressures can lead to pulmonary congestion and edema. Of concern, the compensatory sympathetic stimulation can lead to increased myocardial oxygen consumption in myocardium already rendered ischemic by increased LVEDP and decreased

subendocardial blood flow, and to peripheral constriction, further compromising systemic blood flow.

b. Chronic

(1) Stage 1: Mild mitral regurgitation—asymptomatic with physiologic compensation. During the slow development of chronic mitral regurgitation, eccentric hypertrophy of the left ventricle occurs with the heart shifting eccentrically into the left side of the chest. Both left ventricular dilatation and hypertrophy occur. The dilatation of the left ventricle allows the preservation of a relatively normal left ventricular end-diastolic pressure in spite of a markedly increased end-diastolic volume. The forward cardiac output is preserved by an overall increase in total left ventricular stroke volume (combined forward stroke volume and regurgitant stroke volume). In addition, the left atrium enlarges and becomes distensible. A large distensible left atrium can maintain near normal left atrial pressures in spite of large regurgitant volumes, helping to protect the pulmonary vascular bed. Most of these patients eventually develop atrial fibrillation.

(2) Stage 2: Moderate mitral regurgitation—symptomatic impairment. Left ventricular dilatation and hypertrophy continue to compensate for increasing regurgitation until eventually the forward stroke volume is compromised. In addition, continued left atrial dilatation may lead to further increases in regurgitation owing to stretching of the mitral annulus. At this point, the symptoms of forward heart failure, including increased fatigability and generalized weakness, may intervene. Once the regurgitant fraction is greater than 60%, congestive heart failure occurs. Left ventricular ejection fraction is usually elevated in patients with mitral regurgitation because of the ease of ejecting blood backward into the low-pressure pulmonary circuit. An ejection fraction of 50% or less indicates the presence of significant ventricular dysfunction in these patients.

(3) Stage 3: Severe mitral regurgitation—terminal failure. Continued severe compromise of forward cardiac output leads to increases in pulmonary artery pressure and eventually right ventricular failure. In addition, left ventricular function continues to deteriorate, and the depression of ventricular function becomes irreversible even after cardiac valve replacement.

2. Pressure-volume relationship (Fig. 12-9). In chronic mitral regurgitation the LVEDP may remain relatively normal until the disease is far advanced in spite of major increases in left ventricular end-diastolic and end-systolic volumes. The eccentric hypertrophy of the ventricle allows preservation of forward stroke volume by increasing total stroke volume. Blunting of the left ventricular pressure increase during left ventricular contraction occurs secondary to rapid early run-off of left ventricular volume into the low-pressure left atrium. In acute mitral regurgitation, in contrast, the compensatory increases in left ventricular end-diastolic and end-systolic volumes are attenuated by acute increases in left ventricular end-diastolic pressure until compensatory dilatation can intervene.

3. Calculation of severity. The regurgitant fraction, indicating the severity of mitral regurgitation, can be calculated quantitatively in the same way as in patients with aortic regurgitation using the equation:

$$\text{Regurgitant fraction} = \frac{[(\text{EDV} - \text{ESV}) \times \text{HR}] - \text{CO}}{(\text{EDV} - \text{ESV}) \times \text{HR}}$$

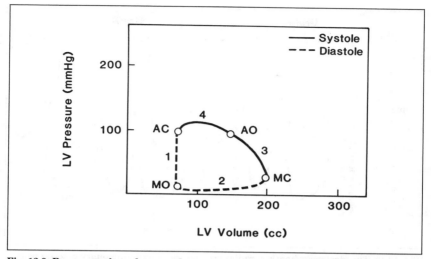

Fig. 12-9. Pressure-volume loop, moderate mitral insufficiency, showing markedly increased left ventricular end-systolic and end-diastolic volumes, along with some increase in left ventricular end-diastolic pressure. AC = aortic valve closure, AO = aortic valve opening, MC = mitral valve closure, MO = mitral valve opening. Phase 1, isovolumetric relaxation; Phase 2, ventricular filling; Phase 3, isovolumetric contraction; Phase 4, ventricular ejection. (Modified from J. M. Jackson, S. J. Thomas, and E. Lowenstein. Anesthetic management of patients with valvular heart disease. *Semin. Anesth.* 1:248, 1982. With permission.)

Mitral regurgitation consisting of less than 30% of total left ventricular stroke volume is considered mild, 30–60% is considered moderate, and greater than 60% is considered severe.

Normally, determination of regurgitant volume is made only semiquantitatively through the use of angiographic dye injection into the left ventricle:

1 + Minimal opacification of the left atrium is rapidly cleared.
2 + Moderate opacification of left atrium is rapidly cleared.
3 + Left atrial opacification is as intense as left ventricular and aortic opacification.
4 + Left atrial opacification is more intense than left ventricular and aortic opacification.

4. Pressure wave disturbances

a. Pulmonary capillary wedge tracing. The size of the regurgitant wave is not directly related to the severity of mitral regurgitation. The size of the regurgitant wave or **"giant V wave"** depends on the compliance of the left atrium, the compliance of the pulmonary vasculature, the amount of pulmonary venous return, and the regurgitant volume. In patients with sudden onset of mitral regurgitation, a relatively noncompliant left atrium leads to large V waves. Patients with chronic mitral regurgitation have a large compliant left atrium that can accept the regurgitant volume without passing the pressure wave on to the pulmonary circuit.

In those patients with giant V waves or regurgitant waves,

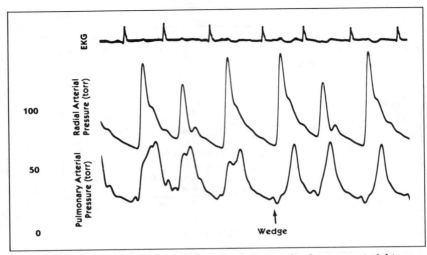

Fig. 12-10. The electrocardiogram, radial arterial trace, and pulmonary arterial trace in the unwedged and unwedged positions for a patient with severe mitral regurgitation. Note that the amplitude of the "giant V wave" or regurgitant wave is actually greater than the peak pulmonary artery pressure. Determination of the wedged position as opposed to the pulmonary arterial position is based on the rightward movement of the upstroke and peak of the pressure trace when in the wedged position. (From R. A. Moore, M. J. Neary, J. D. Gallagher, et al. Determination of the pulmonary capillary wedge position in patients with giant left atrial V waves. *J. Cardiothorac. Anesth.* 1:110, 1987. With permission.)

differentiation between the pulmonary arterial pressure trace and the pulmonary capillary wedge pressure trace can be difficult (Fig. 12–10). One easy way of making this differentiation, however, is by **superimposition of the pulmonary arterial trace and the arterial pressure trace.** Normally, the pulmonary arterial upstroke occurs slightly before the systemic arterial upstroke, but when a wedge position is achieved, an immediate rightward shift is observed in the position of the upstroke and peak to the position of the giant V wave, which occurs later than the arterial pressure upstroke. Therefore, when placing pulmonary artery catheters in patients with mitral regurgitation or patients at risk of having giant V waves, it is imperative to perform simultaneous observation of pulmonary arterial and systemic arterial traces.

C. **Goals of perioperative management**
   1. **Hemodynamic management**

	LV pre-load	Heart rate	Contrac-tile state	Systemic vascular resistance	Pulmonary vascular resistance
Mitral regurgitation	↑,↓	↑, Maintain	Maintain	↓	↓

   a. **Left ventricular preload.** Augmentation and **maintenance of preload** is frequently helpful for ensuring adequate forward stroke volume. Unfortunately, a universal recommendation for preload augmentation cannot be made because in some patients dilatation of the left atrial and left ventricular compartments dilates the mitral valve annulus and increases the regurgitant fraction. A decision about the best level of preload augmentation for an individual patient must be based on that patient's clinical response to a fluid load.

b. **Heart rate.** Bradycardia is harmful in patients with mitral regurgitation because it leads to an increase in left ventricular volume, reduction in forward cardiac output, and an increase in regurgitant fraction. The heart rate should be kept in the normal to elevated range in these patients. Atrial contribution to preload is not as important in patients with mitral regurgitation as in those with stenotic lesions, and many of these patients, particularly those with chronic mitral regurgitation, come to the operating room in atrial fibrillation.

c. **Contractility.** Maintenance of forward stroke volume is dependent on maximal function of the eccentrically hypertrophied left ventricle. Depression of myocardial contractility can lead to major left ventricular dysfunction and clinical deterioration. **Inotropic agents** that increase contractility have a tendency to provide increased forward flow and can actually decrease regurgitation due to constriction of the mitral annulus.

d. **Systemic vascular resistance.** An increase in afterload leads to an increase in regurgitant fraction and reduction in systemic cardiac output. For this reason, **afterload reduction is normally desired,** and alpha-adrenergic agents should be avoided. Typically, sodium nitroprusside will decrease the left ventricular filling pressure and cause a significant increase in forward cardiac index. However, in patients with acute mitral regurgitation secondary to ischemic papillary muscle dysfunction, nitroglycerin might be a more logical choice for a dilating agent.

e. **Pulmonary vascular resistance.** Most patients with extensive mitral regurgitation will develop pulmonary vascular pressure increases and can even present in right heart failure. Extreme caution must be taken to avoid hypercarbia, hypoxia, nitrous oxide, and pharmacologic or other interventions that might lead to pulmonary constrictive responses.

2. **Anesthetic management**

a. **Premedication** should be used **judiciously** because oversedation can lead to hypercarbia and marked increases in pulmonary vascular resistance.

b. **Pulmonary artery catheters** are extremely helpful in guiding fluid management. Also, they help evaluate the changing clinical state and significance of regurgitation for any particular patient as judged by changes in the height of the giant V wave.

c. **Anesthetic agents** leading to decreased contractility should be avoided, and high-dose narcotic relaxant anesthetics are used most commonly.

d. Patients with papillary muscle dysfunction secondary to ischemia are frequently helped by preoperative insertion of an **intraaortic balloon** pump. Inotropic support is also frequently required in the postbypass period.

3. **Surgical intervention.** Surgical intervention is not recommended if the patient can be medically treated with adequate relief of symptoms. However, once significant left ventricular dysfunction occurs, surgery should be performed as soon as possible before the left ventricular failure becomes irreversible. The surgical procedure usually performed is valve replacement using a mechanical or biologic valve, although occasionally annuloplasty can be performed with good results.

4. Postoperative care. Following valve replacement, left atrial and pulmonary arterial pressures should decrease. Patients with long-standing mitral regurgitation will continue to need an elevated left atrial pressure for maintenance of adequate forward flow. A primary concern following valve replacement is the need to maintain left ventricular performance. Once the valve is in place, the left ventricle has to eject a full-stroke volume into the aorta without the protection of a low-pressure pop-off into the left atrium. The result is an increase in left ventricular wall tension that can compromise ejection fraction. Therefore, in the postbypass period, left ventricular performance must frequently be augmented using intraaortic balloon counterpulsation or inotropic support until the left ventricle can adjust to the new hemodynamic state. Also, immediately following weaning from cardiopulmonary bypass, patients who have been in chronic atrial fibrillation may occasionally revert to a sinus rhythm for a short period. An attempt should be made to keep the patient in a sinus rhythm by using overdrive atrial pacing and treatment with procainamide.

VI. Tricuspid stenosis
A. Natural history
1. **Etiology.** The primary cause of acquired tricuspid stenosis is **rheumatic valvulitis.** Other causes for tricuspid stenosis include **systemic lupus erythematosus, endomyocardial fibroelastosis,** and **carcinoid syndrome.**
2. **Symptomatology.** Isolated tricuspid stenosis is manifest by the signs and symptoms of right-sided heart failure, including hepatomegaly, hepatic dysfunction, ascites, edema, and jugular venous distention with giant A waves visible on the central venous pressure recording. As stenosis progresses, cardiac output may be limited, at least during exercise. However, patients with tricuspid stenosis frequently have associated mitral stenosis, which is the primary cause of symptomatology and clinical deterioration.

B. Pathophysiology
1. **Natural progression.** The tricuspid valve area is normally 7–9 cm^2 in the typical adult. Significant impairment to forward blood flow does not occur until the valve orifice decreases to less than 1.5 cm^2. Therefore, there is a long asymptomatic period as stenosis develops. With progression of the stenosis, the right atrial pressure increases, and forward blood flow decreases. Preservation of a sinus rhythm is important for maintaining flow across the tricuspid valve, and rapid clinical deterioration can occur if the sinus rhythm is lost.
2. **Calculation of severity.** Normally the gradient across the tricuspid valve is only 1 mm Hg. A mean gradient of 3 mm Hg across the tricuspid valve indicates significant tricuspid stenosis and usually corresponds to a valve area of 1.5 cm^2. A gradient of 5 mm Hg across the tricuspid valve indicates severe stenosis and corresponds to a valve area of 1.0 cm^2.

C. Goals for perioperative management
1. **Hemodynamic management**

	RV preload	Heart rate	Contractile state	Systemic vascular resistance	Pulmonary vascular resistance
Tricuspid stenosis	↑	↓, Maintain	Maintain	↑	Maintain

a. **Right ventricular preload.** An adequate forward flow of blood across the stenotic tricuspid valve depends on maintenance of adequate preload.

b. Heart rate. Patients with tricuspid stenosis are dependent on maintenance of a sinus rhythm. Supraventricular tachyarrhythmias can cause rapid clinical deterioration and should be controlled either with immediate cardioversion or pharmacologic intervention. At the same time, bradycardia can be harmful because it reduces total forward flow.

c. Contractility. Right ventricular filling is impeded by tricuspid stenosis. Adequate cardiac output is maintained by an increase in right ventricular contractility. A sudden depression in ventricular contractility can severely limit cardiac output and elevate right atrial pressure.

d. Systemic vascular resistance. Changes in systemic afterload have little effect on the hemodynamic state of patients with tricuspid stenosis unless there is associated mitral valve involvement, particularly mitral regurgitation. However, systemic vasodilatation may lead to hypotension in patients with limitation of blood flow across the tricuspid valve.

e. Pulmonary vascular resistance. Because the limitation to forward flow is at the tricuspid valve, reducing pulmonary vascular resistance has little positive effect on improving forward flow. Keeping pulmonary vascular resistance in the normal range is adequate.

2. Anesthetic technique

a. Extensive preoperative preparation including salt restriction, digitalization, and diuretics may reduce hepatic congestion, improve hepatic function, and reduce surgical risks.

b. In patients with coexisting mitral valve disease, anesthetic technique is determined by the mitral valve lesion, as previously described. In patients with isolated tricuspid stenosis, the need to maintain high preload, high afterload, and preoperative contractility favors the use of a narcotic-based anesthetic technique.

c. Passage of a pulmonary artery catheter through the stenotic tricuspid valve may be almost impossible, and the catheter would have to be removed before bypass even if it could be placed. Therefore, use of a central venous pressure catheter, with surgical placement of a left atrial catheter and possibly a pulmonary artery thermistor for cardiac output determination, may represent the best possible monitoring in this setting.

3. Surgical intervention. Commissurotomy of the tricuspid valve is commonly the procedure of choice. However, in cases of extensive calcification, valve replacement with a low profile prosthetic valve may be necessary. In the postcardiopulmonary bypass period, preload augmentation must be continued.

VII. Tricuspid regurgitation

A. Natural history

1. Etiology. Isolated tricuspid regurgitation is most frequently seen in association with drug abuse endocarditis or chest trauma. More commonly, tricuspid regurgitation is associated with other cardiac abnormalities, such as end-stage aortic or mitral valve disease, most often mitral stenosis. With severe aortic or mitral valve disease, elevated pulmonary artery pressure leads to right ventricular strain and eventually right ventricular failure with tricuspid regurgitation. Carcinoid syndrome may produce isolated tricuspid regurgitation. The primary congenital cause of tricuspid regurgitation is Ebstein's anomaly.

B. Pathophysiology

1. Natural progression. Isolated tricuspid regurgitation is well tolerated because the right ventricle can compensate for volume overloading. On the other hand, a pressure load is not well tolerated by the right ventricle. Most symptoms associated with tricuspid regurgitation are directly related to an increased right ventricular afterload. Therefore, when tricuspid regurgitation is associated with pulmonary vascular hypertension, the impedance to right ventricular ejection produces significant clinical deterioration from decreased cardiac output. Most patients with tricuspid regurgitation have associated atrial fibrillation due to distention of the right atrium.

2. **Pressure wave abnormalities.** Central venous pressure tracings may show the presence of giant V waves. However, as with mitral regurgitation, the compliance of the right atrium, filling of the right atrium, and regurgitant volume each help to determine the size of the regurgitant wave.

C. **Goals of perioperative management**
   1. **Hemodynamic management**

	RV pre-load	Heart rate	Contrac-tile state	Systemic vascular resistance	Pulmo-nary vascular resistance
Tricuspid regurgitation	↑	↑, Maintain	Maintain	Maintain	↓

   a. **Right ventricular preload.** To provide adequate forward flow, **preload augmentation** is desirable. A drop in central venous pressure can severely limit right ventricular stroke volume.

   b. **Heart rate. Normal to high heart rates** are beneficial in these patients to sustain forward flow and prevent peripheral congestion. Most of these patients are in **chronic atrial fibrillation,** so maintenance of a sinus mechanism is rarely possible.

   c. **Contractility.** Right ventricular failure is the primary cause of clinical deterioration in patients with tricuspid regurgitation. Because the right ventricle is designed geometrically to accommodate volume but not pressure loads, it may require perioperative inotropic support, especially in the setting of positive pressure ventilation or elevated pulmonary vascular resistance. Any suppression of contractility with myocardial depressants may also induce severe right ventricular failure.

   d. **Systemic vascular resistance.** Variations in systemic afterload have **little effect** on tricuspid regurgitation unless there is concurrent aortic or mitral valve dysfunction.

   e. **Pulmonary vascular resistance.** Since the right ventricle does not tolerate pressure loads, right ventricular function and forward blood flow is improved with decreases in pulmonary vascular resistance. **Hyperventilation is helpful** in reducing pulmonary vascular resistance by producing hypocarbia. However, high airway pressures during pulmonary ventilation and agents such as nitrous oxide that can increase pulmonary arterial pressure should be avoided. If inotropic support is necessary, dobutamine, isoproterenol, or amrinone, which dilate the pulmonary vasculature, should be used.

   2. **Surgical intervention.** Many patients can be successfully treated with tricuspid valvular plication or annuloplasty. If the valve has deteriorated, valve replacement may be necessary. If a prosthetic valve is placed, residual tricuspid stenosis will occur because the valve prosthesis is smaller than the native valve, and postbypass preload augmentation will be necessary. In addition, in the immediate postbypass period the right ventricle will be under increased strain because the entire stroke volume will have to be ejected against

the higher pulmonary vascular resistance, with no low-pressure ejection back into the right atrium. Therefore, right heart failure requiring inotropic support may occur.

VIII. Pulmonic stenosis
A. Natural history
1. **Etiology.** Pulmonic stenosis may be valvular, infundibular, or located in a pulmonary arterial branch (distal pulmonary artery) in location. Nearly all cases of pulmonic stenosis are congenital, although rarely rheumatic heart disease can lead to pulmonic stenosis.
2. **Symptomatology.** Patients with pulmonic stenosis may live for extended periods completely without symptoms and frequently survive past the age of 70 years without surgical intervention. Symptoms, when they do occur, include tachypnea, syncope, angina, or hepatomegaly and peripheral edema. However, intervening bacterial endocarditis or right ventricular failure due to severe stenosis may lead to death.

B. Pathophysiology
1. **Natural progression.** The normal pressure gradient across the pulmonary valve orifice is usually between 5 and 10 mm Hg. Once the gradient increases to more than 15 mm Hg, with an elevation of right ventricular systolic pressure over 30 mm Hg, the diagnosis of pulmonic stenosis can be made (when no intracardiac shunt is present). A stenosis of the valve of more than 60% can occur before any significant obstruction to flow is generated. A peak systolic gradient of 50 mm Hg or less is considered mild pulmonic stenosis, between 50 and 100 mm Hg is considered moderate stenosis, and more than 100 mm Hg is considered severe pulmonic stenosis. As the pulmonic stenosis progresses from mild to moderate, concentric hypertrophy of the right ventricle occurs. The increased muscularization of the right ventricle leads to a situation in which right ventricular subendocardial blood flow no longer occurs throughout the cardiac cycle but only during diastole, similar to the left ventricle. Coronary perfusion pressure must be maintained to provide an adequate right ventricular subendocardial coronary blood supply.
2. **Pressure wave abnormalities**
   a. **Pulmonary arterial pressure trace.** The pulmonary artery pressure upstroke is delayed, and there is a late systolic peak owing to impedance of blood flow through the stenotic pulmonary valve.
   b. **Central venous pressure trace.** A prominent A wave is frequently found in the central venous pressure trace.

C. Goals of perioperative management
1. **Hemodynamic management**

	RV pre-load	Heart rate	Contrac-tile state	Systemic vascular resistance	Pulmonary vascular resistance
Pulmonic stenosis	↑	↑,	Maintain	Maintain	↓, Maintain

a. **Right ventricular preload.** Right ventricular performance depends on adequate preload for the right ventricle. Decreases in central venous pressure will lead to inadequate filling of the right ventricle and decreased right ventricular stroke volume.

b. **Heart rate.** As pulmonic stenosis progresses, the patient becomes increasingly dependent on the **atrial contraction** to provide adequate right ventricular filling. Unfortunately, in severe pulmonic stenosis, tricuspid regurgitation can develop, leading to the occurrence of atrial fibrillation. Because blood flow across the stenotic pulmonary valve occurs primarily during ventricular systole, increases in heart rate are usually beneficial by providing increased flow. Rarely, right ventricular hypertrophy in combination with angina symptoms direct the need for a slower heart rate to allow adequate time in diastole for subendocardial coronary blood flow.

  c. **Contractility.** With severe pulmonic stenosis the right ventricle **hypertrophies** in response to the pressure load. Depression of the contractile state can lead to right ventricular failure and clinical deterioration. Pharmacologic intervention that depresses right ventricular function should be avoided.

  d. **Systemic vascular resistance.** Afterload usually has **little effect** on pulmonic stenosis and can be maintained within normal limits.

  e. **Pulmonary vascular resistance.** Because the primary impedance to forward flow is the pulmonary valve, reducing pulmonary vasculature resistance will do little to enhance the forward flow of blood. However, especially in patients with mild or moderate pulmonary stenosis, major increases in pulmonary vascular resistance can potentially harm forward blood flow and lead to right ventricular dysfunction. Therefore, pulmonary vascular resistance should be kept in the low normal range.

  2. **Surgical intervention.** Any patient developing significant symptomatology, a peak systolic gradient across the pulmonary valve of more than 80 mm Hg, or a peak systolic right ventricular pressure of 100 mm Hg should have surgical intervention. Normally, valvulotomy is all that is necessary. Rarely, the pulmonic valve actually has to be replaced. An attractive alternative to open heart surgery is the use of transluminal balloon angioplasty, which has been used increasingly for congenital pulmonic valvular stenosis.

IX. **Mixed valvular lesions.** For all mixed valvular lesions, management decisions emphasize the most severe, or the most hemodynamically significant lesion.

  A. **Aortic stenosis and mitral stenosis.** The combination of aortic stenosis and mitral stenosis has one positive feature—the mitral stenosis protects the left ventricle from the pressure overload that would normally occur with pure aortic stenosis. Pathophysiologically, the progression of the disease follows a course similar to that seen in patients with pure mitral stenosis with development of pulmonary hypertension and eventually right ventricular failure. Symptomatology is primarily referable to the pulmonary circuit, including dyspnea, hemoptysis, and atrial fibrillation. This combination of valvular heart disease may lead to an underestimation of the severity of the aortic stenosis because the aortic valve gradient may be relatively low owing to low aortic valvular flow. This combination of lesions can be extremely serious owing to **limitations of blood flow at two points.**

  1. **Hemodynamic management**

	LV preload	Heart rate	Contractile state	Systemic vascular resistance	Pulmonary vascular resistance
Mitral stenosis alone	↑	↓	Maintain	↑	↓
Aortic stenosis alone	↑	↓	Maintain	↑	Maintain
Typical management—combined lesion	↑	↓	Maintain	↑	↓

  a. The best hemodynamic management for a patient with both aortic and mitral stenosis includes **preload augmentation, normal to low heart rates, and preservation of contractility.** Due to the high risk of decreased coronary perfusion, systemic vascular resistance must be increased whenever the diastolic perfusion pressure falls. Also, all agents or conditions that might augment pulmonary vascular resistance must be aggressively avoided. PCO_2 should be maintained in the low-normal range, and a high inspired oxygen concentration should be supplied to minimize pulmonary vasoconstriction.

B. **Aortic stenosis and mitral regurgitation.** This combination is relatively rare but should be suspected in patients with aortic stenosis who in addition have left atrial enlargement with atrial fibrillation. Sometimes mitral regurgitation can be exacerbated by left ventricular dysfunction due to severe aortic stenosis. In this situation the mitral valve does not require replacement, and the mitral regurgitation regresses after the aortic valve is replaced.

1. **Hemodynamic management**

	LV pre-load	Heart rate	Contrac-tile state	Systemic vascular resistance	Pulmo-nary vascular resistance
Aortic stenosis alone	↑	↓	Maintain	↑	Maintain
Mitral regurgita-tion alone	↑ , ↓	↑	Maintain	↓	↓
Typical manage-ment—combined lesion	↑	Maintain	Maintain	Maintain	↓

In managing these patients the hemodynamic requirements for aortic stenosis and mitral regurgitation are contradictory. Because aortic stenosis will most frequently lead these patients into deadly intraoperative situations, it should be given priority in managing the hemodynamic variables.

Preload augmentation is normally beneficial and, for coronary perfusion, the maintenance of at least a normal afterload is desirable. Obviously, increased systemic vascular resistance may hurt forward flow, but the stenotic aortic valve provides the primary impedance to forward flow no matter how the systemic vascular resistance is manipulated. Heart rate should be kept at least in the normal range, and tachycardia should be avoided at all costs. Contractility should not be depressed, and conditions or pharmacologic agents that increase pulmonary vascular resistance should be avoided.

C. **Aortic stenosis and aortic regurgitation.** The combination of aortic regurgitation and aortic stenosis is not well tolerated because it provides the left ventricle with both severe pressure and volume overloading. These stresses lead to major increases in myocardial oxygen consumption (MVO_2) and, as might be expected, angina pectoris is an early symptom with this combination. Once symptomatology develops, the prognosis is similar to that of pure aortic stenosis.

1. **Hemodynamic management**

	LV pre-load	Heart rate	Contrac-tile state	Systemic vascular resistance	Pulmo-nary vascular resistance
Aortic stenosis alone	↑	↓	Maintain	↑	Maintain

	LV preload	Heart rate	Contractile state	Systemic vascular resistance	Pulmonary vascular resistance
Aortic regurgitation alone	↑	↑	Maintain	↓	Maintain
Typical management for combined lesion	↑	Maintain	Maintain	Maintain	Maintain

Normally, augmentation of preload is beneficial both for aortic stenosis and aortic regurgitation. However, the hemodynamic requirements for afterload and heart rate for these two lesions are contradictory. Generally, **maintaining a hemodynamic profile consistent with aortic stenosis** is logical because compromise of this lesion intraoperatively is potentially more deadly than increasing the aortic regurgitation. In spite of the risk of decreasing cardiac output, systemic vascular resistance augmentation should be provided whenever systemic pressures begin falling to preserve coronary blood flow. Normalization of heart rate, contractility, and pulmonary vascular resistance will help stabilize the patient.

D. Aortic regurgitation and mitral regurgitation. The combination of aortic and mitral regurgitation occurs frequently, and this combination can cause rapid clinical deterioration.

1. Hemodynamic management

	LV preload	Heart rate	Contractile state	Systemic vascular resistance	Pulmonary vascular resistance
Mitral regurgitation alone	↑ , ↓	↑	Maintain	↓	↓
Aortic regurgitation alone	↑	↑	Maintain	↓	Maintain
Typical management for combined lesion	↑	↑	Maintain	↓	Maintain

There is close matching of the hemodynamic requirements of aortic regurgitation and mitral regurgitation. The primary problem is providing adequate forward flow and peripheral circulation. The development of acidosis leading to peripheral vasoconstriction and an increased impedance to left ventricular outflow can lead to rapid clinical deterioration. Therefore, keeping the systemic vascular resistance relatively low while maintaining an adequate perfusion pressure is the fine clinical balance needed until cardiopulmonary bypass can be initiated.

E. Mitral stenosis and mitral regurgitation. Rheumatic mitral stenosis is rarely pure and commonly exists in conjunction with mitral regurgitation. When dealing with patients with combined mitral stenosis and mitral regurgitation, decisions concerning hemodynamic management must consider which lesion is predominant. As a rule of thumb, **normalization of afterload, heart rate, and contractility,** while avoiding agents or conditions leading to reactive pulmonary constriction and providing adequate preload leads to optimal hemodynamic stabilization.

1. Hemodynamic management

	LV preload	Heart rate	Contractile state	Systemic vascular resistance	Pulmonary vascular resistance
Mitral stenosis alone	↑	↓	Maintain	Maintain	↓

Mitral regurgitation alone	↑,↓	↑	Maintain	↓	↓
Typical management for combined lesion	↑	Maintain	Maintain	↓, maintain	↓

X. Prosthetic cardiac valves

A. History.
The first mechanical prosthetic valve was implanted by Charles Huffnagle and associates in 1952, using a caged acrylic-ball valve prosthesis implanted in the descending aorta for the treatment of aortic insufficiency. This valve was placed without the use of extracorporeal circulatory techniques but had a high incidence of embolization and valve failure. In 1960, Dwight Harken introduced the modern era of cardiac valve replacement with the use of a valve placed in the aortic position under extracorporeal circulatory techniques. Since these early beginnings, the development of prosthetic cardiac valves has been directed toward fulfilling the requirements that Dwight Harken initially listed for the perfect replacement valve. These requirements include the following characteristics:

1. Nonthrombogenic
2. Chemically inert
3. Noninjurious to blood elements
4. Nonresistant to physiologic blood flow
5. Opens and closes promptly
6. Remains closed during the appropriate portion of the cardiac cycle
7. Durable
8. Insertable at the proper anatomic site
9. Capable of being permanently fixed
10. Not annoying to the patient
11. Technically practical to insert

The large number of different prosthetic valves which have been developed means that no ideal valve has yet been found.

B. Types of prosthetic valves

1. **Mechanical.** The primary difficulties associated with the development of early mechanical prosthetic valves were the lack of durability and the high incidence of embolization. Many attempts were made to decrease mechanical valve thrombogenicity without complete success. At present, all patients with mechanical prosthetic valves require anticoagulation therapy for the remainder of their lives. Normally, anticoagulation is provided with warfarin sodium, administered at a dose that will elevate the prothrombin time to 1.5 times over control. There are four basic types of mechanical prosthetic valves.

   a. **Caged-ball valve prosthesis** (Fig. 12-11). The Starr-Edwards valve prosthesis was commercially introduced in 1962 and had the advantage of only a single cage and a sewing ring. Due to the high rate of thromboembolic phenomena, however, improvements were made in this valve, including covering all metal parts with cloth. The cloth-covered metal stimulated the growth of surrounding tissue and allowed the valve to develop a neointima that decreased thrombus formation. Initially, a Dacron-knit was used, which was later changed to a Teflon-knit. The Starr-Edwards valve has been used in the aortic, mitral, and tricuspid positions. Other valves of this type include the Smeloff-Cutter, Braunwald-Cutter, Magovern-Cromie, and the DeBakey-Surgitool.

   b. **Caged-disk valve prostheses** (Fig 12-12). In an attempt to overcome the obstruction to blood flow presented by a bulky caged-

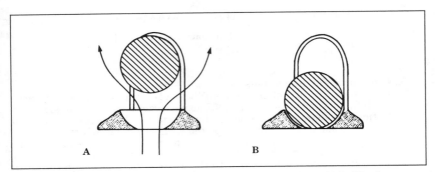

Fig. 12-11. Caged-ball valve prosthesis showing the movement of the ball in the open (A) and closed (B) positions.

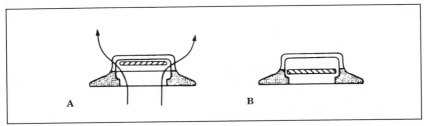

Fig. 12-12. Caged-disk valve prosthesis showing the disk in the open (A) and closed (B) positions.

ball valve, especially during cardiac arrhythmias, a caged-disk valve was developed. The Beall series of caged-disk mitral valve prostheses was introduced in 1967. Due to rapid disk breakdown, which included notching of the disc and even embolization, the disk material was changed from Teflon to carbon pryolite. Though caged-disk valve prostheses are no longer used clinically, the widespread use of these valves in the 1970s has produced a reservoir of patients who may still be encountered with these valves in place. Other caged-disk valve prostheses once used include the Starr-Edwards 6,500 series, Kay-Shiley, Cross-Jones, Harken, and Cooley-Bloodwell-Cutter.

    c. Monocuspid tilting disk valve prosthesis (Fig. 12-13). In an attempt to decrease the postoperative pressure gradient across valves in which a ball or disk occludes the center of the path of blood flow (i.e., caged-ball, caged-disk), the monocuspid, central flow, tilting disk valve was developed. Two valves of this type were the Wada-Cutter and Bjork-Shiley valves developed in 1969. The Bjork-Shiley valve has until recently been widely used in clinical practice. Though flow characteristics are better than those associated with central occluding valves, thromboembolic complications still occur even with adequate anticoagulation. Other monocuspid tilting disk valves that have been clinically used are the Lillehei-Kaster valve, introduced in 1970, and the Medtronic Hall valve, available for use in the aortic or mitral position.

    d. Bi-leaflet tilting disk valve prosthesis (Fig. 12-14). In 1977, a bi-leaflet St. Jude cardiac valve was introduced, followed more

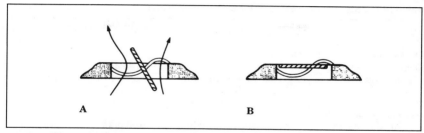

Fig. 12-13. Monocuspid tilting disk valve prosthesis showing the disk in the open *(A)* and closed *(B)* positions.

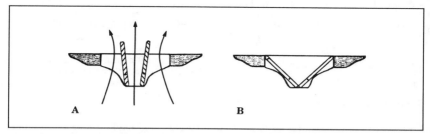

Fig. 12-14. Bileaflet tilting disk valve prosthesis showing disks in open *(A)* and closed *(B)* positions.

recently by the Duromedic valve. These valves are low profile devices that allow central blood flow through two semicircular disks that pivot on supporting struts. The St. Jude valve can be placed in the aortic, mitral, or tricuspid positions. These valves produce low resistance to blood flow and have a lower incidence of thromboembolic complications, though anticoagulation is still necessary.

2. **Bioprosthetic valves.** The high risk of thromboembolic phenomena and the necessity for anticoagulation with mechanical valves led to the search for a bioprosthetic valve that would serve as an adequate substitute. In addition, a bioprosthesis would have the advantage of maintaining a central flow pattern similar to that found in the natural state. Unfortunately, bioprostheses placed in the mitral position continue to show a risk for thromboembolization and require prolonged anticoagulation with warfarin, especially when the patient has a dilated left atrium, atrial fibrillation, or evidence of prior thrombosis. Long-term anticoagulation for bioprostheses placed in the aortic position is usually unnecessary, though aspirin, dipyridamole, or other antiplatelet drugs are often used. The first attempted use of a bioprosthesis was a valve homograft obtained from a cadaver in 1962. Due to the difficulty in procuring these valves and the relatively high failure rate, the Hancock-Porcine aortic bioprosthesis was introduced in 1970, followed by the Ionescu-Shiley bovine pericardial prosthesis in 1974 and the Carpentier-Edwards porcine aortic valve bioprosthesis in 1975. Though there is a low incidence of thromboembolic complications with these valves, durability is still a problem and there is a high late failure rate. As yet, the perfect replacement valve has not been developed.

Table 12-1. Drugs for prevention of bacterial endocarditis

	Dosage for adults	Dosage for children
Dental and upper respiratory procedures		
Oral		
Penicillin V	2 g 1 hr before procedure and 1 g 6 hr later	>60 lb: Adult dosage <60 lb: Half the adult dosage
Penicillin allergy		
Erythromycin	1 g 1 hr before procedure and 500 mg 6 hr later	20 mg/kg 1 hr before procedure and 10 mg/kg 6 hr later
Parenteral		
Ampicillin	2 g IM or IV 30 min before procedure	50 mg/kg IM or IV 30 min before procedure
plus gentamicin	1.5 mg/kg IM or IV 30 min before procedure	2.0 mg/kg IM or IV 30 min before procedure
Penicillin allergy		
Vancomycin	1 g IV infused *slowly over 1 hr* beginning 1 hr before procedure	20 mg/kg IV infused *slowly over 1 hr* beginning 1 hr before procedure
Gastrointestinal and genitourinary procedures		
Parenteral		
Ampicillin	2 g IM or IV 30 min before procedure	50 mg/kg IM or IV 30 min before procedure
plus gentamicin	1.5 mg/kg IM or IV 30 min before procedure	2.0 mg/kg IM or IV 30 min before procedure
Penicillin allergy		
Vancomycin	1 g IV infused *slowly over 1 hr* beginning 1 hr before procedure	20 mg/kg IV infused *slowly over 1 hr* beginning 1 hr before procedure
plus gentamicin	1.5 mg/kg IM or IV 30 min before procedure	2.0 mg/kg IM or IV 30 min before procedure
Oral		
Amoxicillin	3 g 1 hr before procedure and 1.5 g 6 hr later	50 mg/kg 1 hr before procedure and 25 mg/kg 6 hr later

Note: Oral regimens are more convenient and safer. Parenteral regimens are more likely to be effective: They are recommended especially for patients with prosthetic heart valves, those who have had endocarditis previously, or those taking continuous oral penicillin for rheumatic fever prophylaxis.

A single dose of the parenteral drugs is probably adequate because bacteremias after most dental and diagnostic procedures are of short duration. However, one or two follow-up doses may be given at 8- to 12-hr intervals in selected patients, such as hospitalized patients judged to be at higher risk.

Source: From Prevention of bacterial endocarditis. *The Medical Letter* 28:22, February 14, 1986. With permission.

3. **Human valves.** The first use of a bioprosthesis taken from a cadaver occurred in 1962. However, techniques such as irradiation or chemical treatment used to sterilize and preserve the early homografts for implantation led to a shortened life span. More recently, antibiotic solutions have been used to sterilize human valves, which are then frozen in liquid nitrogen until implantation. Using these techniques, weakness of the prosthesis leading to cusp rupture occurs infre-

quently, with more than 75% of prostheses lasting for longer than 10 years regardless of patient age. The incidence of prosthetic valve endocarditis and hemolysis resulting from blood flow through the homograft is very low. When homografts are used in the aortic position, anticoagulation is not required. However, in the mitral position a somewhat higher incidence of thromboembolism makes the use of anticoagulation somewhat more controversial.

Therefore, homografts may be most useful for aortic valve replacement in younger patients and in patients with native valve endocarditis. Homografts would be contraindicated in diseases associated with progressive dilatation of the aortic root, which would stretch the valve prosthesis and lead to early regurgitation, and in patients with poorly controlled hypertension, which would place increased stress on valve leaflets.

XI. Prophylaxis of subacute bacterial endocarditis All prosthetic heart valves, as well as abnormal native valves, provide a nidus for infection. They are not as well protected by the body's immune defenses as are normal heart valves. Therefore, when any invasive procedure puts the patient with valvular heart disease at risk of bacteremia, all precautions should be taken to prevent seeding of an abnormal or artificial valve with bacteria that, once present, are very hard to eradicate. Practically, this concern translates into, first, strict aseptic technique for all procedures performed in patients with valvular heart disease and second, antibiotic prophylaxis before, during, and after invasive procedures. Guidelines for antibiotic prophylaxis of patients with valvular heart disease are shown in Table 12-1.

SUGGESTED READING

Bolen, J. L., and Alderman, E. L., Hemodynamic consequences of afterload reduction in patients with chronic aortic regurgitation. *Circulation* 53:879–883, 1976.

Braunwald, E., Ross, J., and Sonnenblick, E. H. Mechanisms of contraction of the normal and failing heart. *N. Engl. J. Med.* 277:794–800; 277:853–863; 277:910–920, 1967.

Fuchs, R. M., Heuser, R. R, Yin, F. C. P., et al. Limitations of pulmonary wedge V waves in diagnosing mitral regurgitation. *Am. J. Cardiol.* 49:849–854, 1982.

Gorlin, R., McMillan, I. K. R., Medd, W. E., et al. Dynamics of the circulation in aortic valvular disease. *Am. J. Med.* 18:855–870, 1955.

Grossman, W. Aortic and mitral regurgitation. *J.A.M.A.* 252:2447–2449, 1984.

Jackson, J. M., Thomas, S. J., and Lowenstein, E. Anesthetic management of patients with valvular heart disease. *Semin. Anesth.* 1:239–252, 1982.

Kirklin, J. W., and Pacifico, A. D. Surgery for acquired valvular heart disease. *N. Engl. J. Med.* 288:133–140; 288:194–199, 1973.

Mody, M. R. The natural history of uncomplicated valvular pulmonic stenosis. *Am. Heart J.* 90:317–321, 1975.

Selzer, A. Changing aspects of the natural history of valvular aortic stenosis. *N. Engl. J. Med.* 317:91–98, 1987.

Yang, S. S., Bentivoglia, L. G., Maranhao, V., et al. Assessment of Valvular Regurgitation. In S. S. Yang, L. G. Bentivoglia, V. Maranhao, et al. (eds.), *From Cardiac Catheterization Data to Hemodynamic Parameters* (2nd ed.). Philadelphia: F.A. Davis, 1978. Pp. 163–208.

Anesthetic Management for Patients with Congenital Heart Disease

George W. Rung, Paul N. Samuelson, John L. Myers, and John A. Waldhausen

We gratefully acknowledge the assistance of Paul Hickey for reviewing the manuscript and Steve Cyran for reviewing the section on preoperative evaluation of children with congenital heart disease.

I. Introduction

A. Overview. Patients with congenital heart disease (CHD) depend on a delicate balance between their circulatory pathophysiology and compensatory mechanisms. The compensatory mechanisms often decrease the patient's cardiopulmonary reserve, increasing their susceptibility to physiologic insult. This relative lack of a "margin of safety" characterizes the pediatric patient with CHD and dictates the guidelines of care. Physicians involved in the care of these patients must understand the physiology of each cardiac lesion and anticipate the impact of the planned procedure. Maintenance of this delicate homeostasis in CHD patients during anesthesia for a wide variety of procedures (Table 13-1) is the anesthesiologist's challenge.

B. Incidence. The incidence of congenital heart disease is approximately 0.8/100 live births. A multitude of defects have been described, but more than 90% are represented by the most common lesions listed in Table 13-2.

   The patient's age, clinical symptoms, and physiologic parameters determine the timing of operation and whether surgical correction or palliation is indicated. There has been a trend toward early definitive correction rather than staged procedures. The number of patients with CHD requiring noncardiac surgery has increased owing to increased survival secondary to improved anesthetic and surgical techniques. Patients with congenital heart lesions very commonly have another congenital lesion. Table 13-3 lists congenital abnormalities associated with CHD. These anomalies must be suspected and identified preoperatively to properly care for these patients.

C. The pediatric patient. The approach to these patients must emphasize cardiac concerns, but the basic tenets of pediatric anesthesia cannot be overlooked because they form the foundation on which more complex interventions are built. The reader is referred to standard pediatric anesthesia texts for a review of these topics. Important considerations include:

1. The requirement for sufficient premedication to allay separation anxiety and prevent adverse physiologic responses.
2. The immaturity of the central and autonomic nervous systems.
3. The anatomic differences of the pediatric versus adult airway.
4. The need for meticulous attention to volume and composition of intravenous fluids.
5. Pharmacokinetic and pharmacodynamic variations with age.
6. Decreased thermoregulatory control.

Patients with CHD and their parents are often "hospital wise" after enduring multiple interventions including previous surgical procedures, investigations, and cardiac catheterization. Dealing with them requires finesse. An honest and reassuring approach usually is best. Care must be taken to avoid offering promises of outcome or engendering unrealistic goals.

II. Normal neonatal and infant cardiopulmonary physiology

A. Transition from fetal to adult circulation

1. **The fetal circulation** (Fig. 13-1) is characterized by concurrent parallel circulations. Unique features include:

   a. Fetal blood is oxygenated in the placenta and returned to the fetus through the umbilical vein. Most of this oxygenated blood crosses the ductus venosus to the inferior vena cava and right atrium, where the majority is directed through the foramen ovale and ejected from the left ventricle through the aorta to the head vessels. In this way the brain preferentially receives the blood with the highest oxygen tension.

Table 13-1. Spectrum of procedures for CHD patients requiring anesthesia

Cardiac catheterization
  Diagnostic
  Interventional
Open heart procedures
  Palliative
  Corrective
Closed heart procedures
  Palliative
  Corrective
Reoperation
  Early
    Hemorrhage
    Residual defects
  Late
    Residual defects
    Progression of disease
    Planned second stage
Noncardiac surgical procedures

Table 13-2. Frequency of occurrence of cardiac malformations at birth

Disease	Percentage
Ventricular septal defect	30.5
Atrial septal defect	9.8
Patent ductus arteriosus	9.7
Pulmonic stenosis	6.9
Coarctation of the aorta	6.8
Aortic stenosis	6.1
Tetralogy of Fallot	5.8
Complete transposition of the great arteries	4.2
Persistent truncus arteriosus	2.2
Tricuspid atresia	1.3
All others	16.5

Source: From E. Braunwald. *Heart Disease* (3rd ed.). Philadelphia: Saunders, 1988. P. 897. With permission.

    b. Desaturated blood from the superior vena cava is directed to the right ventricle and pulmonary artery, where most is ejected through the ductus arteriosus to the lower body.
    c. Pulmonary vascular resistance (PVR) is high owing to collapsed, fluid-filled lungs.
    d. Systemic vascular resistance (SVR) is low because the placenta is a very low resistance circuit.
  2. The transitional circulation describes the coexistence of parallel (fetal) and series (adult) circuits. This configuration is normal during the first several days after birth. Shunting of blood occurs through the foramen ovale and ductus arteriosus. The transitional circulation may persist in the presence of hypoxemia, acidosis, sepsis, or other stresses. "Persistence of the fetal circulation" is a misnomer. It may be lifesaving in some forms of CHD.

Table 13-3. Syndromes associated with cardiac lesions

Syndrome	Lesion
Heritable	
Ellis–van Creveld syndrome	Single atrium or atrial septal defect
Holt-Oram syndrome	Atrial septal defect
Kartagener's syndrome	Dextrocardia
Noonan's syndrome	Pulmonic valve dysplasia, cardiomyopathy
Familial deafness	Arrhythmias, sudden death
Alagille's syndrome	Pulmonic stenosis
DiGeorge's syndrome	Interrupted aortic arch, tetralogy of Fallot, truncus arteriosus
Friedreich's ataxia	Cardiomyopathy, conduction defects
Muscular dystrophy	Cardiomyopathy
Connective tissue disorders	
Ehlers-Danlos syndrome	Arterial dilatation and rupture, mitral regurgitation
Marfan's syndrome	Aortic dilatation, aortic and mitral incompetence
Pseudoxanthoma elasticum	Coronary artery disease
Inborn errors of metabolism	
Pompe's disease	Glycogen storage disease of heart
Homocystinuria	Aortic and pulmonary artery dilatation
Mucopolysaccharidoses	
Hurler's syndrome, Hunter's syndrome	Multivalvular and coronary and great artery disease, cardiomyopathy
Morquio's syndrome, Scheie's syndrome, Maroteaux-Lamry syndrome	Aortic incompetence
Chromosomal abnormalities	
Trisomy 21	Endocardial cushion defect, atrial septal defect, ventricular septal defect, tetralogy of Fallot
Trisomy 13	Ventricular septal defect, patent ductus arteriosus, double outlet right ventricle
Trisomy 18	Polyvalvular dysplasia, ventricular septal defect, patent ductus arteriosus
Turner's syndrome (XO)	Coarctation of aorta, bicuspid aortic valve
Teratogenic disorders	
Rubella exposure	Patent ductus arteriosus, pulmonary valve–artery stenosis, atrial septal defect
Alcohol abuse	Ventricular septal defect
Dilantin use	Pulmonic stenosis, aortic stenosis, aortic coarctation, patent ductus arteriosus
Lithium use	Ebstein's anomaly, tricuspid atresia

Table 13-3. (continued)

Syndrome	Lesion
Sporadic disorders	
VATER association	Ventricular septal defect
CHARGE association	Tetralogy of Fallot
Williams syndrome	Supravalvular aortic stenosis, peripheral pulmonary stenosis
Cornelia de Lange's syndrome	Ventricular septal defect

Source: Modified from W. F. Friedman. Congenital Heart Disease in Infancy and Childhood. In E. Braunwald (ed.), *Heart Disease* (3rd ed.). Philadelphia: Saunders, 1988. P. 898. With permission.

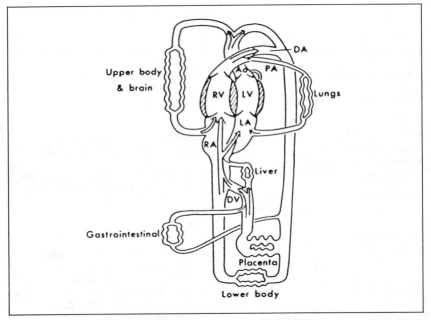

Fig. 13-1. Course of fetal circulation. See text for description. DA = ductus arteriosus; Ao = aorta; PA = pulmonary artery; RV = right ventricle; LV = left ventricle; LA = left atrium; RA = right atrium; DV = ductus venosus. (From J. I. E. Hoffman. The Circulatory System. In A. M. Rudolph [ed.], *Pediatrics* [17th ed.]. Norwalk, CT: Appleton-Century-Crofts, 1982. P. 1232. With permission.)

    a. Right-to-left shunting across the foramen ovale may persist while PVR (and therefore right atrial pressure) is high. As PVR and right-sided pressures decrease, pulmonary blood flow and left atrial pressure increase, functionally closing the foramen ovale.

    b. Bidirectional shunting of blood occurs through the ductus arteriosus while PVR approximates SVR. As PVR decreases, shunting becomes predominantly left to right. Functional ductal closure occurs as ductal tissue constricts in response to normal PaO_2 and falling blood levels of ductal-dilating prostaglandins. Prostaglandin concentration declines because the predominant source (placenta) has been removed from the circulation, and circulating prostaglandins are metabolized by the lung. Anatomic closure occurs at several weeks of age. Functional ductal closure may be delayed (or reversed) by administering prostaglandin E_1 and hastened by indomethacin (a prostaglandin synthesis inhibitor) administration.

    c. In the event of a complete right-sided obstruction to flow (e.g., tricuspid or pulmonary atresia), pulmonary blood flow (and patient survival) is completely dependent on left-to-right ductal shunting.

    d. Ductal patency is also crucial for complete left-sided obstructions (e.g., mitral atresia, critical aortic stenosis, coarctation of the aorta, or hypoplastic left heart syndrome). In this case, systemic flow is dependent on right-to-left shunting through the ductus.

  3. The normal adult circulation is a series circuit in which the entire systemic venous return is ejected into the pulmonary circulation by the right ventricle and all the pulmonary venous return is ejected into systemic circulation by the left ventricle. Although each ventricle pumps approximately the same volume, the left ventricle is much more muscular because it must empty into the high-resistance systemic circuit while the right ventricle ejects into the low-resistance pulmonary circuit.

B. Differences between the neonatal and adult heart

  1. The autonomic innervation of the heart is imbalanced at birth. The parasympathetic nervous system is nearly fully functional, but the sympathetic nervous system is immature. These different rates of maturation contribute to the high vagal "tone" of the infant heart. Sympathetic stimulation of the heart is more dependent on circulating catecholamines than innervation.

  2. At birth the right ventricle weighs approximately the same as the left ventricle. If PVR decreases normally, the left ventricle–to–right ventricle mass ratio of 2:1 is attained by 4 months of age.

  3. The immature ventricles are relatively noncompliant owing to the relative excess of nonelastic tissue and deficiency of contractile tissue compared to a normal adult heart. Cardiac output, therefore, may be less dependent on the Frank-Starling mechanism and more rate dependent if ventricular filling is maintained.

  4. The relative deficiency of contractile tissue in the neonate means that stroke volume is more dependent on afterload than in the adult. This deficiency also contributes to a lower cardiac reserve (versus that in an adult heart) and makes the immature heart more susceptible to myocardial depressants, including anesthetics.

  5. Biventricular failure is more common in neonates because the ventricles are approximately the same size, and failure of one results in dilatation and septal shift, which encroaches on the stroke volume of the other.

C. Development of the pulmonary vasculature

  1. The resistance of the pulmonary vasculature falls rapidly after the neonate's first breath owing to lung expansion, resorption of interstitial lung water, and vascular smooth muscle dilatation secondary to high alveolar PO_2.

  2. After a dramatic fall in PVR during the first 24 hours, PVR approaches adult values at 3 months of age but continues to decrease slowly for several years. The mechanism of this long-term decrease in resistance is the maturation, or arborization, of the pulmonary

Table 13-4. Factors affecting pulmonary vascular resistance (PVR)

Increases PVR
  Hypoxia
  Hypercarbia
  Acidosis
  Atelectasis, collapse
  High airway pressure
  Hypothermia
  Vasoconstrictors
  Polycythemia
  "Light" anesthesia
Decreases PVR
  High inspired oxygen concentration
  Hypocarbia
  Alkalosis
  Vasodilators (although none selective for pulmonary circulation)
  Anemia
  Fentanyl

---

vasculature. As the arteriolar-to-alveolar ratio increases, PVR decreases.

3. The result of pathologically increased pulmonary blood flow (e.g., as seen with a nonrestrictive ventricular septal defect) is persistent high pulmonary artery pressure. This retards normal pulmonary vascular maturation and increases vascular resistance by two mechanisms: (1) Reactive vascular smooth muscle hypertrophy narrows the arteriolar lumen, and (2) arborization is inhibited, resulting in fewer vessels.

4. PVR may also be high in patients with decreased pulmonary blood flow because normal arborization is retarded by the low flow through the vasculature. Therefore, both high and low pulmonary blood flow inhibits pulmonary vascular maturation.

5. The reactivity of the immature or abnormal pulmonary vasculature is more pronounced than it is in adults. Unresponsive pulmonary hypertension is often the lethal event in patients with CHD. Table 13-4 lists the effects of various conditions and drugs on PVR.

III. Clinical classification of congenital heart lesions

A. **Overview.** The enormous variety of congenital heart lesions complicates definitive classification. Several schemes exist today, categorizing lesions on the basis of morphologic or physiologic features. It may be useful to group together patients with similar clinical symptoms despite very different underlying physiologic characteristics. In this way, classification of patient type is facilitated, providing a starting point for planning treatment. Regardless of the classification system used, there is overlap between categories, with some lesions belonging to more than one category simultaneously or to one category at one time and another at a different time. For this reason, it must be stressed that **understanding the underlying pathophysiology is much more important than a classification label.** We have grouped together patients with either predominant **cyanosis** or **congestive heart failure** to simplify classification and facilitate initial treatment and diagnosis. Frequently, asymptomatic patients may also come to surgery for definitive correction of their lesions to circumvent later problems. Their management should mirror that of patients with similar lesions who are symptomatic. The lack of symptoms indicates a compensated circulatory abnormality that may nevertheless benefit from the same interventions and treatment given to symptomatic patients.

B. Cardiac lesion terminology

1. Cardiac lesions may be described as **simple shunts, obstructive lesions,** or **complex shunts** (the combination of a simple shunt and an obstructive lesion). These terms are applicable regardless of whether a congenital cardiac lesion produces clinical cyanosis or congestive heart failure.

2. **Simple shunt lesions**

a. Defects creating a communication between the right and left sides of the heart represent simple shunts. The direction and magnitude of blood flow is dependent on the orifice size and a measure of the "downstream" impedance to flow (e.g., the ratio of right and left ventricular compliance for an atrial septal defect or PVR and SVR for a ventricular septal defect).

b. Small defects are termed **restrictive.** There is a pressure gradient across the defect, and shunt flow is relatively fixed by orifice size. Changes in downstream impedance to flow in restrictive defects have less influence on shunt flow.

c. Large defects are termed **nonrestrictive.** A small pressure gradient (if any) is present across the defect, and flow is largely dependent on the downstream impedance to flow.

d. In the case of a **common chamber** (single ventricle, truncus arteriosus, single atrium), there is **no** pressure gradient between the right and left sides of the heart, and flow direction and magnitude are **entirely** dependent on the balance of downstream impedance to flow.

3. **Obstructive lesions**

a. Adult obstructive lesions are usually valvular. In contrast, congenital obstructive lesions may be subvalvular, valvular, or supravalvular.

b. Subvalvular obstructive lesions may be fixed or dynamic. A dynamic lesion (such as infundibular muscle spasm or asymmetric septal hypertrophy) may be manipulated to improve flow, whereas a fixed lesion is not amenable to manipulation.

c. Obstructive lesions may cause an increase in ventricular pressure and work, possibly progressing to ventricular failure.

d. In cases of complete obstruction to flow (e.g., pulmonary atresia or aortic stenosis-atresia) there must be two shunt pathways: one proximal and one distal to the obstruction to provide blood flow around the obstruction.

4. **Complex shunt lesions (simple shunt plus obstruction)**

a. The magnitude and direction of shunt flow are determined by the communicating orifice size and ratio of downstream impedances to flow, including ventricular compliance, resistance offered by outlet obstruction, and vascular resistance.

b. Dynamic obstructions (e.g., functional obstruction secondary to infundibular spasm) as well as the PVR/SVR ratio may be manipulated to optimize systemic and pulmonary blood flows.

C. Cyanotic patients

1. **Clinical diagnosis**

a. Cyanosis, often most evident in the lips and nail beds, may be present at rest or with exertion. Clinically recognizable cyanosis indicates the presence of more than 5 g reduced hemoglobin/dl of blood. Because the absolute amount of desaturated hemoglobin determines the presence of cyanosis, a child with polycythemia may appear cyanotic at a higher SaO_2 than a normocythemic or anemic child. For example, consider three patients with plasma hemoglobin values of 10, 15, and 20 g/dl. Cyanosis (5 g reduced hemoglobin/dl present) would not be detectable *clinically* until oxygen saturation reached 50%, 67%, and 75% respectively.

b. Tachycardia and tachypnea are effective compensatory mechanisms and are usually present.

c. "Clubbing" of the digits is frequently present.

d. Cyanotic children are often small-for-age due to feeding difficulties.

e. Elevation of the patient's red cell mass helps to maintain adequate peripheral oxygen delivery but increases blood viscosity and risk of cerebral and renal thrombi. Hematocrit, therefore, is a good index of the degree of cyanosis and risk of stroke.

f. Chest x ray and electrocardiographic (ECG) findings are variable, depending on the underlying lesion. These tests provide insight into the cause of cyanosis.

g. No significant improvement in SaO_2 after increasing the inspired oxygen concentration indicates a cardiac rather than pulmonary cause.

h. All cyanotic lesions require surgical repair if possible, although the timing of surgery is variable. The morbidity and mortality of earlier primary repair have decreased and in many instances are preferred to initial palliation followed by later definitive repair.

2. **Mechanism** Table 13-5 lists the mechanisms of several common cyanotic lesions.

There are four mechanisms by which cardiac lesions may cause cyanosis:

a. **Right-to-left shunt.** Because right heart pressures are normally lower than left heart pressures after birth, an obstruction to right heart outflow must be present to produce shunting of blood from right to left (a complex shunt lesion). Tricuspid valve and pulmonary outflow tract stenosis are examples of right-sided obstructions. An atrial septal defect (ASD) or ventricular septal defect (VSD) proximal to the obstruction provides the pathway for shunting to the left side of the heart. The degree of peripheral cyanosis depends on the amount of blood shunted (deoxygenated blood) relative to the amount of pulmonary blood flow (oxygenated blood). The lungs may receive blood flow through alternate pathways (i.e., patent ductus arteriosus [PDA], bronchial collaterals, or surgically created systemic-to-pulmonary shunts) to compensate for the reduced flow through the pulmonary outflow tract.

b. **Mixing lesions.** Lesions that cause variable mixing of deoxygenated and oxygenated blood prior to systemic ejection may occur at the atrial (single atrium), ventricular (single ventricle), or arterial (truncus arteriosus) levels. Because in the "pure" form there is no orifice or obstruction to limit flow, blood flow is entirely dependent on the ratio of downstream impedances to flow (e.g., PVR/SVR for a VSD, or right ventricular/left ventricular compliance for an ASD). Therefore, the shunt flow and direction may be manipulated by pharmacologic and mechanical interventions. In the case of a VSD, a large change in either pulmonary or systemic vascular resistance may decrease or increase blood flow to critical levels.

c. **Transposition of the great arteries.** This unique lesion has two separate parallel circulations, one containing oxygenated blood and the other desaturated blood. Communication between the two circulations is required for survival after birth.

d. **Severely limited cardiac output.** Lesions that severely restrict either pulmonary or systemic blood flow may produce cyanosis. The cyanosis associated with severe pulmonary stenosis is caused by inadequate pulmonary blood flow despite flow by alternate

Table 13-5. Mechanism of cyanosis in congenital heart lesions

Lesion	Lesion classification	CHF*	Pulmonary blood flow	Mechanism
TOF	Complex		↓	Right-to-left shunt
HLHS	Complex	Yes	↑	Right-to-left shunt, mixing
TGA		Yes	↔	Transposition physiology
Truncus arteriosus	Simple	Yes	↑	Mixing
Tricuspid atresia	Complex		↓	Obligatory right-to-left shunt
TAPVC	Simple	Yes	↑	Mixing
DORV with pulmonary stenosis	Simple	Yes	↓, ↔	Mixing
DILV	Simple		↔	Mixing
Single atrium or ventricle	Simple	Yes	↑	Mixing
Pulmonary stenosis	Complex	Yes	↓	Obstruction, right-to-left shunt
Pulmonary atresia	Complex		↓	Obligatory right-to-left shunt

*May also present with congestive heart failure, but primary presentation is cyanosis.
↑ = Increased pulmonary blood flow, ↔ = normal pulmonary blood flow, ↓ = decreased pulmonary blood flow, TOF = tetralogy of Fallot, HLHS = hypoplastic left heart syndrome, TGA = transposition of the great arteries, TAPVC = total anomalous pulmonary venous connection, DORV = double outlet right ventricle, DILV = double inlet left ventricle.

routes (patent ductus arteriosus, bronchial collaterals, and surgical shunts). Conversely, lesions that severely limit systemic cardiac output (e.g., aortic stenosis, hypoplastic left heart syndrome) may produce cyanosis because increased peripheral oxygen extraction causes an increased arteriovenous oxygen gradient. A PDA associated with left heart obstructive lesions often serves as a right-to-left shunt pathway to augment systemic perfusion.

D. Patients with congestive heart failure

1. Clinical diagnosis

   a. The history frequently reveals feeding difficulties and failure to gain weight; however, weight may be maintained owing to retention of water and solutes.

   b. There is often a history of frequent respiratory infections. The etiology of the infections may be focal alveolar collapse secondary to extrinsic small airway compression by engorged pulmonary vasculature. The airway closure may also be associated with expiratory wheezing. In either case, the symptoms may not resolve until the lesion is corrected.

   c. Physical examination often reveals characteristic tachypnea and tachycardia. There may be pallor and diaphoresis due to reduced systemic cardiac output, peripheral vasoconstriction, and high sympathetic tone. Weak peripheral pulses and cool extremities are often found. Peripheral edema is rare; however, hepatomegaly and distended neck veins are hallmarks of congestive heart failure (CHF) in infants and children.

   d. Respiratory function is compromised owing to decreased lung compliance that causes increased work of breathing. Arterial blood gas measurement often reveals an increased alveolar-arterial gradient.

   e. The chest x ray reveals cardiomegaly and pulmonary vascular congestion. ECG findings are variable.

2. Mechanism.
Congenital heart disease commonly causes congestive heart failure by two mechanisms: (1) **left-to-right shunting** of blood, with increased right ventricular and pulmonary blood flow causing ventricular volume overload, and (2) ventricular failure secondary to an **obstructive lesion** causing a pressure overload. In addition, cardiomyopathy is a rare cause of congestive heart failure. Table 13-6 summarizes the pathophysiology of several common congenital heart lesions that may cause CHF.

   a. Left-to-right shunt. Simple shunts, whether intracardiac (e.g., ASD or VSD) or extracardiac (e.g., PDA or anomalous pulmonary venous connection), create an excess of pulmonary blood flow and are the most common causes of CHF in children with CHD. Symptoms increase with larger shunt flow, pulmonary vascular obstructive disease, decreased plasma oncotic pressure, and the presence of downstream left-sided obstructive lesions.

   If the shunting goes uncorrected, the pulmonary vasculature responds with increasing resistance, first by vasoconstriction and then by smooth muscle hypertrophy. The vasoconstriction is reversible, but increased vascular smooth muscle proliferation with thrombosis and sclerosis is usually irreversible. This distinction is very important, because those with reversible pulmonary hypertension respond to perioperative manipulation of PVR and have a better prognosis with surgical repair.

   Those with irreversible pulmonary vascular obstructive changes rarely benefit from surgical repair of the heart defects. Another consequence of elevated pulmonary vascular resistance is that systemic vascular resistance may be exceeded, resulting

Table 13-6. Mechanism of congestive heart failure in congenital heart lesions

Lesion	Lesion classification	Cyanosis[a]	Pulmonary blood flow	Mechanism
ASD	Simple		↑	Left-to-right shunt
VSD	Simple		↑	Left-to-right shunt
PDA	Simple		↑	Left-to-right shunt
Coarctation of the aorta	Obstruction		↔, ↑	Obstruction
Atrioventricular canal	Simple		↑	Left-to-right shunt
Aortic stenosis	Obstruction	Yes[c]	↔	Obstruction
Ebstein's anomaly	Complex	Yes[d]	↓	Tricuspid valve insufficiency or stenosis

[a]May also present with cyanosis, but primary presentation is CHF.
[b]Mixing (if PVR elevated).
[c]If right-to-left shunting through PDA.
[d]Right-to-left atrial level shunt.
↑ = Increased pulmonary blood flow, ↔ = unaffected pulmonary blood flow, ↓ = decreased pulmonary blood flow, ASD = atrial septal defect, PDA = patent ductus arteriosus, VSD = ventricular septal defect, RV = right ventricle.

Table 13-7. Average normal values of pediatric blood pressure and pulse

Age (yr)	Pulse (per min)	Blood pressure (mm Hg)
Newborn	120	70/40
1	120	80/60
2	110	80/60
4	100	85/60
6	100	90/60
8	90	95/60
10	90	100/65

Source: From D. J. Steward, et al. *Manual of Pediatric Anesthesia.* New York: Churchill Livingstone, 1979. Pp. 10–12. With permission.

in reversal of shunt flow and cyanosis (Eisenmenger's reaction). The increased right pressure load may cause ventricular dilatation, decreased function, tricuspid valve annulus dilation, and incompetence.

b. **Obstructive lesions.** Congenital subvalvular, valvular, supravalvular, or great vessel obstruction to flow may cause ventricular failure. The physiologic condition is similar to that characteristic of adult stenotic valvular disease except that right-sided obstructive lesions and right heart failure are more common in children. The similar right and left ventricular size in neonates tends to promote biventricular failure because failure of one ventricle shifts the septum into the other ventricle, which reduces its ejection fraction and cardiac output. If the obstruction is severe, flow may be critically limited and alternate pathways utilized, sometimes producing cyanosis and further ventricular dysfunction.

c. **Cardiomyopathy.** Rarely, ventricular failure may be caused by a cardiomyopthy (viral, idiopathic, or ischemic). Ischemic cardiomyopathy may be secondary to coronary artery anomalies, either congenital or acquired (e.g., Kawasaki disease).

IV. **General perioperative anesthetic and surgical considerations**

A. **Preoperative evaluation**

1. **History.** A thorough history is the most important part of the preoperative evaluation. It is usually underutilized. A complete description of symptomatology, associated anomalies, activity level, feeding patterns, past and current medical and surgical treatment, and known allergies should be sought. A previous anesthetic record is valuable, but unless very recent, it may not accurately predict current behavior under anesthesia. Questions regarding the airway (loose teeth, snoring, respiratory infection) should be asked. In the neonate, maternal history, course of pregnancy, method and problems at delivery, Apgar scores, and treatment should be reviewed.

2. **Physical examination.** General appearance, including color and activity level, should be assessed first, without disturbing the patient. Vital signs are obtained and compared to normal values for age (Tables 13-7 and 13-8).

Examination of the patient's airway, heart, and lungs should be emphasized. The presence and location of surgical scars are clues

Table 13-8. Average normal values of pediatric respiratory rate and tidal volume

Age	Respiratory rate (per min)	Tidal volume (ml)
Newborn	50	21
6 mo	30	45
1 yr	24	78
3 yr	24	112
5 yr	23	270
12 yr	18	480

Source: From R. K. Crone. The Respiratory System. In G. A. Gregory (ed.), *Pediatric Anesthesia*. New York: Churchill Livingstone, 1983. P. 54. With permission.

to identifying previous surgical procedures. The quality of peripheral pulses should be determined and ease of vascular access estimated.

3. **Electrocardiogram.** There is a wider range of normal ECG patterns in infants and children compared with adults, and the normal range changes with age. It is important to note that a normal ECG does not rule out CHD. Conversely, there are very few ECG tracings that are considered diagnostic of a particular lesion. Some ECG findings associated with common lesions are listed in Table 13-9.

4. **Chest x ray.** The chest x ray should be examined preoperatively for evidence of increased or decreased pulmonary blood flow, heart size, and impingement of vascular structures on the airway. Malposition of the heart or abnormal heart shape should be noted. The location of the aortic arch may be identified. Noncardiac findings include visceral situs and presence of pulmonary infiltrates.

5. **Laboratory investigations.** Routine tests include complete blood count, urinalysis, electrolytes, and urea nitrogen. Others may be ordered as indicated.

6. **Echocardiography.** Noninvasive two-dimensional (2-D) echocardiographic imaging and color Doppler flow determination techniques yield a wealth of information and in many cases may obviate the need for invasive cardiac catheterization. Two-dimensional echocardiography reveals both anatomic and dynamic features of extracardiac and intracardiac structures in real time. M-mode echocardiography shows an "ice pick" view of the heart that is useful for measuring vessel and chamber diameters, ventricular function (by measuring diastolic versus systolic chamber size), and estimating pressure. Doppler flow echocardiography receives signals reflected from moving red blood cells. Flow direction and velocity and pressure gradients may be determined. Transesophageal and surface techniques have been extended into the operating room and may be useful in guiding surgical management.

7. **Cardiac catheterization.** Cardiac catheterization delineates anatomy and yields important physiologic information, including shunt flow (location, direction, and magnitude), chamber pressures, and pulmonary and systemic vascular resistances. Qualitative information may be obtained from axial views of contrast cineangiograms. The ability to access and visualize the central circulation also provides an opportunity to perform interventional maneuvers.

Table 13-9. Electrocardiogram findings in congenital heart disease

Lesion	Findings
VSD	High-voltage equiphasic QRS in midprecordial leads (in 50–75%), LVH, RVH, or both.
ASD	rSR' pattern in V_1. Right atrial enlargement in some. First-degree AVB and atrial arrhythmias in a few.
PDA	Similar to VSD, but left atrial enlargement and first-degree AVB are more common.
AS	Normal in 25% of patients with significant obstruction. LVH by voltage criteria only in most. LVH with ST and T-wave changes in those with more severe obstruction.
ASH	Prominent Q waves, especially in I, III, F, V_5–V_6, with tall R waves in left chest leads (septal hypertrophy), LVH.
COARC	Normal or LVH. An rSR' pattern is occasionally seen in V_1.
PS	RVH with upright T waves or qR in V_1 (RV pressure ≥ LV) with Rs or rR in V_1 (LV pressure < RV). In severe PS, R waves are dominant and T waves upright in V_1–V_3.
TOF	RVH with dominant R and upright T waves in right precordial leads.
TGA	RVH, qR, or rSR' in V_1 suggests intact ventricular septum.
Endocardial cushion defect	LAD and incomplete RBBB. First-degree AVB occasionally.
Ebstein's anomaly	Right atrial enlargement without RVH. Low amplitude, atypical RBBB. WPW in 10%. First-degree AVB in 15–20%. Atrial tachycardia common.
TA	LVH or LAD in 80–90%. RA enlargement.

VSD = Ventricular septal defect, LVH = left ventricular hypertrophy, ASH = asymmetric septal hypertrophy, RVH = right ventricular hypertrophy, ASD = atrial septal defect, AVB = atrioventricular block, PDA = patent ductus arteriosus, COARC = aortic coarctation, RBBB = right bundle branch block, AS = aortic stenosis, PS = pulmonary stenosis, RV = right ventricle, LV = left ventricle, TOF = tetralogy of Fallot, TGA = transposition of the great arteries, LAD = left axis deviation, WPW = Wolf-Parkinson-White syndrome.
Source: Modified from H. J. L. Marriott. *Practical Electrocardiography* (7th ed.). Baltimore: Williams & Wilkins, 1983. Pp. 449–453. With permission.

a. **Shunts.** The presence and location of left-to-right shunts may be determined by advancing a catheter through a large vein to the right atrium, right ventricle, and pulmonary artery while collecting serial blood samples for oximetry. The presence of a "step-up" in oxygen saturation indicates a left-to-right intracardiac shunt at that level. Pulmonary and systemic blood flows may be calculated by the Fick principle if oxygen consumption, oxygen saturation, and hemoglobin are known:

$$PBF\ (Qp) = \frac{\text{oxygen consumption}}{PV\ O_2\ \text{content} - PA\ O_2\ \text{content}}$$

$$SBF\ (Qs) = \frac{\text{oxygen consumption}}{AO\ O_2\ \text{content} - MV\ O_2\ \text{content}}$$

Where PBF = pulmonary blood flow
SBF = systemic blood flow
PV = pulmonary venous
PA = pulmonary arterial
AO = aortic
MV = mixed venous

Because standard values for oxygen consumption based on age and heart rate may be inaccurate, it is useful to express pulmonary and systemic blood flows as a ratio. Notice that hemoglobin concentration and oxygen consumption are not required:

$$\dot{Q}p/\dot{Q}s = \frac{AO \text{ oxygen saturation } - MV \text{ oxygen saturation}}{PV \text{ oxygen saturation } - PA \text{ oxygen saturation}}$$

A $\dot{Q}p/\dot{Q}s$ ratio of greater than 1.0 indicates a left-to-right shunt, and less than 1.0 indicates a right-to-left shunt.
   b. **Pressure and resistance measurements.** Intracardiac and vascular pressure measurements are important for determining absolute pressures as well as pressure gradients across valves, obstructions, and shunt orifices. Elevated pulmonary artery pressure due to irreversible elevated pulmonary vascular resistance secondary to medial smooth muscle hypertrophy is a very poor prognostic sign. For this reason, it is important to determine whether pulmonary hypertension is caused by high flow or high resistance. One technique is to administer 100% oxygen (a potent pulmonary vasodilator) and monitor the response. Pulmonary hypertension associated with high pulmonary blood flow (elevated $\dot{Q}p/\dot{Q}s$) has a better prognosis than pulmonary hypertension with low flow (normal or decreased $\dot{Q}p/\dot{Q}s$) because the latter indicates increased pulmonary vascular resistance. Frequently, there is a combination of increased pulmonary blood flow and elevation of pulmonary vascular resistance. Pulmonary vascular resistance may be calculated by the following equation:

$$PVR = (PAP - LAP \text{ [or PCWP]})/PBF$$

Where PAP = pulmonary artery pressure
LAP = left atrial pressure
PBF = pulmonary blood flow
PCWP = pulmonary capillary wedge pressure

If pulmonary vascular resistance is elevated it is important to know whether there is a reversible component.
   c. **Cineangiography.** Qualitative and quantitative assessments of ventricular function may be made by this method. Vascular obstructions and shunts may be visualized. Although the coronary ostia are not commonly injected directly, coronary anatomy may be discerned by aortic root injections. The presence of anomalous coronary anatomy may alter surgical technique (e.g., tetralogy of Fallot with anomalous origin of the left coronary artery).
   d. **Interventions.** Patients with lesions that isolate the systemic and pulmonary circuits (e.g., transposition of the great arteries with

intact ventricular septum) or decrease pulmonary blood flow (e.g., tricuspid atresia) improve with greater mixing of blood. This may be accomplished in the catheterization laboratory by enlarging the foramen ovale and tearing the septum primum. A balloon-tipped catheter may be passed from the right atrium through the foramen ovale, inflated, and then pulled back abruptly into the right atrium, creating an atrial septal defect (Rashkind balloon atrial septostomy). In older children this procedure is usually preceded by a Park blade septotomy.

Other interventions at catheterization include embolizing silicone balloons or coils to occlude bronchopulmonary collaterals, occluding a patent ductus arteriosus or ASD with an umbrella occlusion device, and performing balloon angioplasty of stenotic valves.

e. **Limitations.** The measurements obtained at catheterization must be interpreted in view of the fact that they are obtained under artificial conditions and represent only one point in time. Sedation or general anesthesia may cause or aggravate preexisting hypoxia, hypercarbia, and pulmonary hypertension. Anesthetics, contrast dye, and acid-base abnormalities may affect ventricular performance.

B. **Patient preparation**

1. **Fasting interval, intravenous fluid, and blood availability guidelines.** The risk of dehydration associated with a prolonged fast must be weighed against the need for an empty stomach at the time of anesthetic induction. Standard guidelines for fasting interval based on age must be adjusted according to the individual patient. Cyanotic patients with polycythemia (especially those with a hematocrit of >60) are at increased risk of cerebral and renal thrombi if not adequately hydrated. Conversely, those with congestive heart failure may require fluid restriction to prevent further deterioration in ventricular function may tolerate a longer fasting interval.

The use of intravenous (IV) fluid therapy preoperatively allows precise fluid management and increases the likelihood of an empty stomach at the time of anesthetic induction. Those with severe cyanosis may have 1–1½ times maintenance fluids, whereas patients with congestive heart failure may only need ¼–½ maintenance. In either case, the presence of a functional IV line on the day of surgery may be useful for anesthetic induction.

Cross-matched blood should be available for transfusion perioperatively. In cases of reoperation, patients with anemia, and those cyanotic patients with multiple chest wall collaterals, blood must be ready to administer at the start of surgery. Blood replacement therapy must be more liberal for infants compared to adults (in whom blood administration is avoided to minimize the risk of blood-borne infections) because the immature heart is less well equipped to deal with the physiologic stress of anemia, and bone marrow erythrocyte production is very low for several months after birth.

2. **Premedication.** The drugs and dosages used for premedication depend on the patient's age, cardiac lesion, and general medical status as well as on institutional tradition. The advantages of premedication (easier separation from parents, calm and cooperative patient, smooth anesthetic induction, and decreased anesthetic requirement) must be weighed against the disadvantages (respiratory depression, loss of airway reflexes, and cardiac depression).

Patients with cyanotic lesions usually benefit from preoperative sedation because it reduces their baseline oxygen consumption and the likelihood of an acute rise in oxygen demand due to crying or struggling. One standard regimen is pentobarbital 2 mg/kg, morphine 0.2 mg/kg, and atropine 0.02 mg/kg. In patients with congestive heart failure, the pentobarbital may be omitted. Some physicians suggest avoiding morphine for patients with reactive pulmonary vasculature. Dosages may also be decreased for patients in poor general condition. Standard formulas serve only as a starting point; the premedication used should reflect consideration of the individual patient's condition.

C. Preparation of the operating room

  1. **Standard equipment.** The equipment requirements for a pediatric cardiac case are similar to those for an adult cardiac case (see Chap. 2 for details of operating room setup for an adult). The differences between pediatric and adult equipment will be presented here.

   a. **Anesthesia circuit.** The Bain modification of the Mapleson D circuit offers several advantages for children weighing less than 10 kg. There are no valves and therefore less resistance to breathing, the inspired anesthetic concentration may be rapidly changed, and the single, lightweight airway tubing is practical and convenient.

   b. **Endotracheal tube size.** Large tubes are desirable because pulmonary toilet is facilitated, plugging by secretions is less likely, and kinking is resisted. A smaller than usual tube may be necessary for a patient with generalized edema (i.e., the airway may be involved).

   c. **IV setups.** The importance of meticulous removal of air from all intravenous administration sets cannot be overemphasized. This is especially true for patients with right-to-left shunts, but patients with left-to-right shunts are also at risk because right-to-left shunting may occur during certain phases of the cardiac cycle, cardiopulmonary interventions (positive pressure ventilation, manual manipulation of the heart), or coughing. A graduated, volume-limited delivery system (e.g., buretrol) or volumetric infusion pump should be used to administer fluids accurately. The use of dextrose-containing solutions intraoperatively has been criticized because they may contribute to hyperglycemia, which, in the case of an ischemic event, may result in adverse neurologic outcome. It is our feeling that the stress of anesthesia and surgery may be expected to maintain an adequate level of blood glucose without administration of exogenous dextrose, but serum glucose concentration should be determined as indicated.

   d. **Drugs.** Routine and emergency drugs should be drawn into appropriate sized syringes (1-ml syringes for patients <10 kg, 3-ml for patients 10–20 kg), and dosages should be calculated so that they may be given quickly and accurately. Likewise, drugs for continuous infusion should be prepared in a concentration that allows a wide range of doses to be administered without fluid overload (see Chap. 3). Table 13-10 lists drugs that should be available for all pediatric cardiac cases.

  2. **Special monitors**

   a. **Arterial catheter.** The insertion of an arterial catheter in the radial or femoral artery provides beat-to-beat blood pressure determinations and access to arterial blood. A 22-gauge radial artery catheter may be inserted percutaneously or by cutdown for patients less than 10 years old, and an "adult" (20-gauge) catheter is appropriate for older patients.

   b. **Central venous catheter (CVC).** Access to the central circulation

Table 13-10. Drugs commonly used for pediatric cardiac surgery

Drug	Dose
To be administered as an intravenous bolus	
Atracurium	0.4 mg/kg (intubation), 0.2 mg/kg (maintenance)
Atropine	0.02 mg/kg
Calcium chloride	5–15 mg/kg
Diazepam	0.05–0.2 mg/kg
Edrophonium	0.5–1.0 mg/kg
Epinephrine	0.05–10.0 µg/kg
Fentanyl	0.25–100 µg/kg
Glycopyrrolate	0.01 mg/kg
Heparin	3 mg/kg
Ketamine	1–5 mg/kg
Lidocaine	1–2 mg/kg
Midazolam	0.01–0.1 mg/kg
Morphine	0.05–0.5 mg/kg
Neostigmine	0.05 mg/kg
Pancuronium	0.1–0.2 mg/kg (intubation), 0.02 mg/kg (maintenance)
Phentolamine	0.25–0.5 mg/kg
Phenylephrine	0.05–0.1 µg/kg
Propranolol	0.01–0.05 mg/kg
Protamine	1.5 mg/1.0 mg heparin
Sodium bicarbonate	1 mEq/kg
Sufentanil	0.05–10.0 µg/kg
Thiopental	3–6 mg/kg
Vecuronium	0.1–0.2 mg/kg (intubation), 0.02 mg/kg (maintenance)
To be administered as an infusion	**Infusion rate**
Amrinone	0.75 mg/kg (load), 5–10 µg/kg/min
Dobutamine	2.5–10.0 µg/kg/min
Dopamine	2.5–15.0 µg/kg/min
Epinephrine	0.05–0.5 µg/kg/min
Isoproterenol	0.05–0.5 µg/kg/min
Prostaglandin	0.05–0.4 µg/kg/min

is valuable for measuring right ventricular filling pressure, administering vasoactive drugs, and rapidly infusing intravascular volume expanders. The simultaneous performance of all these functions is facilitated by the use of multiple-lumen catheters.

A suggested guide to the size and type of heparin-coated catheters for various ages is:

Premature	3 Fr, 5 cm, single lumen
< 1 yr	3 Fr, 8 cm, single lumen
1– 2 yr	5 Fr, 8 cm, double lumen
3– 8 yr	5 Fr, 12 cm, double lumen
> 8 yr	5 Fr "adult" introducer

Size may be modified if the patient is small for age.

   c. Additional invasive pressure monitors. Additional transducers should be available to measure pressures intraoperatively through a surgeon's exploring needle or catheters placed directly in the right or left atrium or pulmonary artery.

   d. Other. As the use of sophisticated monitoring increases, we will have the advantages of mass spectrometric analysis of inspired and expired gases, transesophageal and surface echocardiography, and processed electroencephalogprahy (EEG).

3. Environment. The room temperature is usually prewarmed for closed heart procedures to avoid the deleterious effects of hypothermia on the pulmonary vasculature and myocardium and to preserve the opportunity to extubate the patient at the end of the procedure. For procedures requiring hypothermic cardiopulmonary bypass (especially with circulatory arrest), the advantages of surface cooling may be utilized by precooling the operating room and allowing the patient's temperature to "drift" downward prior to bypass. This practice may not be ideal if the start of bypass is delayed.

D. Anesthetic strategies for congenital heart disease

  1. General. The goal is to induce and maintain anesthesia in a controlled fashion without upsetting the balance between the patient's pathophysiology and compensatory mechanisms. The anesthetic plan, although important, cannot cover all possibilities, and the anesthetist must be prepared to change course as the anesthetic progresses.

   a. Cyanosis. The effect of anesthetics on cyanotic patients is dependent on the mechanism of cyanosis. The anesthetic plan differs, therefore, based on the etiology of the cyanosis.

    (1) Right-to-left shunt. These patients usually benefit from maneuvers that increase pulmonary blood flow, which decreases the amount of blood shunted.

     (a) Reactive pulmonary vasculature. The pulmonary arterial vasculature may be the site of right-sided resistance to flow. In these cases (e.g., acute pulmonary hypertensive episode), pulmonary vascular resistance may be decreased by hyperventilation (which lowers $PaCO_2$), 100% oxygen administration, and alkalosis.

     (b) Fixed pulmonary outflow obstruction. Pulmonary blood flow may be severely limited by a fixed resistor (e.g., valvular pulmonic stenosis). In this case, changes in pulmonary vascular resistance will have little effect on pulmonary blood flow. Infusion of PGE_1 (0.10 μg/kg/min) supports ductal patency and pulmonary blood flow until definitive measures can be taken.

     (c) Variable pulmonary outflow tract stenosis. Hypertrophy of the right ventricular infundibulum may obstruct pulmonary blood flow in a dynamic fashion. In this case (e.g., tetralogy of Fallot), a negative inotropic agent may relax infundibular spasm and increase pulmonary blood flow.

    (2) Mixing lesions. In general, these lesions (e.g., single ventricle, truncus arteriosis) are associated with increased pulmonary blood flow, and management is aimed at decreasing the excessive flow. Further increases in pulmonary blood flow may precipitate congestive heart failure or a "pulmonary steal" phenomenon in which the increased pulmonary flow occurs at the expense of systemic flow, resulting in hypoperfusion of vital organs and metabolic acidosis. Specific measures to decrease pulmonary blood flow (and concurrently increase systemic flow) include maintenance of normocarbia and limiting inspired oxygen tension.

b. **Congestive heart failure.** Myocardial depressants should be avoided and preoperative inotropic support continued. Management of valvular lesions may be guided by the same principles as those governing adult valvular disease. Patients with CHF secondary to left-to-right shunting usually benefit from maintenance of normal PCO_2, limitation of inspired oxygen concentration, and positive pressure ventilation. Patients with CHF secondary to critical left-sided stenosis (e.g., aortic stenosis, hypoplastic left heart syndrome) may benefit from infusion of PGE_1 (0.10 μg/kg/min) to maintain ductal patency and systemic flow by right-to-left flow through the ductus arteriosus.

2. **Induction**
   a. **Intravenous.** A wide variety of intravenous induction agents, including thiopental, ketamine, fentanyl, and sufentanil, have been used successfully in patients with CHD. Selection of the appropriate agents depend on the patient's age and pathophysiology.
      (1) **Cyanosis.** Agents that increase SVR (e.g., ketamine) or inhibit rises in PVR (e.g., fentanyl) are good choices for lesions that cause right-to-left shunting. Intravenous drugs reach the systemic circulation (and brain) faster in the presence of right-to-left shunting but attain a lower peak plasma concentration compared to normal (Fig. 13-2). This effect results in a clinically noticeable speeding of anesthetic induction.
      (2) **CHF.** Negative inotropes (thiopental) should theoretically be avoided. Opioids and ketamine have been shown to have minimal hemodynamic effects. Ketamine's mild negative inotropic activity is usually balanced by increasing sympathetic tone, but a severely debilitated infant (with maximal preexisting sympathetic stimulation) may be unable to respond further to the sympathetic stimulating properties of ketamine. Left-to-right shunts dilute intravenous agents prior to systemic ejection, which results in normal (or only slightly delayed) appearance time but a prolonged systemic concentration curve (Fig. 13-2). This does not seem to be clinically important.
   b. **Inhalation.** The advantages of inhalation induction include the ability to titrate anesthetic depth and rapidly eliminate the drug through the lungs. A cooperative (or sleeping) patient is ideal. This technique also allows reduction of myocardial oxygen consumption and contractility and the possibility of early postoperative extubation. The unique features of each inhalation agent (e.g., increased vagal tone with halothane, vasodilation with isoflurane) may be used to advantage depending on the situation. Mask inductions are very effective for patients who arrive in the operating room asleep from their premedication.
      (1) **Cyanosis.** Inhalation anesthetic induction is associated with a decrease in total body oxygen consumption and an increase in mixed venous oxygen saturation (an increase in oxygen supply and a decrease in demand). Another possible mechanism of improved oxygenation in the presence of right ventricular

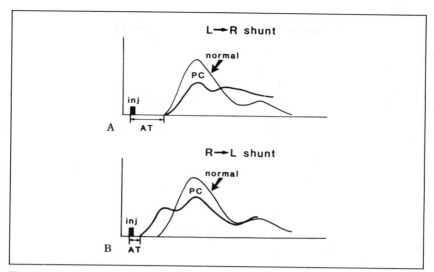

Fig. 13-2. Diagrammatic cardiac output curves for patients with left-to-right *(A)* and right-to-left *(B)* shunts. A normal cardiac output curve in each graph is indicated by an arrow. inj = time of intravenous indicator injection; PC = peak blood concentration of indicator; AT = appearance time in arterial circulation after intravenous injection. See text for complete discussion. (From F. W. Campbell and A. J. Schwartz. Anesthesia for noncardiac surgery in the pediatric patient with congenital heart disease. *Am. Soc. Anesthesiol.* 14:94, 1986. With permission.)

infundibular spasm is relaxation of the infundibulum (and increased pulmonary blood flow) secondary to the negative inotropic effects of inhalation agents (including nitrous oxide).

A theoretical concern is that the negative inotropic property may decrease cardiac output, lower systemic blood pressure, and increase right-to-left shunting. Clinically, at lower concentrations of potent inhalational agents, improvement in oxygenation, for the reasons mentioned above, usually results.

Right-to-left shunts may theoretically delay induction of anesthesia with inhalation agents because shunted blood bypasses the lungs (Fig. 13-3). This is clinically unimportant.

(2) **CHF.** The negative inotropic effects of inhalation agents make them undesirable for patients with congestive heart failure.

c. **Intramuscular ketamine (2–5 mg/kg).** This technique works well for patients who will not cooperate with anesthetic face mask application or intravenous cannula insertion. It may be used for most patients with CHD lesions (both cyanotic and CHF) because ketamine's sympathetic stimulating properties support the circulation in patients with CHF and increase SVR, which improves cyanosis caused by right-to-left shunting. Cyanosis usually improves even when sympathetic stimulation is theoretically detrimental (e.g., in tetralogy of Fallot), probably due to decreased total body oxygen consumption.

d. **Intranasal sufentanil (1–3 μg/kg).** This new method of "preinduction" may be useful for the uncooperative or nonpremedicated

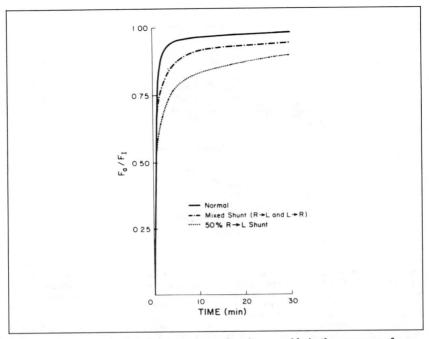

Fig. 13-3. Computer-simulated uptake curves for nitrous oxide in the presence of a normal circulation, a right-to-left (R→L) shunt, and a mixed shunt (R→L and L→R). Anesthetic uptake is slightly delayed in the presence of a R→L shunt, but this seems to be unimportant clinically. (From G. E. Tanner, D. G. Angers, P. G. Barash, et al. Effects of left-to-right, and mixed left-to-right and right-to-left shunts on inhalational anesthetic induction in children. *Anesth. Analg.* 64:105, 1985. With permission.)

child without an IV. Its safety in pediatric cardiac anesthesia has not been evaluated. Clinical studies in noncardiac patients have described the advantages of an easy separation from parents, co-operation with application of a face mask, and insertion of an intravenous catheter. The disadvantages include a variable incidence of chest wall rigidity and an unknown effect on pulmonary vascular resistance. Further evaluation is needed prior to widespread application of this technique.

3. **Maintenance.** The technique chosen for maintenance of anesthesia depends on the patient, procedure, and plan for timing of extubation. High-dose opioid techniques provide hemodynamic stability, minimal myocardial depression, and decreased reactivity of the pulmonary vasculature. Administration of additional opioid is often the only treatment needed for labile pulmonary artery pressure. A disadvantage of this technique is that these patients are committed to postoperative ventilation.

Maintenance of anesthesia with inhalation agents offers the advantages of the individual agent's hemodynamic effects, the ability to titrate anesthetic depth to match the level of surgical stimulation, and rapid elimination through the lungs to allow the possibility of "early" tracheal extubation at the end of the case.

E. Management of cardiopulmonary bypass for congenital heart disease. The reader is referred to Chapter 7 for a complete discussion of the anesthetic management of cardiopulmonary bypass (CPB). This section will emphasize the unique aspects of CPB for the pediatric patient.

1. Surgical procedures. A median sternotomy incision is made, anticoagulation is achieved with heparin, and the arterial and venous cannulae are inserted. The small vessel size demands accurate cannula positioning to avoid obstruction of vascular branches or misdirecting flow. The superior and inferior vena cavae are usually cannulated separately, and external caval tourniquets are applied to divert systemic venous return completely to the heart-lung machine. A single venous cannula may be used for left heart procedures or if deep hypothermic circulatory arrest is employed with venous cannula removal. Occasionally, (e.g., for repair of an interrupted aortic arch), two arterial cannulae must be inserted for adequate perfusion of the entire body. Previous systemic-to-pulmonary surgical shunts and visible bronchopulmonary collaterals are ligated to prevent systemic hypoperfusion and excessive pulmonary blood flow with left heart filling during CPB. After repair and rewarming are complete, myocardial function and integrity of suture lines may be tested by occluding the venous cannula(e) transiently, allowing the heart to fill and eject. If satisfactory, CPB is discontinued after adequate de-airing, hemostasis is obtained, and the chest is closed.

2. Perfusion technique. The high morbidity and mortality of CPB in infants in the past was due in part to amplification of the deleterious effects of CPB (e.g., hemodilution and damage to blood elements) in pediatric patients. For example, the ratio of pump prime to intravascular volume in an adult is usually about 0.25:1. In contrast, the same ratio in an infant may be 3:1. Therefore, the composition of the circulating volume during bypass is dominated by the composition of the pump prime. This is why erythrocytes must be added to pediatric prime solutions. Newer surfaces and equipment with smaller prime volumes have minimized these problems.

Because an infant's vascular tree is generally free of occlusive disease, it offers little resistance to flow. A manifestation of this low resistance is the low arterial pressures (20–40 mm Hg) seen while on bypass despite high flow rates (up to 150 ml/kg/min compared to adult flows of 50–70 ml/kg/min). These low pressures are usually well tolerated. Increased vigilance is indicated, however, because the combination of low arterial pressure and even a slight increase in central venous pressure (e.g., caused by a misplaced or obstructed venous cannula) may greatly reduce tissue perfusion pressure and cause ischemia.

3. Monitoring CPB. Parameters monitored during CPB include:

a. Anticoagulation. Anticoagulation is done with heparin (3 mg/kg) prior to cannulae insertion. Adequate anticoagulation is determined by an activated coagulation time (ACT) of more than 480 seconds. An ACT should be measured at least every 30 minutes on CPB. Heparin activity is reversed with protamine (1.5 mg/mg heparin) after CPB. Hypotension secondary to protamine administration is less frequent and severe in children than in adults.

b. Arterial pressure. Adequate arterial pressure is required for organ perfusion. Low arterial pressure may indicate low SVR, the presence of bronchopulmonary collaterals, or misplacement of the arterial cannula. High arterial pressure may indicate cannula malposition, high SVR, or light anesthesia.

c. **Central venous pressure.** The central venous pressure may be positive, zero (atmospheric) when the right heart is open, or negative due to the siphon effect of the venous return reservoir. High pressure may indicate hypervolemia, cannulae malposition, or venous line occlusion.

d. **Temperature.** Hypothermia is the cornerstone of organ preservation. Surface cooling promotes uniform hypothermia. Cardiopulmonary bypass with pulsatile flow and the administration of vasodilators (e.g., phentolamine) speed the rate of core cooling. The progress of cooling and rewarming is monitored by thermistors placed at various points to reflect core (nasopharyngeal, tympanic membrane) and shell (rectal, abdominal wall) temperatures. The core temperature changes more quickly than the shell; the rate of change is a measure of tissue perfusion.

e. **Organ perfusion.** The adequacy of perfusion is reflected in the urine output (although it may be normally low during moderate hypothermia), mixed venous oxygen saturation, and acid-base status.

f. **Gas exchange.** The efficiency of respiration may be monitored by measuring PaO_2 and $PaCO_2$. Frequent intermittent or continuous on-line determinations should be made.

g. **Depth of anesthesia.** Although hypothermia decreases anesthetic requirements, anesthetic agents (opioids, amnestic agents, and muscle relaxants) must be administered. The dose of these agents must reflect the increased volume of distribution. The pharmacology of many drugs during bypass remains unknown. Volatile anesthetics may be administered through the bypass circuit.

4. **Specific techniques of myocardial preservation.** Although the mechanism is poorly understood, immature hearts may better withstand ischemic insult, possibly in part due to an increased capacity to produce adenosine triphosphate (ATP) via glycolytic pathways.

a. Cardiopulmonary bypass with systemic hypothermia, aortic crossclamping, and infusion of cold (4°C) cardioplegia solution is the most common technique. Topical cardiac hypothermia is employed by adding iced saline or slush in the pericardial well or a cold jacket with recirculating cold water.

b. Deep hypothermia with circulatory arrest (DHCA) may be used for infants less than 1 year of age (usually <10 kg) or for repair of specific cardiac abnormalities (e.g., aortic arch repair). Advantages of circulatory arrest include a bloodless operating field to permit precise surgical repair, enhanced myocardial preservation by reducing noncoronary blood flow, and decreased blood trauma due to shorter bypass time.

Specifically, core cooling on cardiopulmonary bypass is established until the rectal temperature is 18–20°C and the nasal temperature is 15–17°C. This process usually takes 25–30 minutes and may be speeded by the use of a vasodilator such as phentolamine 0.5 mg/kg. Surface cooling is also employed, including a lowered room temperature and ice applied to the head. The perfusion pump is then stopped, and the body is exsanguinated through the single venous cannula before it is removed. Because circulation is arrested, drugs may not be administered during this time. It is our practice to give additional muscle relaxants just prior to circulatory arrest. Resumption of bypass involves reinsertion of the arterial and venous cannulae and de-airing of the cannulae and heart.

See Chapter 24 for a complete discussion of the conduct of DHCA including use of hemodilution, alpha-stat pH management, avoidance of glucose-containing intravenous or pump prime solutions, and adjuncts such as steroids, mannitol, nimodipine, and thiopental.

c. Continuous coronary perfusion on CPB with cardiac fibrillation is a simple technique for short procedures rarely used today.

5. Separation from CPB

a. Criteria for initiation of separation from bypass must be met prior to attempting to discontinue CPB. The use of a checklist such as the one described in Chapter 8 may be helpful.

b. In pediatric patients, problems with separation from bypass are usually not due to myocardial failure. First check for:

(1) Adequacy of surgical repair. Inspect suture line integrity, graft patency, and valve competence.

(2) Residual shunts. Intracardiac shunting of blood may impede separation from bypass. The residual shunt may be the result of an inadequate repair (e.g., ASD or VSD) or an undiagnosed VSD (muscular VSDs are often multiple).

(3) Arterial outflow or venous inflow obstruction

(a) Arterial outflow obstruction may involve a residual anatomic obstructive lesion, inadequate surgical repair or arterial cannula position. It should be suspected when the heart is distended and cardiac output is low.

(b) Venous inflow obstruction may be a complication of atrial surgery (e.g., total anomalous venous connection, Fontan procedure, and so on) or venous cannula position; it causes systemic or pulmonary venous congestion and underfilling of the heart.

(4) Pulmonary hypertension. High pulmonary vascular resistance is a common problem during separation from bypass. It may be diagnosed by low systemic output, high right-sided pressures, and right heart failure.

(5) Inadequate alveolar ventilation. Normal myocardial function is dependent on adequate oxygenation. As bypass is discontinued, the lungs must assume the role of respiration. If alveolar ventilation is inadequate, hypoxia and hypercarbia may cause heart failure.

(6) Iatrogenic causes. Unknown or excessive administration of myocardial depressants or vasodilators may deter separation from bypass.

(7) Myocardial failure. If present, look for treatable causes such as hyperkalemia or presence of myocardial depressants. Inotropic support is indicated and sometimes continued perfusion or CPB until ventricular function is optimized.

F. Post bypass management

1. Hemodynamic management. The maintenance of hemodynamic stability after CPB often involves continuation of inotropic and vasodilator therapy required for CPB discontinuation and careful volume management. The rapid weaning of these drugs in the operating room gains little and may subject the patient to additional hemodynamic insult. We recommend a slow wean from these drugs in the ICU. Volume is usually replaced with a colloid (blood if required, otherwise an expander such as 5% albumin). The freshest whole blood available should be used to take advantage of functioning platelets and clotting factors.

2. Extubation in the operating room. If extubation is planned prior to transport, the criteria in Table 13-11 must be met. Early extubation avoids the hazards of continued intubation and muscle paralysis (airway trauma or apnea from a circuit disconnection or an

Table 13-11. Criteria for extubation in the operating room

1. Patient must be awake, strong, and warm.
2. Spontaneous ventilation is present with normal blood gas tensions.
3. Cardiopulmonary bypass is not utilized or, if used, aortic cross clamp time is less than 30 minutes.
4. Normal pulmonary artery pressure and reactivity are present.
5. Hemodynamic parameters are stable without pharmacologic support.
6. Hemostasis is adequate.

obstructed endotracheal tube) and positive pressure ventilation (increased airway pressure, elevated PVR, decreased venous return, pneumothorax, and so on). If the patient fails (even marginally) to meet standard extubation criteria, plans should be made for postoperative mechanical ventilation. Our practice is to electively change the endotracheal tube of all infants who require continued mechanical ventilation because small endotracheal tubes can easily become occluded with secretions and blood, and the results of uncontrolled emergency reintubation may be disastrous.

3. **Prior to ICU transport.** Additional muscle relaxant and opioid should be given to intubated patients to smooth the transition to ICU care and prevent the metabolic demands of shivering until the patient is fully rewarmed. Transport from the operating room is not begun until the anesthesiologist and surgeon are satisfied with the patient's condition, emergency drugs are ready, and transport monitors are functional.

V. **Anesthetic management of patients with specific lesions requiring cardiopulmonary bypass.** A general anesthetic plan for surgery requiring CPB is offered in Table 13-12. Modifications to this basic plan are indicated for individual lesions.

A. **Management of cyanotic patients.** The overriding consideration in these patients is optimizing oxygen delivery to the tissues. This requires adequate oxygenation of blood and systemic perfusion (oxygen supply) and depression of oxygen consumption (oxygen demand). It is the rule rather than the exception for oxygenation to improve under anesthesia compared to the awake state. Strategies vary according to lesion.

1. **Tetralogy of Fallot**

a. **General hemodynamic considerations.** Fallot's tetralogy describes a VSD, pulmonary outflow tract obstruction, right ventricular hypertrophy, and an "overriding aorta" (Fig. 13-4). The spatial relationship of the aorta and ventricular septal defect is such that the aorta receives ejected blood from the right ventricle as well as from the left ventricle. Because right ventricular outflow is obstructed, blood is shunted right-to-left through the VSD. The amount of blood shunted depends on the degree of pulmonary outflow tract obstruction, the systemic vascular resistance, and, to a lesser extent, pulmonary vascular resistance. The pulmonary vasculature is "protected" from hypertensive changes by the stenotic right ventricular outflow tract, but it may be of congenital small caliber. Palliative systemic-to-pulmonary surgical shunts increase pulmonary blood flow to improve oxygenation as well as stimulate pulmonary vascular development. The presence of reasonably normal sized pulmonary vessels allows the possibility of complete repair.

b. **Surgical procedure for complete repair**

Table 13-12. General anesthetic plan for surgery requiring CPB

Preoperatively
1. Premedicate as indicated by age. May omit barbiturate if CHF is present.
2. Consider intravenous fluid administration prior to surgery for polycythemic patients.

Prebypass
1. Precool operating room.
2. Supplement the premedication with intravenous opioid, thiopental, benzodiazepine, or ketamine, intramuscular ketamine, or intranasal sufentanil as required to avoid the increased oxygen consumption due to crying and struggling.
3. Place noninvasive monitors, including ECG, BP cuff, precordial stethoscope, and pulse oximeter probe (right arm reflects preductal [brain] saturation). Do not use arm with surgically altered blood flow (e.g., Blalock shunt).
4. Induction may be intravenous or by inhalation. See text under specific lesion.
5. Intravenous catheters may be inserted after induction.
6. Pancuronium 0.15 mg/kg is given, and the patient is intubated. Intravenous fluids (hemodilution) decrease peripheral resistance and may increase pulmonary blood flow.
7. Controlled ventilation is established and adjusted according to the lesion.
8. Central venous, arterial, and urinary bladder catheters are inserted.
9. The patient is positioned for surgery, and final preparations are performed (e.g., insertion of rectal and nasopharyngeal temperature probes, placement of EEG electrodes and ice on the head if circulatory arrest is planned, etc.) while the patient is prepared.
10. An arterial blood specimen is obtained for blood gas tension and baseline ACT measurements.
11. Blood availability is checked, especially for reoperation, or cyanotic patients with extensive collateral vessels.
12. Heparin 3 mg/kg is given by the surgeon after aspiration of blood from right atrium. Nitrous oxide, if used, is discontinued. Anticoagulation is verified by ACT of > 480 sec.

During bypass
1. Ventilation is stopped when left heart ejection ceases.
2. The head is examined for suffusion from misdirected arterial cannula or obstruction to venous drainage.
3. Adequacy of CPB perfusion is monitored by arterial and venous pressures, urine output, rate of temperature changes, pH status, and mixed venous SaO_2.
4. Inotropes, pacemaker, protamine (1.5 mg/mg heparin), and fresh blood are prepared. An airway humidifier is added, and warm IV fluids are prepared. Pressure transducers are recalibrated.
5. On rewarming, additional opioid, sedative, and muscle relaxant are given as indicated. Ice, if used, is removed from the head, warming blanket is turned on, and room temperature is elevated.

Postbypass
1. Separation from CPB may be attempted when the repair is complete, the rectal temperature is greater than 32.5°C, adequate cardiac rhythm is present, and electrolytes, acid-base status, and hemoglobin are within acceptable ranges. The lungs are ventilated with 100% oxygen, and breath sounds are checked.
2. After patient has been weaned from CPB and is hemodynamically stable, protamine is given, hemostasis is obtained, and the chest is closed.

CHF = congenital heart failure, BP = blood pressure, EEG = electroencephalogram, ACT = activated clotting time.

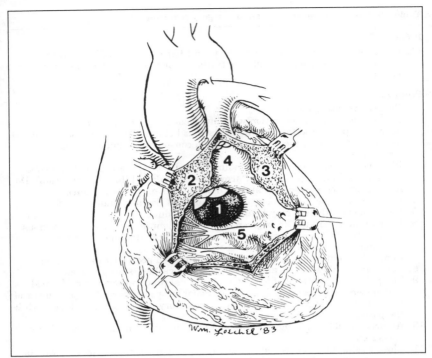

Fig. 13-4. Tetralogy of Fallot showing ventricular septal defect (VSD) with overriding aorta *(1)*, hypertrophied parietal *(2)* and septal *(3)* bands. The infundibular septum *(4)* is hypoplastic and deviated anteriorly. The papillary muscle of the conus *(5)* inserts along the lower margin of the VSD. (From E. Arciniegas [ed.], *Pediatric Cardiac Surgery.* Chicago: Year Book, 1985. P. 204. With permission.)

(1) Ligation of previous systemic-to-pulmonary shunt.
(2) Excision of parietal and septal muscle band in right ventricular outflow tract.
(3) Patch closure of VSD.
(4) Right ventricular outflow tract patch (subannular or transannular).
(5) Right ventricle (RV) to pulmonary artery (PA) conduit for pulmonary atresia or anomalous course of the left anterior descending coronary artery.

c. **Anesthetic considerations**

(1) **Preoperative.** Important information to be obtained preoperatively includes the degree and frequency of symptoms ("tet spells"), history of previous palliative procedure, and evidence of heart failure. Useful catheterization data include size of the pulmonary arteries, presence of an anomalous left anterior descending coronary artery that crosses the right ventricular infundibulum, ventricular function, and size of the pulmonary valve annulus.

(2) **Intraoperative.** Intraoperative prebypass management includes maintaining intravascular volume, minimizing PVR (although the major impedance to pulmonary blood flow is the

stenotic right ventricular outflow tract), and maintaining SVR. Negative inotropic agents (halothane or, rarely, propranolol or esmolol) may be useful to relieve infundibular "spasm" and increase pulmonary blood flow. Intravenous induction has been recommended as the induction of choice in the past, but inhalation induction with halothane has recently been shown to increase arterial oxygenation uniformly. This result, despite theoretical disadvantages including slow rate of change of blood anesthetic tension, myocardial depression, and possibly decreased SVR and increased shunting, is probably due to decreased total body oxygen consumption and increased pulmonary blood flow due to relaxation of the pulmonary outflow tract (infundibulum). If an intravenous induction is preferred, a technique that maintains SVR would be appropriate (e.g., opioid or ketamine). Hypotension prebypass is usually due to hypovolemia and responds well to intravenous fluids. The hemorrheologic effects (decreased viscosity, increased pulmonary blood flow, and cardiac output) associated with even mild hemodilution may also be clinically useful. Postbypass management includes support of right ventricular function, if necessary, and maneuvers to decrease PVR. Successful weaning from CPB depends on the adequacy of surgical repair, right ventricular function, pulmonary artery size and reactivity, and myocardial preservation. An inotropic agent (e.g., dopamine 5–10 µg/kg) may be necessary, especially if a right ventriculotomy was performed. Occasionally, transient atrioventricular conduction disturbance necessitates temporary atrioventricular sequential pacing.

 d. Problems and complications
  (1) Residual right ventricular outflow obstruction
  (2) Dysrhythmias
  (3) Right ventricular failure (especially if ventriculotomy performed)
  (4) Heart block
  (5) Excessive pulmonary flow via bronchopulmonary collaterals or residual VSD

2. Transposition of the great arteries
 a. General hemodynamic considerations. Transposition of the great arteries (TGA) creates two independent parallel circulations (Fig. 13-5A). One circuit carries blood to the lungs and back (LA-LV-PA), and the other carries blood to the periphery and back (RA-RV-AO). This condition is incompatible with life if there is no communication between the two circulations. Mixing of the two circulations may take place at the atrial, ventricular, or arterial (ductus arteriosus) level. If the ductus arteriosus is the only communication, ductal closure is rapidly fatal. A VSD is present in about 15% of patients. If the arterial switch operation is planned for patients with an intact ventricular septum, surgery should be performed early in the neonatal period before PVR falls and the left ventricle (LV) loses muscle mass.

 b. Surgical procedures
  (1) Atrial redirection operations, such as the Senning or Mustard procedure, use an intra-atrial baffle to direct systemic venous return to the left ventricle (and pulmonary artery) and the pulmonary venous return to the right ventricle (and aorta).
  (2) The arterial switch (Jatene) operation (Fig. 13-5B–D) involves transection of the aorta above the coronary ostia, which are excised with a "button" of surrounding aortic wall. The aorta

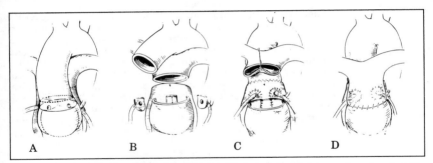

Fig. 13-5. Transposition of the great arteries *(A)*. Arterial switch operation showing division of the great arteries and excision of the coronary ostial buttons *(B)*. Transfer of the coronary arteries to the neoascending aorta and anastomosis of the neoascending aorta to the distal ascending aorta *(C)*. Anastomosis of the neomain pulmonary artery to the distal main pulmonary artery. (From E. Arciniegas [ed.], *Pediatric Cardiac Surgery.* Chicago: Year Book, 1985. P. 275. With permission.)

is passed behind the pulmonary arteries, the proximal pulmonary artery is transected, and the coronary ostia are reimplanted in the proximal pulmonary artery. The aorta is then sewn to the proximal pulmonary artery above the transplanted coronary ostia to complete the left-sided circulation. The pulmonary artery is brought forward and attached to the right ventricular outflow tract. A large patch of pericardium is used to repair the defects created by removal of the coronary buttons.

(3) The Rastelli repair is well suited for patients with TGA and associated VSD and left ventricular outflow tract obstruction. The repair involves patching the VSD so that left ventricular blood is directed to the aorta and connecting the right ventricle to the pulmonary artery by a valved external conduit.

c. **Anesthetic considerations**

(1) **Preoperative.** If hypoxia is severe (owing to inadequate mixing of blood from the separate pulmonary and systemic circulations), a balloon atrial septostomy (Rashkind) should be performed at the time of cardiac catheterization. This procedure creates a large interatrial communication and thereby improves mixing at the atrial level. The use of PGE_1 to maintain patency of the ductus in neonates may also be lifesaving. Premedication in neonates is usually not necessary.

(2) **Intraoperative.** Induction may be intravenous or inhalational, taking care not to provoke an increase (or large decrease) in pulmonary vascular resistance. This may be accomplished by maintaining normal $PaCO_2$, pH balance, oxygenation, and adequate anesthesia. PGE_1 in neonates is discontinued after bypass has been instituted. Myocardial preservation and continuity of the coronary circulation are important.

Specific points for the Jatene procedure include consideration of starting a nitroglycerin infusion (1μg/kg/min) after removing the aortic cross-clamp. ST-segment elevation may occur, especially in the inferior leads because the nondependent position of the right coronary ostia favors embolism of air. If coronary artery air embolism is suspected, intermittent transient occlusion of the aorta distal to the aortic cannula will "hyperperfuse" the coronaries and help push any air through the myocardial circulation. The ability of the left ventricle to accept systemic vascular resistance is readily apparent.

Postoperative ventilation is used for 24 hours. Continuation of the nitroglycerin infusion should be considered. Myocardial ischemia that is more than transient may require cardiac catheterization to delineate coronary abnormalities. Treatment of infarction parallels that of adult patients (supplemental oxygen, ECG monitoring, nitroglycerin, afterload reduction, and arrhythmia management).

d. Problems and complications
   (1) Mustard or Senning operation
      (a) Atrial arrhythmia (sick sinus syndrome)
      (b) Systemic or pulmonary venous inflow obstruction (secondary to the atrial baffle)
      (c) Right (systemic) ventricular failure
      (d) Systemic (tricuspid) valve insufficiency
      (e) Residual atrial shunt
   (2) Arterial switch operation
      (a) Myocardial ischemia
      (b) Left (systemic) ventricular failure
      (c) Supravalvular pulmonary stenosis (late)
      (d) Supraventricular aortic stenosis (rare)
   (3) Rastelli
      (a) Conduit obstruction
      (b) Persistent atrial shunt

3. Tricuspid atresia
a. General hemodynamic considerations.
The flow of blood from the right atrium to the right ventricle is prevented by the atretic tricuspid valve (Fig. 13-6); thus all systemic venous blood must cross the atrial septum into the left atrium through a patent foramen ovale or an ASD (obligatory right-to-left shunt). The left atrium and left ventricle are enlarged owing to the increased volume. Pulmonary blood flow is dependent on the presence of a VSD or PDA. With normally related great arteries, pulmonary blood flow may occur through a VSD into the hypoplastic right ventricle and then into the pulmonary arteries. A large VSD without associated pulmonic stenosis results in unrestricted pulmonary blood flow, whereas pulmonic stenosis or a restrictive VSD reduces pulmonary blood flow. Transposition of the great arteries (the aorta arises from the hypoplastic RV) is present in about 30% of cases.

b. Surgical procedures.
The Fontan procedure (Fig. 13-7) represents a "reparative" procedure in which the right atrium is isolated and anastomosed to the pulmonary artery. Pulmonary blood flow is entirely dependent on the pressure gradient across the lung (CVP–LAP) because there is no ventricle in the right-sided circulation. Ideal criteria for the Fontan operation include PAP of less than 20 mm Hg, PVR of less than 4 Wood units, sinus rhythm, LVEF of more than 0.6, LVEDP of less than 10, PA/AO diameter more than 0.75, normal systemic venous drainage, and no systemic atrioventricular valve dysfunction. Recent experience has shown that the major preoperative risk factors are distorted pulmonary arteries and elevated pulmonary vascular resistance.

c. Anesthetic considerations
   (1) **Preoperative.** Chest x ray, echocardiography, and cardiac catheterization data are important to determine whether there is associated TGA and to assess the pulmonary outflow tract. Preoperative inotropic support may be required for left ven-

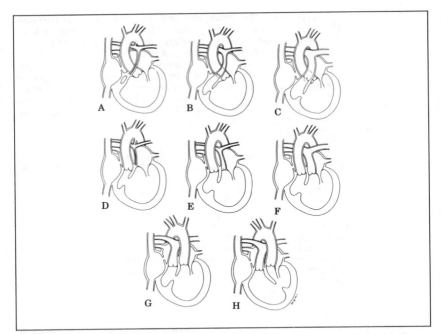

Fig. 13-6. Type I tricuspid atresia: without transposition of the great arteries. *A.* Type Ia, pulmonary atresia with virtual absence of the right ventricle. *B.* Type Ib, pulmonary hypoplasia with subpulmonary stenosis, diminutive right ventricle, and small ventricular septal defect *C.* Type Ic, no pulmonary hypoplasia. There is a diminutive right ventricle. Type II tricuspid atresia: with D-transposition of the great arteries. *D.* Type IIa, pulmonary atresia, aorta arises from the right ventricle. *E.* Type IIb, pulmonary or subpulmonary stenosis. *F.* Type IIc, normal or enlarged pulmonary artery. Type III tricuspid atresia: with I-transposition of the great arteries. *G.* Type IIIa, pulmonary or subpulmonary stenosis. *H.* Type IIIb, subaortic stenosis. There is ventricular inversion. (From E. Arciniegas [ed.], *Pediatric Cardiac Surgery.* Chicago: Year Book, 1985. Pp. 298–300. With permission.)

tricular cardiomyopathy due to chronic volume overload. In neonates with reduced pulmonary blood flow, PGE_1 (0.1 µg/kg/min) should be started to maintain ductal patency, and balloon atrial septostomy may be performed at catheterization if the atrial septal defect or patent foramen ovale (PFO) is small. Premedicate as heavily as tolerated.

(2) **Intraoperative.** Intraoperative management is centered around maneuvers to maintain optimal intravascular volume and decrease pulmonary vascular resistance and left atrial pressure to promote pulmonary blood flow. Induction of anesthesia may be inhalational if the airway is carefully maintained to prevent rises in pulmonary vascular resistance and hypotension is avoided (ductal flow is dependent on arterial pressure). For patients with compromised ventricular function (requiring preoperative inotropic support) an intravenous induction with an agent that has minimal negative inotropic effect and maintains SVR (opioid or ketamine) may be preferable. If the patient underwent a previous palliative procedure, increased bleeding

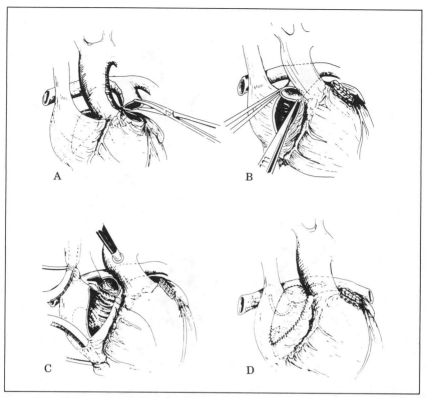

Fig. 13-7. Modified Fontan operation. The main pulmonary artery is divided *(A)* and then passed behind the aorta and sutured to the superior aspect of the right atrium *(B)*. The pulmonary artery incision is extended into the right pulmonary artery, and the atrial septal defect is closed *(C)*. A large patch of pericardium is used to ensure a large anastomosis *(D)*. (From J. E. Molina, Y. Wang, R. Lucas, et al. The technique of the Fontan procedure with posterior right atrium-pulmonary artery connection. *Ann. Thorac. Surg.* 39(4):372–373, 1985. With permission.)

before bypass should be anticipated from pericardial collaterals and adhesions.

Bronchopulmonary collaterals may allow blood to reach the myocardium during bypass and inhibit hypothermic myocardial preservation by rewarming the heart even though the aorta is cross-clamped. The preexisting ventricular dysfunction and relatively long bypass time sometimes required for repair make the use of inotropes and vasodilators likely on separation from bypass. Starting these agents during partial bypass will increase the success rate of the first attempt to discontinue CPB. It is important to maintain an adequate CVP (12–15 mm Hg) while minimizing LAP.

Positive pressure ventilation decreases pulmonary blood flow and should be discontinued postoperatively as soon as practical. Despite this disadvantage, positive pressure ventilation may be required to prevent rises in $PaCO_2$ and pulmo-

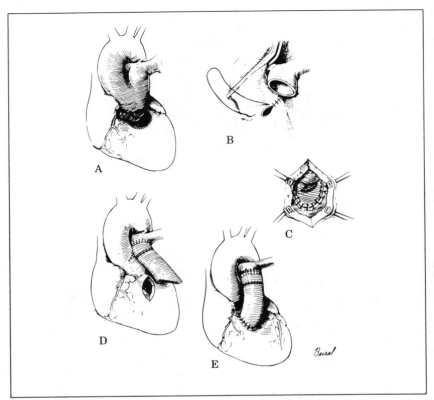

Fig. 13-8. *A.* Truncus arteriosus. *B.* The pulmonary trunk is separated. *C.* The ventricular septal defect is closed with a prosthetic patch. *D.* A valved conduit (usually pulmonary allograft) is used to establish right ventricle to pulmonary artery continuity. *E.* The complete repair. (From J. A. Waldhausen and W. S. Pierce, *Johnson's Surgery of the Chest* [5th ed.]. Chicago: Year Book, 1985. P. 397. With permission.)

nary hypertension in younger patients with reactive pulmonary vasculature. If positive pressure ventilation is necessary, the inspiratory time should be shortened and mean airway pressure minimized.

  d. Problems and complications
  (1) Systemic venous hypertension (hepatomegaly, ascites, pleural and pericardial effusions)
  (2) Atrial dysrhythmias
  (3) Residual left-to-right shunt through bronchopulmonary collaterals
  (4) Residual right-to-left atrial level shunt causing systemic arterial desaturation.

4. Truncus arteriosus
  a. General hemodynamic considerations. The truncus arteriosus is a single great vessel that gives rise to the coronary, pulmonary, and systemic circulations (Fig. 13-8*A*). It represents the failure of the conotruncal ridges to separate the embryologic truncus arteriosus into the aorta and pulmonary artery. The main pulmonary

artery may arise from the truncus, or one or both branch pulmonary arteries may arise separately from the truncus. A VSD is invariably present, straddled by the truncus. Cyanosis results from the mixing of systemic and pulmonary blood at the level of the VSD-truncus. The truncal valve may have two to six cusps, and insufficiency may be present. Pulmonary blood flow is excessive, especially after pulmonary vascular resistance decreases early in life.

b. Surgical procedures. Repair should be accomplished in the first several months of life, after pulmonary vascular resistance decreases but before the increased pulmonary blood flow induces obstructive vascular changes. Repair is attained by patching the VSD and then separating the pulmonary circulation from the truncus (Fig. 13-8B–D). This may be done by placing a valved conduit between the right ventricle and the pulmonary artery. Truncal valve replacement may be necessary for valve insufficiency.

c. Anesthetic considerations. Maneuvers to decrease pulmonary blood flow are helpful during the prebypass period. These include limitation of inspired oxygen concentration, maintenance of normocarbia, intubating only after an adequate level of anesthesia is obtained, and mechanical compression of the pulmonary artery by the surgeon if necessary, after the chest is open. Conversely, efforts should be directed at increasing pulmonary blood flow after repair and weaning from bypass. Use of 100% inspired oxygen, hyperventilation, and correction of acidosis are the mainstays of treatment. Right ventricular failure postoperatively may be secondary to elevated pulmonary vascular resistance or obstructed conduit. Inotropes or vasodilators may be required for separation from bypass. Postoperative mechanical ventilation is employed to maintain hypocarbia and PaO_2 at over 100 to reduce PVR.

d. Problems and complications

(1) Pulmonary hypertension or conduit obstruction and right ventricular failure.

(2) Truncal valve regurgitation and left ventricular failure.

(3) Persistent VSD and left-to-right shunt.

5. Total anomalous pulmonary venous connection

a. General hemodynamic considerations. Pulmonary venous blood drains into the right side of the heart and mixes with desaturated systemic venous blood. Some of this partially saturated blood crosses an associated patent foramen ovale or atrial septal defect, which causes systemic cyanosis when ejected systemically. The pulmonary veins may drain into the superior vena cava and its branches (supracardiac type) (Fig. 13-9A, top), the inferior vena cava and its branches or the portal venous system (infracardiac type) (Fig. 13-9A, middle), or the coronary sinus or right atrium (intracardiac type) (Fig. 13-9A, bottom). There is enlargement of the right atrium, volume overload of the right ventricle, and increased pulmonary blood flow. Pulmonary vascular congestion is worsened by the presence of pulmonary venous obstruction. With the typical supracardiac type, a vertical vein attaches the pulmonary confluence to the innominate vein, which drains into the right atrium. The intracardiac type describes a connection between the pulmonary confluence and the RA or the coronary sinus. A descending vertical vein traverses the diaphragm to drain the pulmonary confluence into an abdominal vein (often hepatic) in the infracardiac type.

b. Surgical procedures. Treatment involves restoring the pulmonary venous return directly into the left atrium and closing the ASD (Fig. 13-9B). The pulmonary venous confluence is anasto-

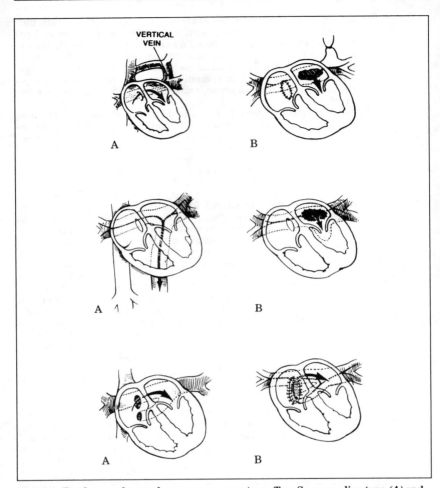

Fig. 13-9. Total anomalous pulmonary venous return. *Top.* Supracardiac type *(A)* and surgical correction *(B)*. *Middle.* Infracardiac type *(A)* and surgical correction *(B)*. *Bottom.* Intracardiac type *(A)* and surgical correction *(B)*. (From J. A. Waldhausen and W. S. Pierce, *Johnson's Surgery of the Chest* [5th ed.]. Chicago: Year Book, 1985. Pp. 355, 357, 359. With permission.)

mosed to the posterior aspect of the left atrium, and the anomalous vein is often ligated. For intracardiac communications, the coronary sinus is incised into the left atrium, and a patch is used to direct pulmonary venous return through the ASD into the left atrium.

c. **Anesthetic considerations**

(1) **Preoperative.** Interventions emphasize maintaining normal PVR and supporting ventricular function. Treatment of pulmonary edema secondary to increased pulmonary blood flow or pulmonary venous obstruction may require positive pressure

ventilation and inotropes. Increases in pulmonary blood flow may be minimized by avoiding hyperventilation and high inspired concentrations of oxygen.

(2) **Intraoperative.** An opioid technique is often used because myocardial depression is minimal and early extubation (day of surgery) is unlikely. Increased pulmonary blood flow and pulmonary venous congestion are often associated with increased pulmonary vascular reactivity. Separation from bypass may be facilitated by taking steps to decrease pulmonary vascular resistance (by initiating hyperventilation, 100% FIO_2, alkalosis) prior to weaning from bypass. If inotropes were required preoperatively they are usually utilized to facilitate weaning from CPB. Postoperative mechanical ventilation is usually required, and adequate sedation (e.g., fentanyl infusion) is advisable to blunt pulmonary vascular reactivity.

d. Problems and complications

(1) Pulmonary venous obstruction

(2) Increased pulmonary vascular reactivity

(3) Pulmonary parenchymal disease

6. Hypoplastic left heart syndrome (HLHS)

a. General hemodynamic considerations. There is an obligatory left-to-right shunting of blood at the atrial level (and complete mixing) because the mitral valve, left ventricle, and ascending aorta are hypoplastic or atretic (Fig. 13-10*A*). Systemic blood flow is entirely dependent on right-to-left shunting through the ductus arteriosus. Coronary blood flow is maintained by retrograde flow through the hypoplastic ascending aorta. Systemic perfusion is severely limited by ductal closure or, if the ductus is kept open, by "pulmonary steal" as the PVR decreases. Metabolic acidosis and organ dysfunction are consequences of chronic systemic hypoperfusion.

b. Surgical procedures. The Fontan operation is the definitive surgical correction, but it requires low pulmonary vascular resistance. Because PVR is elevated at birth and decreases during the first year of life, a staged approach is necessary. The first stage involves atrial septectomy and reconstruction of the aortic arch using a pulmonary allograft and incorporating the proximal main pulmonary artery (Norwood procedure) (Fig. 13-10*B–F*). Pulmonary blood flow is supplied by a separate surgical shunt (e.g., modified central or Blalock-Taussig shunt). The second stage is undertaken between 1 and 3 years of age when PVR has declined. A modified Fontan procedure separates the pulmonary from the systemic circulation, restoring the normal series arrangement of the circulation.

c. Anesthetic considerations. The delicate balance of pulmonary and systemic vascular resistances must be maintained to provide adequate oxygenation as well as systemic perfusion. For example, a systemic saturation of 75–80% represents a $\dot{Q}p/\dot{Q}s$ ratio of approximately 1–2:1 (assuming an SvO_2 of 50%). If interventions that decrease PVR (hyperventilation, high inspired oxygen) are employed, the SaO_2 may increase to 85–90%, but this increase in pulmonary blood flow necessarily decreases systemic flow ($\dot{Q}p/\dot{Q}s$ increases to 4–5:1) and may cause hypoperfusion and metabolic acidosis (Fig. 13-11). An SaO_2 of approximately 80% is desirable.

The myocardium may require inotropic support and may be irritable if coronary blood flow is borderline. Renal failure may

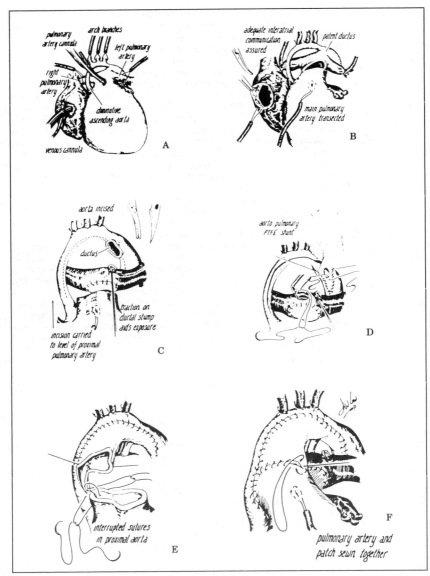

Fig. 13-10. *A.* Hypoplastic left heart anatomy. *B.* Atrial septectomy and division of main pulmonary artery. *C.* Patch closure of distal main pulmonary artery, ligation, and division of patent ductus arteriosus. *D.* Incision of the entire hypoplastic aortic arch and homograft patch enlargement and central aortopulmonary shunt. *E.* Anastomosis of proximal main pulmonary artery reconstructed aortic arch. *F.* Completed repair. (From L. H. Edwards et al. *Atlas of Cardiothoracic Surgery.* Philadelphia: Lea & Febiger, in press. With permission.)

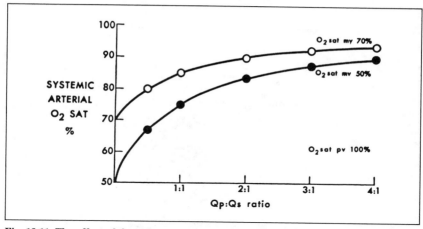

Fig. 13-11. The effect of the pulmonary-systemic blood flow ($\dot{Q}p/\dot{Q}s$) ratio on the systemic arterial oxygen saturation when there is complete admixture of both systemic and pulmonary venous returns. (From A. M. Rudolph [ed.], *Congenital Diseases of the Heart.* Chicago: Year Book, 1974. P. 125. With permission.)

be present, complicating management. No premedication is necessary. Induction and maintenance of anesthesia are usually accomplished with an opioid agent to minimize myocardial depression. After repair, hyperventilation is maintained initially to promote pulmonary blood flow. The FIO_2 is reduced to the lowest concentration that maintains SaO_2 at 80–85 percent. The PCO_2 may then be slowly normalized (while monitoring effect on SaO_2) by reducing mechanical ventilation to prevent excessive pulmonary blood flow. Sedation is recommended to prevent pulmonary hypertensive episodes.

d. Problems and complications
(1) Persistent myocardial ischemia related to distortion of ascending aortic anastomosis
(2) Myocardial failure and low output syndrome
(3) Tricuspid (systemic atrioventricular valve) regurgitation
(4) Decreased or excessive pulmonary blood flow (depends on surgical shunt size and PVR/SVR ratio)
(5) Pulmonary hypertensive crisis

B. Management of patients with congestive heart failure.
The anesthetic management of patients with congestive heart failure, whether secondary to left-to-right shunting, obstruction to ventricular ejection, or primary cardiomyopathy, is based on maintaining myocardial contractility, afterload reduction, and manipulation of pulmonary vascular resistance. In lesions with associated cyanosis, arterial hypoxemia further compromises ventricular function. Judicious volume replacement is required to avoid further fluid overload while maintaining the higher filling pressures required by the failing ventricle.

1. VSD
a. General hemodynamic considerations.
Although the defect may be located anywhere in the ventricular septum, the most common location is the perimembranous region. Other sites include the muscular septum and infundibulum (Fig. 13-12). Shunting of blood from left to right occurs through the VSD (simple shunt), increas-

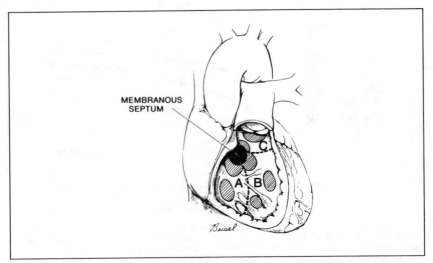

Fig. 13-12. The location of ventricular septal defects in the membranous inlet *(A)*, trabecular *(B)*, and infundibular *(C)* septa. (From J. A. Waldhausen and W. S. Pierce [eds.], *Johnson's Surgery of the Chest* [5th ed.]. Chicago: Year Book, 1985. P. 335. With permission.)

ing pulmonary blood flow, left atrial volume, and left ventricular work. If the VSD is large, the amount of shunt flow is dependent on the PVR/SVR ratio. Small VSDs are termed *restrictive* because a pressure gradient is present between the two ventricles. Shunt flow is then limited by VSD orifice size and is less dependent on PVR/SVR ratio. High pulmonary blood flow reduces pulmonary compliance, increases the work of breathing, and may precipitate respiratory failure. Pulmonary hypertension associated with high pulmonary flows (e.g., $\dot{Q}p/\dot{Q}s = 2$–$4{:}1$) and normal to moderately elevated PVR is more likely to normalize after repair than pulmonary hypertension at lower flows (which reflects pulmonary vascular obstructive changes). Irreversible pulmonary vascular change may occur with time in patients with moderate to large VSDs, and therefore surgical closure of the VSD is recommended during the first year of life.

b. Surgical procedures. Repair is usually accomplished with a Dacron patch, approaching the ventricular septal defect through the right atrium and tricuspid valve. A ventriculotomy may be needed for defects located in the ventricular apex or in the right ventricular outflow tract.

c. Anesthetic considerations. Premedication is dependent on the degree of ventricular dysfunction that is present. The goal is to have a sleeping child on arrival in the operating room. Crying or struggling will only further stress a compromised circulatory system. The preoperative opioid dose should be reduced in patients with severe pulmonary hypertension because the rise in PCO_2 secondary to respiratory depression may elevate PAP further and reduce pulmonary blood flow. Supplemental oxygen administration should be considered at the time of premedication.

Anesthesia may be induced with ketamine or an opioid for

patients with poor ventricular function, or an inhalational agent for those who can tolerate the additional myocardial depression. Supplemental intravenous volume may be useful after induction as discussed earlier. If the VSD is nonrestrictive and pulmonary blood flow is increased, ventilation should be adjusted to maintain normocarbia and inspired oxygen limited to prevent reduction of pulmonary vascular resistance and further increases in pulmonary blood flow ("pulmonary steal").

Separation from bypass may be more difficult for patients with preexisting pulmonary hypertension and right ventricular dysfunction and those who required a ventriculotomy for repair. Heart block occurs infrequently and is usually related to edema around the conduction system from surgical traction or suture placement. Improper suture technique can also injure the conduction system. Atrioventricular pacing is utilized in these instances. Efforts should be directed toward lowering PVR prior to termination of bypass to minimize right ventricular afterload. If there is unusual difficulty in weaning the patient from bypass, the possibility of another VSD (often muscular) or shunt (PDA) should be considered.

  d. Problems and complications
  - **(1)** Right ventricular failure and arrhythmias may be caused by increased PVR or ventriculotomy.
  - **(2)** Respiratory failure may be seen in patients with large VSDs and increased lung water.
  - **(3)** Heart block may occur.
  - **(4)** Right ventricular volume overload may occur if there is a persistent left-to-right shunt.
  - **(5)** Rarely, there may be right ventricular outflow tract obstruction due to patch malposition, or aortic regurgitation after repair of a subaortic VSD due to traction and distortion of the septal cusp.

2. ASD
  a. General hemodynamic considerations. There are three types of ASD(Fig. 13-13).
  - **(1)** Secundum defects (the most common) are located in the mid-atrium and are a deficiency in septum primum.
  - **(2)** Primum defects are located adjacent to the atrioventricular valves (an endocardial cushion defect).
  - **(3)** Sinus venosus defects are located at the caval-atrial junction and are often associated with partial anomalous pulmonary venous connections.

There is a left-to-right shunt at the atrial level and right ventricular volume overload. The amount of shunt flow depends on the defect size and ratio of ventricular compliance (simple shunt physiology). Early in life the shunt flow is small, and symptoms rare because the right ventricle is relatively noncompliant. As the left ventricle becomes less compliant and PVR decreases, shunt flow increases. It is rare for pulmonary vascular changes to be induced by shunting from an ASD because pulmonary artery pressures are usually only slightly elevated, but repair is indicated because there is an increased incidence of endocarditis and paradoxical emboli.

  b. Surgical procedures. Repair is performed through the right atrium. Small defects may be closed primarily, but more commonly a patch is used. For patients with a sinus venosus defect with partial anomalous pulmonary venous connection, a patch is fashioned to divert the anomalous pulmonary venous flow through the

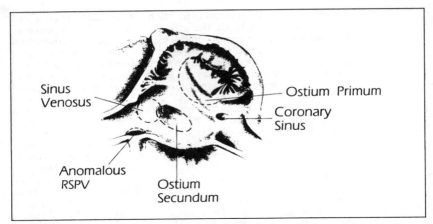

Fig. 13-13. Artist's depiction of the opened right atrium showing the anatomic location of atrial septal defects. RSPV = right superior pulmonary vein. (From D. B. Doty. *Cardiac Surgery.* Chicago: Year Book, 1985. ASD P. 1. With permission.)

ASD and into the left atrium. A cleft anterior mitral valve leaflet, which is almost always present with primum defects, is repaired if regurgitation occurs through the cleft. Patch sutures must avoid the atrioventricular node and penetrating bundle.

- c. **Anesthetic considerations.** Because these patients are usually minimally symptomatic, they are premedicated as indicated for age. Anesthesia may be induced with almost any agent, including thiopental. In the choice of maintenance anesthetic the possibility of extubation at the end of the case should be considered.

   Although the predominant shunt is left-to-right, extreme care should be taken to avoid venous air embolism because "paradoxical" arterial embolism may occur. Several anesthetic interventions (positive airway pressure, Valsalva maneuver, and so on) may create right atrial pressures higher than left atrial pressures and transiently reverse the direction of shunt flow.

   The duration of cardiopulmonary bypass is usually less than 1 hour. Separation from bypass is usually without incident. Difficulty with weaning from bypass should alert the operating room team to the possible existence of another lesion. Supplemental opioids given after bypass should be limited to permit the possibility of extubation at the end of the case. The patient may be extubated in the operating room if the usual criteria are met.

   Postoperative atrial dysrhythmias may be treated with verapamil or digoxin.
- d. **Problems and complications**
   - (1) Atrial dysrhythmias and persistent left-to-right shunt from patch dehiscence may occur with any type of ASD.
   - (2) Heart block and atrioventricular valve regurgitation may occur after ASD primum repair.
3. **Atrioventricular septal defect (atrioventricular canal)**
   - a. **General hemodynamic considerations.** This lesion includes defects of the inferior atrial septum (primum ASD), inlet ventricular septum, and the atrioventricular valves (Fig. 13-14A). A complete atrioventricular canal has a single common atrioventricular valve. A partial atrioventricular canal can have one of a continuum of

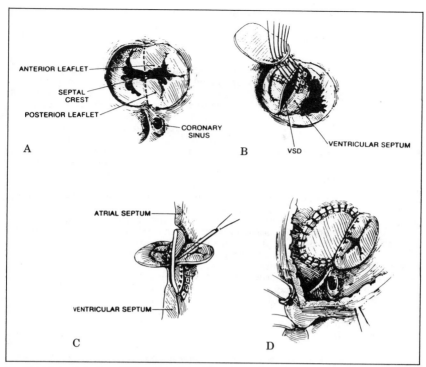

Fig. 13-14. *A.* Artist's depiction of complete atrioventricular canal as viewed from above. *B.* The pericardial patch is attached to the rightward aspect of the ventricular septum. *C.* The valve leaflets are attached to the pericardial patch. *D.* The completed repair from the right atrial view. (From J. A. Waldhausen and W. S. Pierce [eds.], *Johnson's Surgery of the Chest* [5th ed.]. Chicago: Year Book, 1985. P. 349. With permission.)

atrioventricular valve types from a common valve to the usual two-valve arrangement. There is communication between all four chambers of the heart and usually increased pulmonary blood flow. The defect is most commonly nonrestrictive, so the direction and magnitude of shunting are entirely dependent on the ratio of systemic and pulmonary vascular resistances and the differences in diastolic filling of the ventricles. The atrioventricular valve is usually competent, and insufficiency worsens the prognosis. Approximately 50 percent of patients with this lesion have Down's syndrome.

b. **Surgical procedures.** Repair (Fig. 13-14*B–D*) is carried out through the right atrium, first patching the VSD, then attaching the "midline" atrioventricular valve leaflets to the VSD patch to form two atrioventricular valves, then closing the ASD. To prevent damage to the conduction system, the suture line should avoid the area of the atrioventricular node and penetrating bundle. The atrial patch is sutured around the right side of the coronary sinus to avoid the conduction system and as a result of this, the coronary sinus drains into the left atrium. A mitral or tricuspid annuloplasty may be required to establish valve competence.

c. Anesthetic considerations. Premedication should reflect the often exaggerated effect of sedatives in patients with Down's syndrome. Intravenous induction may be preferable to minimize myocardial depression and systemic hypotension. Maneuvers to minimize excess pulmonary blood flow are useful before bypass. Abrupt rises in systemic vascular resistance must be avoided to prevent further increases in pulmonary blood flow. In infants, deep hypothermia with circulatory arrest or low flow CPB is utilized. Separation from bypass may be difficult because of ventricular dysfunction, high pulmonary vascular resistance, and possible atrioventricular valve regurgitation. Inotropic support and measures to decrease PVR are indicated. Atrioventricular conduction problems may require atrioventricular pacing. Continued sedation and mechanical ventilation are necessary for patients with increased pulmonary vasculature reactivity (especially Down's patients).

d. Problems and complications

(1) Persistent pulmonary hypertension may cause right ventricular failure.

(2) Mitral regurgitation worsens pulmonary hypertension.

(3) Long-term atrioventricular conduction problems are surprisingly rare (91 percent of patients are free of heart block at 1 year postoperatively).

VI. Anesthetic management of patients for procedures not requiring cardiopulmonary bypass. Pediatric cardiac surgical procedures that do not require CPB may be palliative (e.g., systemic-to-pulmonary or cavopulmonary shunts, pulmonary artery banding, and atrial septectomy) or curative (e.g., PDA ligation or division, aortic coarctation repair, and division of a vascular ring). These procedures avoid the detrimental effects of CPB but require maintenance of circulatory stability without mechanical support. Anesthetic management must consider the cardiac lesion's pathophysiology and the impact of thoracotomy and vascular manipulation. Symptomatology varies widely in this diverse group of patients, ranging from asymptomatic older patients undergoing elective closure of a patent ductus arteriosus to very ill neonates.

A. Procedures to relieve cyanosis

1. Systemic-to-pulmonary shunt

a. General hemodynamic considerations. Cyanosis caused by inadequate pulmonary blood flow may be palliated by providing systemic arterial blood to the pulmonary vasculature (Fig. 13-15). The oxygen saturation of partially saturated systemic arterial blood should improve on this "second pass" through the lungs but must mix with desaturated systemic venous return prior to systemic ejection. The resulting systemic SaO_2 therefore depends on the ratio of pulmonary-to-systemic blood flow ($\dot{Q}p/\dot{Q}s$) and the saturation of mixed venous blood ($S\bar{v}O_2$). If $S\bar{v}O_2$ is 50%, $\dot{Q}p/\dot{Q}s$ must be 3–4:1 to attain a systemic SaO_2 higher than 85%. This could result in ventricular volume overload, pulmonary vascular obstructive changes, and systemic hypoperfusion. The shunt size must be chosen very carefully to allow adequate but not excessive pulmonary blood flow.

In addition to improving arterial oxygen content, the increased pulmonary blood flow stimulates pulmonary artery growth, a prerequisite for later reparative surgery.

b. Surgical procedures

(1) **Systemic-to-pulmonary shunts.** There are a variety of surgical procedures available, some not requiring a synthetic graft (Blalock-Taussig, Potts, Waterston), and some that do (modified Blalock). The advantage of using a synthetic tube graft is

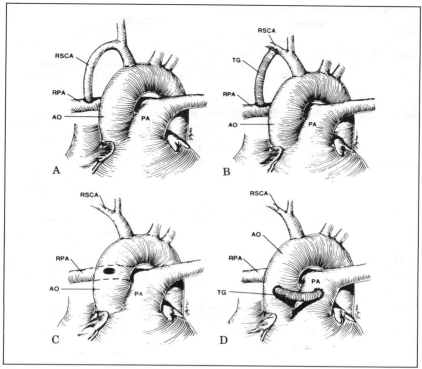

Fig. 13-15. Types of systemic-to-pulmonary artery anastomoses. *A.* Classic Blalock-Taussig anastomosis. *B.* Modified Blalock-Taussig shunt using prosthetic graft. *C.* Direct aortopulmonary (Waterston) anastomosis. *D.* Central aortopulmonary shunt with prosthetic graft. RSCA = right subclavian artery, RPA = right pulmonary artery, AO = aorta, TG = tube graft, PA = main pulmonary artery. (From P. R. Hickey and D. L. Wessel. Anesthesia for Treatment of Congenital Heart Disease. In J. A. Kaplan [ed.], *Cardiac Anesthesia* [2nd ed.]. Philadelphia: Grune & Stratton, 1987. P. 683. With permission.)

the ability to choose shunt size. The Blalock-Taussig anastomosis has a good record of long-term patency and a low incidence of complications. The surgical approach for all these procedures is through a lateral thoracotomy, usually on the side of the aortic arch. The ductus arteriosus is ligated if present, after the shunt is open. Various shunts and their connections are listed in Table 13–13.

(2) **Cavopulmonary shunts.** The Glenn anastomosis is an example of a cavopulmonary shunt in which the superior vena cava is sutured to the right pulmonary artery (RPA), and the proximal RPA and right atrium are oversewn. The advantages of a cavopulmonary shunt (e.g., Glenn) compared to a systemic-to-pulmonary shunt include more efficient oxygenation (desaturated systemic blood is rerouted to the lungs instead of systemic arterial blood), a reduced volume load for the left

Table 13-13. Systemic-to-pulmonary shunts

Shunt	Anastomosis	Complications
Classic Blalock-Taussig	Right subclavian artery to right pulmonary artery (with left aortic arch)	Kinking of right pulmonary artery, right arm ischemia, excessive pulmonary flow
Modified Blalock-Taussig	Tube graft from right (or left) subclavian artery to right (or left) pulmonary artery	Kinking of pulmonary artery, tube graft does not allow for growth, chylothorax
Waterston	Ascending aorta to right pulmonary artery	Kinking of right pulmonary artery, amount of blood flow difficult to control
Potts	Descending aorta to left pulmonary artery	Rarely used, difficult to control shunt size, and difficult take-down at later repair
Central (aortic-pulmonary shunt)	Anastomosis between aorta and pulmonary artery with tube graft	Distortion of main pulmonary artery, excessive pulmonary flow
Glenn	Superior vena cava to right pulmonary artery	Thrombosis, superior vena cava syndrome, insufficient pulmonary blood flow, pulmonary arteriovenous fistula

ventricle, and the ability to serve as the first stage of a definitive procedure (Fontan procedure). The Glenn shunt cannot be used in the neonatal period because pulmonary vascular resistance is elevated.

   c. Anesthetic considerations

      (1) Preoperative. Efforts to decrease pulmonary vascular resistance should include supplemental O_2 administration and hyperventilation. PGE_1 infusion (0.1 μg/kg/min) inhibits ductal closure and decreases PVR. Balloon atrial septostomy may be performed at catheterization if right-sided obstruction is severe and the patent foramen ovale or ASD is small to improve mixing and hence oxygenation. If cyanosis is severe, with peripheral lactate production, acidosis should be corrected with sodium bicarbonate. Patients often are neonates, and no premedication is required.

      (2) Intraoperative. Inhalation induction is usually well tolerated in the absence of ventricular dysfunction and may relax infundibular spasm if present (e.g., tetralogy of Fallot) and increase pulmonary blood flow. Endotracheal tube leak should not be less than 20 cm H_2O to enable adequate ventilation after one lung is packed away from the surgical field. Limiting the dose of opioids may allow extubation of older infants at the end of the procedure.

         Hypoxemia usually worsens intraoperatively secondary

to one lung ventilation and distortion and clamping of the central vasculature. It is important to note that end-tidal carbon dioxide measurement underestimates $PaCO_2$ when a branch pulmonary artery is clamped (carbon dioxide excretion occurs only in the perfused lung), and therefore arterial blood gas measurements should be made serial to assess $PaCO_2$, oxygenation, and acid-base status.

Maneuvers to decrease pulmonary vascular resistance are helpful to increase pulmonary blood flow and minimize hypoxemia but should be discontinued at the time of assessment of shunt size after lung reexpansion (the size might appear adequate with these maneuvers but could actually be too small when these maneuvers are withdrawn). The shunt size may be too large or too small, and both conditions may require shunt revision. Small or obstructed shunts are manifest by continued hypoxemia. Large shunts and excessive pulmonary blood flow may be diagnosed by systemic hypotension, low diastolic pressure, wide pulse pressure, pulmonary edema, and acidosis. Many patients may be extubated in the operating room to avoid decreased pulmonary blood flow secondary to positive pressure ventilation, but neonates with reactive pulmonary vasculature may benefit from postoperative controlled ventilation.

Pulmonary blood flow usually increases during the first 24 hours postoperatively. This may be due to the absence of positive pressure ventilation, decreased pulmonary vascular resistance secondary to improved oxygenation or "recruitment" of vasculature from increased flow, decreased sympathetic tone, or a combination of these factors.

  d. **Problems and complications**
    (1) Common problems include inadequate or excessive pulmonary blood flow.
    (2) Other problems are specific to the type of shunt and are listed in Table 13–13.
2. **Blalock-Hanlon atrial septectomy.** This procedure is rarely performed as a separate procedure because of the success of percutaneous balloon atrial septostomy (Raskind procedure) and blade septotomy techniques and the trend toward primary repair in infancy.
3. **Vascular rings.** Respiratory and feeding difficulties may be due to extrinsic compression of the trachea and esophagus by vascular structures.
  a. **General hemodynamic considerations.** Vascular rings involve duplication or an aberrant location of the great arteries and their branches that encircle the trachea or esophagus. Patients may be asymptomatic or have respiratory complaints (stridor, frequent upper respiratory tract infections [URIs], cyanosis) or dysphagia. There is an increased incidence of apnea and respiratory arrest.

The most common forms of vascular rings are double aortic arch, aberrant right subclavian artery, and pulmonary artery sling. Other forms exist (Fig. 13-16). The double aortic arch surrounds the esophagus and trachea, compromising both. The aberrant right subclavian artery arises distal to the left subclavian and travels posteriorly to the right, compressing the esophagus and trachea against the aortic arch. Pulmonary artery sling describes an abnormality in which the left pulmonary artery arises from the right pulmonary artery and courses behind the tracheal bifurcation. Pulmonary artery sling is often associated with primary tracheobronchial malformations.

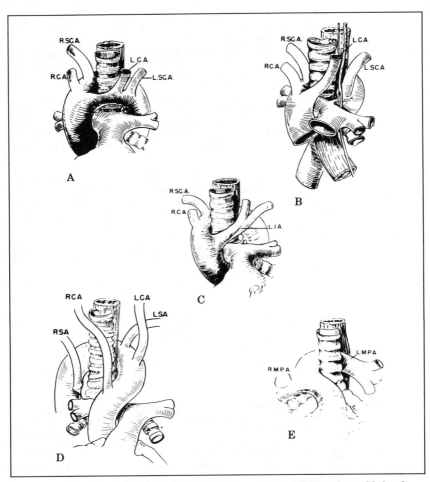

Fig. 13-16. *A.* Double aortic arch. *B.* Right aortic arch with retroesophageal left sub-clavian artery. *C.* Right aortic arch with mirror-image branching and left ligamentum arteriosum. *D.* Left aortic arch with retroesophageal right subclavian artery and right ligamentum arteriosum. *E.* Anomalous left pulmonary artery from right pulmonary artery. RCA, LCA = right and left carotid arteries; RSCA(RSA), LSCA(LSA) = right and left subclavian arteries, LMPA = left main pulmonary artery, RMPA = right main pulmonary artery. (From E. Arciniegas [ed.]. *Pediatric Cardiac Surgery.* Chicago: Year Book, 1985. Pp. 119, 122, 123. With permission.)

    b. Surgical procedures. The approach is usually through a left thoracotomy. The technique varies with the specific lesion, but in many cases the offending duplication may simply be ligated and divided. Repair of pulmonary artery sling is more difficult because the left pulmonary artery must be clamped and reattached to the main pulmonary artery.

    c. Anesthetic considerations. Atropine should be given preoper-atively to decrease airway secretions and inhibit vagal reflexes during airway manipulation. Inhalation induction may be preferred owing to the collapsibility of the airway. Halothane and oxygen are usually well tolerated. Upper airway obstruction during induction may be treated by administering gentle positive pressure breaths to support airway patency. Muscle relaxants should be avoided until the airway is secured. Hypoxemia and hypotension may occur during periods of surgical dissection. Early extubation should be contemplated only in patients with minimal symptoms without evidence of tracheomalacia.

d. Problems and complications.

(1) Some neonates require long-term ventilation until the tracheal rings mature.

(2) Patients with pulmonary artery sling are often only marginally better after repair because of the associated tracheomalacia.

B. Procedures to relieve congestive heart failure

1. PA banding

a. General hemodynamic considerations. Congenital heart lesions that cause high pulmonary blood flow and elevated pulmonary artery pressure induce pulmonary vasculature changes. If primary repair of the lesion is not technically feasible, the excessive pulmonary flow may be attenuated and sequelae avoided by placing a constrictive band around the main pulmonary artery. The band increases resistance to right ventricular ejection, decreases left-to-right shunting (e.g., through a VSD), and increases systemic perfusion. In other words, the shunt physiology is changed from simple to complex.

b. Surgical procedures. The size of the band (Fig. 13-17) is chosen to minimize hypoxemia (too small) and systemic hypoperfusion (too large). Pulmonary artery pressure after band replacement may serve as a guide. A pulmonary artery pressure that is one-half of the systemic pressure usually indicates the proper size. Pulse oximetry is also a useful tool and may identify systemic hypoxemia when the band is too tight.

c. Anesthetic considerations. These patients are often less than 6 months old and have complex lesions that cannot be repaired until they are older. The high pulmonary vascular resistance that occurs during the first few months of life limits blood flow initially, but as PVR decreases and pulmonary flow increases, the infant becomes symptomatic. Limitation of supplemental oxygen and medical closure of PDA, if present, are indicated preoperatively. Premedication is usually not required. Induction of anesthesia may be intravenous or by inhalation, care being taken to avoid abrupt increases in SVR or decreases in PVR, which may further increase pulmonary blood flow. If severe ventricular failure is present, inhalational agents should be avoided. Extubation may be possible at the end of the procedure if the infant was not intubated preoperatively.

d. Problems and complications

(1) Pulmonary blood flow may be excessive or inadequate.

(2) Distortion of the main branch pulmonary arteries has been reported.

2. PDA ligation

a. General hemodynamic considerations. Failure of the ductus arteriosus to close allows bidirectional shunting between the main pulmonary artery and the descending aorta while PVR is high, then predominantly left-to-right shunting as PVR decreases. The increased pulmonary blood flow results in pulmonary hyperten-

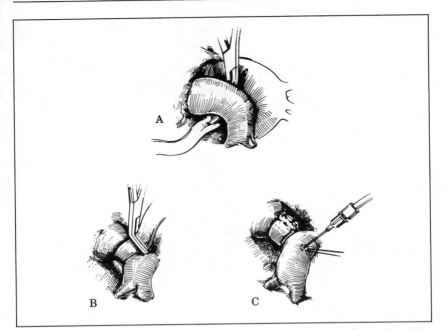

Fig. 13-17. Pulmonary artery banding. Band is passed around main pulmonary artery (A). The band is snugged down (B), and pulmonary artery pressure measurements are obtained (C) to verify proper "tightness" of the band. (From J. A. Waldhausen, and W. S. Pierce [eds.]. *Johnson's Surgery of the Chest.* **Chicago: Year Book, 1985. P. 345. With permission.)**

   sion, increased lung water, and elevated work of breathing (Fig. 13-18).

b. **Surgical procedure.** The ductus is ligated through a left thoracotomy. Ligation and division may be required in older children because recanalization can occur with ligation alone. A calcified ductus complicates repair and may require CPB.

c. **Anesthetic considerations.** These patients are often premature with hyaline membrane disease. Hypoxemia due to lung disease retards ductal closure. Conservative measures (fluid restriction, supplemental oxygen) and medical therapy (indomethacin) are utilized first. Cerebral intraventricular hemorrhage contraindicates use of indomethacin. Neonates are often intubated preoperatively and require only an opioid and muscle relaxant for the procedure. Older children may be extubated at the end of the case. Monitoring may be limited to an automated blood pressure cuff, ECG, oximetry, capnography, and temperature. Supplemental oxygen administration is indicated for hypoxemia, which may occur with lung retraction but should be titrated to maintain SaO_2 at 85–90 percent to minimize the risk of retrolental fibroplasia. Ligation of the ductus is usually accompanied by an increase in systemic diastolic pressure, a decrease in pulse pressure, and an "autotransfusion" as blood that formerly recirculated through the lungs is redistributed to the periphery.

d. **Problems and complications**

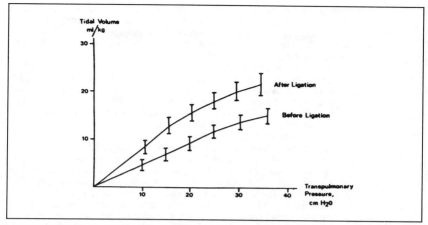

Fig. 13-18. Pressure-volume (compliance) curves immediately before and after ligation of a large PDA in seven infants. Compliance improves after ligation. (From T. Gerhardt, and E. Bancalari. Lung compliance in newborns with patent ductus arteriosus before and after surgical ligation. *Biol. Neonates* 38:101, 1980. With permission.)

(1) There may be left ventricular dysfunction due to elevation in afterload caused by removal of the low-resistance pulmonary circuit.

(2) Because vessel diameters are similar, the left pulmonary artery or the descending aorta have been mistakenly ligated, causing hypoxemia or systemic hypoperfusion, respectively.

(3) Recurrent laryngeal nerve damage and ductal recanalization have also been reported.

3. **Coarctation of the aorta**

a. **General hemodynamic considerations.** The position of the aortic coarctation, or narrowing, is variable but is usually juxtaductal, distal to the origin of the left subclavian artery. In neonates it is most commonly preductal and in older children usually postductal. The symptomatology varies greatly, with neonates often presenting with severe congestive heart failure whereas older children are usually asymptomatic.

The aortic narrowing causes a relative increase in blood flow and pressure in the head and upper extremity and hypoperfusion distal to the coarctation. In the neonatal period, the constriction impedes left ventricular ejection and may precipitate CHF, and the hypoperfusion distally may create a metabolic acidosis. The formation of collateral blood vessels around the site of narrowing, often through the thyrocervical trunk, and retrograde flow through the intercostal arteries are required to provide adequate blood flow to the lower extremities and decrease LV afterload. In the absence of collateral flow, hypertension may be severe, with left ventricular failure and pulmonary hypertension. In neonates with preductal coarctation or pulmonary hypertension, there may be right-to-left ductal flow, resulting in "differential cyanosis" (pink preductal, blue postductal). In older patients the only symptoms may be upper extremity hypertension, with decreased lower extremity pulses, systolic murmur, and rib "notching" on chest x ray if the patient is older than 6 or 7 years.

b. **Surgical procedures.** The surgical approach is through a left thoracotomy. Patients less than 1 year of age usually undergo subclavian flap aortoplasty, and older patients have coarctectomy with end-to-end anastomosis. Interposition grafts are required in some older children and adults.

c. **Anesthetic management**

(1) **Preoperative.** Neonates with left ventricular failure and right-to-left shunting will benefit from PGE_1 infusion to maintain postductal blood flow and minimize metabolic acidosis. Administration of sodium bicarbonate and hyperventilation, if the patient is intubated, are also beneficial. Antihypertensive medications should be continued.

(2) **Intraoperative.** Monitors should include right radial arterial catheter, ECG, oximetry, capnography, and temperature. Aortic cross-clamping may be associated with upper extremity hypertension with left ventricular strain, elevated intracranial pressure, distal hypoperfusion, acidosis, and spinal cord ischemia. Use of vasodilators to control this hypertension should be tempered by the need for adequate perfusion pressure to supply distal flow through collaterals. Lowering body temperature to 32°–34°C may decrease the incidence of neurologic deficits. Early extubation eliminates the endotracheal tube as a cause of hypertension.

d. **Problems and complications**

(1) Hypertension often persists, requiring medical treatment for a few weeks to months in most cases.

(2) Abdominal pain occurs occasionally and is thought to be secondary to reactive mesenteric vasoconstriction and ischemia.

(3) Paralysis of the lower extremities is a tragic and fortunately very rare consequence of spinal cord ischemia during cross-clamping.

VII. **Noncardiac surgery for patients with congenital heart disease**

A. **General**

1. Caring for patients with congenital heart disease outside of the cardiac operating room is, in many ways, more difficult than managing them for cardiac surgery. A few reasons are:

a. The preoperative evaluation may not be as extensive as that for a cardiac procedure.

b. The procedure may be emergent, with no time to obtain medical records.

c. Intraoperative monitoring may be less extensive.

d. The chest is not open to allow direct visualization and access to the heart.

e. The operating surgeon (and anesthesiologist) may not be familiar with cardiac pathophysiology and surgical corrective repair.

2. In general, patients with CHD may require noncardiac surgery:

a. **Before the congenital lesion is diagnosed.** Undiagnosed disease may present as an unexpected complication during anesthesia such as cyanosis, arrhythmia, or ventricular dysfunction. Treatment consists of resuscitation as indicated and termination of surgery as soon as possible. Diagnostic studies may be performed postoperatively. A useful exercise in this circumstance may be a review of the preoperative data for suggestions of cardiac disease that may serve as a predictor for future cases.

b. **After diagnosis, before surgical intervention.** These patients have the advantages of a previous cardiac workup and the care of a cardiologist. The reason why surgery has not been done is important. If the noncardiac surgery is elective, and the cardiac surgery is due to be performed, then thought should be given to performing the cardiac surgery first. For asymptomatic patients (small ASD or minimal aortic coarctation), anesthetic management in these procedures may differ very little from the routine. Sicker patients require invasive monitoring and management as indicated.

c. After surgical palliation. All records concerning the patient's previous procedure and current status should be reviewed. The timing of corrective surgery, if planned, should be coordinated with the noncardiac procedure. Monitoring and postoperative management depends on the degree of symptoms, exercise tolerance, presence of pulmonary hypertension, and extent of the planned surgical procedure.

d. After surgical correction. It is important to keep in mind that there are variable degrees of surgical "repair." An otherwise healthy patient who has had a patch closure of a small ASD may be treated as completely normal, but a patient presenting for the same noncardiac procedure with a history of pulmonary hypertensive episodes after repair of a large VSD may need special attention. Problems that occur after "repair" of congenital heart lesions are ventricular dysfunction, dysrhythmias, residual shunts, and persistent obstructions.

e. Inoperable cardiac lesion. Patients with cardiac lesions that are deemed inoperable (e.g., pulmonary vascular disease with right-to-left shunting) who present for noncardiac surgery are at high risk for morbidity and mortality. The decision to proceed should be made only after consultation with the parents, cardiologist, and surgeon. Consideration should be given to declining intervention. If surgery is elected, even a minimally invasive procedure demands full invasive monitoring and postoperative care.

B. Specific points

1. The interaction of the lesion, anesthesia, and surgery. It is crucial to understand not only the pathophysiology of the underlying lesion but also the changes that may come (or be prevented) with the stresses of anesthesia and surgery. This may require the anesthesiologist to review the surgical plan in detail with the surgeon to anticipate hemodynamically stressful manipulations.

2. All available information must be reviewed. Often there are echocardiograms and catheterization reports in addition to routine laboratory test results, chest X ray, and ECG. A recent cardiac consultation report should be obtained from the cardiologist caring for the patient.

3. Avoid outpatient surgery. As indicated above, there is increased potential for cardiac dysfunction in these patients, even after surgical "cure." All patients but those with the most insignificant lesions undergoing trivial procedures should stay in the hospital postoperatively.

4. Subacute bacterial endocarditis (SBE) prophylaxis. Abnormal endocardium, cardiac valves, or prosthetic material may serve as a nidus for infection by intraoperative bacteremia. See Chap. 12 for current recommendations for perioperative antibiotic therapy to prevent SBE.

5. Regional anesthesia. Regional anesthesia may be contemplated as a technique for these patients, but it is not without risk. The decrease in systemic vascular resistance may not be tolerated by patients with "mixing lesions" in whom the balance of PVR and SVR determines the amount of pulmonary blood flow or those with borderline coronary perfusion (e.g., aortic stenosis). There is also less control of the patient's airway and ventilation. Finally, one must avoid the tendency to monitor patients undergoing regional anesthesia less extensively (intraoperatively and postoperatively) than those undergoing general anesthesia.

6. The conduct of noncardiac anesthesia for patients with CHD should be governed by the same considerations as those governing cardiac procedures. The reader is referred to the applicable portions of this chapter.

SUGGESTED READING

Campbell, F. W., and Schwartz, A. J. *Anesthesia for Non-Cardiac Surgery in the Pediatric Patient with Congenital Heart Disease.* ASA Refresher Course (14th ed.). Philadelphia: J. B. Lippincott, 1986. Pp. 75–98.

Hickey, P. R., and Wessel, D. L. Anesthesia for Treatment of Congenital Heart Disease. In J. A. Kaplan (ed.), *Cardiac Anesthesia* (2nd ed.). New York: Grune & Stratton, 1987. Pp. 635–724.

Lake, C. *Pediatric Cardiac Anesthesia.* Philadelphia: Grune & Stratton, 1988.

Marriott, H. J. L. The Heart in Childhood and Congenital Lesions. In H. J. L. Marriott (ed.), *Practical Electrocardiography* (7th ed.). Baltimore: Williams & Wilkins, 1983. Pp. 442–455.

Moss, F. H., and Emmanouilides, G. C. *Moss' Heart Disease in Infants, Children and Adolescents* (3rd ed.). Baltimore: Williams & Wilkins, 1983.

Stark, J., and deLeval, M. *Surgery for Congenital Heart Defects.* Philadelphia: Grune & Stratton, 1983.

Waldhausen, J. A. Congenital Heart Disease. In J. A. Waldhausen and W. S. Pierce (eds.). *Johnson's Surgery of the Chest* (5th ed.). Chicago: Year Book, 1985. Pp. 287–430.

Anesthetic Management for Cardiac Transplantation

William R. Camann and Frederick A. Hensley, Jr.

Cardiac transplantation has become an increasingly common (Fig. 14-1) and successful procedure (Fig. 14-2) in the United States and worldwide as a treatment of end-stage heart disease. Cardiac transplantation is no longer considered experimental, a fact reflected in the increasing number of third-party payers providing reimbursement for this procedure. Consequently, a cardiac anesthesiologist today must be familiar with anesthetic management for cardiac transplantation. Likewise, all anesthesiologists, even those practicing in centers that do not perform transplants, may be faced with the prospect of anesthetizing a patient with a transplanted heart for noncardiac surgery.

I. Preoperative evaluation of the heart transplant recipient

A. **Hemodynamics.** Patients presenting for cardiac transplantation are gravely ill with end-stage cardiac failure. Regardless of the cause of cardiac failure, cardiac dilatation is a common feature. This dilatation is usually global, involving all four cardiac chambers, although some patients may initially present with predominantly left ventricular failure. The term **dilated cardiomyopathy** has been applied to this end-stage heart failure. These patients are almost always New York Heart Association Class IV and invariably have ejection fractions (EF) of less than 20%. Consequently, these individuals have fixed, low stroke volumes and depend on an adequate preload for marginal ventricular performance. Although the upper range of stroke volume is "fixed" and insensitive to further increases in preload, maneuvers that increase afterload may dramatically decrease stroke volume, as depicted in the pressure-volume curves (Fig. 14-3).

Inadequate preload and depressed contractility will also further depress a marginal stroke volume. These patients compensate for their low cardiac output by increased sympathetic activity leading to an increased heart rate and activation of the renin-angiotensin-aldosterone axis with resultant vasoconstriction and sodium and water retention.

B. **Etiology of pump failure.** Today, idiopathic (largely viral) cardiomyopathy and ischemic cardiomyopathy are the two most common causes of pump failure in the transplant recipient. Rheumatic, congenital, or valvular heart disease may be the cause in a small percentage of patients.

C. **Selection criteria for cardiac transplantation.** Absolute and relative contraindications for cardiac transplantation exist (Table 14-1). Certain relative contraindications preclude cardiac transplantation in some institutions but not others. Advanced age represents one prior absolute contraindication that is now a relative contraindication at most major transplant centers because of the recent excellent survival results in older recipients. Cardiac transplantation is now being performed in patients well into their sixth decade[3]. There are two consequences of this trend toward older patients. First, the major indication for transplant becomes heavily weighted in favor of ischemic cardiomyopathy, and second, the size of the potential recipient pool increases dramatically while the size of the donor pool remains the same. At the other extreme of age, neonatal transplants are being successfully performed. Hence, because of the changes in and liberalization of indications for transplantation in general, a severe donor organ shortage is present that will only increase in severity in the future.

D. **Unique preoperative considerations.** The preoperative evaluation of a patient for cardiac transplantation should include the standard criteria involved in evaluating any patient for cardiac surgery. However, some special considerations exist:

1. **Pulmonary hypertension.** Although left ventricular impairment is a hallmark of this patient population, the status of the right ventricle and pulmonary vasculature should be assessed preoperatively. Severe, fixed pulmonary hypertension (greater than 8 Wood units) is still regarded as an ominous sign for failure of transplantation

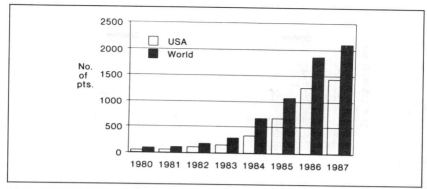

Fig. 14-1. Number of heart transplantations performed in the United States and worldwide from 1980 through 1987. (From L. S. Fragomeni and M. P. Kaye. The Registry of the International Society for Heart Transplantation: Fifth Official Report–1988. *J. Heart Trans.* 7:249, 1988. With permission.)

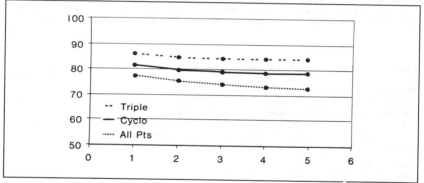

Fig. 14-2. Five-year actuarial survival in persons with heart transplants involving different treatment regimens. Triple = cyclosporine, azathioprine, and steroid immunotherapy; Cyclo = cyclosporine; All pts = all types of immunotherapy. (From L. S. Fragomeni, and M. P. Kaye. The Registry of the International Society for Heart Transplantation: Fifth Official Report–1988. *J. Heart Trans.* 7:251, 1988. With permission.)

and is a contraindication to transplantation in most centers. Those patients with pulmonary vascular resistance (PVR) of 6–8 Wood units should have a decrease in PVR when challenged with vasodilators in the catheterization laboratory to be considered candidates for orthotopic heart transplantation. Recatheterization in this patient subgroup should be performed every 3 months while the patient is awaiting transplantation to document that PVR is less than 8 Wood units and is responsive to vasodilators.

2. **Organ function (other than cardiac).** The cardiac transplant patient has near normal function of other vital organs, otherwise transplantation would not be indicated. However, the following dysfunction may be apparent:

a. **Reversible renal dysfunction.** Chronic systemic hypoperfusion (left ventricular failure) may produce some element of reversible renal insufficiency as reflected in borderline elevation of BUN and

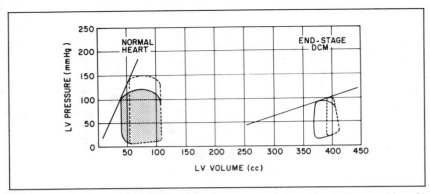

Fig. 14-3. Pressure-volume (P-V) loops from a normal heart *(left)* and a heart with end-stage dilated cardiomyopathy (DCM) *(right)*. In each case, superimposed on the resting P-V loop is the P-V loop *(dotted line)* created when peak systolic pressure is elevated. The straight, inclining lines depict the slopes of the respective end-systolic pressure-volume relations. Note the marked decrease in stroke volume of the myopathic heart when its peak systolic pressure is mildly elevated. LV = left ventricular. (From N. J. Clark, and R. D. Martin. Anesthetic considerations for patients undergoing cardiac transplantation. *J. Cardiothorac. Anesth.* 2:523, 1988. With permission.)

Table 14-1. Selection criteria for cardiac transplantation

Absolute contraindications
  Uncontrolled malignancy
  Severe pulmonary hypertension > 8 Wood units
  Active infection (including patients infected with HIV)
  Irreversible severe hepatic, renal, or pulmonary dysfunction
Relative contraindications
  Advanced age
  Insulin-dependent diabetes mellitus
  Mental or psychological defects
  Unfavorable socioeconomic factors
  Severe peripheral vascular disease
  Pulmonary infarction

creatine. BUN may be proportionately higher compared to creatine secondary to hypoperfusion and the concomitant prerenal effects of high-dose diuretics.

b. Reversible hepatic dysfunction. Chronic systemic hypoperfusion (left ventricular failure) *and* hepatic venous congestion (right ventricular failure) are additive and lead to a decrease in hepatic perfusion pressure, with subsequent reversible hepatic dysfunction. This dysfunction may be evidenced by mild to moderate elevations of hepatic enzymes, bilirubin, and prothrombin time.

c. Generalized atherosclerosis. Those patients whose symptoms arise from ischemic cardiomyopathy should be examined for end-organ sequelae of generalized vascular disease, particularly chronic hypertension and cerebral-carotid atherosclerosis. Such patients may also have had one or more previous coronary artery bypass procedures. Precise prebypass control of coronary perfusion and hence maintenance of marginal ventricular performance will aid in averting hemodynamic compromise and consequent aggravation of preexisting end-organ dysfunction.

3. **Preoperative medications.** Preoperative medications may include digitalis-diuretic combinations; hence an increased risk of dysrhythmias due to hypokalemia may ensue. The chronic use of antiarrhythmics may reduce ventricular contractility, and orally administered chronic afterload reducing agents may decrease peripheral vascular resistance. Likewise, warfarin (Coumadin) therapy for prophylaxis of thromboemboli may increase the need for vitamin K and fresh frozen plasma in the perioperative period.

4. **Circulatory support.** Patients with severe cardiac decompensation presenting for cardiac transplantation may require preoperative circulatory support. Most institutions performing transplants utilize intravenous inotropic agents preoperatively in selected patients as well as to a lesser degree, the intraaortic balloon pump (IAPB) [4]. Ventricular assist devices (univentricular and biventricular) and total artificial hearts have been used as a "bridge" to transplantation. Refer to Chapter 22 for a detailed discussion of mechanical devices used for bridging to transplantation.

5. **Previous cardiac surgery.** Occasionally, patients may require transplantation after one or more previous cardiac operations. If such a history is obtained, appropriate preoperative preparations in anticipation of hemorrhage should be undertaken.

II. **Donor selection and management.** The process of donor heart procurement is extremely important for the success of cardiac transplantation. Often little care is taken in the anesthetic management of the donor. An anesthesiologist from the heart transplant team may accompany the surgeon for organ harvesting at a distant institution. This practice currently occurs in less than 10% of institutions performing heart transplants but may increase as donor supply becomes more limited.

A. **Donor selection criteria**

1. **General.** Motor vehicle accidents leading to irreversible brain damage supply the largest number of cardiac transplant donors. Severe trauma, malignancy, and systemic infections are contraindications to donor acceptance. Donors range in age from birth–53 years (mean, 25 years) [3]. Most transplant centers generally do not accept female donors over 45 years of age and males over 35 years of age. However, as indicated, the upper age of donors at some centers is increasing.

2. **Cardiac evaluation.** Prior to acceptance of a donor for cardiac transplantation, a thorough cardiac evaluation is performed consisting of cardiac history and physical examination, electrocardiogram, chest x ray, echocardiogram, and cardiology consultation. If any question exists about myocardial function or coronary disease, cardiac catheterization is performed.

   Contraindications to donor acceptance include prolonged hypotension or cardiac arrest, cardiac trauma, or a requirement for high doses of inotropes (equivalent to > 10 µg/kg/min of dopamine) with a CVP of more than 12 mm Hg (i.e., inadequate preload).

3. **Size requirements.** Most centers do not allow a weight differential of greater than 20 kg to exist between donor and recipient. Indeed, in recipients with pulmonary hypertension, attempts are made to obtain a larger heart to handle the increased impedance to right ventricular outflow ejection.

4. **Immunologic evaluation.** ABO blood type matching of donor and recipient is mandatory. In the pretransplant workup the recipient's

blood is tested against a standard antigen panel with the following criteria:

    a. Less than 10–15% reactivity on the panel. Proceed with the transplant on the basis of ABO typing,

    b. Greater than 10–15% reactivity on the panel. A lymphocyte cross-match (i.e., recipient serum (antibodies) tested against donor lymphocytes) is needed. If lysis of lymphocytes occurs, the donor is not suitable. An additional 6 hours are required for a complete lymphocyte cross-match. Also, time is required to transport the donor blood sample to the transplant center immunology laboratory. Thus a lymphocyte cross-match can add considerable delay to the start of the transplant procedure.

B. Pathophysiology related to irreversible brain damage. Many physiologic abnormalities are associated with brain death.

    1. Cardiovascular instability is a common feature, secondary to loss of neurologic control of the myocardium and vascular tree.

    2. Volume depletion frequently occurs secondary to diabetes insipidus and the use of diuretics to treat patients with increased intracranial pressure.

    3. Loss of thermoregulatory control occurs.

    4. Neurogenic pulmonary edema may be present.

C. Perioperative management of the heart transplant donor. It is imperative that excellent perioperative therapy be given to the donor patient. Loss of normal hemodynamic control mechanisms require careful attention to prevent damage to the myocardium. Continuous monitoring of arterial blood pressure and central venous pressure (CVP) is necessary for perioperative management of these patients. Volume repletion under monitored conditions is crucial for the reasons outlined above. The CVP should be maintained around 10 mm Hg. If hypotension exists with a high or normal central venous pressure, inotropic support is indicated. Diabetes insipidus should be treated with vasopressin. Arterial hypertension is treated with vasodilators (e.g., sodium nitroprusside). Warming-cooling blankets are utilized for thermal control, and intravenous fluids can be warmed if necessary. Acid-base status and electrolytes must be maintained within a normal range. Pulmonary dysfunction may exist secondary to neurogenic pulmonary edema and may require positive end-expiratory pressure for normal oxygenation.

    Hypertensive responses may occur during surgical stimulation in cadaver donors [9], probably through spinal-mediated mechanisms. These responses do not indicate cerebral function or perception of pain.

D. Logistics of organ removal. The actual harvest procedure can be quite lengthy, particularly if multiple organs are to be obtained. The perfusion-sensitive organs (kidneys and liver) are removed prior to cessation of pump function by cardiectomy. The donor heart is excised en bloc via a median sternotomy incision after dissection of its pericardial attachments. The superior and inferior vena cavae are ligated first, allowing exsanguination of the donor organ. The aorta is then cross-clamped, and cold cardioplegia is administered. The aorta and pulmonary arteries are then transected, leaving as much native donor length on these segments as possible. The last remaining attachments are the pulmonary veins, which are individually divided after lifting the donor organ out of the thoracic cavity.

III. Anesthetic and surgical management of the transplant recipient

    A. Preinduction preparation

        1. Timing and coordination of personnel. The great majority of cardiac transplant procedures are performed between 6 P.M. and 6 A.M. [4], often placing a burden on anesthesiologists and other operating room personnel. Most cardiac anesthesiologists feel that a transplant procedure requires considerably more time and effort than a routine coronary artery bypass procedure [4]. Close communication must be maintained between the transplant center and the donor retrieval team regarding timing of the recipient's OR arrival, line placement, and induction of anesthesia. Approximately half of all institutions surveyed in 1986 [4] reported an average of 2 hours from arrival of the recipient in the operating room to induction of anesthesia. The arrival time of the donor heart must be carefully estimated. Anesthesia should not be induced long before arrival to avoid a prolonged prebypass and bypass period in a patient with a failing heart. Conversely, induction should not be needlessly delayed, thus resulting in a longer ischemic time for the donor organ before implantation.

2. **Premedication.** Premedication should be administered with caution to these preload-dependent individuals because vasodilation could be deleterious. Intravenous sedation can be administered to the anxious patient in the monitored environment of the operating room.

3. **Invasive monitoring controversy—central venous catheter versus pulmonary artery catheter.** Access to the central vasculature is necessary for any procedure involving cardiopulmonary bypass, both for measurement of central venous pressures and for infusion of potent vasoactive medications. However, a controversy in cardiac transplantation involves whether to merely place a central venous monitoring line (CVC) or a pulmonary artery catheter (PAC).

   a. **Arguments for the use of a PAC include**
      (1) Ability to measure cardiac output.
      (2) Ability to measure left-sided filling pressures.
      (3) Ability to measure right-sided filling pressures and pulmonary artery pressures.
      (4) Ability to calculate systemic and pulmonary resistances.
      (5) Facilitation of titration of inotropes and vasodilators.
      (6) Ability to measure mixed venous oxygen saturation (fiberoptic PAC).

   b. **Arguments against a PAC are as follows:**
      (1) Most patients undergoing cardiac transplantation do not have marked pulmonary hypertension, hence hemodynamics can often be sufficiently assessed by CVC alone.
      (2) The PAC must be withdrawn from the surgical field during bypass.
      (3) The PAC may be a source of infection.
      (4) There are complications of PAC insertion in any patient, regardless of the procedure.
      (5) The PAC may be difficult to pass in patients with large, dilated native ventricles and low cardiac outputs, and catheter placement may be more prone to induce dysrhythmias.
      (6) There is a danger of passage of the PAC across fresh surgical suture lines.

         The advent of sterile introducer sheaths for PACs allows manipulation of the catheter to and from the heart during the surgical procedure; however, the sterile barrier of such sheaths is not inviolable. The risks of introduction of an intracardiac catheter in the presence of immunosuppression must always be carefully weighed against the benefits obtained from the information that such a catheter provides.

         Most cardiac anesthesiologists agree that a PAC is most useful in assessment of postbypass hemodynamic function and offers little in prebypass management [4]. Consequently, a PAC may be placed by means of an introducer sheath to the superior vena cava position before bypass and advanced into the pulmonary artery after bypass. This approach minimizes manipulation of the catheter with its associated prebypass arrhythmogenesis but still subjects the patient to an intracardiac foreign body that must be passed across a surgical suture line.

Still another issue is whether to place the chosen catheter in the internal jugular on the left or right side. Institutional preference usually prevails, although many institutions will place the catheter on the left side, preserving the right internal jugular (IJ) as a route for future myocardial biopsies. Those who choose to place a PAC must consider the difficulty in floating the balloon from the left neck, particularly in a patient with elevated central pressures versus the increased trauma to the IJ (owing to the larger introducer apparatus) if a right-sided approach is taken.

4. **Sterility.** All patients undergoing transplantation will receive immunosuppressive drugs, which are often begun preoperatively. Hence, meticulous care must be exercised to reduce contamination in the operating room. Operating room personnel should be kept to the minimum level required for safe patient care, and onlookers and operating room traffic should be discouraged.

Anesthesia equipment should include a clean breathing circuit and airway instruments and a sterile supply of freshly opened and drawn drugs. All vascular access catheters (intravenous, arterial, and central) should be placed in a sterile fashion only after a skin preparation with a bacteriocidal agent (e.g., Betadine), and all lines should be promptly dressed with sterile occlusive dressings. Consideration should be given to the use of sterile gowns for central venous access procedures.

B. Anesthetic induction

1. **Aspiration precautions.** Because there is often little advance notice preceding a transplant procedure, patients may have eaten a recent meal. In addition, oral cyclosporine may be administered (along with a significant amount of liquid) preoperatively. Precautions to minimize the risk and consequences of aspiration should be taken. Thirty milliliters of a nonparticulate antacid (e.g., Bicitra) can be given orally shortly before induction, and an H_2-receptor antagonist (e.g., cimetidine or ranitidine) can be given parenterally. Metoclopramide, 10 mg IV, will promote antiemesis and gastric emptying. The induction sequence itself can be carried out with the patient in a slightly head-up position and with maintenance of cricoid pressure.

2. **Anesthetic induction agents.** Although concerns about aspiration are important, a true "rapid-sequence" induction is not likely to be well tolerated in this patient population. A slow, controlled induction with narcotic (fentanyl, 50–75 μg/kg, or sufentanil, 5–8 μg/kg), oxygen, muscle relaxants, and maintenance of cricoid pressure with positive pressure ventilation is ideal. Preinduction application of topical local anesthetic agents to the upper airway may allow early placement of an oral airway or endotracheal tube with minimal hemodynamic consequences. Small doses of a benzodiazepine, ketamine, or scopolamine will enhance amnesia in a patient receiving high-dose narcotic anesthesia. However, combining benzodiazepine with narcotics will decrease systemic vascular resistance and blood pressure and may enhance myocardial depression in a patient with poor contractility.

Potent inhalation agents are generally contraindicated for induction in this class of patients. Although subanesthetic doses may be appealing for their amnestic properties in selected patients, these agents are rarely used before cardiopulmonary bypass during cardiac transplantation.

With adequate preload, induction with narcotic and relaxant is surprisingly well tolerated in most individuals. However, inotropic agents should be mixed and ready to administer should decompensation occur during induction. In patients with ischemic cardiomyopathy meticulous care is taken to avoid variation from baseline hemodynamics so that myocardial oxygen supply-demand relationships remain favorable so that acute decompensation and emergent institution of bypass are avoided.

3. **Induction muscle relaxant.** The choice of a muscle relaxant depends on the hemodynamic and autonomic needs of the individual patient. However, maintenance of cardiac output is largely dependent on heart rate in a patient with failing ventricles and fixed low stroke volumes. Thus, pancuronium is the most common agent used [4], because its vagolytic properties will tend to counteract the vagotonic effects of a narcotic induction. Conversely, the danger of extreme tachycardia and ventricular arrhythmias in patients on high-level inotropic support may warrant the use of an agent like vecuronium, which has minimal cardiovascular side effects.

4. **Maintenance of preoperative circulatory support.** Any patient who is receiving preoperative circulatory support of any kind (pharmacologic or mechanical) should generally continue to receive the same level of support during induction of anesthesia. The dose of intravenous inotropes, however, may need to be increased during and after induction as the patient's endogenous catecholamine levels fall.

C. **Anesthetic maintenance.** The main goal during the prebypass period is to maintain adequate end-organ perfusion. A narcotic-based technique is most common, with benzodiazepine supplementation as tolerated until institution of cardiopulmonary bypass (CPB). However, the precarious hemodynamic status of these patients before bypass often requires the use of subanesthetic levels of narcotic and other agents. Use of a narcotic-based anesthetic in young patients may result in a different incidence of recall than that occurring in an older group with a similar anesthetic. Therefore, administration of additional narcotic and amnestic agents during CPB is indicated to avoid an underanesthetized patient during rewarming and termination of CPB.

D. **Surgical technique of implantation**

1. **Orthotopic heart transplantation.** The operative technique for orthotopic heart transplantation (OHT) was first described by Shumway in 1960 and remains essentially unchanged today [5] (Fig 14-4). The majority of cardiac transplantations performed are orthotopic.

   The recipient is placed on cardiopulmonary bypass in a standard fashion, and a pulmonary artery catheter, if passed, is withdrawn to the tip of the introducer sheath. Aortic cannulation is performed as distally on the aorta as possible, and bicaval cannulae are placed with snares around the venae cava, thus allowing complete exclusion of the heart from the native circulation. The aorta and pulmonary arteries are clamped and divided. The atria are transected to preserve the atrioventricular grooves, but the atrial appendages are discarded, because they may serve as sites of postoperative thrombus formation.

   The left atria of donor and recipient are anastomosed first, followed by the right atria. The donor and recipient aortas are then joined. The aortic cross-clamp is removed with the patient in the

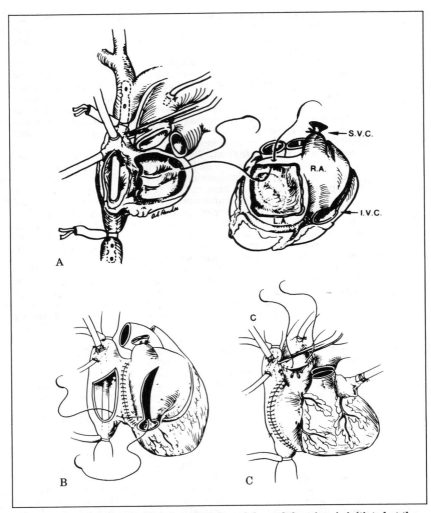

Fig. 14-4. *A.* The anastomosis of the recipient and donor left atrium is initiated at the level of the appendage. *B.* The left atrial anastomosis is completed, and the right atrial anastomosis commences. Note the curvilinear excision in the donor right atrium that protects the SA node from the proximity of the suture line. *C.* The atrial anastomoses are completed, and the aortic anastomosis is in the process of completion. The cannula in the left atrial appendage is in place to afford cooling of the heart and displacement of air. The pulmonary artery anastomosis is sutured last. RA = right atrium; LA = left atrium; SVC = superior vena cava; IVC = inferior vena cava. (From A. A. Raney, E. B. Stinson, P. E. Oyer, et al. The Technique of Cardiac Transplantation. In J. W. Hurst, R. B. Logue, C. E. Rackley, et al. [eds.], *The Heart* [Vol. 2, 5th ed.]. New York: McGraw-Hill, 1982. P. 1924. With permission.)

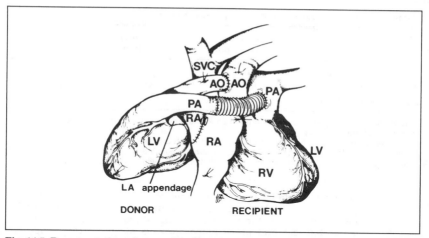

Fig. 14-5. Representation of a completed surgical implantation of a donor heart in the heterotopic position. SVC = superior vena cava; AO = aorta; PA = pulmonary artery; LV = left ventricle; RV = right ventricle; RA = right atrium; LA = left atrium. (From D. Novitzky, D. K. C. Cooper, and C. N. Barnard. The surgical technique of heterotopic heart transplantation. *Ann. Thorac. Surg.* 36:481, 1983. With permission.)

head-down position. Finally, the pulmonary artery anastomosis is completed, de-airing is performed, and attempts to wean from CPB are begun.

2. **Heterotopic heart transplantation.** The technique of heterotopic heart transplantation (HHT) has been advocated for recipients with severely elevated PVR, for situations in which a small donor heart is procured, and for a donor heart exposed to prolonged ischemia. This more complex procedure connects the donor heart in a parallel circulation with the recipient's own heart, which is not excised [6] (Fig. 14-5).

   HHT is performed by anastomosing respectively the right and left atria and aortas of the donor and recipient. The pulmonary arteries are usually joined by an artificial conduit. Thus the ventricles are not joined primarily, but both right ventricles empty into the native main pulmonary artery, and both left ventricles supply the native aortic trunk. Although different heart rates may ensue, this does not seem to interfere with the total cardiac output. The contribution to cardiac output of each organ will depend on the relative compliance of donor versus recipient ventricle. Although the bulk of the cardiac workload will be carried by the donor heart, the contribution of the native organ may be lifesaving during the immediate postischemic period (after CPB) or during any episode of acute rejection. Major disadvantages of HHT are its lower survival record [3] compared to OHT, the necessity to still treat the failing native heart medically, and the possibility that the native heart may be a site of thromboembolism.

E. **Termination from CPB and the postbypass period**

1. **Unique aspects of the donor heart.** Once the donor heart has been implanted into the recipient's chest, the anesthesiologist will, in many respects, be treating a different patient than the one cared for prebypass. The level of inotropic support required by the recipient native heart prebypass should be disregarded. Instead, the anesthe-

Table 14-2. Effects of pacing in the transplanted heart*

	Increase in HR (bpm)	Stroke volume	Cardiac output
Ventricular pacing	40	↓	NC
Atrial pacing	40	sl ↓	sl ↑ or NC
Isoproterenol infusion	40	↑ ↑	↑ ↑

*Effects of electrical pacing or isoproterenol on stroke volume and cardiac output of the acutely transplanted human heart.
HR = heart rate, bpm = beats per minute, NC = no change, sl = slight.
Source: From N.J. Clark, and R.D. Martin. Anesthetic considerations for patients undergoing cardiac transplantation. *J. Cardiothorac. Anesth.* 2(4):533, 1988. With permission.

siologist should be aware of any inotropic support given to the donor prior to harvest because that same degree of support, or possibly more, may be required during weaning from CPB. Although the donor harvest and procurement process attempts to provide the healthiest possible heart for implantation, the process itself may introduce variable degrees of dysfunction in the donor organ. This dysfunction may be based on:

a. **Donor inotropic support.** If the donor received any degree of prolonged inotropic support, theoretically the donor organ could manifest the phenomenon of down-regulation of beta-receptors and thus may require a relatively large dose of beta-agonist support during weaning from CPB.

b. **Ischemic interval.** The interval between harvest and implantation should be as short as possible to minimize ischemic damage to the donor organ. The upper limit of an acceptable ischemic interval is 4 hours. With more than a 1½-hour interval, 30-day mortality progressively and proportionately increases.

c. **Myocardial preservation.** The mode of preservation during the ischemic interval may affect post-CPB function. Although an initial dose of cardioplegia is administered prior to organ removal from the donor, repeat doses are not given during transport. Thus, the benefits of multiple dose cardioplegia are lost.

d. **Subclinical myocardial damage.** The donor screening process may fail to detect any subclinical damage to the potential donor organ.

e. **Denervation.** The hallmark of the transplanted heart, however, is denervation, and it is thus unresponsive to any interventions mediated through the recipient's autonomic nervous system. If bradycardia is noted after either electrical or spontaneous defibrillation of the donor heart, only direct-acting chronotropes such as isoproterenol are useful for increasing heart rate. A heart rate between 90 and 120 bpm is sought. Atropine or pancuronium, whose effects are mediated through vagolytic mechanisms, have no influence on the rate of a transplanted heart.

Infusion of isoproterenol is almost universally required post-CPB. In addition to its salutary chronotropic effects, this pure beta-agonist will provide a significant degree of inotropic support as well [8]. Temporary pacing is also effective to maintain heart rate post-CPB. However, it may not increase cardiac output as much as isoproterenol (Table 14-2).

f. **Pulmonary hypertension.** Transplant recipients often have mild degrees of pulmonary hypertension owing to preexisting chronic elevation of left heart filling pressures, and isoproterenol may aid in relaxing the pulmonary vasculature, thus easing right heart strain on the donor heart.

2. Problems during weaning and the postbypass period

  a. Right heart failure. The most important and common cause of cardiac decompensation during weaning from CPB is acute right heart failure (RHF) [4].

    (1) Etiology. The etiology of right ventricular failure is usually pretransplant elevation in pulmonary vascular resistance in the recipient and may be compounded by dysfunction of the donor right ventricle. A donor heart of small size may be incapable of overcoming the pulmonary resistance to ejection even if only mild to moderate elevations of pulmonary vascular resistance exist. Hence, efforts are made to provide a larger "oversize" donor heart for these patients.

    (2) Diagnosis of right heart failure. In addition to visual examination of the right ventricle when the chest is open, elevation of both central venous pressure and pulmonary artery pressure and narrowing of the mean pulmonary artery–CVP pressure gradient all indicate right ventricular failure. PAC monitoring with cardiac output determinations and calculation of pulmonary vascular resistance will help guide drug therapy and hyperventilation in these cases. Mixed venous saturation (fiberoptic PAC) measurements may be beneficial in following trends as well as sudden changes in right ventricular function.

    (3) Treatment

      (a) Hyperventilation. Hyperventilation to an arterial PCO_2 of 25–30 mm Hg is always the **first line** treatment in patients with pulmonary hypertension and should be considered before pharmacologic intervention. It is essential to continue hyperventilation throughout the postbypass period for possibly as long as 24 hours in the intensive care unit to avoid rapid increases in pulmonary vascular resistance.

      (b) Pharmacologic and mechanical support. Pharmacologic support for RHF includes inotropic support of the right ventricle and/or pulmonary vasodilatation. Isoproterenol is a particularly appealing drug to use when RHF is secondary to increases in PVR because beta-receptor activity not only increases cardiac inotropy and chronotropy but also leads to pulmonary vasodilatation. Prostaglandin (PGE_1), a pulmonary vasodilator, has been extremely beneficial in the treatment of severe pulmonary hypertension. Table 14-3 lists treatments available for pulmonary hypertension leading to RHF. Refer to Chapter 3 for more detailed pharmacologic information. Pharmacologic therapy in combination with right ventricular assist devices has been reported to be effective in the treatment of right heart failure in the cardiac transplant patient.

        Aggressive intervention is justified because moderate degrees of pulmonary hypertension before transplantation have been shown to normalize 1–2 weeks postoperatively and remain normal at 1-year followup [1].

  b. Other causes of inability to wean from CPB. Biventricular dysfunction, left ventricular dysfunction, and systemic vascular collapse account for the remainder of patients unable to be separated from cardiopulmonary bypass. Pulmonary artery catheter monitoring may be beneficial in sorting out the differential di-

Table 14-3. Agents used for treatment of right ventricular failure associated with pulmonary hypertension

Pharmacologic
    Nitroglycerin, 0.1–7.0 μg/kg/min
    Nitroprusside, 0.1–8.0 μg/kg/min
    Isoproterenol, 0.05–0.50 μg/kg/min; upper range for adults is ≤ 20 μg/min
    Dobutamine, 2–20 μg/kg/min
    Dopamine, ≤5 μg/kg/min
    Prostaglandin (PGE$_1$), 0.05–0.4 mg/kg/min
Mechanical
    Hyperventilation (a first-line treatment!)
    Right ventricular assist device
    ? Pulmonary artery balloon counterpulsation

agnosis of systemic hypotension, especially when the chest is closed and visual inspection of the heart is not possible.

Although most patients are weaned from CPB uneventfully with the use of a CVC alone, those that prove recalcitrant to separation from CPB will probably be managed more effectively with a PAC. The risks, however, of a PAC are not to be taken lightly. Proof that PAC monitoring affects outcome in cardiac transplant procedures remains lacking, and the decision must be based on institutional and personal preferences.

   c. **Hemostasis.** Hemostasis may be more problematic postbypass in transplant procedures other than in other cardiac surgical procedures for two reasons. First, the extensive bi-atrial suture line may be disrupted. Meticulous attention must be directed toward ensuring competency of the cardiac anastomosis, particularly on the less visible posterior aspect of the atria, prior to chest closure. Second, coagulopathy owing to chronic passive hepatic congestion or preoperative coumadin may require administration of fresh frozen plasma or cryoprecipitate to ensure satisfactory hemostasis. Any question of the adequacy of heparin reversal with protamine should be resolved by some measure of circulating heparin activity (e.g., Hepcon) and coagulation studies.

   d. **Renal dysfunction.** Oliguria is common in the post-CPB bypass period. The etiology of this problem is often multifactorial:
      (1) Preexisting renal impairment secondary to chronic low output state
      (2) Chronic diuretic use
      (3) Cyclosporine renal toxicity
      (4) Effects of cardiopulmonary bypass
         Treatment consists of maintaining adequate preload and cardiac output and possibly continuing preoperative diuretics.

IV. **Anesthesia for surgical procedures after transplantation.** As the frequency of cardiac transplantation and survival rates increase, patients with transplanted hearts will become more common visitors to the operating room for noncardiac procedures. Such patients will present for a wide variety of surgical procedures.

   A. **Types of procedures.** Although patients may present for procedures unrelated to their cardiac disease, most post-transplant operations are either secondary to the patient's intrinsic disease, such as peripheral vascular reconstruction due to atherosclerosis, or a direct result of either the transplant itself (e.g., retransplant for acute rejection, me-

Table 14-4. Common surgical procedures performed after transplantation

Emergency exploration for mediastinal bleeding
Complications caused by infection (usually abscess drainage)
  Laparotomy
  Craniotomy
  Mediastinotomy/thoracotomy
  Extremity abscess drainage
  Bronchoscopy
Complications caused by steroid treatment
  Total hip arthroplasty or pinning
  Laparotomy for perforated viscus
  Cataract excision
  Vitrectomy
  Scleral buckle
Vascular surgery
  Aortic
  Peripheral
  Amputations
Elective surgical procedures, especially biliary tract surgery

Source: Modified from J. Wyner, and E.L. Finch. Heart and Heart-Lung Transplantation. In S. Gelman (ed.), *Anesthesia and Organ Transplantation*. Philadelphia: Saunders, 1987. P. 123. With permission.

diastinal exploration for bleeding) or the sequelae of immunosuppression (e.g., orthopedic or ophthalmologic procedures owing to steroid use and surgical exploration related to infection). Table 14-4 lists the common surgical procedures performed after transplantation.
  B. **Physiology of the denervated heart.** The unique characteristic of patients after transplantation is cardiac denervation. All post-transplant patients will manifest this phenomenon because no histologic evidence for cardiac reinnervation in humans has been demonstrated, even in long-term survivors [7].
    1. **Hemodynamics.** Baseline hemodynamic alterations are noted in patients with transplanted hearts, although in general, the denervated, nonrejecting donor organ demonstrates excellent functional capability [2,8]. Of note is that intrinsic control systems of the heart are intact despite denervation. Cardiac impulse formation and conduction (and the Treppe effect) are normal. The Frank-Starling effect is intact, as is the response to circulating catecholamines. Finally, metabolic regulation of coronary blood flow is preserved. The majority of patients receiving cyclosporine immunosuppression manifest mild to moderate hypertension, and most require antihypertensive medications. In contrast, azathioprine-treated heart transplant patients rarely manifest hypertension. The baseline, resting heart rate of transplant recipients will be relatively high, owing to absence of vagal tone [7].
         The response to stress in denervated hearts is different from that in normal patients. Stress-induced increases in cardiac output in the cardiac patient are initially due to increases in stroke volume (Frank-Starling mechanism), whereas stress-induced increases in heart rate are delayed and result from rising circulating catecholamine levels. Therefore, maintenance of preload is crucial to ensure

Table 14-5. Hemodynamic changes after transplantation

1. Normal to high-normal filling pressures
2. Mild to moderate abnormalities include systemic hypertension (usually secondary to cyclosporine) with resultant vasoconstriction and afterload stress
3. Low-normal to normal cardiac output
4. Increased basal heart rate
5. Normal intrinsic contractility and reserve in a nonrejecting heart
6. No evidence of reinnervation despite excellent long-term functional capacity
7. Increased response to beta agonists (increased beta-receptor density)
8. Resolution of moderate pulmonary hypertension (within 2 weeks)
9. Increased incidence of dysrhythmias (first 6 mos)
10. Response to exercise:
    First few minutes of exercise—increased stroke volume (augmented by increased venous return, hence increased end-diastolic volume)
    Later—increased catecholamines (from adrenal medulla) leading to increased heart rate, increased cardiac output
11. Intact intrinsic control systems (see sec. **IV.B.1**)

adequate cardiovascular responses to physiologic stressors, such as anesthesia. Table 14-5 summarizes the hemodynamic changes that occur in the patient after transplantation.

2. **Drug effects.** Any maneuver or drug acting solely through the autonomic nervous system will be ineffective in a post-transplant patient; for example, vagolytic agents (atropine or glycopyrrolate) will not cause a rise in heart rate, and acetylcholinesterase inhibitors (e.g., neostigmine) will not result in slowing of the heart rate. Likewise, carotid sinus massage or ocular pressure (the oculocardiac reflex) will not result in changes in heart rate because both of these maneuvers operate by way of a vagal efferent pathway. Changes in heart rate, however, may be affected by direct-acting circulating agents. Isoproterenol, a direct-acting beta-agonist, will exert a positive chronotropic effect, whereas β-blockers such as propranolol will provide negative chronotropy. It should be noted that beta-agonists may have an exaggerated effect on denervated, transplanted hearts compared to normal, innervated hearts. This has been shown to be due to increased beta-receptor density (up-regulation) with no change in beta-receptor sensitivity in transplanted hearts [10]. Important drug effects are summarized in Table 14-6.

C. **Anesthetic management**
   1. **Preoperative evaluation**
      a. **History and physical examination.** The patient's activity level and exercise tolerance should be noted. Transplant patients will not manifest symptoms of angina, and transplanted hearts can undergo accelerated graft atherosclerosis. These patients are thus at risk for silent coronary artery disease (see sec. **d.** below). Steroid use may predispose to pressure ulcerations and fragile skin and bones. Such sequelae should be known to provide safe patient positioning intraoperatively. The upper airway should be examined for any alterations secondary to "cushingoid" features (see also sec. **4.** below).
      b. **Laboratory studies** should include measurements of electrolytes, and particularly renal and hepatic panels, to assess any effect of immunosuppressive therapy on these organ systems. Chest radiographs should be examined for evidence of subclinical infectious processes. Electrocardiograms may demonstrate multiple P waves,

Table 14-6. Drug effects on the denervated heart

Anesthetic drugs
    Pancuronium—No ↑ HR
    Neostigmine, edrophonium, and so on—No ↓ HR, but peripheral (noncardiac)
        cholinergic properties intact
    Fentanyl—No ↓ HR secondary to vagotonic effects
    Demerol—No ↑ HR secondary to vagolytic effects
Cardiac drugs
    Isoproterenol—Potent inotropy and chronotropy (↑ beta-receptor density)
    Digoxin—With inotropy, initial vagotonic effect is absent; chronic ↓
        atrioventricular nodal conduction is present as in innervated myocardium
    Atropine, glycopyrrolate—No ↑ HR, peripheral vagolytic properties intact
    Ephedrine—Has decreased effect (both direct and indirect agent; only direct
        effect remains intact)

because both donor and recipient sinus nodes are present (although only the donor sinus node is functional—the native node will not be able to conduct an electrical impulse across a surgical suture line).

   c. **Echocardiography** can be performed if there is suspicion of a rejection episode. A decrease in exercise tolerance or new onset of dysrhythmias may signal such an episode.
   d. **Cardiac catheterization** is usually performed electively on a yearly basis. This may be the only way to assess development of coronary artery disease; as noted above, anginal symptoms will be absent! Obtaining the data from the most recent catheterization report, if time permits, may be helpful.
   e. **Immunosuppressive therapy.** All the agents used will increase the incidence of infection, and all have nonimmunologic side effects (Table 14-7). The three most common agents are cyclosporine, azathioprine, and prednisone. Triple therapy is common to decrease the side effects of each. Recently, antithymocyte serum (a lymphotoxic agent) and OKT$_3$ (a monoclonal antibody that decreases circulating T cells and interferes with T-cell antigen recognition) are gaining popularity for treatment of rejection episodes.
2. **Asepsis.** Strict adherence to asepsis is essential in these immunocompromised patients. Airway instrumentation and intravenous access should be kept to a minimum and accomplished with rigid adherence to clean technique. For example, a pretracheal stethoscope is a reasonable, noninvasive alternative to an esophageal stethoscope. Likewise, unless a procedure is lengthy or involves large fluid shifts, omission of invasive (i.e., nasopharyngeal) temperature monitoring is acceptable provided that ability to institute such monitoring is available if needed.
3. **Monitoring.** Electrocardiographic monitoring for ischemia and dysrhythmias is essential. Atrial and ventricular dysrhythmias are common in the first 6 months after transplantation and may represent cardiac rejection.
   Central venous or pulmonary artery monitoring should be used only if absolutely necessary to avoid introduction of catheter-related infectious agents. However, such monitoring should not be withheld if a procedure involving moderate blood loss or fluid shifts is anticipated, or if the patient exhibits congestive heart failure during a rejection episode. In such situations, maintenance of adequate preload and therefore monitoring of central venous pressures is crucial

Table 14-7. Immunosuppressive agents

Agent	Mechanism	Side effects

Cyclosporine A	Decreased helper T-cell activity
	Impaired interleukin-II production[a]
		Neuroectodermal
		  Hypermycosis[b]
		  Gingival hyperplasia
		  Tremors
		  Burning paresthesias
		Mesenchymal
		  Nephrotoxicity
		    Vasoconstriction
		    Platelet adhesion
		  Hepatotoxicity
		  Systemic hypertension

Azathioprine	Purine antimetabolite	Leukopenia/thrombocytopenia Hepatotoxicity Antagonizes nondepolarizing neuromuscular blockade
Steroids *(prednisone)*	Inhibits inflammatory response Inhibits PMN leukocyte margination	Infection Hypertension Insulin resistance Cataracts Avascular necrosis of bone Obesity Peptic ulcer disease ? Accelerated graft atherosclerosis

[a]Interleukin II stimulates T-cell proliferation and enhances differentiation of activated T cells
[b]A preponderance of fungal infections

Table 14-8. Indications for invasive monitoring

Surgical procedures with large fluid shifts
Rejection crisis with decreased ejection fraction
Known coronary disease
Sepsis
Pulmonary hypertension

for optimal cardiovascular performance. The same considerations hold true for invasive arterial blood pressure monitoring. Table 14-8 lists indications for invasive monitoring.

4. **Steroid use** (see Table 14-7). These patients will probably be receiving chronic steroid therapy. "Stress" steroid coverage should therefore be administered. Care should be exercised with patient positioning because fragile bones may be easily injured in patients with chronic steroid use. Likewise, paper tape should be used on their delicate skin, and automated blood pressure cuffs should be used with caution because high inflation pressures can result in skin abrasions. Symptoms of peptic ulcer disease should be sought, and perioperative antacid therapy is warranted.

5. **Anesthetic agents and techniques.** Virtually all agents and types of anesthesia have been used successfully in patients with transplanted hearts. The key to successful management of these patients

is **avoidance of rapid vasodilation** because compensatory heart rate changes will be delayed. Any anesthetic intervention should therefore be done slowly, allowing time for the patient's cardiovascular system to adapt. Rapid administration of a large bolus of thiopental or induction of high spinal anesthesia should be done with caution, if at all. Certainly such maneuvers should be preceded by adequate volume loading, and the immediate availability of a direct-acting vasopressor such as phenylephrine and a chronotropic agent such as isoproterenol (not atropine) should be ensured before induction of anesthesia. Although neostigmine will not cause bradycardia, **reversal of nondepolarizing neuromuscular blockade must nevertheless be accompanied by an anticholinergic agent** because peripheral (noncardiac) muscarinic effects of the acetylcholinesterase inhibitors must still be blocked.

Depth of general anesthesia may be difficult to assess because chronically elevated heart rates (absence of vagal tone) provide little or even misleading information about anesthetic depth. Appropriate doses of anesthetic agents should be administered and overdosage avoided by using blood pressure, not heart rate, as an end point for anesthetic titration.

REFERENCES

1. Bhatia, S. J. S., Kirshenbaum, J. M., and Shemin, R. J., et al. Time course of resolution of pulmonary hypertension and right ventricular remodeling after orthotopic cardiac transplantation. *Circulation* 76:819–826, 1987.
2. Borow, K. M., Neumann, B. S., and Arensman, F. W. Left ventricular contractility and contractile reserve in humans after cardiac transplantation. *Circulation* 71:866–872, 1985.
3. Fragomeni, L. S., and Kaye, M. P. The registry of the International Society for Heart Transplantation: Fifth Official Report—1988. *J. Heart Trans.* 7(4):249–253, 1988.
4. Hensley, F. A., Jr., Martin, D. E., and Larach, D. R., et al. Anesthetic management for cardiac transplantation in North America—1986 Survey. *J. Cardiothorac. Anesth.* 1:429–437, 1987.
5. Lower, R. R., and Shumway, N. E. Studies on orthotopic transplantation of the canine heart. *Surg. Forum* 11:18–19, 1960.
6. Novitzky, D., Cooper, D. K. C., and Barnard, C. N. The surgical technique of heterotopic heart transplantation. *Ann. Thorac. Surg.* 36:476–482, 1983.
7. Schroeder, J. S. Hemodynamic performance of the human transplanted heart. *Transplant. Proc.* 11:304–308, 1979.
8. Stinson, E. B., Caves, P. K., and Griepp, R. B., et al. Hemodynamic observations in the early period after human heart transplantation. *J. Thorac. Cardiovasc. Surg.* 69:264–270, 1975.
9. Wetzel, R. C., Setzer, N., Stiff, J. L., et al. Hemodynamic responses in brain dead organ donor patients. *Anesth. Analg.* 64:125–128, 1985.
10. Yusuf, S., Theodoropoulos, S., and Mathias, C. J. Increased sensitivity of the denervated transplanted human heart to isoprenaline both before and after β-adrenergic blockade. *Circulation* 75:696–704, 1987.

SUGGESTED READING

Clark, N. J., and Martin, R. D. Anesthetic considerations for patients undergoing cardiac transplantation. *J. Cardiothorac. Anesth.* 2(4):519–542, 1988.
Gay, W. A., Jr. Cardiac transplantation: A surgical perspective. *J. Cardiothorac. Anesth.* 2(4):513–518, 1988.
Renlund, D. G., Bristow, M. R., Lee, H. R., et al. Medical aspects of cardiac transplantation. *J. Cardiothorac. Anesth.* 2(4):500–512, 1988.

Wyner, J., and Finch, E. L. Heart and Heart-Lung Transplantation. In Gelman, S. (ed.), *Anesthesia and Organ Transplantation*. Philadelphia: Saunders, 1987. Pp. 111–137.

Anesthetic Management for Thoracic Aneurysms and Dissections

Thomas M. Skeehan and John R. Cooper, Jr.

The anesthetic management of thoracic aortic surgery may call for a variety of responses from the anesthesiologist because of the marked variability in the problems associated with etiology, type, and anatomic location of the surgical procedure. This chapter will give a concise overview of the pathophysiology, an understanding of the surgical approaches and results, and a rational approach to the management of the patient undergoing thoracic aortic surgery.

I. Classification and natural history

A. Dissections.
An **aortic dissection** occurs when blood penetrates the aortic intima and forms an expanding hematoma within the vessel wall, usually separating the intima and media to create a so-called false lumen or dissecting hematoma. The intima is not dilated and in fact is often compressed by the advancing hematoma. In contrast, an **aortic aneurysm** involves dilatation of all three layers of the vessel wall and has a very different pathophysiology and implications for management. The term **dissecting aneurysm,** though very commonly used, is often a misnomer.

1. Incidence and pathophysiology

a. Incidence.
Aortic dissections have been estimated to be the cause of 1 per 10,000 hospital admissions. In large autopsy series, aortic dissection has been found in 1 in 600 cases, and it was felt that dissections may have caused or contributed significantly to the mortality in up to 1% of these autopsy cases.

b. Predisposing conditions.
The medical conditions predisposing to aortic dissection are listed in Table 15-1 in their order of importance. Interestingly, **atherosclerosis** by itself may not contribute to the risk of subsequent dissection.

c. Inciting event.
The onset of aortic dissections has been associated with increased physical activity or emotional stress. Dissections have also been associated with blunt trauma to the chest; however, the temporal relationship of blunt trauma and subsequent dissections has not been well established. Dissections can occur without any physical activity. They may also occur during cannulation for cardiopulmonary bypass.

d. Mechanism of aortic tear.
An intimal tear must be the initial event in aortic dissection. The intimal tear of aortic dissections usually occurs in the presence of a weakened aortic wall, predominantly involving the middle and outer layers of the media. In this area of weakening, the aortic wall is more susceptible to shear forces produced by pulsatile blood flow in the aorta. The most frequent locations of intimal tears are the areas experiencing the greatest mechanical shear forces, as listed in Table 15-2.

In large autopsy series, however, up to 4% of dissections had no identifiable intimal disruption. In these cases, rupture of the **vasa vasorum,** the vessels that supply blood to the aortic wall, have been implicated as an alternative cause of dissections. These thin-walled vessels are located in the outer third of the aortic wall, and their rupture would cause the formation of a medial hematoma and propagation of a dissection in the presence of an already diseased vessel, without formation of an intimal tear.

e. Propagation.
Propagation of an aortic dissection can occur within seconds. The factors that contribute to propagation are the hemodynamic forces inherent in pulsatile flow: (1) pulse pressure, and (2) ejection velocity of blood.

f. Exit points.
Exit points of dissections are found in a relatively small percentage of cases. Exit point tears usually occur distal to the intimal tear and represent points at which blood from the false

Table 15-1. Aortic dissections—predisposing conditions

History of hypertension	Present in ≈90% of patients
Advanced age	>60 years
Sex	Male preponderance under age 60
Arachnodactyly (Marfan's syndrome)	Also other connective tissue diseases
Congenital heart disease	Coarctation of aorta, bicuspid aortic valve
Pregnancy	Uncommon
Other causes	Toxins and diet

Table 15-2. Sites of primary intimal tears in acute dissections of the aorta (398 autopsy cases)

Site	Percent incidence
Ascending	61
Descending Isthmus (16%) Other (8%)	24
Arch	9
Abdominal	3
Other	1

Note: The ascending and isthmic (just distal to the left subclavian artery) segments of the aorta are relatively fixed and thus cause the greatest amount of mechanical shear stress. This explains the high incidence of intimal tears in these areas.
Source: Modified from A. E. Hirst Jr., V. J. Johns Jr., and W. Kime Jr. Dissecting aneurysm of the aorta: A review of 505 cases. *Medicine* 37:243, 1958.

lumen reenters the true lumen. The presence or absence of an exit point does not appear to have an impact on the clinical course.

- **g. Involvement of arterial branches.** The origins of the major branches of the aorta, including the coronary arteries, may be involved in aortic dissections. Their involvement may include occlusion of their lumens by compression by the aorta false lumen as well as propagation of the dissecting hematoma into the arterial branch. The incidence of involvement of arterial branches from a large autopsy series is outlined in Table 15-3.

2. **DeBakey classification of dissections** (Fig. 15-1). This classification comprises three different types, depending on (1) where the intimal tear is located, and (2) which section of the aorta is involved.

- **a. Type I.** The intimal tear is located in the ascending portion, but the dissection involves all portions (ascending, arch, and descending) of the thoracic aorta.
- **b. Type II.** The intimal tear is in the ascending aorta, but the dissection involves the ascending aorta only, stopping before the takeoff of the innominate artery.
- **c. Type III.** The intimal tear is located in the descending segment, and the dissection almost always involves the descending portion of the thoracic aorta only, starting just distal to the origin of the left subclavian artery. By definition, type III dissections can propagate proximally into the arch, but this is rare.

Table 15-3. Involvement of major arterial branches in aortic dissections

Artery	Percent incidence
Iliac	25.2
Common carotid	14.5
Innominate	12.9
Renal (either)	12.0
Left subclavian	10.9
Mesenteric	8.2
Coronary (either)	7.5
Intercostal	4.0
Celiac	3.2
Lumbar	1.6

Source: Modified from A.E. Hirst Jr., V.J. Johns Jr., and W. Kime Jr. Dissecting aneurysm of the aorta: A review of 505 cases. *Medicine* 37:243, 1958.

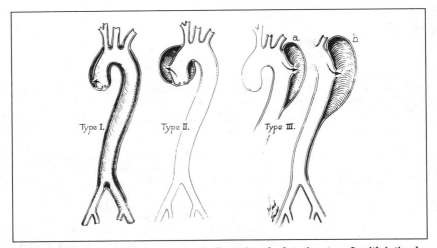

Fig. 15-1. DeBakey classification of aortic dissections by location: type I, with intimal tear in the ascending portion and dissection extending to descending aorta; type II, ascending intimal tear and dissection limited to ascending aorta; type III, intimal tear distal to left subclavian, but dissection extending for a variable distance. (From M. E. DeBakey, W. S. Henly, et al. Dissecting aneurysms of the aorta. *J. Thorac. Cardiovasc. Surg.* 49:131, 1965. With permission.)

3. **Stanford (Daily) classification of dissections** (Fig. 15-2). This classification is simpler than the DeBakey classification and also has more clinical relevance.
   a. **Type A.** Type A dissections are those that have any involvement of the ascending aorta, regardless of where the intimal tear is located and regardless of how far the dissection propagates. Clinically, type A dissections run a more virulent course.
   b. **Type B.** Type B dissections are those that involve the aorta distal to the origin of the left subclavian artery.

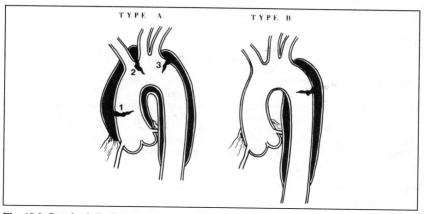

Fig. 15-2. Stanford (Daily) classification of aortic dissections: Type A describes a dissection involving the ascending aorta regardless of site of intimal tear; in type B, both the intimal tear and the extension are distal to the left subclavian. (From D. C. Miller, E. B. Stinson, et al. Aortic dissections. *J. Thorac. Cardiovasc. Surg.* 78:367, 1979. With permission.)

4. **Natural history**
   a. **Mortality—untreated.** The survival rate of untreated patients with aortic dissections is dismal, with a 2-day mortality of up to 50% in some series, and a 6-month mortality approaching 90%. The usual cause of death is rupture of the false lumen and fatal hemorrhage. Other causes of death include progressive cardiac failure (aortic valve involvement), myocardial infarction, stroke, irreversible coma, and bowel gangrene (mesenteric artery occlusion).
   b. **Surgical mortality.** The overall surgical mortality is approximately 30%, but surgical therapy is often the only viable option for most of these patients.

B. **Aneurysms**
   1. **Incidence.** Thoracic aortic aneurysms comprise 1–4% of aneurysms seen at autopsy. Currently, approximately 60% involve the ascending aorta, and 30% are localized to the descending aorta. Aneurysms involving the aortic arch exclusively are more rare, making up less than 10% of the total.
   2. **Classification by location and etiology.** In general, the etiology and pathophysiology of aortic aneurysms are site dependent. The most common causes by region are medionecrosis in the ascending aorta and atherosclerosis in the arch and descending aorta. Other etiologies are listed in Table 15-4.
   3. **Classification by shape**
      a. **Fusiform.** Fusiform aneurysmal dilatation involves the entire circumference of the aortic wall.
      b. **Saccular.** Saccular aneurysms involve only one portion of the aortic wall. **Aortic arch aneurysms** are commonly of this type.
   4. **Natural history.** The usual history of aortic aneurysm is that of progressive dilation and, in more than 50% of cases, rupture. The untreated 5-year survival is approximately 13%, depending on the size of the aneurysm at diagnosis. Other complications include mycotic infection, atheroembolism to peripheral vessels, and dissection. This last complication is rare, probably occurring in less than 10%

Table 15-4. Etiology of aneurysms based on location in the aorta

Ascending	
Medionecrosis	Accumulation of mucoid material between elastic elements in the outer third of aortic wall, eventually involving the entire media
Syphilis	Major cause before 1950, distinguished by invasion of the aortic wall by *Treponema pallidum*
Congenital	Secondary to inborn errors in metabolism (Marfan's syndrome, Ehrlos-Danlos syndrome) leading to generalized defect of connective tissue
Post-stenotic dilation	Secondary to longstanding aortic stenosis
Atherosclerosis	Not a major cause in ascending pathology
Arch	
Isolated	Atherosclerosis
Associated with ascending disease	Same etiologies as for disease in ascending aorta
Descending	
Atherosclerosis	Begins as intimal disease; major cause of thoracoabdominal and abdominal aneurysms
Congenital	See above under Ascending
Trauma	Causal relationship difficult to prove; history of blunt trauma may be distant
Infection	Syphilis, *Salmonella,* tuberculosis

Etiologies are listed in order of frequency.

of cases. Some predictors of poor prognosis are large size (greater than 10 cm maximum transverse diameter), presence of symptoms, and associated cardiovascular disease, especially coronary artery disease, myocardial infarction, or cerebral vascular accident.

C. Thoracic aortic rupture (tear)

1. Etiology. The overwhelming majority of thoracic ruptures are secondary to trauma and almost always involve a **deceleration injury** in a motor vehicle accident. Sudden deceleration places large mechanical stresses on the aortic wall at points where the aorta is relatively immobile. Rupture of the aorta in many cases leads to immediate exsanguination and death. However, in approximately 10–15% of cases, the integrity of the lumen is maintained by the adventitial covering of the aorta, and these patients are able to reach emergency care. Surgical treatment of these survivors is often successful.

2. Location. The location of most ruptures of the thoracic aorta is the area just distal to the origin of the left subclavian artery (isthmus), owing to the relative fixation of the aorta at this point by the ligamentum arteriosum (Fig. 15-3). The aorta is also fixed in the ascending portion just distal to the aortic valve, and this is the second most common site of rupture.

II. Diagnosis

A. Clinical signs and symptoms

1. Dissections. The clinical presentation of aortic dissection is usually characterized by a dramatic onset and a fulminant course. Differences and clinical presentation of Stanford types A and B are outlined in Table 15-5.

2. Aneurysms. Aneurysms of the ascending, arch, or descending thoracic aorta are often asymptomatic until late in their course. In many circumstances, the presence of an aneurysm is not diagnosed until

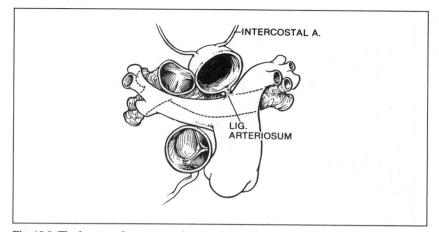

Fig. 15-3. The heart and great vessels are relatively mobile in the pericardium, whereas the descending aorta is relatively fixed by its anatomic relations. The attachment of the ligamentum arteriosum enhances this immobility and increases the risk of aortic tear due to deceleration injury. (From D. A. Cooley [ed.], *Surgical Treatment of Aortic Aneurysms.* Philadelphia: Saunders, 1986. P. 186. With permission.)

medical evaluation is conducted for an unrelated problem or for a problem related to a complication of the aneurysm.

3. **Traumatic rupture.** Ruptures most commonly occur just distal to the left subclavian artery. In this setting, signs and symptoms are similar to those seen for aneurysms of the descending thoracic aorta if the patient survives the initial event.

B. **Laboratory diagnosis**
   1. **Electrocardiogram (ECG).** A common finding for many patients with aortic disease is that of **left ventricular hypertrophy,** which correlates with a history of hypertension that is often present. The ECG may also show a pattern associated with ischemia or pericarditis caused by coronary artery occlusion or hemopericardium, respectively in the setting of ascending aortic dissection.
   2. **Chest x ray.** A **widened mediastinum** is a classic x-ray finding in the presence of thoracic aortic pathology. Widening of the aortic knob is often seen, with **disparate ascending** to **descending diameter.** A double shadow has been described in the setting of aortic dissection, in which the false lumen is actually visualized.
   3. **Serum chemistries.** There are no specific laboratory findings with asymptomatic aneurysm. Dissection or rupture will produce a fall in hemoglobin, and dissections may also cause elevation of cardiac enzymes (coronary artery occlusion), elevation of BUN and creatine (renal artery occlusion), and acidosis (low cardiac output or bowel ischemia).
   4. **Computed tomography scans (CT scans).** CT is a useful tool for diagnosing aneurysm size and has replaced angiography in some instances.
   5. **Angiography.** This remains the "gold standard" for determining the severity and extent of aneurysm and dissection. It can be used to determine the site of an intimal tear in the setting of dissecting hematoma, assess aortic valve function, and the distal and proximal spread of the lesion. In the case of ascending aortic pathology that

Table 15-5. Presenting clinical signs and symptoms by location and type of aortic pathology

	Aneurysm	Dissection	Aortic tear
General presentation	Chronic symptoms, but leaking or ruptured aneurysm can lead to fulminant course (see aortic tear for symptoms and signs)	Dramatic onset and fulminant course. Symptoms depend on location (type A or type B). Patient presents in shock, anxious, diaphoretic	History of deceleration injury; usually fulminant course (good chance of survival if patient gets to treatment center). Patient can present in hypovolemic shock
Symptoms and signs			
Ascending and arch			
Location of pain	Anterior chest pain secondary to compression of: (1) coronary arteries (2) sensory mediastinal nerves	**Type A dissection[a]** Anterior chest pain secondary to: (1) extension of dissection (ripping or tearing sensation) (2) angina, from dissection of coronaries	Chest pain secondary to compression of structures by enlarging adventitia (the only structure maintaining aortic integrity)
Cardiovascular	CHF[b] symptoms secondary to aortic annular enlargement (1) widened pulse pressure (2) diastolic murmur Facial and upper trunk venous congestion secondary to superior vena cava compression Blood pressure usually elevated chronically	CHF symptoms: (1) murmur of aortic valve insufficiency (2) narrowing of true lumen (increased afterload) systolic ejection murmur Blood pressure (1) hypotension secondary to rupture into the retroperitoneum, intraabdominal, intrathoracic, or pericardial spaces (2) hypertension secondary to pain, anxiety Assymmetry of pulses, or pulseless extremity	Blood pressure (1) Hypotension from hypovolemia (2) Hypertension from pain

Respiratory	Hoarseness secondary to compression of recurrent laryngeal nerve Dyspnea or stridor due to tracheal compression Hemoptysis due to erosion into trachea Rales secondary to CHF	Hoarseness secondary to compression of recurrent laryngeal nerve Dyspnea and stridor due to tracheal compression Hemoptysis due to erosion into trachea (chronic) Rales secondary to CHF	Lung contusion if chest trauma is significant
Gastrointestinal	Not usually affected	See Descending Dissection[a]	Not usually affected
Renal	Not usually affected	See Descending Dissection[a]	Decreased function secondary to hypotension
Neurologic	Possible due to emboli from aortic valve	Hemiparesis or hemiplegia secondary to involvement of single carotid artery Reversible or progressive coma	Symptoms related to hypoperfusion
Descending		**Type B dissection**	
Location of pain	Chronic back pain may occur	Located in back, midscapular region	Located in midscapular region
Cardiovascular	Blood pressure—usually normal or elevated (chronic hypertension)	Blood pressure (1) Elevated secondary to pain (common) (2) Hypotension if rupture of aneurysm has occurred	Blood pressure (1) Elevated secondary to pain (esp. with other injuries from trauma) (2) Hypotension if hypovolemic
Respiratory	Dyspnea from left mainstem obstruction Hemoptysis due to erosion into left bronchus Hemorrahgic pleural effusion	Dyspnea due to left mainstem obstruction Hemorrhagic pleural effusion	Sequelae of lung contusion or rib fracture

Table 15-5. (continued)

	Aneurysm	Dissection	Aortic tear
Gastrointestinal	Usually not abnormal	Mimics an acute abdomen Pain, rigid abdomen, nausea and vomiting Gastrointestinal bleeding Bowel ischemia secondary to: Compression or dissection of mesenteric or celiac artery	Usually normal
Renal	Renal insufficiency or renovascular hypertension if occlusive aortic disease develops	Ischemia due to involvement of renal arteries in dissection: (1) infarction and renal failure (2) renal insufficiency	Renal hypofunction from hypoperfusion or hypovolemia
Neurologic	Usually not affected	Paraparesis or paraplegia possible	Paraplegia possible

aType A dissections may involve the entire aorta; therefore, symptoms of both ascending and descending pathology may be present.
bCHF = Congestive heart failure.

will require cardiopulmonary bypass, the coronary anatomy can be delineated. Patients with disease of the thoracic aorta usually have concurrent coronary disease; bypassing significant lesions would help to improve ventricular function for weaning from cardiopulmonary bypass. Aortography can diagnose the involvement of major vessels but can rarely identify the critical intercostal vessels that provide blood supply to the spinal cord (see sec. **IV.G.**).

C. Indications for surgical correction

1. Ascending aortic pathology

a. Dissections. Currently, any acute type A dissection should be corrected surgically, given the virulent course and high mortality if left untreated.

b. Aneurysms. Surgical indications for resection include:

(1) The presence of persistent pain despite a small aneurysm.

(2) Involvement of the aortic valve producing aortic insufficiency.

(3) The presence of angina due either to left ventricular strain from aortic valve involvement or coronary artery involvement by the aneurysm.

(4) A rapidly expanding aneurysm or an aneurysm greater than 10 cm in diameter, because the chance of rupture increases with increasing size.

2. Aortic arch pathology

a. Dissections. An acute dissection limited to the aortic arch is also an indication for surgery (rare).

b. Aneurysms. Because even elective surgical treatment for these types of aneurysms is more difficult and is associated with a higher morbidity and mortality, management tends to be more conservative. Surgical indications include:

(1) Persistence of symptoms

(2) An aneurysm of greater than 10 cm in transverse diameter

(3) Progressive expansion of an aneurysm

3. Descending aortic pathology

a. Dissection. Some controversy remains concerning the best treatment for an acute type B dissection. Owing to similar mortality statistics for medical or surgical intervention, type B dissections are often treated medically in the acute phase, especially if a patient's concurrent disease would make surgical mortality prohibitively high. However, patients with a type B dissection who develop any of the following complications should be treated surgically:

(1) Failure to control hypertension medically

(2) Continued pain (indicating progression of the dissection)

(3) Enlargement on chest x ray, CT scan, or angiogram

(4) Development of a neurologic deficit

(5) Evidence of renal or gastrointestinal ischemia

(6) Development of aortic insufficiency

It should also be noted, as shown in Table 15-6, that 10-year survival for patients with type B dissections managed medically is similar to surgical survival for types A and B dissections together. Both of these managements compare favorably to the 10-year survival of patients with untreated aortic dissections.

b. Aneurysm. Surgical indications include:

(1) A chronic aneurysm of the descending thoracic aorta that causes persistent pain or other symptoms

(2) An aneurysm greater than 10 cm in diameter

(3) An expanding aneurysm

(4) A leaking aneurysm (more fulminant symptoms)

Table 15-6. Aortic dissections: surgical vs medical therapy

	Percent hospital mortality	
	Surgical	Medical
Type A	32	72
Type B	32	27
10-yr survival	20–25 (A and B)	33 (B only)

Source: Modified from D.C. Miller, E.B. Stinson, P.E. Oyer. et al. Operative treatment of aortic dissection. *J. Thorac. Cardiovasc. Surg.* 78:365, 1979.

III. **Preoperative management of patients requiring surgery of the thoracic aorta.** Emergency preoperative management of **aortic dissections** is discussed below. However, emergency preoperative management for a **leaking thoracic aneurysm** and a **contained thoracic rupture** would be similar.

A. **Prioritizing making the diagnosis versus controlling blood pressure.** In the setting of a suspected dissecting hematoma, aortic tear, or leaking aneurysm, the first priority must always be to control the blood pressure. **Making the diagnosis with chest x ray or angiogram should occur only when proper monitoring, IV access, and therapy have been established.** During the diagnostic procedure the patient should be closely monitored with a physician present as the clinical situation dictates. The anesthesiologist should become involved as early as possible to lend expertise in monitoring and in airway and hemodynamic management should clinical deterioration occur before the patient reaches the operating room.

B. **Blood pressure control.** Not only systolic and diastolic pressures but also the ejection velocity must be reduced because both of these factors have been shown to be important in the propagation of dissecting hematomas.

1. **Monitoring.** It is imperative that these patients have the following: an ECG for detection of ischemia and dysrhythmias, two large-bore intravenous catheters, an arterial catheter in the proper location (to be discussed), and, if time permits, a central venous catheter or pulmonary artery catheter to follow filling pressures and to allow drug infusion.

2. **Agents**

a. **Vasodilators**

(1) **Nitroprusside** has emerged as the agent of choice for controlling the blood pressure, since it is effective and also easily regulated owing to its short duration of action. It is given as an intravenous (IV) infusion, and central administration is optimal. The usual starting dose is 0.5–1 µg/kg/min, titrated to effect. Doses of 8–10 µg/kg/min have been associated with toxicity (see Chap. 3).

(2) **Trimethaphan** has also been used with success. However, it is considered to be a second-line agent owing to its unwanted side effects (such as pupil dilation) and the tachyphylaxis that is seen commonly with continuous infusions. Due to ganglionic blocking effects, trimethaphan decreases ejection velocity (see also sec. **b.** below) and lowers blood pressure. Bolus adminis-

tration should be in small increments (1–2 mg initially), with a continuous infusion starting at 1 mg/min and titrated to effect.

b. Decreasing ejection velocity. Decreasing ejection velocity becomes an important therapeutic consideration, especially if nitroprusside is used as the agent to lower blood pressure. Nitroprusside will increase ejection velocity by increasing dP/dt and heart rate. For this reason, beta-adrenergic blockade should be employed with nitroprusside not only to decrease tachycardia but also to decrease contractility (see Chap. 3).

(1) Propranolol can be administered in an IV bolus of 1 mg, and doses of up to 4–8 mg may be required until the effect is seen.

(2) Labetalol, a combined α- and β-blocker, may offer a single alternative to the nitroprusside-propranolol combination. It should be given initially as a 20-mg loading bolus, allowing several minutes for its effect to be seen. If no effect is seen, the dose should be doubled and several minutes allowed again for onset of effect. This process should be repeated up to a maximum dose of 40–80 mg every 10 minutes until a total dose of 300 mg is reached or until blood pressure is controlled. A continuous infusion starting at 1 mg/min may be used, or a small bolus dose can be repeated every 10–30 min to maintain blood pressure control.

(3) Esmolol is a new short-acting beta-blocking agent with a very short half-life that may also be useful. It is administered as a bolus loading dose of 500 μg/kg over 1 minute and then continued as an infusion starting at 50 μg/kg/min, titrated to effect. This drug is particularly advantageous in someone with obstructive lung disease because its action can be terminated quickly if respiratory symptoms ensue.

3. Desired end points. Blood pressure should be lowered to approximately 105–115 mm Hg systolic, and heart rate should be kept at 60–80 beats/min. If a pulmonary artery catheter is in place, the cardiac index may be lowered to the $2–2.5$ liters $\cdot$ min^{-1} $\cdot$ m^{-2} range because a hyperdynamic myocardium may promote the progression of a dissecting hematoma.

C. Transfusion. A total of 8–10 units of blood should be typed and cross-matched prior to surgery. Use of blood scavenging devices has decreased the amount of banked blood used, but the logistics of processing scavenged blood, plus the clinical situation, may require that homologous transfusion still be used.

D. Assessment of other organ systems

1. Neurologic. The patient should be followed closely to detect signs of any change in neurologic status, since deterioration in function is an indication for immediate surgical intervention.

2. Kidneys. Renal function should be followed closely after insertion of a urinary catheter. If aortic dissection has been diagnosed, the development of anuria or oliguria in the setting of euvolemia is an indication for immediate surgical intervention.

3. Gastrointestinal. Serial abdominal examinations should be performed. In addition, blood gas analysis should be done routinely to assess changes in acid-base status, since ischemic bowel can produce significant acidosis.

E. Use of pain medications. Patients with aortic dissections may be very anxious and may be in quite severe pain. Pain relief should be given not only to lessen suffering but also to aid in control of blood pressure. It is important to avoid obtundation; otherwise, important

Table 15-7. Incidence of coexisting diseases in patients with aortic pathology presenting for surgery

Coronary artery disease	66%
Hypertension	42%
Chronic obstructive pulmonary disease	23%
Peripheral vascular disease	22%
Cerebrovascular disease	14%
Diabetes mellitus	8%
Other aneurysms	4%
Chronic renal disease	3%

Source: Modified from A. Romagnoli and J.R. Cooper Jr. Anesthesia for aortic operations *Cleve. Clin. Q.* 48:148, 1981.

changes in patient status will be missed. Worsening of back pain or abdominal pain may indicate expansion of the lesion or further dissection and is regarded by many surgeons as an emergent situation. In addition, propagation of a dissection into a head vessel may lead to a change in mental status that may be undetected if the patient is oversedated.

IV. Surgical and anesthetic considerations

A. Goal of surgical therapy (for dissections, aneurysms, aortic rupture).
The first major goal in treating acute aortic disruption must be to control hemorrhage. Once control is achieved, the objectives of management of both acute and chronic lesions are similar: (1) to repair the diseased aorta, and (2) to restore relationships of major arterial branches.

Elective repair of a thoracic aneurysm is most often accomplished by replacing the diseased segment of aorta with a synthetic graft and then implanting major arterial branches into the graft. With a dissection, in contrast, the major goal is to resect the segment of aorta containing the intimal tear. When this segment is removed, it is then possible to obliterate the false lumen and interpose graft material. It may not be possible or necessary to replace *all* of the dissected portion of the aorta because, if the origin of dissection is controlled, the reexpansion of the true lumen may compress and obliterate the false lumen. With contained aortic tears, the objective is to resect the area of the tear and either (1) reanastomose the natural aorta to itself in an end-to-end fashion, or (2) use graft material for the anastomosis if there is insufficient natural aorta remaining.

B. Overview of intraoperative anesthetic management (for dissections, aneurysms, aortic rupture)

1. Key principles

a. Managing blood pressure. Blood pressure control must be maintained during the transition from the preoperative to the intraoperative period. Such control is very important in light of the surgical and anesthetic manipulations that will profoundly affect blood pressure.

b. Monitoring of organ ischemia. The following organs must be monitored continuously for adequacy of perfusion: central nervous system, heart, kidney, and lungs. The liver and gut cannot be continuously monitored, but their metabolic functions can be periodically checked.

c. **Treating coexisting disease.** Patients with aortic pathology often have associated cardiovascular and systemic diseases, as outlined in Table 15-7.

d. **Controlling bleeding.** Achieving hemostasis after cardiopulmonary bypass or with graft material in place poses special challenges, especially when the native tissue is damaged or diseased. Coagulation abnormalities and their treatment are discussed in Chapter 18.

2. **Induction and anesthetic agents.** Because many of these patients come to surgery emergently, most are considered to have a full stomach and require rapid securing of the airway. On the other hand, these patients also require a smooth induction, since wide swings in hemodynamics may worsen the clinical situation. Usually a compromise is made using a controlled induction with cricoid pressure and manual ventilation. This "modified" rapid-sequence induction allows some airway protection and expeditious titration of anesthetic drugs to control blood pressure, the main goal being to secure the airway as quickly as possible with a minimum of hemodynamic perturbation. Use of nonparticulate antacids, H_2 blockers, and metaclopramide should be considered prior to induction of anesthesia. Anesthetic considerations and agents are described more fully in sec. **IV.D.** Despite all precautions, marked changes in hemodynamics are common and should be expected.

3. **Importance of site of lesion** (Table 15-8). Although the principles of anesthetic induction and choice of anesthetic agents are similar for all aortic lesions, practical intraoperative management depends almost entirely on the site of the lesion.

C. **Surgical considerations for ascending aortic surgery**

1. **Surgical approach.** The approach used for ascending aortic surgery is a midline sternotomy.

2. **Cardiopulmonary bypass (CPB).** Because of the proximal involvement of the aorta and because the repair often includes repair or replacement of the aortic valve, cardiopulmonary bypass is required for this type of surgery.

a. If the aneurysm ends in the proximal or midportion of the ascending aorta, the arterial cannula for CPB can be placed in the upper ascending aorta or arch.

b. The usual site of cannulation, however, is the femoral artery. This is required if the entire ascending aorta is involved because an aortic cannula **cannot be placed distal to the pathology without jeopardizing perfusion to the great vessels.**

c. Venous cannulation can usually be performed through the right atrium; however, femoral venous cannulation may be necessary if the aneurysm is especially large.

3. **Aortic valve involvement.** Frequently, either aortic valvuloplasty or aortic valve replacement is necessary with ascending aortic dissections or aneurysms. Which procedure is used depends on the degree of involvement of the sinuses of Valsalva and the aortic annulus.

4. **Coronary artery involvement.** With an acute dissecting hematoma, the coronary arteries may be involved. Coronary occlusion usually takes the form of compression of the coronary lumen by the expanding false lumen and will require bypass grafting. Also, displacement of the coronary arteries from their normal position with enlargement of the aortic annulus will demand reimplantation of their orifices into the graft wall or a vein bypass.

Table 15-8. Anesthetic and surgical management for thoracic aortic surgery

	Surgical site		
	Ascending	Arch	Descending
Surgical approach	Median sternotomy	Median sternotomy	Left thoracotomy
Perfusion	CPB—aortic cannula distal to lesion, or in femoral artery	CPB—femoral artery cannula	Simple cross-clamp Heparinized Gott shunt ECC with cannulae proximal and distal to lesion
Involvement of			
Aortic valve	Sometimes	No	No
Coronary arteries	Sometimes	No	No
Pericardium	Sometimes	No	No
Invasive monitoring	Left radial or femoral arterial catheter PA catheter[b]	Arterial catheter—either arm, or femoral[a] PA catheter[b]	Proximal arterial (right radial or brachial) Distal arterial (femoral)[b] PA catheter[b]
Special techniques	Renal preservation EEG	Deep hypothermic circulatory arrest Cerebral protection Renal preservation EEG	Somatosensory evoked potentials[b] One lung ventilation Renal preservation CSF drainage[b]
Common complications	Bleeding Cardiac dysfunction	Bleeding Hypotension from cerebral protective doses of thiopental Neurologic deficits	Bleeding Paralysis Renal failure Cardiac dysfunction

CPB = Cardiopulmonary bypass, ECC = extracorporeal circulation, PA = pulmonary artery, EEG = electroencephalogram, CSF = cerebral spinal fluid.
[a]Depends on whether the left subclavian or innominate arteries are involved in the pathologic process. If there is uncertainty preoperatively, use a femoral artery catheter.
[b]Optional, depending on physician's preferences.

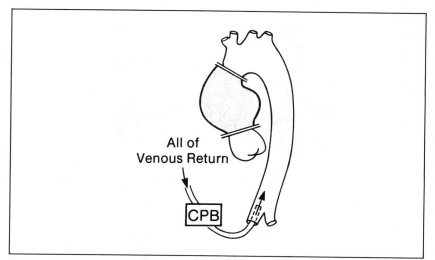

Fig. 15-4. Circulatory support and clamp placement for surgery of the ascending aorta. Femoral arterial cannula is usually required, and distal clamp must be beyond the extent of pathology. Proximal clamp would be needed to provide cold cardioplegia to the aortic root, but placement of this clamp is not possible if the proximal aorta is involved. (From J.L. Benumof. Intraoperative Considerations for Special Thoracic Surgery Cases. In J. L. Benumof [ed.], *Anesthesia for Thoracic Surgery*. Philadelphia: Saunders, 1987. P. 384. With permission.)

5. **Surgical techniques.** An example of the usual cross-clamp placement used in surgery of the ascending aorta is shown in Fig. 15-4. Note that placement of the distal clamp is more distal than would be the case for simple cross-clamping for coronary surgery and at times might even include a part of the innominate artery. If aortic insufficiency is present, a large portion of the cardioplegic solution infused into the aortic root will flow through the incompetent aortic valve instead of the coronaries, causing distention of the left ventricle and loss of the myocardial preservative effects of cardioplegia. For these reasons, an immediate aortotomy must be performed and the coronary vessels infused individually with cold cardioplegia.

If the aortic valve and annulus are both normal, the diseased section of aorta is replaced with graft material. If the annulus is normal and the valve is incompetent, the valve may be resuspended or replaced. If both valve incompetence and annular dilatation are present, either a composite graft (i.e., a tube graft with an integral artificial valve) or an aortic valve replacement with a graft sewn to the native annulus can be used. The coronary arteries must be reimplanted into the wall of the composite graft and may or may not require reimplantation when separate aortic valve replacement and grafts are used, depending on whether enough of the native sinus of Valsalva remains (Fig. 15-5). The posterior wall of the old aneurysm can then be wrapped around the graft material and sewn in place to maximize hemostasis.

In patients with ascending dissections, the aortic root is opened and the site of the intimal tear is located. A section of the aorta that includes the intimal tear is excised, and the edges of the true and

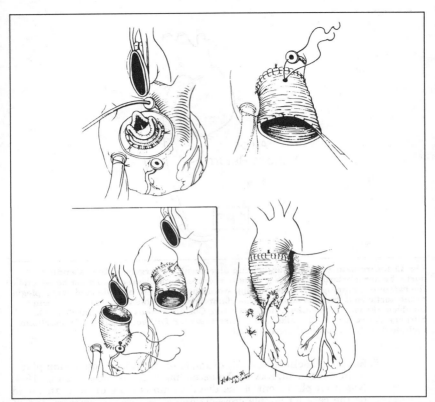

Fig. 15-5. Surgical repair of ascending aortic aneurysm or dissection. *Upper left,* Aortic valve has been replaced, aorta is transected at native annulus, leaving "buttons" of aortic wall around coronary ostia. *Upper right,* Graft material anastomosed to annulus, with left coronary reimplantation. *Lower left,* Completion of left and beginning of right coronary reimplantation. *Lower right,* Completion of distal graft anastomosis. (From D. C. Miller, E. B. Stinson, P. E. Oyer, et al. Concomitant resection of ascending aortic aneurysm and replacement of the aortic valve—operative results and long-term results with "conventional" techniques in ninety patients. *J. Thorac. Cardiovasc. Surg.* 79:394, 1980. With permission.)

false lumens are sewn together. A section of graft is used to replace the excised portion of the aorta.

6. **Complications.** Complications are those that occur with any case involving cardiopulmonary bypass and an open ventricle. These include:

a. Air emboli

b. Atheromatous or clot emboli

c. Left ventricular dysfunction secondary to ischemia

d. Myocardial infarction or myocardial ischemia secondary to technical problems with reimplantation of coronaries

e. Renal or respiratory failure

f. Clotting abnormalities

g. Surgical hemostasis; bleeding from suture lines can be especially difficult to control

D. Anesthetic considerations for ascending aortic surgery

1. Monitoring

a. Arterial catheter placement. Because the right subclavian artery may be involved in either the disease process or the surgical repair, a left radial or femoral arterial catheter is inserted for monitoring blood pressure.

b. ECG. Five-lead, calibrated electrocardiography should be used to monitor both leads II and V_5.

c. Pulmonary artery catheter. Because of the advanced age of many of these patients and the presence of severe systemic disease, a pulmonary artery catheter can be a useful aid in management preoperatively and postoperatively but is not mandatory.

d. Valvular function and two-dimensional echocardiography. Although transesophageal echocardiography may be an option to aid in assessing aortic valve function, due caution should be exercised in placing this probe in the presence of a large ascending aortic aneurysm. In the setting of preexisting esophageal dysfunction due to aneurysmal compression, placement of an esophageal echoprobe should be avoided.

e. Neurologic monitors

(1) Electroencephalogram (EEG). For evaluating brain function, either raw or processed EEG data may be helpful for judging the adequacy of cerebral perfusion during CPB.

(2) Temperature. A nasopharyngeal temperature probe, when correctly placed, gives the anesthesiologist an approximation of brain temperature. Rectal temperature should also be monitored.

f. Renal monitors. As with all cases involving bypass, urine output should be monitored.

2. Induction and anesthetic agents. See Table 15-9.

3. Cooling and rewarming. Hypothermic CPB is used in most cases of ascending aneurysms. Deep hypothermia and circulatory arrest are needed if the proximal arch is involved. If femoral cannulation is used and the femoral artery is small, a smaller cannula may be needed. This will probably delay cooling and rewarming, since lower blood flows are used to avoid excessive arterial line pressures. Extra time for cooling and rewarming must be allowed in this setting.

E. Aortic arch surgery

1. Surgical approach. The aortic arch is approached through a median sternotomy.

2. Cardiopulmonary bypass. CPB is required, and femoral cannulation must be used in almost all cases.

3. Cerebral protection. Resection of aortic arch aneurysms involves interruption of the cerebral flow. To avoid or prevent cerebral ischemia various surgical techniques have been used.

a. Temporary placement of an artificial aortic arch was the first method used but was very time consuming and technically very demanding.

b. Individual cannulation and perfusion of cerebral vessels was next used with some success. However, the technical considerations in performing this were extensive and subject to significant complications. This technique remains in use in some centers with good success.

c. Deep hypothermic circulatory arrest has been adopted by most surgeons as the best technical way to repair aortic arch pathology. Deep hypothermic circulatory arrest requires core cooling to 15–22°C, depending on the exact technique employed. Turning off the pump and partially draining the patient's blood volume into the

Table 15-9. Anesthetic considerations and choice of anesthetic agent for surgery of the aorta

Patient variables	Opioids[a]	Volatile agent[b]	Other IV agents[c]
Full stomach	Rapid acting (especially sufentanyl, alfentanyl)	Prolonged induction	Rapid acting if tolerated
Hemodynamic instability	Minimal myocardial depression Potent analgesics useful for treating intraoperative hypertension	Dose-dependent myocardial depression Indicated if hypertensive with adequate cardiac output	T: Myocardial depression D, E: Minimal myocardial depression K: Worsens hypertension
Ventricular function (VF)	Indicated with poor VF	Use only in patients with good VF	D, E, and K maintain VF Avoid T if VF is poor
Neurologic function	Decrease $CMRO_2$[d]	Decrease $CMRO_2$, especially isoflurane. Unclear in vivo protective effects	T decreases $CMRO_2$, probably protective, used with hypothermic arrest or open ventricle
Myocardial ischemia (coronary involvement)	Oxygen balance: increase supply and demand and therefore will have adverse effects in presence of hypertension	Decrease supply and demand but will have negative effect in presence of hypotension	T: Adversely affects supply secondary to hypotension K: Increases oxygen demand, decreases supply (secondary to tachycardia)

[a]Refers to fentanyl, sufentanyl, and alfentanyl.
[b]Halothane, enflurane, and isoflurane.
[c]T = thiopental, E = etomidate, K = ketamine, D = diazepam.
[d]Cerebral metabolic rate of oxygen consumption.
VF = ventricular function.

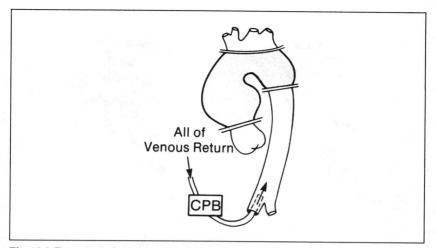

Fig. 15-6. Representation of cannula and clamp placement for surgery of the aortic arch. Femoral bypass is used. Proximal clamp is placed to arrest the heart. Distal clamp isolates the arch so that the distal anastomosis can be performed. Middle clamp on major branches isolates the head vessels so that en bloc attachment to graft is possible. (From J. L. Benumof. Intraoperative Considerations for Special Thoracic Surgery Cases. In J. L. Benumof [ed.], *Anesthesia for Thoracic Surgery*. Philadelphia: Saunders, 1987. P. 384. With permission.)

     pump provides a bloodless field with hypothermic brain protection. This has improved results but is associated with longer bypass runs.

  4. Technique. Typical placement of clamps for this procedure is shown in Fig. 15-6. Note that the surgical technique dictates that the cerebral vessels be clamped to resect the aneurysmal or dissected section of aortic arch.

     The attachments of the cerebral vessels are usually excised en bloc; such that all three vessels are located on one "button" of tissue, as shown in Fig. 15-7. This facilitates a rapid reimplantation of vessels and reestablishment of blood flow. Once the distal anastomosis is completed, the surgeon then sutures the button of cerebral vessels to the graft material. The clamp can then be replaced more proximally, the arch portion of the graft de-aired, the distal aortic clamp removed, and flow reestablished to the cerebral vessels from the femoral CPB aortic cannula. Thus the time of brain ischemia is minimized. The proximal anastomosis is then completed.

  5. Complications. Complications of this operation are similar to those with any procedure employing CPB. Irreversible cerebral ischemia is a distinct possibility with this type of surgery. Hemostatic difficulties may be increased secondary to the multiple suture lines and long bypass time.

F. Anesthetic considerations for aortic arch surgery
  1. Monitoring
    a. Arterial blood pressure. An intraarterial catheter can be placed in either the right or left radial artery for prebypass management if the innominate or left subclavian arteries, respectively, are not involved. If both are involved, the femoral artery should be catheterized.

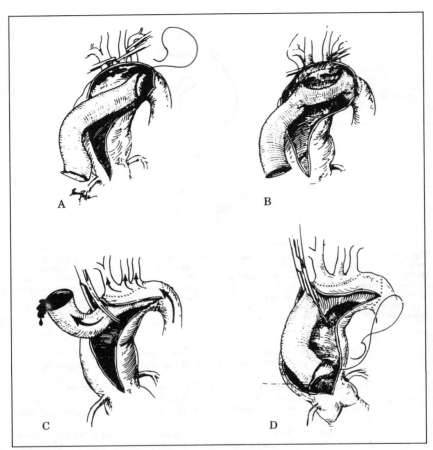

Fig. 15-7. Aortic arch replacement. In *A,* the distal suture line is completed first, followed by *B,* reattachment of the arch vessels. Flow is then reestablished to these vessels by moving the clamp more proximally, as in *C.* The proximal suture line is then completed *D.* (From E. S. Crawford and S. A. Saleh. Transverse aortic arch aneurysm—improved results of treatment employing new modifications of aortic reconstruction and hypokalemic cerebral circulatory arrest. *Ann. Surg.* 194:186, 1981. With permission.)

b. Neurologic monitors

    (1) EEG can be useful not only for ensuring that adequate cooling has been achieved but also for titration of the thiopental dose for brain protection.

    (2) Nasal temperature will also verify adequate brain cooling.

2. Choice of anesthetic agents. See Table 15-9.

3. Management of hypothermic circulatory arrest. The technique involves core cooling to 15–20°C, packing the head in ice, utilizing other cerebral protective agents, avoiding glucose-containing solutions, and utilizing proper monitoring. More detail is supplied in Chap. 24.

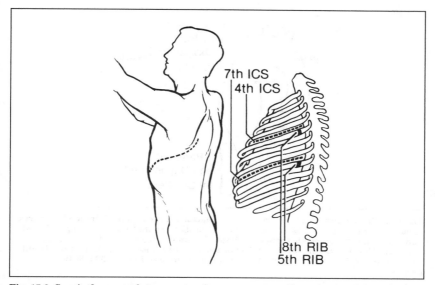

Fig. 15-8. Surgical approach to an extensive aneurysm or dissection involving the descending thoracic aorta. A single musculocutaneous incision and a double intercostal incision are used. The standard proximal and distal intercostal incisions are made through the fourth and seventh intercostal spaces (ICS), respectively. A traumatic aortic rupture at the isthmus can usually be reached through a single intercostal incision. (From D. A. Cooley [ed.], *Surgical Treatment of Aortic Aneurysms.* Philadelphia: Saunders, 1986. P. 63. With permission.)

4. **Complications.** Complications related to anesthesia for this procedure are uncommon. One is myocardial depression secondary to the use of thiopental for cerebral protection, and inotropic agents may be needed to wean the patient from cardiopulmonary bypass.

G. **Descending thoracic aortic surgery**

1. **Surgical approach.** Exposure of the descending aorta is accomplished through a left thoracotomy incision, usually between the fourth and fifth ribs. A double intercostal incision may be necessary for complete exposure (Fig. 15-8). The patient is placed in a full right lateral decubitus position with the hips slightly rolled to the left to allow access to the femoral vessels. When positioning the patient, it is important to provide protection to pressure points, including use of axillary roll, pillows between the knees, and pads for the head and elbows. It is also important to maintain the occiput in line with the thoracic spine to prevent traction on the brachial plexus.

2. **Surgical techniques.** The surgical technique used, whether for treating an aneurysm, dissection, or rupture, involves placing crossclamps above and below the lesion, opening the aorta, and replacing the diseased segment with a graft.

a. **Simple cross-clamping.** Many groups report success with crossclamping the aorta above and below the lesion without adjuncts to maintain distal perfusion. This technique has the advantage of simplifying the operation and reducing the amount of heparin needed (Fig. 15-9).

Clamping the descending aorta produces marked hemodynamic changes: profound **hypertension** in the proximal aorta and

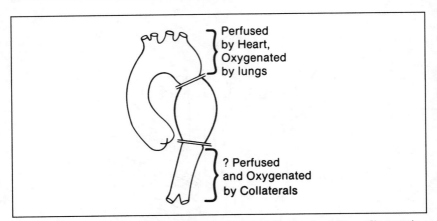

Perfused
by Heart,
Oxygenated
by lungs

? Perfused
and Oxygenated
by Collaterals

Fig. 15-9. Illustration of simple cross-clamp placement for repair of descending aortic aneurysm or dissection. Distal clamp placement dictates that flow to the spinal cord and major organs proceeds through collateral vessels. (From J. L. Benumof. Intraoperative Considerations for Special Thoracic Surgery Cases. In J. L. Benumof [ed.], *Anesthesia for Thoracic Surgery*. Philadelphia: Saunders, 1987. P. 384. With permission.)

hypotension below the distal clamp. The increase in afterload that occurs when the majority of the cardiac output goes only to the great vessels causes acute elevations in left ventricular filling pressures and a progressive fall in cardiac output. The presumption is that left ventricular failure will result if this afterload is maintained for any significant length of time. Also, the acute increase in pressure proximal to the clamp can precipitate a catastrophic cerebral event (e.g., rupture of a cerebral aneurysm).

Mean arterial pressure distal to the cross-clamp decreases to less than 10–20% of control. This decrease is paralleled by a decrease in renal blood flow and spinal cord blood flow. The presence of a chronic obstruction to flow and the resultant well-developed collateral flow (i.e., coarctation) will lessen the hemodynamic changes that are usually seen. Examples of blood pressures above and below a cross-clamp are shown in Table 15-10.

b. Shunts. A method that provides decompression of the proximal aorta and perfusion of the distal segment involves placement of a heparin-bonded (Gott) extracorporeal shunt from the left ventricle, aortic arch, or left subclavian artery to the femoral artery. Systemic heparinization is not required. The advantage with this technique is that distal perfusion can be maintained while decompression of the proximal aorta is achieved. The major problems with this technique are technical difficulties with placement and kinking with inadequate distal flows (Fig. 15-10).

c. Extracorporeal circulation (ECC). Historically the first method used for distal perfusion and proximal decompression, this technique is being used more often recently after a period of being out of favor at many centers. There are several ways to perform ECC; all involve removal of blood, passage of blood to an extracorporeal pump, and reinfusion of blood into the femoral artery to perfuse the aorta below the distal cross-clamp (Fig. 15-11). Blood may be returned to the pump from the femoral vein, which is technically

Table 15-10. Simple aortic clamp: proximal versus distal blood pressures

	Proximal systolic/diastolic (mm Hg)	Distal mean (mm Hg)
Coarctation	160/85	23
	145/80	54
	150/85	18
	155/80	36
Average	152/82	33
Thoracic aneurysm	260/160	12
	240/135	8
	245/150	24
	235/140	4
	240/155	10
	255/160	6
Average	245/150	10

Source: Modified from A. Romagnoli and J. R. Cooper, Jr. Anesthesia for aortic operations. *Cleve. Clin. Q.* 48:150, 1983.

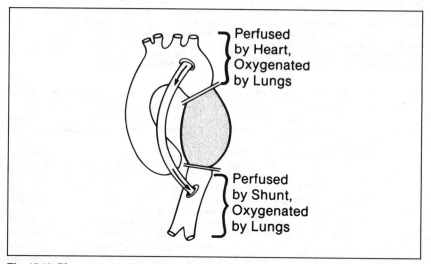

Fig. 15-10. Placement of a heparin-coated vascular shunt from proximal to distal aorta during repair of descending aneurysm or dissection. (From J. L. Benumof. Intraoperative Considerations for Special Thoracic Surgery Cases. In J. L. Benumof [ed.], *Anesthesia for Thoracic Surgery*. Philadelphia: Saunders, 1987. P. 384. With permission.)

the easiest site to use. However, this site requires placement of an oxygenator in the circuit. Alternatively, the left atrium or left ventricular apex may be cannulated for blood return to the pump. The pump may be a standard double roller (positive displacement) or a centrifugal (kinetic) type.

Each of these variations has disadvantages. Use of an oxygenator demands complete systemic heparinization, which is associated with increased incidence of hemorrhage, especially into

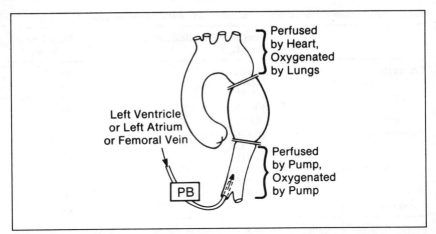

Fig. 15-11. Partial bypass (PB, or extracorporeal circulation [ECC]) method for maintaining distal perfusion pressure and avoiding proximal hypertension. Oxygenated blood can be taken directly from the left ventricle or atrium (or aortic arch) and pumped either by roller-head or centrifugal pump into the femoral artery. Alternatively, unoxygenated blood can be taken from the femoral vein, passed through a separate oxygenator, and pumped into the femoral artery. Use of an oxygenator dictates the use of a full heparinizing dose. (From J. L. Benumof. Intraoperative Considerations for Special Thoracic Surgery Cases. In J. L. Benumof [ed.], *Anesthesia for Thoracic Surgery*. Philadelphia: Saunders, 1987. P. 384. With permission.)

the left lung. Left atrial or ventricular cannulation without an oxygenator may allow use of less heparin but does carry an increased risk of air embolism. Table 15-11 summarizes the possible cannulation sites and major differences between heparinized shunts and ECC for distal perfusion.

4. **Complications of repair**

   a. **Cardiac.** Cardiac disorders (myocardial infarction, dysrhythmia, or low-output syndrome) are a significant (20–40%) cause of death in patients with all types of descending aortic repair.

   b. **Hemorrhage.** This also is a significant cause of death in all types of repair (20–30%) of the descending aorta.

   c. **Renal failure.** The incidence of renal failure ranges from 4–9% among survivors, with a much higher incidence among nonsurvivors. The etiology is presumed to be a decrease in renal blood flow during cross-clamping. However, renal failure may occur in the presence of apparently adequate perfusion (heparinized shunt or ECC). Preexisting impairment of renal blood flow from a dissection involving the renal arteries increases the incidence of renal failure.

   d. **Paraplegia.** This is probably the most feared complication not associated with death because it is irreversible. The cause is usually interruption or prolonged hypoperfusion (> 15 minutes) of the blood supply to the anterior spinal artery. The anterior spinal artery is formed from the vertebral arteries rostrally and, as it descends, also receives blood from radicular arteries. These arise from the intercostal arteries (Fig. 15-12). In a majority of patients, one of these radicular arteries, the great radicular artery (of Adamkiewicz), contributes a major portion of the supply to the midportion of the anterior spinal artery. Unfortunately, this vessel

Table 15-11. Descending aortic surgery: options for increasing distal perfusion

Blood removed from	Blood infused into	Heparinized shunt	Perfusion apparatus		Extracorporeal bypass	
			Roller	Centrifugal	Oxygenator	Heparin (ACT)[a]
LV, AoA, LSA	FA, DAo	Yes	No	No	No	None (nl)
FV	FA, DAo	No	Either		Yes	Full (>480)
LA, AoA, LSA, LV	FA, DAo	No	Yes	No	No	Partial (250–480)
LA, AoA, LSA, LV	FA, DAo	No	No	Yes	No	Minimum (nl–250)[b]

LV = left ventricle; FA = femoral artery, FV = femoral vein, LSA = left subclavian artery, AoA = aortic arch, DAo = descending aorta, LA = left atrium.
[a]Refers to the activated clotting time, in seconds; if used, optimum ACT is controversial.
[b]Some groups will not use heparin when using a centrifugal pump.

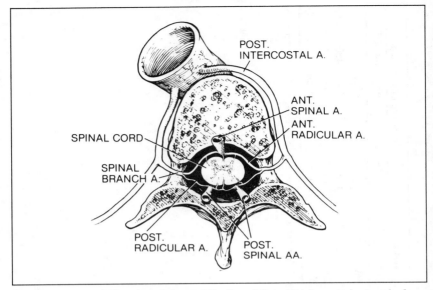

Fig. 15-12. Anatomic drawing of the contribution of the radicular arteries to spinal cord blood flow. If the posterior intercostal artery is involved in a dissection or is sacrificed to facilitate repair of aortic pathology, critical blood supply may be lost, causing spinal cord ischemia. (From D. A. Cooley [ed.], *Surgical Treatment of Aortic Aneurysms.* Philadelphia: Saunders, 1986. P. 92. With permission.)

is almost impossible to identify angiographically or by inspection at operation. It may arise anywhere from T5 to below L1. These anatomic considerations place blood flow in this artery at higher risk intraoperatively and postoperatively. Interruption of flow in this vessel may or may not lead to paraplegia depending on the contribution available from other collaterals. An anterior spinal syndrome can result, in which motor function is lost (anterior horns), but some sensation remains intact (posterior columns).

e. **Miscellaneous.** Many other complications may arise. Some are a function of the type of pathology. For instance, death from multiple organ trauma is a major factor in patients who survive traumatic rupture. Respiratory failure alone and as a component of multiple organ failure is more common with thoracic aortic disease than with abdominal aortic disease. Cerebrovascular accidents are seen in a small number of patients, as is left vocal cord paralysis due to recurrent laryngeal nerve damage.

H. **Anesthetic consideration in descending aortic surgery**
   1. **Monitoring**
      a. **Arterial blood pressure.** A right radial or brachial arterial catheter is needed to monitor pressures above the cross-clamp because the left subclavian artery may be compromised by the cross-clamp. Many anesthesia and surgical teams prefer to monitor pressure below the clamp also, which requires placement of a femoral arterial catheter. Should a partial bypass technique be employed, the left femoral artery is cannulated for distal perfusion, and the right femoral artery is used for blood pressure monitoring.

b. Ventricular function. Some operative teams prefer to monitor left ventricular function during proximal cross-clamping and therefore insert a pulmonary artery catheter to follow filling pressures and cardiac output.

c. Other monitors. Additional monitors used are similar to those listed for other thoracic procedures: electrocardiogram (standard lead V_5 cannot be used because of the surgical approach), pulse oximetry, core temperature, and urine output.

2. **One lung anesthesia.** Double-lumen endobronchial tubes are recommended not only to improve surgical exposure but also to provide an element of patient safety. By collapsing the left lung, trauma to that lung is decreased, and if manipulation during surgery does lead to hemorrhage, the contralateral (right) lung is protected from blood spillage. A left-sided tube is technically easier to place and is often used but may be impossible to insert in some patients because of aneurysmal distortion of the trachea or left main stem bronchus. Patients with aortic rupture may also have a distorted left mainstem bronchus. Right-sided tubes may be used, but proper alignment with the right upper lobe bronchus should be checked with a fiberoptic bronchoscope. A detailed description of double-lumen tube placement and single lung ventilation is beyond the scope of this chapter.

3. **Conduct of anesthesia before and during cross-clamping.** Before the aorta is cross-clamped, mannitol (0.5g/kg) should be infused to provide some renal protection during clamping. Despite the fact that a shunting procedure will be used, changes in the distribution of renal blood flow make mannitol administration prudent. In addition, sodium nitroprusside should be mixed and ready for infusion.

After the clamp is applied, it is important to monitor acid-base status closely with serial arterial blood gas measurements. It is common for metabolic acidosis to develop owing to hypoperfusion of critical organ beds, and this should be treated aggressively if the patient is normothermic. If simple cross-clamping without adjuncts is employed, proximal hypertension should be controlled, again with the realization that distal organ flow may be diminished. In treating proximal hypertension, regional blood flow studies have shown that nitroprusside infusion may decrease renal and spinal cord blood flow in a dose-related fashion. Ideally, cross-clamp time (regardless of technique) should be under 30 minutes, because the incidence of complications, especially paraplegia, begins to increase above this limit.

If a heparinized shunt has been placed and proximal **hyper**tension cannot be treated without producing subsequent distal **hypo**tension (less than 60 mm Hg), the surgeon should be made aware that there may be a technical problem with shunt placement. If partial bypass (ECC) is employed, the pump speed or venous return can be adjusted so that control of proximal hypertension can be maintained by adequate unloading while the lower body is simultaneously perfused. Usually little or no pharmacologic intervention is necessary in this case because the pump speed and manipulation of venous return provide rapid control of proximal and distal pressures. Table 15-12 highlights the treatment options for several clinical scenarios during ECC.

Prior to removal of the cross-clamp, a vasopressor should be available. The anesthesiologist must be constantly aware of the stage of operation so that major events such as clamping and declamping may be anticipated.

4. **Declamping shock.** When **simple cross-clamping** of the aorta is used, subsequent unclamping can lead to serious and even life-

Table 15-12. Management of extracorporeal circulation for surgery of the descending aorta

Proximal pressure	Distal pressure	Wedge pressure	Treatment
↑	↓	↓	Volume; ↑ pump flow
↑	↓	↑	↑ Pump flow
↑	↑	↓	Volume; vasodilator
↑	↑	↑	Vasodilator; diuretic; maintain pump flow, hold volume in pump reservoir (if in use)
↓	↓	↓	Volume; look for partial occlusion of arterial outflow cannula (if reservoir in use)
↓	↓	↑	↑ Pump flow; inotrope
↓	↑	↑	↓ Pump flow; inotrope; diuretic
↓	↑	↓	↓ Pump flow; may need volume

threatening consequences. These usually consist of severe hypotension or myocardial depression. There are several theoretical causes of this declamping syndrome, including washout of acid metabolites, vasodilator substances, sequestration of blood in the lower extremities, and reactive hyperemia. The usual cause, however, is relative or absolute hypovolemia. To attenuate the effects of clamp removal, in the 10–15 minutes prior to unclamping of the thoracic aorta the volume status of the patient should be optimized. This includes elevating filling pressures by infusing blood products, colloid, or crystalloids. Prophylactic bicarbonate administration is advocated by some just prior to clamp removal to minimize the myocardial depression caused by the acidosis that occurs following cross-clamp removal. It is also advisable for the surgeon to release the cross-clamp slowly over a period of 1–2 minutes to allow enough time for compensatory changes to occur.

Vasopressors may be needed to compensate for hypotension but must be used with care because even transient hypertension may result in significant bleeding. With a volume-loaded patient and slow clamp release, any significant hypotension is usually short lived and well tolerated. If hypotension is severe, the easiest maneuver is reapplication of the clamp to allow further volume infusion.

If shunts or ECC are used, declamping hypotension is usually attenuated because the vascular bed below the clamp is less "empty." ECC also provides a means of very rapid volume infusion, if a reservoir is used.

5. **Fluid therapy and transfusion.** Even patients undergoing elective repair of a descending aneurysm may be relatively hypovolemic, and fluid therapy should have the following aims: correct this fluid deficit, provide maintenance fluids, compensate for evaporative and "third space" losses, decrease red cell loss by mild hemodilution (hematocrit in 30s), and replace blood loss as needed.

Despite proximal and distal control of the aorta, blood loss can be considerable in these cases due to back-bleeding from the intercostal arteries. These collateral vessels are often ligated on opening the aorta. Use of cell scavenging devices has become quite common and has reduced the need for banked blood, but because massive losses may occur, banked blood may often still be needed. As long as liver perfusion is adequate, even with a large blood loss, citrate toxicity is not usually a problem because of rapid "first pass" metabolism in the liver. Repair of a thoracic aneurysm with simple clamping, however, presents a unique situation—the liver is not perfused. In this circumstance, transfusion of large amounts of banked blood may rapidly produce citrate toxicity, resulting in myocardial depression that requires calcium chloride infusion.

6. **Spinal cord protection.** Several methods have been espoused to provide protection of the spinal cord during cross-clamping in addition to ECC, shunts, and expeditious surgery.

    a. Maintaining perfusion pressure. Some groups prefer to maintain perfusion pressure of the distal aorta in the range of 40–60 mm Hg to increase blood flow to the mid and lower spinal cord. This statement should be regarded as controversial because at present there are few data on outcome to support this position. **No method used to maintain blood flow to the distal aorta (i.e., shunt or partial bypass) guarantees that spinal cord blood flow, and therefore function, will be maintained.** Proximal and distal clamp placement to isolate the diseased aortic segment may include critical intercostal vessels that provide flow to the cord and whose loss is not compensated by distal perfusion. In addition, distal perfusion may be hindered by the presence of atherosclerotic disease in the abdominal aorta, which may prevent significant flow to the kidneys and spinal cord. Last, these crucial vessels may be disrupted in gaining surgical exposure. One should never assume that the cord and kidneys are absolutely "protected" because a shunt or partial bypass have been used. In fact, the largest studies have shown no difference in incidence of paraplegia regardless of the surgical adjunct employed.

    b. Somatosensory-evoked potentials (SEP). SEP have been promoted as a means of assessing functional status of the spinal cord during periods of possible ischemia. Briefly, SEP monitor spinal cord function by stimulating a peripheral nerve and monitoring the response in the brainstem and cerebral cortex. Normal SEP would seem to ensure the integrity of the posterior (sensory) columns. However, during aortic surgery it is the *anterior* (motor) horns that are more at risk. Perhaps for this reason, there have been reports of patients who had normal SEP during cross-clamping and who subsequently were found to have paraplegia. SEP must be regarded as an unproved technique at this writing.

    c. Hypothermia. Allowing the core temperature to be reduced to approximately 33–34°C will lower the metabolic rate of the spinal cord tissue and may provide some protection from reduced or interrupted blood flow. If employed, this technique can be done with topical cooling agents (cooling blankets, bags of crushed ice). Iced saline gastric lavage may also be used. Administration of even 1 or 2 units of cool banked blood (only if indicated) will also lower the core temperature. Precise control of temperature is difficult, and, at temperatures below 32°C, the myocardium may become more irritable and prone to ventricular arrhythmias. These facts, plus the lack of improved outcome data, have resulted in sparse use of this technique.

    d. Spinal drains. Experimental data show that spinal cord damage may be mediated through the increase in cerebrospinal fluid (CSF) pressure that accompanies the reduction in spinal cord blood flow during cross-clamping. CSF pressure may be increased to as high as the mean distal **arterial** pressure. Since spinal cord blood flow is proportional to the mean arterial pressure minus the higher of the CSF or venous pressure, perfusion in this circumstance may be reduced to zero. A spinal drain would allow not only for measurement of the intraspinal pressure but also for therapeutic removal of cerebrospinal fluid. However, removal of CSF in the presence of an elevated intraspinal pressure may provide a gradient for herniation of cerebral structures. In addition, the placement of a spinal drain followed by systemic heparinization may lead to the formation of an epidural hematoma as a rare complication. To date, there has been no controlled study that has demonstrated a reduction in morbidity associated with the use of spinal drains.

  e. Other. Additional "protective" measures such as intravenous steroids, pharmacologic suppression of spinal cord function, or free radical scavengers are not widely used or are frankly experimental.

7. Prevention of renal failure. The etiology of renal failure is thought to be ischemia from interruption of blood flow by clamping, although embolism remains another possibility. Use of CPB or a shunt may be protective, but superior outcome data are still lacking, and renal failure still occurs despite these surgical adjuncts. Adequate volume loading should certainly be used and is probably most important in renal protection. Mannitol may also help, and because its use is innocuous in most patients, it is recommended.

SUGGESTED READING

Cooley, D. A. *Surgical Treatment of Aortic Aneurysms*. Philadelphia: Saunders, 1986.

Crawford, E. S., and Crawford, J. L. *Diseases of the Aorta: Including an Atlas of Angiographic Pathology and Surgical Technique*. Baltimore: Williams & Wilkins, 1984.

Cunningham, J. N., Jr., Laschinger, J. C., and Spencer, F. C. Monitoring of somatosensory evoked potentials during procedures on the thoracoabdominal aorta. IV: Clinical observations and results. *J. Thorac. Cardiovasc. Surg.* 94:275–285, 1987.

Romagnoli, A., and Cooper J. R., Jr. Anesthesia for aortic operations. *Cleve. Clin. Q.* 48:147–152, 1981.

Roseberg, J. N., Shine T., and Nugent, M. Thoracic Aortic Disease. In J. A. Kaplan (ed.), *Cardiac Anesthesia*. (2nd ed.). Philadelphia: Grune & Stratton, 1987. Pp. 725–750.

Anesthesia for Patients with Electrophysiologic Disorders

Mark W. Stull, Jerry C. Luck, and Donald E. Martin

More than 500,000 patients in the United States now have permanent cardiac pacemakers. About 100,000 new pacemakers are implanted each year. With developing technology pacemakers are becoming increasingly complex in their circuitry, making them more versatile and at the same time more susceptible to electrical interference. Thus, newer pacemakers are both more useful and more dangerous to the anesthetized patient.

I. **Indications for permanent pacemaker insertion** [3]

 A. **Bradydysrhythmias.** The insertion of a permanent pacemaker is necessary whenever (1) bradydysrhythmias refractory to medical therapy actually compromise cardiac output, or (2) bradydysrhythmias are likely to develop or progress to the point where they may compromise cardiac output.

   Dysrhythmias in the following categories *may* require insertion of a permanent pacemaker as shown in Table 16-1.

  1. **Acquired atrioventricular (AV) block in adults**
    a. **First-degree** (prolonged PR interval without dropped beats)
    b. **Second-degree** (intermittent conduction)
      (1) **Type I.** Progressive PR prolongation before dropped beat
      (2) **Type II.** Dropped beats without progressive PR prolongation
      (3) **Advanced.** Block of two or more successive P waves
    c. **Third-degree or complete** (no conduction)
  2. **Acquired AV block following myocardial infarction**
  3. **Chronic bifascicular and trifascicular block**
  4. **Sinus node dysfunction**
  5. **Hypersensitive carotid sinus syndrome**
  6. **Bradydysrhythmias in children**

 B. **Tachycardia.** The indications for a permanent pacemaker may include treatment of some tachycardias. The pacemaker may be combined with other agents, such as the automatic implantable cardioverter defibrillator, to treat these rhythms.

  1. **Definitely indicated.** Symptomatic supraventricular tachycardia (atrial flutter, AV nodal reentry tachycardia) not responsive to medical treatment.
  2. **Probably indicated**
    a. Drug-resistant ventricular tachycardia, accelerated idioventricular rhythm, and torsade de pointes.
    b. For tachycardia prevention in patients in whom tachydysrhythmia develops during periods of bradycardia.

II. **Indications for temporary pacemaker insertion following an acute myocardial infarction.** In the setting of an acute myocardial infarction (MI), particularly an anterior MI, incomplete infranodal block is likely to progress. Therefore, in this situation any of the following rhythms are an indication for **temporary** pacemaker insertion, whether or not they are symptomatic:

 1. Type II second-degree or third-degree AV block.
 2. Right bundle branch block (RBBB) and either left anterior (LAFB) or left posterior (LPFB) fascicular block (new or indeterminate onset).
 3. RBBB or left bundle branch block (LBBB) and either first-degree or Mobitz type I second-degree AV block.
 4. Alternating RBBB and LBBB, regardless of time of onset.
 5. RBBB with alternating LAFB and LPFB, regardless of time of onset.

III. **Preoperative and postoperative pacing**

 A. **Preoperative.** When a patient who has indications for a permanent or temporary pacemaker requires surgery, at least a temporary pacemaker should be placed preoperatively. In addition, because of the tendency for surgical stimuli or anesthetic agents to exacerbate brady-

Table 16-1. Indications for permanent cardiac pacing and temporary pacing for bradycardia in the perioperative period

Rhythm disturbance	Subacute acquired	After myocardial infarction	Congenital
Atrioventricular block			
Third-degree—complete			
Symptomatic	+ +	+ +	+ +
Asymptomatic	+ (rate <50 bpm or if patient is taking drugs that may suppress ventricular escape)	+ +	−
Second-degree—advanced			
Symptomatic	+ +	+ +	+ +
Asymptomatic	+ + (after cardiac surgery) + (rate <50 bpm)	+ +	−
Second-degree—Mobitz II			
Symptomatic	+ +	+ +	+ +
Asymptomatic	+ (rate <50 bpm or if patient is taking drugs that may suppress ventricular escape)	+ +	−
Second-degree—Mobitz I			
Symptomatic	+ +	+ +	+ +
Asymptomatic	− (supra-His)	−	−
First-degree			
Asymptomatic	−	+ (if associated with new bundle branch block)	−
Reversible or transient AV block	−	+ (if associated with new intraventricular block)	−
Intraventricular conduction defects			
Bifascicular or trifascicular AV block with:			
Permanent or intermittent complete			

Table 16-1. (continued)

Rhythm disturbance	Subacute acquired	After myocardial infarction	Congenital
AV block			
Symptomatic	++	++	++
Asymptomatic	++	++	—
Alternating bundle branch block			
Symptomatic	++	++	++
Asymptomatic	++	++	—
His ventricular prolongation			
Symptomatic	+	—	—
Asymptomatic	—	—	—
Pacing-induced	+	—	—
First-degree AV block			
Symptomatic	+	+ (with new bundle branch block)	—
Asymptomatic	—	+ (with new bundle branch block)	—
Intraventricular conduction delay or fascicular block alone	—	—	—
Sinoatrial dysfunction			
Documented symptomatic irreversible bradycardia	++	++	++
Recurrent rate < 40 bpm or asystole > 3 sec with symptoms not clearly associated with bradycardia	+	+	—
Asymptomatic sinus node dysfunction	—	—	—

Carotid sinus hypersensitivity		
Hyperactive cardioinhibitory response		
Symptomatic	++	++
Asymptomatic	—	—
Hyperactive vasodepressor syncope	—	—

++ = definitely indicated (Class I), + = probably indicated (Class II), — = not indicated (Class III).

dysrhythmias or conduction disturbances, a transcutaneous pacemaker should be at least available in the following situations:
1. Extreme **sinus bradycardia.**
2. Poorly controlled **supraventricular dysrhythmias.**
3. **Bifascicular block in a comatose patient.** There is a possibility that transient progression to third-degree AV block could have resulted in a syncopal episode and subsequent head injury and coma.
4. **Bifascicular block and first-degree AV block without symptoms.** Some authors have strongly suggested use of temporary pacing for major vascular or extended surgery.

B. **Postoperative antitachycardia pacing**
1. Postoperative noncardiac patients rarely require pacing unless preoperative indications and signs were initially overlooked.
2. Postoperative patients with heart disease may experience paroxysmal episodes of bradycardia but frequently have nonsustained or sustained tachycardias. Pacing techniques can be used therapeutically to terminate, suppress and possibly prevent some tachycardias.
3. **Pacing techniques**
   a. **Termination.** Tachycardias that are based on reentry can generally be initiated and terminated by critically timed depolarizations. These **loop** or **circus movement** tachycardias have some area of the circuit that is responsive to critically timed depolarization. If a critically timed depolarization enters the circuit or loop in the **termination zone,** it can terminate the tachycardia. The pacing techniques used consist of single capture methods, such as underdrive pacing or programmed single extrastimuli, multiple capture methods, such as programmed multiple extrastimuli, and overdrive burst pacing. Supraventricular tachycardias that are easily terminated by atrial pacing include atrial flutter and atrioventricular reentrant and atrioventricular nodal reentrant tachycardias. Sustained ventricular tachycardia (VT) caused by reentry in a zone of old infarction can be terminated by a multiple capture technique. Sustained VT secondary to acute ischemia, electrolyte imbalance, and drug intoxications may be difficult to terminate by pacing. Attempts at termination by pacing may fail and can accelerate the VT to ventricular fibrillation.
   b. **Suppression.** Temporary ventricular pacing at rates slightly above the normal range (100–130 bpm) may suppress recurrence of VT for transient conditions such as acute infarction and drug-induced VT. Atrial pacing at these higher rates may be equally effective and better tolerated because AV synchrony is maintained. The clinically recognized form of VT termed **torsade de pointes** is frequently suppressed by this overdrive pacing technique. Permanent pacing at rates above 100 bpm is uncomfortable and impractical for suppression of ventricular tachycardia.
   c. **Prevention.** Generally pacing patients with bradycardia-dependent tachycardias at normal rates will prevent these tachycardias. These are rare and generally associated with either heart block or sinus node dysfunction.
4. The use of antitachycardia pacing techniques requires a correctly diagnosed dysrhythmia, understanding of the theory of paced termination of tachycardias, the presence of temporary pacing electrodes, and a versatile programmable stimulator.

IV. **Hemodynamic effects of pacing for bradycardia.** Pacemakers are designed to provide electrical stimulation of the atria, ventricles, or both. Pacemakers simulate as closely as possible normal heart rate and rhythm. Dual chamber pacemakers coordinate atrial and ventricular depolarization and maximize cardiac output. Variable rate pacemakers are available to increase heart rate to meet the metabolic demands of the body.

A. Pathophysiology of bradycardia

1. As heart rate changes, cardiac output (CO) generally changes on the basis of the relationship: CO = heart rate (HR) × stroke volume (SV). The usual response to exercise in the patient with intact cardiac innervation is expressed by the formula: ↑ HR × ↑ SV = ↑ CO. Heart rate is more important than stroke volume in this relationship. Commonly, heart rate is responsible for 75% of an increase in cardiac output, whereas stroke volume accounts for only 25%. Thus, during profound bradycardia an increase in stroke volume rarely increases cardiac output enough to meet metabolic demands. How much the output falls during bradycardia depends in part on the ability of the ventricle to increase the stroke volume. **In patients with ventricular dysfunction stroke volume may be fixed,** and cardiac output will drop significantly.

2. **Emergence of lower pacemakers.** There is a hierarchy of subsidiary pacemakers below the sinus node. In the presence of sinus node dysfunction or AV block, an escape focus emerges below the level of the block. The AV junctional escape foci are somewhat responsive to metabolic demands, but ventricular foci rarely respond to changing demand.

3. Bradycardia may allow appearance of ectopy and dysrhythmias.

B. Compensatory mechanisms

1. The ventricle will dilate as much as possible to provide a greater stroke volume and preserve cardiac output. This will, however, increase wall stress and result in ventricular hypertrophy.

2. A rise in mean atrial pressure, pulmonary peak systolic pressure, and systemic and pulmonary resistance follows.

C. Effect of artificial cardiac pacing

1. There are two possibilities: fixed rate pacing and variable rate pacing.

   a. If pacing is at a **fixed rate,** cardiac output can increase only as much as stroke volume, as shown by the following formulas:

   (1) Normal ventricular function: Fixed HR × ↑ SV = ↑ CO

   (2) Abnormal ventricular function: Fixed HR × fixed SV = fixed CO

   b. **Variable rate** pacing may be one of two types:

   (1) **"P" synchronous,** triggered by the P wave in patients with normal sinus node function

   (2) **Rate responsive** to a physiologic parameter. Electronic sensors have been designed to respond to catecholamines, respiratory rate, Q–T interval, muscle activity, and small increases in temperature.

2. **Ventricular pacing**

   a. Ventricular pacing results in an **abnormal pattern of ventricular activation.** This pattern may result in a less efficient ventricular contraction and therefore a reduction in stroke volume.

   b. Loss of AV synchrony has two results:

   (1) Increased mean atrial pressure and decreased left ventricular end-diastolic volume (LVEDV) and pressure (LVEDP) with **decreased cardiac output.**

   (2) **Retrograde ventriculoatrial (VA) conduction** may occur. With VA conduction, atria will contract against closed AV valves, resulting in systemic and pulmonary venous congestion.

   c. Although ventricular pacing has been quite satisfactory in many patients, these drawbacks to ventricular pacing are manifest clinically by the **"pacemaker syndrome"** (Table 16-2). The incidence of this syndrome is reported to be about 7.3%.

Table 16-2. The pacemaker syndrome

Symptoms
  Jugular venous distention and pulsations
  Weakness, dizziness, near-syncope
  Hypotension
  Precordial distress
Physiology
  "Cannon waves" in the jugular venous system
  "Cannon waves" in the pulmonary venous system
  Cyclic variation in cardiac output, arterial pressure, peripheral vascular
    resistance
Etiology
  Loss of AV synchrony
  Intact VA conduction with activation of atrial stretch receptors

Source: From S. Furman, D. L. Hayes, and D. R. Holmes. *A Practice of Cardiac Pacing.* Mount Kisco, NY: Futura, 1986. P. 88. With permission.

3. **Atrial pacing**
   a. Atrial pacing allows atrial contribution to cardiac output in patients with intact AV conduction.
   b. Atrial contribution can be up to 20–40% of cardiac output as a result of two effects:
      (1) Mean atrial pressure is decreased and venous return facilitated.
      (2) Ventricular filling is increased, especially in patients with distended or noncompliant ventricles.
   c. Atrial pacing improves hemodynamics in patients with [2] and without [8] heart disease. In postoperative heart patients, atrial pacing increases cardiac output an average of 14% and ejection fraction an average of 10–12% above fixed-rate ventricular pacing [5].
   d. Heart rate is fixed and not variable.
4. **AV sequential pacing**
   a. This mode of pacing allows for atrial contribution to cardiac output in patients with sinus node dysfunction and abnormal AV conduction.
   b. In most sequential pacemaker units, the AV interval, or the time between atrial and ventricular contraction, ranges from 50–250 msec. The normal AV interval is usually 110–140 msec in children and 120–200 msec in adults and is usually shorter at faster heart rates. A 50-msec variation from an individual's optimal AV interval could drop cardiac output.
   c. Ventricular depolarization still occurs through an abnormal pathway.
V. **Pacemaker technology**
   A. **Definitions**
      1. **Response mode**
         a. **Triggered.** Pulse generator senses a spontaneous atrial or ventricular depolarization and delivers a stimulus.
         b. **Inhibited.** Sensing of a spontaneous depolarization inhibits pacemaker output and resets the pacemaker's internal clock to inhibit pacing for a preset interval (so-called noncompetitive pacing).
      2. **Output**
         a. Pacemaker output may be defined in terms of:
            (1) Current = voltage/resistance
            (2) Energy = current × voltage × pulse width

    b. If resistance is constant, then: Energy is proportional to voltage^2 $\times$ pulse width.

3. Programmability. Ability to reset pacemaker's parameters transcutaneously by means of programmed electromagnetic signals.

4. Asynchronous. Pacemaker that fires at a fixed rate, regardless of intrinsic cardiac activity. This type of pacemaker may compete with intrinsic electrical activity.

5. Demand. Pacemaker that is activated only when the intrinsic heart rate falls below a present lower limit (see sec. **9** and **10** below). Demand pacemakers are much less likely than asynchronous pacemakers to compete with intrinsic cardiac rhythm.

6. Sensitivity. The pacemaker's ability to sense intrinsic cardiac activity to prevent competition between the pacemaker and intrinsic activity. Proper sensing involves sensing a specific amplitude, rate, and duration of this intrinsic activity.

7. Refractory period. Period of time the pacemaker will not respond to sensed electrical activity.

8. Blanking period. Short refractory period for both atrial and ventricular circuits in a dual chamber pacemaker to ensure that each circuit will not sense the pacing artifact of the other as intrinsic electrical activity. The term **crosstalk** applies specifically to the ventricular circuit that senses the atrial stimulus artifact, resulting in ventricular asystole.

9. Lower rate limit. The rate at which the pacemaker is preset to pace. The escape interval or the time the pacemaker will wait for an intrinsic heart beat before beginning to pace may be either the present lower rate limit or the hysteresis interval, whichever is longer.

10. Hysteresis. A preset escape interval that is longer than that of the preset pacing rate to allow maximum utilization of the intrinsic cardiac conduction system.

11. Antitachydysrhythmic functions

    a. Pacing. Treatment of tachydysrhythmia by underdrive pacing or overdrive pacing (in older terminology, **normal rate competition** and **bursts** respectively).

    b. Shock. Internal cardioversion-defibrillation.

    c. Scanning (old terminology). Use of timed extrasystoles to eliminate tachydysrhythmia.

    d. External (old terminology). Tachydysrhythmic control by use of external maneuvers in concert with the implanted pacemaker (e.g., magnets, radio frequency).

12. Pacemaker hardware

    a. Generator. Contains power source and circuitry of pacemaker. May be external or implanted.

    b. Electrode. The terminal portion of the pacemaker in contact with the myocardial surface.

    c. Lead. The conductor of the electrical impulses to and from the electrode and generator.

13. Types of pacemaker lead

    a. Unipolar. Active electrode located at the end of the pacemaker lead while ground electrode is located on the pulse generator case.

    b. Bipolar. Both active and ground electrodes located on the pacemaker lead.

14. Location of pacemaker electrode

    a. Endocardial pacing. Most common form of permanent pacing in which leads are passed transvenously into the right atrium or right ventricle to contact the endocardium. The generator is most commonly then placed on the anterior chest wall below the clavicle with access to the heart through the subclavian vein.

      b. Epicardial pacing. In this type of pacing the electrodes are placed directly on the epicardial surface of the heart, usually under direct vision. The pacemaker generator is usually placed in the epigastric area.

B. Nomenclature. A five-letter code is used to identify pacemaker type. This system has recently been revised [1], and the resulting code is listed in Table 16-3. Positions 1, 2, and 3 are specifically related to pacing for bradycardia. Position 4 describes programmable features of the pulse generator. Position 5 describes the antitachydysrhythmia function of the pacemaker.

C. Specific pacemaker modes. Several examples of common modes of pacemaker function are shown in Table 16-4; their mode of operation is defined using the Generic Pacemaker Code.

D. Perioperative temporary pacing techniques

    1. Transvenous endocardial pacing. If temporary pacing is indicated perioperatively, a transvenous endocardial electrode is most commonly placed under fluoroscopic guidance in the preoperative period.

        a. When transporting a patient with a transvenous electrode in place, it is necessary to stabilize the arm if the electrode is floated through an antecubital vein because pacing can be lost or right ventricular perforation can occur with arm movement. If a transvenous pacemaker is placed through the jugular vein, the patient should avoid excessive movement of the head.

        b. Controls of external pulse generators should be easily accessible to the anesthesiologist at all times.

        c. Dislodgement of leads of temporary endocardial pacemakers has been reported with positive pressure ventilation. Therefore, consideration should be given either to a trial of positive pressure ventilation before muscle relaxants are administered or to the use of regional anesthesia.

    2. Transcutaneous pacing

        a. Clinical efficacy. Transcutaneous pacing performed noninvasively by means of two conductive pads placed on the chest wall is effective and has a high likelihood of capture in patients who are hemodynamically stable. Usually a pacemaker output of 50–200 mA at 10–40 msec pulse duration is required for capture. In the cardiac arrest situation, however, early intervention is necessary to ensure pacemaker capture. Hemodynamically, transcutaneous pacing has been shown to be as effective as transvenous pacing in animal studies [10].

        b. Safety. The major side effect for the conscious patient is pain with electrical stimulation, which is intolerable for 10–20% of patients but may be amenable to treatment with parenteral analgesics. Anesthetized patients of course do not experience pain during pacing but may later complain of muscle soreness that could be attributed to pacing. Dysrhythmias are unlikely. In anesthetized dogs the ventricular fibrillation threshold was found to be 12 times the pacing threshold. After pacing in dogs, microscopic lesions consistent with electrically induced myocardial damage were found, but they were not extensive and were felt not to produce clinically detectable changes in cardiovascular status [6].

        c. Uses in the cardiac operating room. The transcutaneous pacemaker is very useful for situations in which temporary pacing may be needed for a short time preoperatively or before cardiopulmonary bypass. Patients with left bundle branch block, in whom passage of a Swan-Ganz catheter could induce complete heart block, are one good example.

Table 16-3. The generic pacemaker code

Category	I Chamber(s) paced	II Chamber(s) sensed	III Response to sensing	IV Programmability, rate modulation	V Antitachyarrhythmia function(s)
	O = None	O = None	O = None	O = None	O = None
	A = Atrium	A = Atrium	T = Triggered	P = Simple programmable	P = Pacing (antitachyarrhythmia)
	V = Ventricle	V = Ventricle	I = Inhibited	M = Multiprogrammable	S = Shock
	D = Dual (A + V)	D = Dual (A + V)	D = Dual (T + I)	C = Communicating	D = Dual (P + S)
				R = Rate modulation	
Manufacturer's designation	S = Single (A or V)	S = Single (A or V)			

Note: Positions I through III are used exclusively for antibradyarrhythmia function.
Source: From A. D. Bernstein, A. J. Camm, R. D. Fletcher, et al. The NASPE/BPEG generic pacemaker code for antibradyarrhythmia and antitachyarrhythmia devices. *PACE* 10:795, 1987. With permission.

Table 16-4. Modes of pacemaker operation

Generic pacer code	Definition	Indication	Advantages	Disadvantages
AOO	Asynchronous atrial	Post-CPB Presence of EMI	Independent of EMI Simple circuitry	Dysrhythmias Competes with intrinsic rhythm Shorter battery life
VOO	Asynchronous ventricular	Post-CPB Presence of EMI	Simplest circuit	Dysrhythmias Competes with intrinsic rhythm No atrial contribution to CO
AAI	Atrial demand pacer	Post-CPB Sick sinus syndrome Symptomatic sinus bradycardia	Single lead Allows intrinsic AV conduction	Ventricle not paced if AV block develops
VVI	Ventricular demand pacer	Post-CPB Temporary pacer after cardiac surgery	Simple Long battery life	Atrial contribution to CO would be lost Not rate responsive No AV synchrony
VDD	Atrial-ventricular (or "P") synchronous	Normal sinus function with AV block	AV synchrony Rate responsive	Two leads Cannot pace atria Can lead to pacemaker-mediated tachycardia
DVI	AV sequential pacemaker	Atrial bradycardia with AV block Patients with pacemaker-mediated tachycardia	Maintains AV synchrony in atrial bradycardia Useful in pacer-mediated tachycardia	Two leads Not synchronous if atrial rate greater than paced rate

DDD	Optimal sequential universal pacer	Atrial bradyarrhythmia Normal sinus rhythm with AV block	Most physiologic Maintains AV synchrony	Not rate responsive Competing atrial rhythms Two leads Complex circuitry Can lead to pacer-mediated tachycardia With sinus node dysfunction no response to metabolic needs

AV = atrioventricular, CO = cardiac output, CPB = cardiopulmonary bypass, EMI = electromagnetic interference.

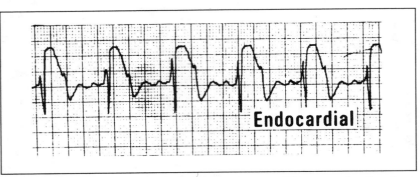

Fig. 16-1. QRS complex showing the "current of injury" or ST-segment elevation characteristic of contact of the pacing electrode with the endocardium. (From K. A. Mansour, E. R. Dorney, and S. B. Kisig. Techniques for Insertion of Pervenous and Epicardial Pacemakers. In J. W. Hurst, R. B. Logue, C. E. Rachley, et al. [eds.], *The Heart, Arteries and Veins* [5th ed.]. New York: McGraw Hill, 1982. P. 1759. With permission.)

      d. Conclusion. The transcutaneous pacemaker appears to be a reliable alternative to transvenous pacing in the management of intraoperative bradydysrhythmias. It does not require extensive training to use. Its efficacy does seem to decrease markedly with longer periods of hemodynamic instability (as do other forms of pacing) and as such needs to be readily available.

3. Pacing through a modified Swan-Ganz catheter

  a. Swan-Ganz catheters are commercially available with

    (1) Bipolar pacing electrodes mounted directly on the catheter. In this catheter electrodes are positioned on the catheter so that, when the catheter reaches a wedge position in the average adult, the electrodes will be in the right atrium or right ventricle. Thus, with this catheter, which contains both atrial and ventricular electrodes, either atrial, ventricular, or AV sequential pacing is possible. Catheter position may, however, have to be manipulated to allow the electrodes to contact the myocardium.

    (2) A catheter orifice through which a pacing electrode can be inserted. With this catheter, the orifice is positioned so that in the average adult it is inside the right ventricle when the catheter is in the wedge position. Only the pacing electrode must be maneuvered into position contacting the endocardium.

        The pacing electrode may be properly positioned by observing the position at which a pacemaker best causes ventricular depolarization or the position at which the characteristic electrocardiogram (ECG) pattern can be seen with the active lead placed on the pacing electrode (Fig 16-1).

  b. Pacing current required

    (1) Capture is usually achieved with less than 2 mA.

    (2) No capture with a current of 5 mA indicates poor electrode position.

  c. Complications

    (1) Perforation of a ventricle with a pacing electrode can occur, especially when the **heart is empty** or is manipulated during cardiopulmonary bypass (CPB).

       **(a) Pacing wire, if present in the ventricle, should be with-
drawn during cardiopulmonary bypass.**

       (2) Ventricular dysrhythmias may occur.

       (3) Pacing can be lost with changes in electrode position.

    d. Uses in the cardiac operating room. Temporary pacing for either AV block or sinoatrial (SA) node dysfunction, primarily in the prebypass period.

  4. Epicardial pacing in the cardiac operating room

    a. Before termination of cardiopulmonary bypass, the surgeon most commonly places epicardial ventricular pacing electrodes and often atrial electrodes as well.

    b. These leads may be connected to an external pulse generator to provide temporary ventricular, atrial, or AV sequential pacing.

    c. Most external pacemakers used for this purpose have an adjustable

      (1) Heart rate

      (2) Current output

      (3) Sensing threshold

      (4) AV interval (for AV sequential pacemakers)

    d. Before terminating CPB, the pacemaker should be adjusted for emergency response to asystole as follows:

      (1) Heart rate—90–100 bpm

      (2) Current output—maximum

      (3) Sensing threshold—asynchronous

      (4) AV interval—150 msec.

    e. When the patient is hemodynamically stable after cardiopulmonary bypass and a majority of the electrocautery is completed, pacemaker output can be decreased to a level that just allows reliable capture and pacemaker sensitivity increased to convert pacemaker to demand mode.

    f. Heart rate can be adjusted to meet physiologic demand at any one time.

IV. Perioperative management of the pacemaker patient

  A. Preoperative evaluation of the patient with a pacemaker in place

    1. Evaluation of the patient's dysrhythmia

      a. What were the **indications** for pacemaker implantation?

      b. What were the patient's **symptoms** before implantation? Are they ever still present?

      c. What is the **present rhythm?**

    2. Evaluation of pacemaker function—history and physical examination

      a. What are the manufacturer and model number of the pacemaker, as well as its programmed settings? There are presently 25–30 separate pacemaker manufacturers, each with its own electronic programmer. The patient should have an identification card on which should be noted the above information and the name of the implanting physician or primary cardiologist.

        (1) The chest film can show whether the pacemaker is:

          (a) Single or dual chamber (one versus two separate leads)

          (b) Unipolar or bipolar (one or two electrodes at the end of each pacing lead)

        (2) With the aid of charts provided by pacemaker manufacturers, each pacemaker model can be identified by its characteristic x-ray appearance.

      b. When was the pacemaker placed? The most common battery in use is the lithium cell. The usual life span of lithium cells is 6–12 years. More than 95% of lithium generators exceed a 5-year survival time. Other battery types are far less common and include the obsolete mercury zinc cell, which had a 2-year battery life; the plutonium-238 nuclear cell, which is still in use today and does have an extremely long duration of more than 25 years; and the promethium-147, which has only a 2- to- 3-year half-life.

c. **Are there any symptoms suggestive of pacemaker malfunction?**
   (1) Palpitations
   (2) Syncope
   (3) Weakness
   (4) Chest pain
   (5) Orthostasis
   (6) Pain or pectoral muscle contraction with pacing

d. **Cardiac ausculatory findings.** Often there may be a variable intensity of the first heart sound, a paradoxically split S_2, and right ventricular depolarization preceding left ventricular depolarization with an endocardial pacemaker. With a left ventricular epicardial pacemaker, however, a widely split S_2 will result from left ventricular depolarization preceding right ventricular depolarization. Systolic clicks and murmurs may be secondary to valve-lead interactions, and there may be a systolic whoop secondary to movement of the lead in the ventricle itself. Tricuspid insufficiency secondary to presence of the endocardial pacemaker lead is the most common valvular lesion seen. Usually, however, this lesion is hemodynamically insignificant. Presence of a pericardial rub should raise the question of possible ventricular perforation of the pacemaker lead.

e. **Loss of pacing.** Loss of pacing may occur with gentle manipulation of the generator in its pocket; this may indicate a loose connection or partial lead fracture.

f. **Is there swelling of the ipsilateral neck, face, and extremities?** Swelling indicates a possible venous obstruction and even superior vena cava syndrome. Rarely, recurrent pulmonary emboli can result and may cause pulmonary hypertension.

g. Lead breaks, but not insulation breaks, can be seen on the chest film.

3. **Evaluation of pacemaker function—The surface electrocardiogram**

a. In general, a transvenous pacemaker with endocardial leads in the right ventricle will have a left bundle branch configuration. If the ECG shows a right bundle branch configuration, left-sided pacing is probably occurring. Possible causes include (1) right ventricular perforation with left ventricular epicardial stimulation, (2) catheter in the distal coronary sinus, (3) fusion of paced heart beat and spontaneous heart beat of right bundle branch block configuration.

b. Left ventricular epicardial leads will show a right bundle branch block configuration.

c. Unipolar pacing spikes tend to be larger than bipolar pacing spikes.

d. A comparison of the frequency of paced and intrinsic beats will give an index of the extent to which the patient depends on the pacemaker.

e. ECG configuration should be stable; if changes are present from earlier ECGs an investigation is warranted.

4. **Specialized evaluation of pacemaker function**

a. If longer than 1 year has elapsed since the pacemaker has been evaluated, or if there is any evidence of pacemaker malfunction, specialized evaluation or interrogation of the pacemaker preoperatively by a cardiologist is warranted to examine the unit and evaluate battery life.

b. In general, a 10% decrease in paced rate below the programmed rate may indicate impending battery failure.

c. Generally, as a pacemaker battery ages, the **sensing function is lost before the pacing function.**

d. If paced stimulation is the only pattern evident on ECG, reprogramming to a slower paced rate may allow evaluation of the patient's spontaneous rhythm. Then one can identify the patient's back-up rhythm in case of pacemaker failure and evaluate ECG evidence for ischemia or infarction.

  (1) Determination of the patient's blood pressure with both the paced and intrinsic rhythm can indicate the effects of the paced rhythm on stroke volume.

  (2) If the patient's blood pressure is significantly lower (>30 mm Hg systolic) with a paced rhythm, symptoms of the pacemaker syndrome are likely.

e. If spontaneous rhythm inhibits pacing activity, paced rhythm can be evaluated by

  (1) Slowing the patient's spontaneous rhythm by the Valsalva maneuver, ocular pressure, or carotid sinus massage (care must be taken in patients with potential cerebrovascular disease to avoid cerebral emboli).

  (2) Increasing the programmed pacemaker rate.

  (3) Applying a magnet over the pacemaker generator.

  (a) Generally, magnet application eliminates sensing function and results in delivery of stimuli in a fixed asynchronous mode for as long as the magnet remains in place. With asynchronous stimulation, competing rhythms can develop, and the possibility of dysrhythmia generation must be kept in mind.

  (b) Different generators may respond to magnet application in different ways. Some pacemakers may be reprogrammed by magnet application. **The characteristics of the patient's pacemaker should be known before the magnet is applied!!**

  (c) Magnet rate may differ from the programmed paced rate.

  (d) Moving a magnet around a VVI pacemaker may actually inhibit pacemaker output by changing the magnetic fields.

  (e) With the VDD-DDD pacemaker, application of a magnet can be used to interrupt pacemaker-mediated tachycardia (PMT). However, PMT may occur upon removal of the magnet.

  (f) Absence of pacemaker spikes at magnet application may be due to

  (i) Pacemaker in which the magnet mode function has been turned off or is absent.

  (ii) Pacemaker battery voltage is exhausted.

  (iii) Other component failure exists (lead fracture, generator failure, etc.).

f. Determination of threshold. Generally, threshold will increase slowly after placement of electrodes. Peak increase occurs at 2–4 times the threshold at placement, approximately 2–6 weeks after acute placement. Subsequently values will then decrease to an intermediate level. Generally accepted thresholds in the acute placement period include a current of less than 2 mA, a voltage of less than 1.25 volts at a simulus duration of 0.5 milliseconds. Common causes of threshold changes are shown in Table 16-5.

Table 16-5. Factors affecting myocardial stimulation threshold

Factor(s)	Increase in threshold	Decrease in threshold	No change in threshold
Physiologic	↓ Sympathetic tone Sleeping Eating	↑ Sympathetic tone Exercise Postural change	
Metabolic	Hyperglycemia (> 600 mg/dl) Hypoxemia Hypercarbia Metabolic alkalosis Metabolic acidosis Hyperthyroidism	Hyperventilation ↑ PO_2	Hypoglycemia

Drugs	Type I antidysrhythmics
	  Quinidine
	  Procainamide
	  Disopyramide
	Beta blockade
	  Propranolol
	Lidocaine (+/−)
	Flecainide
	Tricyclic
	  antidepressants (?)
	Mineralocorticoids
		Isoproterenol
		Corticosteroids
		  Prednisone
		  Prednisolone
			Amiodarone
			Atropine
			Acetylcholine
			Succinylcholine
			Volatile
			  anesthetics
			  Enflurane
			  Isoflurane
			  Halothane

Electrolytes	Hyperkalemia (>7.0 mEq/liter)	Hypernatremia	
Other	Myocardial infarction Ischemia		

Source: From M. L. Dohrmann and N. F. Goldschlager. Myocardial stimulation threshold in patients with cardiac pacemakers: Effect of physiologic variables, pharmacologic agents and lead electrodes. *Cardiol. Clin.* 3:528, 1985. With permission.

5. Related cardiovascular diseases
   a. Does the patient have **angina,** a prior **myocardial infarction,** or signs or symptoms of **coronary artery disease** or **congestive heart failure?**

Pacemaker patients

   50% have coronary artery disease
   20% have hypertension
   10% have diabetes mellitus [7]

   b. What is the patient's present and past drug therapy? Digoxin and antiarrhythmics, in particular, may interact with the conducting system.
B. Anesthetic management of the patient with a preexisting pacemaker
   #### 1. Monitoring
   a. Monitoring should be based on the patient's underlying disease and surgical procedure.
   b. During anesthesia on all patients with pacemakers, **pulsatile per-**

fusion should be monitored on a beat-to-beat basis with a finger on the pulse, a precordial or esophageal stethoscope, Doppler probe, pulse oximeter, or arterial catheter.

c. A pulmonary artery catheter can be placed despite the presence of an endocardial (transvenous) pacemaker. However, if the pacemaker is less than 4 weeks old there is danger of dislodging the fresh pacing electrode. In this situation, if a pulmonary artery catheter is required, consideration should be given to passing a pace-port Swan-Ganz catheter or having available other means of temporary pacing such as a transcutaneous pacemaker.

   (1) The Swan-Ganz catheter should be placed under fluoroscopy whenever possible, and a chest film should be obtained before **Swan-Ganz removal** to detect knots or loops around the pacemaker lead.

2. Anesthetic technique

a. Regional anesthesia, volatile anesthetic, and narcotic relaxant techniques have all been used without problems. Three-fourths of the minimum alveolar concentration (MAC) of enflurane, isoflurane, or halothane does not affect pacing thresholds in patients undergoing cardiac surgery with baseline diazepam, narcotic, and pancuronium anesthesia.

b. Unipolar pacemakers can be inhibited by sensing muscle biopotentials from either voluntary muscular activity, fasciculations, or shivering.

   (1) Use succinylcholine only if indicated and with preceding administration of a nondepolarizing defasciculant in patients who have a unipolar pacemaker in place.

   (2) Minimize postoperative shivering.

c. Positive pressure ventilation could cause loss of endocardial contact and intraoperative pacemaker failure. Positive pressure ventilation should be tested, if feasible, before muscle relaxants are administered in patients who have had a pacemaker lead in place less than 4 weeks. Further, inflation pressures should be kept as low as possible to minimize stretching of the thorax.

3. Intraoperative pacemaker complications.
Causes of intraoperative pacemaker malfunction are shown in Table 16-6.

a. The most common source of intraoperative pacemaker complications is electromagnetic interference (EMI), primarily due to electrocautery.

b. EMI causes pacemaker malfunction primarily by interfering with the sensing and pacing functions of the pacemaker but may also actually damage the generator itself.

c. EMI can be transferred from the pacemaker to the electrodes, causing thermal damage to the electrode-myocardial interface and increasing the capture threshold or actually stimulating dysrhythmias.

d. **Recommendations concerning EMI due to electrocautery**

   (1) Bipolar cautery should be utilized. If unipolar cautery is essential, the ground should be as far away from the pacemaker generator as possible with the current path from the cautery probe to ground directed away from the generator-lead system and if possible perpendicular to it.

   (2) Because cautery will distort ECG data, a monitor of pulsatile perfusion is paramount.

   (3) Cautery, if used, should be applied for 1-second bursts with 5–10 seconds between bursts if the patient has inadequate native rhythm.

Table 16-6. Causes of intraoperative pacemaker malfunction

Cause	Failure category	Mechanism	Comments
Electrical			
Electromagnetic interference (EMI; electrocautery)	Failure to sense Failure to pace Reprogram generator Damage generator	Electrical current surges	Most common cause of failure
Cardioversion-defibrillation	Failure to sense Failure to pace Erratic pacing pattern	Electrical current surges Thermal damage at myocardium/interface	Defibrillate with minimum energy Place paddles as far as possible from pacer Interrogate or reprogram pacer after use
Electrical cross-talk	Failure to pace	Ventricular sensing of atrial paced beat	Dual chamber pacemakers
Generator failure	Failure to pace Failure to sense	Electronic or battery malfunction	Include generator programmer error
Physical			
Lead dislodgement	Loss of capture Loss of sensing	No myocardial contact	Common with cardiac manipulation
Incorrect lead	Failure to sense	Inadequate voltage detected from the intracardiac electrogram	
Lead fracture or insulation failure	Failure to pace	Incomplete circuit	May be visible on chest x ray
Fibrosis at electrode site	Failure to capture	Increased resistance	
Myocardial perforation	Failure to capture or sense	Loss of contact	Visible on chest x ray
Shivering	Pacer inhibition	Myopotential inhibition	
Radiation therapy	Unpredictable	Damage generator circuitry	Shield generator

Nitrous oxide	Failure to pace	Expansion of residual air in pocket	Newly implanted unipolar pacer
		Loss of electrical contact	
Positive pressure ventilation	Failure to capture/sense	Loss of endocardial pacer contact	Thoracic expansion
			Important within first 4 weeks of pacer placement
Drug effects			
Succinylcholine	Pacer inhibition	Myopotential inhibition	Fasciculations
Propranolol	Failure to capture	Increased pacer threshold	
Procainamide			
Quinidine			
Verapamil			
Digoxin			
Lidocaine			
Flecainide			
Metabolic			
Hypokalemia	Loss of capture	Decreased pacer threshold	
Hyperkalemia	Dysrhythmia	Increased pacer threshold	
		T-wave sensing	
		Large T waves	
Hypothermia	Failure to capture	Increased pacer threshold	
Hypoxia	Failure to capture	Increased pacer threshold	
Hypercarbia			

(4) The anesthesiologist should be aware of the "default" program of the pacemaker in case of interference because the program may vary from unit to unit (consult the manufacturer if necessary).

(5) During cardiothoracic surgery, the generator may be disconnected and the permanent lead(s) connected to an external pulse generator to prevent damage to the implanted pacemaker generator.

(6) If a nonprogrammable demand pacemaker is implanted, a magnet may be used for conversion to asynchronous mode.

(7) In programmable pacemakers consider preoperative programming to a fixed asynchronous mode as an option to minimize the effects of EMI.

(8) In a programmable pacemaker, the programming unit for that pacemaker model and the ability to utilize it should be available intraoperatively, especially in patients who are pacemaker dependent.

e. Cardioversion-defibrillation. Pacemakers are fairly resistant to external direct current cardioversion. Electrodes for defibrillation should be placed at least 12 cm from the pacemaker, and the lowest energy possible should be utilized for defibrillation. The pacemaker should be reinterrogated after defibrillation or cardioversion to rule out reprogramming.

f. Electroconvulsive therapy should cause no significant risk due to its distance from the pacemaker.

g. X rays can cause damage to silicon chips in the pacemaker circuitry. Although diagnostic x rays are considered safe, radiation therapy could cause an unpredictable pacing pattern. During radiation therapy the pacemaker generator should be shielded or operative relocation of the generator considered.

h. Magnetic resonance imaging (MRI) with its high magnetic field strength can cause pacemaker reprogramming, and permanent **pacemaker patients should not undergo MRI.**

i. Extracorporeal shock wave lithotripsy is very unlikely to damage conventional pacemakers. At present motion sensors in some variable rate pacemakers may be damaged. Dual chamber pacemakers, although not damaged, may need to be reprogrammed to single chamber mode to avoid oversensing.

j. Failure to sense may be due to:

(1) Inadequate electrogram amplitudes (recommended minimal implant values for the ventricle are more than 4 mV and for the atrium more than 2 mV). Adequate sensing depends on both amplitude and slew rate (i.e., rate of change in voltage with respect to time of the intrinsic deflection of the signal). The slew rate of 0.6–0.8 volt/second is generally adequate. Typically, there will be a less than 15% change in amplitude after implantation and a less than 50% change in slew rate after implantation.

(2) Malposition of the lead.

(3) Magnetic interference.

4. Microshock. Because of the direct connection of the leads to the myocardium, the exposed leads of temporary endocardial or epicardial pacemakers should always be handled with gloves and covered with gloves when not in use. This minimizes the likelihood of transmission of extraneous electrical activity to the heart with subsequent danger of microshock and generation of dysrhythmia.

5. Treatment of intraoperative pacemaker failure

a. Ensure adequate **oxygenation** and ventilation.

b. Begin cardiopulmonary resuscitation (**CPR**) if spontaneous rate is absent or hemodynamically ineffective.

c. If an **external pacemaker** generator is in place:

    (1) Turn pacemaker to maximal output in asynchronous mode.

    (2) Check all **connections.**

    (3) **Replace** external generator unit or batteries.

    (4) With an external bipolar pacemaker, attempt pacing with reversal of lead polarity. When the failure occurs in a pacemaker with a temporary transvenous wire, attempt to advance the transvenous pacing wire slowly.

d. If a programmable permanent pacemaker is in place, reprogram it using the "panic button" on the programming unit, or, with a ventricular demand pacemaker, place a magnet to allow asynchronous mode functioning.

e. Administer **atropine** and **isoproterenol** to attempt to stimulate intrinsic rhythm and, in the case of the latter drug, to lower the pacemaker threshold.

f. If the pacemaker does not begin to capture with the above maneuvers within several minutes, a **temporary pacemaker** should be considered. Possibilities include placement of a fresh transvenous pacing wire under fluoroscopy or application of an external transcutaneous pacemaker.

C. Anesthetic management of permanent pacemaker insertion

1. Route of placement, transvenous or epicardial. More than 90% of pacemakers are implanted through the transvenous route. Local anesthesia with light sedation should be adequate for comfort. Often placement of an epicardial pacemaker will require the use of a general anesthetic. If general anesthesia is necessary, the patient should have a temporary or transcutaneous pacemaker immediately available before induction.

2. As with any patient with conduction disturbances or a pacemaker in place, **temporary pacing** capabilities, **monitoring** of **pulsatile blood flow,** and **chronotropic agents** such as atropine or isoproterenol should be available.

3. Potent inhalational anesthetics have been shown to increase AV nodal conduction time in chronically instrumented dogs anesthetized with controlled ventilation. Isoflurane has been demonstrated to have a weaker effect than enflurane or halothane in this regard, but it too will prolong conduction in clinically relevant concentrations. It is important to note, however, that this effect is indirect, mediated by changes in autonomic tone. In animals with previous autonomic blockade, neither halothane, enflurane, nor isoflurane produced significant slowing of conduction [1].

    Potent inhalational agents should therefore be used with caution in a patient with AV nodal disease and conduction block who requires a general anesthetic for pacemaker placement. Further, if conduction block does develop during induction of anesthesia with these agents, it should respond to adrenergic agents.

4. Pacemaker generator replacement. Usually replacement of the pacemaker generator can be performed under local anesthesia. Knowledge of the patient's underlying rhythm is extremely important because the patient can be without pacing for short periods during the procedure, and asystole can result unless temporary pacing is immediately available.

5. Immediate pacemaker complications with insertion of a permanent transvenous pacemaker

    a. Dysrhythmia. Asystole, atrial or ventricular tachydysrhythmias, or fibrillation are common. Immediate antidysrhythmic therapy and defibrillator capability should be available.

    b. Hemorrhage. Bleeding may occur, especially if surgery involves the internal jugular venous system. Adequate venous access is required preoperatively because access to a peripheral vein is usually not available intraoperatively.

    c. Pneumothorax or hemothorax.

    d. Cardiac perforation with possible acute cardiac tamponade.

    e. Air embolism with inspiration.

VII. Resection of dysrhythmogenic foci

A. Indications

1. Present surgical therapy of tachycardias focuses on the ablation of ventricular dysrhythmogenic foci and the interruption of ventricular reentrant loops and accessory AV conduction pathways. Surgical ablation of dysrhythmogenic foci is recommended for tachycardia that is refractory to medical therapy.

2. Patients undergoing surgery for supraventricular tachycardia tend to be young and otherwise healthy. Patients with ventricular tachycardia tend to be older, have impaired ventricular function due to prior myocardial infarction or ventricular aneurysm, and have multisystem disease.

B. Ablative procedures

1. Ablative procedures may be either surgical or accomplished through a transvenous catheter.

    a. Transvenous catheter ablation of the atrioventricular junction is routinely performed for uncontrollable supraventricular tachycardias and generally results in complete AV block that frequently requires subsequent pacing. High-energy direct current shocks have been used to ablate atrial and ventricular tachycardia foci as well as some accessory pathways.

    b. Direct surgical ablative procedures are designed to offer a curative rather than a palliative solution to symptomatic tachycardia. Present surgical techniques use encircling ventriculotomy, myotomy, endocardial resection, cryoablation, and laser photocoagulation singularly or in combination to destroy the dysrhythmogenic focus. These procedures are performed at normothermia without cardioplegia. Combining different approaches and individualizing the procedure to the pathophysiologic findings appear to produce satisfactory results. Surgical therapy results in an average 10% operative mortality with a 90% cure rate for ventricular tachycardia.

2. For the ablative approaches, **preoperative catheter endocardial ECG mapping** is performed in an attempt to ascertain the anatomic origin of a dysrhythmogenic focus (including an accessory pathway). Epicardial mapping at surgery allows one to visualize anatomic landmarks in relation to the earliest epicardial sites of activation of the abnormal focus. Simultaneous computer-assisted ECG recordings from multiple sites on the heart (minimum 50–60) is rapidly replacing single-point mapping of tachycardia. Single-point intraoperative mapping is laborious and time-consuming and requires excessive cardiac manipulation.

3. Multipoint intraoperative mapping systems allow computerization and rapid analysis of activation sequences. Mapping is performed through a median sternotomy and after cannulation for cardiopulmonary bypass. Intraoperative mapping is performed at normothermia and prior to any cardioplegia; the tachycardia is induced by pacing through electrodes on the right or left ventricle. Normo-

thermic cardiopulmonary bypass is frequently required to support the patient through point-by-point mapping during ventricular tachycardia and to maintain normothermia during mapping of AV accessory pathways. Today's automated mapping systems allow speedier interpretation of the earliest site of activation, the presumed location of the abnormal dysrhythmogenic focus

C. Anesthetic management

1. Patients undergoing ablative surgery fall into two distinct groups, those with supraventricular tachycardias and those with ventricular tachycardias.

2. **Supraventricular tachycardia**

   a. **Patient population.** Patients are usually young and otherwise in good health with good ventricular function and a low perioperative mortality rate (1%).

   b. **Preoperative drug therapy.** Drug therapy should be discontinued preoperatively, if possible under monitored conditions, to make the dysrhythmia more inducible.

   c. **Perioperative monitoring**

      (1) In these otherwise healthy patients, arterial and central venous pressure (CVP) monitoring is often sufficient. If a Swan-Ganz catheter is placed, it should not be advanced beyond the sheath until after bypass to avoid disrupting conduction pathways, causing dysrhythmias, or temporarily suppressing the bypass tract.

      (2) Monitoring temperature and maintaining normothermia are essential in these patients because hypothermia may alter conduction. Room temperature, therefore, should be elevated to maintain the patient's temperature at 37°C or greater.

      (3) External defibrillator-cardioverter pads should be placed prior to induction of anesthesia to treat dysrhythmias that appear before the chest is open.

   d. **Anesthetic techniques.** Any combination of opiates, benzodiazepines, thiopental, volatile anesthetics, and nitrous oxide may be used because these will not adversely affect conduction or inducibility of the supraventricular tachycardia. In this group of patients, it is often possible to use lower doses of opiates and higher doses of thiopental and volatile anesthetic agents in order to extubate them early in the postoperative period. For muscle relaxation, vecuronium and atracurium seem to have little if any effect on conduction. One should avoid droperidol because it affects both antegrade and retrograde conduction velocities in the atrium in a dose-dependent manner [4].

   e. **Mapping and bypass procedure**

      (1) The patient will be cannulated with two atrial cannulae and one aortic cannula. Often, however, the inferior vena cava cannula is not inserted until mapping is complete for right-sided pathways.

      (2) Mapping will occur after cannulation but usually before bypass. For left-sided foci, correction will take place with the patient on bypass with cardioplegic arrest. Right-sided foci will be corrected on bypass with the heart beating so that the His bundle will be found and marked.

      (3) Bypass may be required to maintain normothermia during mapping.

         (a) During normothermic bypass, heparin requirements are increased because of increased metabolism.

         (b) During a rapid rhythm, the heart's oxygen requirements are very high.

     f. At the conclusion of cardiopulmonary bypass, the mapping procedure may be repeated.

     g. After all mapping procedures are concluded, the Swan-Ganz catheter, if present, should be floated into the pulmonary artery.

     h. A stable postbypass period and short period of postoperative intubation can normally be anticipated.

3. Ventricular tachycardia (VT)

  a. Patient population. These patients tend to be older, have impaired ventricular function (average ejection fraction 30–36%) due to prior myocardial infarction or ventricular aneurysm, and have multisystem disease. Operative mortality is often greater than 10%. Many patients who represent poor surgical risks for resection of ventricular dysrhythmogenic foci with CPB are candidates for implantation of an automatic implantable cardioverter defibrillator (AICD), a much simpler procedure that does not require CPB.

  b. Preoperative drug therapy

     (1) Negative inotropes: β blockers

     (2) Vasodilators

       (a) Nitrates

       (b) Calcium channel blockers

       (c) Angiotensin-converting enzyme inhibitors

     (3) Antidysrhythmics

       (a) Procainamide—potent negative inotrope and vasodilator

       (b) Lidocaine

       (c) Amiodarone

         (i) Half-life of approximately 4 weeks

         (ii) Potent vasodilator; refractory to vasopressors

         (iii) Associated with intractable bradydysrhythmias in patients undergoing noncardiac surgery

         (iv) May be associated with inability to wean from cardiopulmonary bypass

     (4) In this patient population, it may be impossible to discontinue all drug therapy preoperatively.

  c. Perioperative monitoring

     (1) Standard monitoring will include the routine noninvasive monitors plus an arterial catheter and a pulmonary artery catheter inserted only to the end of the introducer sheath (10–12 cm). Because of long bypass times, poor ventricular function, and, in some cases, a history of amiodarone use, all patients undergoing surgery for ventricular tachycardia probably should have a pulmonary artery catheter ready to advance into the pulmonary artery. The PA catheter may be advanced in VT patients after the chest is open (patients with catheter-induced VT may not respond to drugs or electrical therapy) and after cannulation for bypass. Lidocaine for skin infiltration should be used in as small a dose as possible for vascular access.

     (2) Femoral arterial lines will be placed in most patients needing VT surgery because many of them will require an intraaortic balloon pump to be weaned from bypass.

     (3) The two-dimensional transesophageal echocardiogram may be useful in VT surgical patients for assessment of regional wall motion abnormalities and valvular problems caused by a change in ventricular geometry. Occasionally valvular dysfunction may be secondary to injury of one or both of the papillary muscles. Precautions must be taken to prevent esophageal damage during external defibrillation.

     (4) External defibrillator-cardioverter pads should be placed prior to induction for use before the chest is open.

(5) Temperature should be closely monitored, and all efforts should be made to maintain normothermia.

d. Anesthetic techniques. Generally these patients will tolerate only a high-dose opiate technique. They should not receive intravenous, oral, or intratracheal lidocaine because this may prevent dysrhythmia induction.

e. Dysrhythmias that occur before bypass should be treated with cardioversion or defibrillation without the use of pharmacologic agents whenever possible.

f. Mapping and bypass procedures

(1) To locate the dysrhythmogenic focus, VT must be induced during mapping while the patient is supported by cardiopulmonary bypass. Most of these foci will be left-sided. After inducing VT, these foci are mapped endocardially (with transmural probes) as well as epicardially. The lesions are corrected with the heart beating and with normothermic bypass. **The left ventricle will be open and the aorta is not cross-clamped.** It is essential to maintain the mean arterial pressure both to keep the aortic valve competent (to prevent bleeding and air emboli) and to maintain subendocardial blood flow during VT. Blood pressure may be maintained with a phenylephrine drip.

(2) The surgical procedure usually combines cryosurgical ablation and surgical resection.

(3) These patients, especially those with VT, will be subjected to a fairly long period of normothermic bypass, and a membrane oxygenator will be used. These patients will also have a fairly high heparin requirement.

(4) After resection, attempts at reinduction of VT are performed before weaning from bypass. If a ventricular focus cannot be resected, an AICD device will be placed. Generally, several pacing leads will be placed also.

(5) If the heart is opened, normal de-airing procedures are undertaken prior to the termination of bypass.

(6) Ablation of an ectopic ventricular focus often requires ventriculotomy and resection of at least some ventricular tissue. Although precise mapping techniques can limit the extent of the resection, any ventriculotomy is associated with depressed ventricular function and possible difficulty in weaning from cardiopulmonary bypass.

g. After the completion of all mapping procedures but before termination of CPB, the Swan-Ganz catheter should be advanced into the pulmonary artery if it is not already in this position.

h. After CPB, these patients often require inotropic support, an intraaortic balloon, and prolonged postoperative ventilation. Coagulation status should be monitored closely because of the potential for destruction of platelets and coagulation factors during prolonged normothermic bypass.

VIII. Automatic implantable cardioverter defibrillator (AICD)

A. Description of the AICD

1. The present AICD generator weighs 292 g and is bulky in size at $11.2 \times 7.1 \times 2.5$ cm. The device has receptacles to receive two patch electrodes (or one patch and one spring electrode) and each pole of a bipolar transvenous or epicardial pacing electrode. The device is designed to sense ventricular electrical activity and emit an electrical countershock within 35 seconds of sensing a tachydysrhythmia (Fig. 16-2).

2. The present device can sense tachydysrhythmias by two methods.

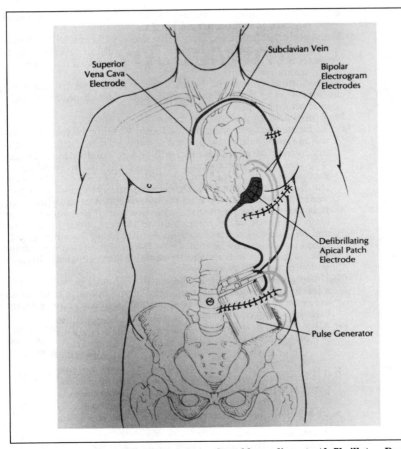

Fig. 16-2. Components of the automatic implantable cardioverter/defibrillator. Device may include either one (as shown) or two defibrillating epicardial patch electrodes. The "bipolar electrogram electrodes" may be either epicardial (as shown) or transcutaneous. (From R. A. Winkle. The implantable defibrillator in ventricular arrhythmias. *Hosp. Prac.* 18:150, 1983. With permission.)

    a. **Probability density function (PDF).** The probability density function algorithm measures the sinusoidal character of the transcardiac ECG signal (patch-to-patch QRST signal). Ventricular fibrillation will always fulfill this criterion, as will nearly any wide QRS tachycardia.

    b. **Heart rate.** A generator manufactured prior to August 1989 has a predetermined rate cut-off (range 120–200 bpm). The rate-detection criterion is enabled by any tachycardia including sinus tachycardia that exceeds the preset rate cut-off of the device. In the present generator the heart rate criterion is programmable noninvasively.

    c. In the present AICD dysrhythmia sensing requires either rate only or both sensing functions to be satisfied (i.e., both heart rate and PDF). Once the device is triggered, it charges and delivers a discharge. Generally, the device requires 5–10 seconds to sense VT or ventricular fibrillation (VF).

3. The present AICD has fixed energy settings. The standard device delivers a 25-joule discharge. If this is unsuccessful at terminating VT or VF, a second discharge of 30 joules is delivered. The device can deliver four or five discharges, after which it must sense a period of sinus rhythm before it can be triggered again. The high-energy device delivers a 30-joule first shock. It delivers 30 joules at the second, third, fourth, and fifth discharges if necessary. In the future, energy settings will be programmable. The AICD usually requires 5–15 seconds to charge its storage capacitors.

4. The generator is delivered from the manufacturer in the inactive mode and must be activated either by a donut magnet or programmer. When inactive, the application of a magnet causes the generator to produce a constant tone. When active and disconnected, the generator is silent when the magnet is removed. The implanted generator produces an audible tone synchronous with the ventricular rate (heart rate) when the magnet is applied. If the magnet is applied to the generator before implantation and it is silent (i.e., active mode), the magnet should be left in place for at least 30 seconds until the constant tone is produced (inactive mode). Conversely, the generator can be activated by leaving the magnet applied for about 30 seconds, until the constant tone stops. The device also has an electrophysiology (EP) test mode in which it will neither sense nor shock.

B. **Surgical techniques.** The surgical approaches for AICD insertion include:

1. **Median sternotomy.** The median sternotomy allows the best visualization and must be performed when implantation is combined with other cardiac surgical procedures, such as coronary artery bypass grafting. This technique allows easy placement of one or two epicardial patch electrodes and two epicardial pacing electrodes for bipolar detection of the rhythm. All leads are tunneled to a subcutaneous pocket that is made in the left upper abdominal quadrant (see Fig. 16-2).

2. **Left thoracotomy.** The left thoracotomy approach is good for placement of the AICD electrodes and patches only. It does not allow a combined procedure (i.e., concomitant coronary artery bypass grafting) and is not ideal for resuscitation.

3. The **subxiphoid approach** requires use of the transvenous spring electrode because only a single patch can be applied to the epicardial surface.

4. The **subcostal approach** is a modification of the subxiphoid technique. A longer left subcostal incision allows more exposure and use of two epicardial patches.

5. When indicated, coronary bypass grafting or valve replacement is carried out prior to placement of the AICD patch and sensing electrodes.

C. **Intraoperative testing.** After the sensing and defibrillation electrodes are implanted, the device is tested with the chest open but without the benefit of cardiopulmonary bypass.

1. **Testing sensing function.** The QRS complex on the unfiltered signals from the bipolar sensing electrodes and the defibrillation electrodes (patches) should be 5 mV in amplitude and less than 120 msec in duration. The AICD has a short refractory period of about 150 msec. Thus, to avoid double sensing of a single ventricular electrogram, the QRS duration must be less than 150 msec and the T wave must be sufficiently small.

2. **Testing defibrillation function.** An external cardioverter defibrillator (ECD) is used to deliver test shocks of 1–40 joules. VT and VF are induced using standard temporary electrodes. Ideally, defibrillation thresholds should be at or below 20 joules because the present device has a **maximum energy output** of about 30 joules. It is desirable to have defibrillation thresholds at least 10 joules below the first shock energy setting of the device. If the defibrillation threshold is over 25 joules, move the pads and change their polarity to improve the threshold. If there is no success, close the wound with the defibrillator leads in place and return in about 1 week to see if the threshold has decreased below 25 joules with healing.

After the external test shocks are complete, the AICD generator is attached to the four electrodes, and VF is again induced to determine the functional integrity of the system. Note that the AICD generator is handed to the surgeon in an inactive mode. Once connected, the surgeon activates the unit. The defibrillator is deactivated once it has been tested, and the generator is placed subcutaneously in the abdominal pocket. In the early postoperative stages the unit is left deactivated because many of these patients are prone to supraventricular tachycardia (atrial fibrillation, atrial flutter) with a rate that frequently exceeds the rate cut-off of the device. Once the patient's condition is stabilized, usually in 1–3 days, the device is activated.

D. **Anesthetic management**

1. **Antiarrhythmic agents.** Many of the patients who are having an AICD implanted will be taking oral antidysrhythmic agents at the time of surgery. In theory, the device and defibrillation thresholds should be tested while the patient is on the drug regimen that is planned after the procedure. Patients should not be given excessive amounts of lidocaine while cannulas and catheters are being inserted, nor should lidocaine be given intravenously for ventricular ectopy. However, patients on chronic antidysrhythmic therapy must often continue their therapy until the operative morning. Of major concern is the antidysrhythmic agent amiodarone, which is a negative inotropic agent and vasodilator but nevertheless must often be continued preoperatively. In combination with other potent vasodilators and myocardial depressants, amiodarone may cause refractory bradycardia or may precipitate a profound and prolonged hypotensive state postoperatively. Thus, the selection of anesthetic agent becomes crucial when amiodarone is present.

2. **Congestive heart failure.** Ventricular dysrhythmias often occur in association with ischemic heart disease, ventricular failure, or a ventricular aneurysm. Patients often present for AICD placement, therefore, with poor preoperative ventricular function.

3. **Intraoperative monitoring**

   a. Implantation of an AICD is a limited procedure but does involve induction of ventricular fibrillation. Therefore, standard noninvasive monitoring plus at least an arterial catheter to monitor blood pressure continuously and a central venous catheter to administer vasoactive drugs are mandatory

   b. Use of a Swan-Ganz catheter depends solely on the patient's preoperative cardiovascular status and the estimated risk of inducing ventricular dysrhythmias during catheter insertion

4. **Anesthetic technique**

   a. A low-dose nitrous oxide, narcotic relaxant anesthetic is effective and allows early extubation without predisposing the patient to dysrhythmias.

b. In patients with poor ventricular function, a narcotic anesthetic may be required. The use of a short-acting narcotic such as alfentanil may allow extubation relatively soon postoperatively.

5. Postoperative dysrhythmia detection and management

a. A major concern following defibrillation is the status of sinus node recovery. On occasion, patients may need to be paced temporarily for asystole following cardioversion by the AICD (or during threshold testing). Therefore, temporary pacing must be readily available, probably using temporary epicardial wires inserted surgically.

b. Ventricular tachycardia or fibrillation may occur after the procedure when the newly implanted AICD is in the inactive mode. An external device is mandatory, and monitoring must be constant until the AICD can be activated.

c. New-onset atrial fibrillation with a rapid ventricular rate is not uncommon. Standard agents or external direct current cardioversion should be used to correct this rhythm. The AICD is generally in the inactive mode postoperatively until this somewhat proarrhythmic phase subsides. It should be remembered that atrial fibrillation with a rapid rate can exceed the rate cut-off of the device and trigger the AICD to discharge, especially if the device is not equipped with PDF.

Monitoring is necessary postoperatively until the patient's condition is stabilized and the device has been activated.

REFERENCES

1. Atlee, J. L., III, Brownlee, S. W., and Burstrom, R. E. Conscious state comparisons of the effects of inhalation anesthetics on specalized atrioventricular conduction tissues in dogs. *Anesthesiology* 64:703–710, 1986.

2. Bernstein, A. D., Camm, A. J., Fletcher, R. D., et al. The North American Society of Pacing and Electrophysiology/British Pacing and Electrophysiology Group generic pacemaker code for antibradyarrhythmia and adaptive-rate pacing and antitachyarrhythmia devices. PACE 10:794–799, 1987.

3. Cohen, S. I., and Frank, H. A. Preservation of active atrial transport: An important clinical consideration in cardiac pacing. *Chest* 81:51–54, 1982.

4. Frye, R. L., Collins, J. J., DeSanctis, R. W., et al. Guidelines for permanent cardiac pacemaker implantation. *J. Am. Coll. Cardiol.* 4:434–442, 1984.

5. Gomez-Arnau, J., Marquez-Montes, J., and Avello, F. Fentanyl and droperidol effects on the refractoriness of the accessory pathway in the Wolff-Parkinson-White syndrome. *Anesthesiology* 58:307–313, 1983.

6. Hartzler, G. O., Maloney, J. D., Curtis, J. J., et al. Hemodynamic benefits of atrioventricular sequential pacing after cardiac surgery. *Am. J. Cardiol.* 40:232–236, 1977.

7. Kicklighter, E. J., Syverud, S. A., Dalsey, W. C., et al. Pathological aspects of transcutaneous cardiac pacing. *Am. J. Emerg. Med.* 3:108–113, 1985.

8. Panidis, I., Dreifus, L. S., and Michelson, E. L. Hemodynamic effects of cardiac pacing. Pacemaker therapy. *Cardiovascular Clin.* 14(2):1–11, 1983.

9. Samet, P., Castillo, C., and Bernstein, W. H. Hemodynamic consequences of sequential atrioventricular pacing: Subjects with normal hearts. *Am. J. Cardiol.* 21:207–212, 1968.

10. Syverud, S. A., Hedges, J. R., Dalsey, W. C., et al. Hemodynamics of transcutaneous cardiac pacing. *Am. J. Emerg. Med.* 4:17–20, 1986.

SUGGESTED READING

Ausubel, K., and Furman, S. The pacemaker syndrome. *Ann. Intern. Med.* 103:420–429, 1985.

Cannom, D. S., and Winkle, R. A. Implantation of the automatic implantable cardioverter defibrillator (AICD): Practical aspects. *PACE* 9:793–809, 1986.

Parsonnet, V. Pacemaker Implantation. In D. B. Essler (ed.), *Blades' Surgical Diseases of the Chest* (4th ed.). St. Louis: Mosby, 1978. Pp. 699–758.

Saksena, S., Lindsay, B. D., and Parsonnet, V. Developments for future implantable cardioverters and defibrillators. *PACE* 10:1342–1358, 1987.

Winkle, R. A., Stinson, E. B., Echt, D. S., et al. Practical aspects of automatic cardioverter/defibrillator implantation. *Am. Heart J.* 108:1335-1346, 1984.

Management of Cardiothoracic Surgical Emergencies

David B. Campbell and David R. Larach

Emergency is a relative term. For the endocrinologic, plastic, or opthalmologic surgeon, an emergency may require operative intervention within hours. In cardiothoracic surgery, in contrast, emergencies require surgical intervention within minutes or seconds. Cardiothoracic emergencies are precipitated by (1) intractable myocardial ischemia, (2) obstruction to forward cardiac output, (3) hemorrhage from the heart or great vessels, or (4) obstruction to air flow to the lungs. Each can kill within minutes. This chapter will discuss emergencies in each of these categories, emphasizing throughout an appropriate sense of urgency and clinical priority.

I. The heart
A. Acute pericardial tamponade
1. **Pathophysiology.** The steps in the development of pericardial tamponade are:
   a. Fluid accumulation in the pericardial (potential) space.
   b. Impaired diastolic ventricular filling, leading to small, underfilled ventricles. **The primary problem is reduced ventricular preload,** not failure of myocardial contractility.
   c. Increased central venous (CVP) and right atrial (RA) pressure as venous return is impeded from entering the right ventricle (RV).
   d. Reduced stroke volume, compensatory tachycardia, and vasoconstriction are attempts to preserve cardiac output and blood pressure.
   e. Patients with moderate tamponade may **decompensate precipitously.** As the pericardial fluid volume increases, pericardial compliance decreases until a critical point is reached. Beyond this, addition of only small extra amounts of fluid can cause marked increases in pericardial pressure with ventricular compression.
   f. End-stage tamponade is marked by hypotension with shock and myocardial ischemia, a nearly obliterated ventricular cavity with minimal cardiac contraction, an electrocardiogram (ECG) with diffuse low voltage, and distant heart sounds with a quiet precordium. Vagally mediated bradycardia may occur, further reducing cardiac output.
2. **Clinical setting**
   a. After open heart surgery
   b. Myocardial infarction
   c. After cardiac catheterization, Swan-Ganz catheter, or pacemaker insertion
   d. Thoracic trauma
   e. Malignant, idiopathic, or uremic pericarditis (usually chronic); following radiation therapy; anticoagulated patients
   f. Aortic dissection
2. **Diagnosis**
   a. **Clinical presentation.** The presence of **hypotension with elevated filling pressures** should always prompt the physician to consider pericardial tamponade. A **low stroke volume** is usually seen, which often prompts a reflex **tachycardia** in an attempt to maintain **cardiac output.** However, cardiac output eventually does decrease in more advanced tamponade. Recognize, too, that other causes for these signs exist (e.g., severe heart failure, tension pneumothorax, massive pulmonary embolism).
   b. Chest x ray shows a globular heart, with change in cardiac silhouette.
   c. ECG often shows diffusely low voltage, and **electrical alternans** may be present owing to variation in conduction of the ECG through shifting pericardial fluid (Fig. 17-1).

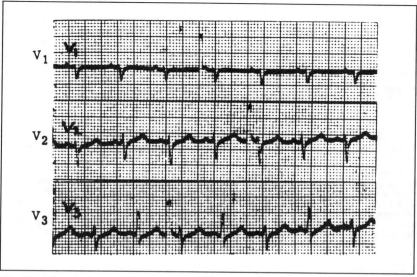

Fig. 17-1. Electrical alternans with cardiac tamponade. Lead V_3 demonstrates the variation in R-wave axis in alternate beats. Note that this phenomenon is not seen in all ECG leads. (From J. M. Goldman. *Principles of Clinical Electrocardiography* [11th ed.]. Los Altos: Lange, 1982. P. 305. With permission.)

    d. Pulsus paradoxus. A decrease of more than 10 mm Hg in systolic arterial pressure with inspiration (not a specific finding—also seen with airway disease and right ventricular infarction).

    e. Distended neck veins, with a diminished or absent y descent, may be present.

    f. Tamponade characteristically involves loss of the y descent from the RA pressure waveform because RA pressure remains elevated during diastole even after the tricuspid valve opens (Fig. 17-2). If a pulmonary artery catheter is present, nearly **equal mean right atrial, RV diastolic, and pulmonary wedge** pressures usually will be present.

    g. Echocardiography usually provides a definitive diagnosis non-invasively. A characteristic echo-free space is seen between the epicardium and the pericardium. However, clotted blood in the pericardial space can complicate accurate echocardiographic diagnosis.

4. Initial (temporizing) management

    a. Pericardiocentesis should be performed immediately in the presence of life-threatening tamponade when the patient is in extremis or fluid infusion is ineffective. Dramatic improvement may be produced by withdrawal of small amounts of pericardial fluid.

        (1) Technique (Fig. 17-3). A needle electrogram can be obtained during pericardiocentesis by using the needle as the V lead on the ECG. When the needle tip contacts the epicardium, an "injury" pattern with ST segment elevation is seen (see Fig. 16-1). A drain can be left in the pericardial space.

        (2) Complications. Puncture of RA or RV, laceration of a coronary artery, pneumothorax, and exacerbation of blood leak into the

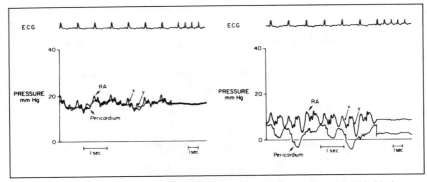

Fig. 17-2. Right atrial and pericardial pressures in cardiac tamponade. *Left.* Notice equal RA and pericardial pressure and the diminished *y*-descent of RA waveform. *Right.* After removal of 100 ml of fluid, the pericardial pressure is now lower than RA pressure, and the normal large *y*-descent has returned. (From B. H. Lorell, and E. Braunwald. Pericardial Disease. In E. Braunwald [ed.], *Heart Disease.* Philadelphia: Saunders, 1984. P. 1481. With permission.)

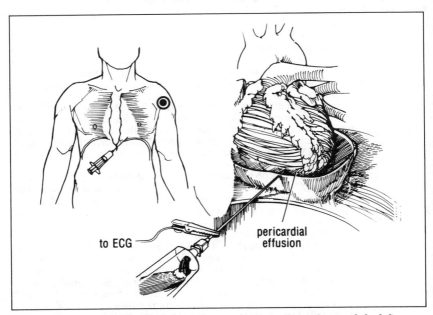

Fig. 17-3. Technique of pericardiocentesis. The needle is directed toward the left shoulder. Needle electrogram permits identification of contact between needle tip and epicardium (causes ST elevation). (From R. C. Polomano and S. E. Miller. *Understanding and Managing Oncologic Emergencies.* Colombus: Adria Laboratories, 1987. P. 22. With permission.)

pericardial space may occur. If fluid is withdrawn too rapidly, pulmonary edema has been reported.

b. Volume infusion causes the RA pressure to rise, increasing the diastolic pressure gradient for RV filling. Right-sided filling pressures should be kept high for any patient with significant tamponade until the tamponade is relieved.

c. Vasoconstrictor and inotropic drugs provide, at best, only temporary benefit. Venous constriction may increase RA pressure; alpha-adrenergic agonists may increase coronary perfusion pressure and ameliorate hypotension-related ischemia for a short period.

d. Avoid lowering the heart rate because the stroke volume is fixed, and a reduction in cardiac output would immediately ensue.

e. Maintain spontaneous ventilation as long as possible because positive-pressure ventilation may further reduce cardiac filling.

5. Definitive surgical management

a. Following cardiac surgery, immediate reopening of the sternotomy incision should be performed under sterile conditions to relieve tamponade.

b. Subxiphoid pericardiotomy. A small subxiphoid incision is made, and dissection under the xiphoid permits the pericardium to be incised, usually without entering the pleural or peritoneal cavity.

c. Pericardiectomy. Through a sternotomy or thoracotomy incision, a large area of pericardium is excised. As a more limited procedure, a "window" can be opened between the pericardial and pleural spaces.

6. Anesthetic considerations

a. Because anesthetic induction may directly or indirectly cause vasodilation and reduced cardiac performance, consideration should be given to performing pericardiocentesis or a subxiphoid pericardiotomy initially under **local anesthesia.** This technique should be considered even if extensive surgery is planned because initial relief of tamponade will substantially reduce the risk of subsequent induction of general anesthesia. Communication with the surgeon in the key in such cases.

b. Maintenance of high filling pressures and an elevated heart rate as well as avoidance of significant myocardial depression can help prevent severe hemodynamic decompensation with general anesthetic induction.

c. Once in the operating room, the patient should be prepped and draped **prior** to anesthetic induction to minimize the time interval between onset of positive-pressure ventilation and relief of tamponade.

d. Potent vasoconstrictor and inotropic drugs (e.g., epinephrine) may be needed to counteract anesthetic-induced vasodilation or myocardial depression. Cardiovascular depression may be caused by direct anesthetic actions, or may result from withdrawal of sympathetic tone with loss of consciousness.

e. The use of **ketamine** as an induction agent may help preserve heart rate and vascular tone in the presence of severe tamponade.

f. Consider the use of a spontaneous-ventilation anesthetic technique when a subxiphoid pericardiotomy is performed, provided the pleural space is not entered.

g. After relief of tamponade, right-sided cardiac output increases dramatically and can induce **pulmonary edema** if the left ventricle (LV) cannot handle the sudden rise in preload. This risk may be increased if a very high CVP is required preoperatively, or if the LV afterload is high. Therefore, the anesthesiologist should be prepared to administer diuretics and vasodilators (especially venous-acting drugs such as nitroglycerin) after the tamponade is removed. Knowledge of the pretamponade hemodynamics is useful for management following surgical intervention.

B. Emergency coronary artery bypass surgery. This section discusses the complications of myocardial ischemia.

1. Pathophysiology

a. Myocardial ischemia may result in myocardial necrosis if not rapidly treated.

b. Myocardial ischemia presents clinically as unstable or unrelenting angina pectoris ("preinfarction angina") that does not respond adequately to medical therapy.

c. Inadequate coronary perfusion may result in significant regional wall motion abnormalities, causing "papillary muscle dysfunction" and mitral regurgitation. Manifestations of acute left ventricular failure such as "flash pulmonary edema" are believed to be due to this mechanism.

2. Clinical setting

a. The difficulty lies in achieving adequate myocardial protection before and during the surgical procedure. The longer the interval between the onset of ischemia and either reestablishment of perfusion or achievement of good myocardial protection, the less muscle will be saved.

b. The indications for emergent coronary bypass grafting include

(1) Ongoing, acute myocardial ischemia (such as occurs with complications of coronary angioplasty).

(2) Truly unstable angina pectoris, in spite of maximal medical therapy, particularly in the setting of left main coronary disease and with or without evidence of left ventricular failure.

(3) "Salvage" operations (myocardial revascularization for acute infarcts more than a few hours old) are **not** accepted in practice.

3. Surgical management

a. All members of the team should work together (in "parallel" rather than in "series") to minimize the time interval between the decision to operate and the achievement of control of myocardial perfusion.

b. The **goal of the operation** is to provide satisfactory and complete myocardial revascularization in an expeditious manner; spending the extra time required for takedown of internal mammary arteries may not be prudent. Saphenous vein grafting, therefore, is performed swiftly, and the most critical lesions are bypassed first with cardioplegia given down the grafts as they are completed.

c. The technical aspects of the surgical procedure differ little from those used in elective coronary artery bypass grafting. However, several **adjunctive measures** may be of particular use in such an emergency setting, including:

(1) Lower systemic perfusion temperatures.

(2) Intensified efforts to achieve (local) myocardial hypothermia, including cooling pads, electrolyte slush or irrigation solutions, bicaval cannulation with snares, and venting. The latter two techniques reduce the rewarming of the arrested heart that occurs when the warmer systemic venous blood returns to the heart.

(3) Retrograde coronary sinus cardioplegia in an attempt to achieve better cardioplegic distribution and hypothermia.

(4) A period of "controlled reperfusion" of the nonworking heart following completion of the revascularization (see Chap. 21).

(5) Reducing myocardial workload both before and after cardiopulmonary bypass (CPB) by use of an intraaortic balloon pump.
4. **Anesthetic management**
   a. **Time is of the essence.** The sooner the patient can be placed on CPB, the fewer myocytes will die. Steps to hasten surgery may be most beneficial in these patients.
   b. **History.** Usually these patients will be transported directly from the cardiac catheterization laboratory to the operating room. It is important for the anesthesiologist to understand the nature of the coronary anatomy, the interventions performed (i.e., angioplasty, transluminal perfusion catheter), and medications administered. Often an intraaortic balloon pump has been placed, and some patients may be on partial femoral bypass. High doses of nitroglycerin and calcium channel blockers are the rule to help control ischemia, and frequently inotropic and antidysrhythmic drugs have been started to maintain blood pressure. Patients may still be partially heparinized from their catheterization.
   c. **Monitoring.** The cardiologist may have inserted **femoral arterial and venous lines** during catheterization. These should remain in place for two reasons: They can be extremely useful for patient management in the operating room (OR), and profuse bleeding will occur from the cannulation sites after heparinization if they are removed. For unstable, severely ischemic patients, it may be prudent to forgo preinduction insertion of a pulmonary artery (PA) catheter or a neck CVP line. The femoral artery line can be used for invasive blood pressure monitoring, the femoral vein line becomes the patient's volume infusion line, and the surgeon can provide transthoracic left atrial (LA) and right atrial (RA) monitoring lines before termination of CPB. Indeed, in any difficult patient it can be extremely useful to monitor femoral arterial pressure (to avoid artificially low radial artery pressure readings immediately after CPB) and LA pressure directly. For cardiac output monitoring after CPB, either green dye may be used, or a surgically placed transthoracic pediatric thermistor catheter may be inserted directly into the PA through the wall of the right RV outflow tract. At the conclusion of surgery, a conventional jugular or subclavian PA catheter can be inserted.
   d. **Technique.** As with any myocardial ischemia patient, anesthetic technique must address maintenance of a favorable myocardial oxygen supply/demand balance. Additionally, for patients in shock, brain perfusion and kidney function should be optimized. It must be recognized, however, that pharmacologic measures to improve cardiac output and blood pressure may worsen myocardial ischemia by increasing oxygen demand. Therefore, often it is necessary to compromise and temporarily accept lower cardiac output values to reduce myocardial work until CPB can be performed.
C. **Surgery for complications of myocardial necrosis**
   1. **Pathophysiology.** Severe complications of myocardial infarction (MI) most often occur within the first 2 weeks after the event. Surgically amenable conditions include papillary muscle rupture, free wall ventricular "rupture," and acquired ventricular septal defect (VSD). These may result from acute occlusion of blood flow to a region of myocardium with inadequate collateral perfusion. The risk and severity of these complications depend on the coronary artery or arteries involved in the acute infarction, as well as the nature of any preexisting myocardial disease.

2. Clinical setting. Sudden deterioration of cardiopulmonary function during the early recovery phase of myocardial infarction should prompt immediate suspicion and investigation:

a. Physical examination should focus on:

(1) The presence of new cardiac murmurs due to papillary muscle rupture or development of a VSD.

(2) Evidence of right ventricular failure due to a VSD.

(3) Evidence of cardiac tamponade (rupture of ventricular free wall).

b. Placement of a **Swan-Ganz catheter** and taking vena caval and pulmonary arterial blood samples will establish the presence of a shunt (VSD) with left-to-right shunting.

c. An **echocardiogram** will allow precise diagnosis of pericardial effusion, overall ventricular function, regional wall motion abnormalities, and mitral valve pathology. Doppler imaging can quantify regurgitant mitral flow and flow across a VSD.

3. Management. All these disease processes present particular challenges to the surgical team, and they represent tests of the quality and efficiency of the operating "machine." There are few "standard recipes" for achieving good results, and the reported series of such patients are notable for consistently high mortality and morbidity figures. Again, the primary objectives in management are swift transport to the operating room and initiation of CPB, and arrest of the heart with good myocardial preservation techniques.

4. Ventricular rupture

a. Urgent operation is the patient's only hope for survival.

b. Surgical management. Pericardiocentesis may provide the patient just enough time to permit transport to the operating room. After establishing control with CPB and cardioplegia, the necrotic ventricular wall is identified, debrided, and reconstructed, most often using a prosthetic patch. The mitral valve (especially the papillary muscles and subvalvular apparatus) is carefully analyzed, and the reconstruction is designed to preserve mitral function and minimize the size of the patch. Viable myocardium must support the numerous sutures required to accomplish the reconstruction, which often is not simple in the presence of infarction.

c. Anesthetic management. Pericardial tamponade should be considered the most immediate problem (see sec. **A.** above); therefore, management includes augmentation of preload as required and pericardial drainage if effusion and shock are present. Anesthetic techniques should avoid excessive vasodilation and myocardial depression while maintaining adequate coronary perfusion pressure. Often it is not advisable to delay surgical treatment to insert central monitoring lines in the presence of shock, although adequate venous access for transfusion is essential. Weaning from bypass after the repair requires careful titration of vasodilator and inotropic drugs to minimize ventricular wall tension (which can jeopardize the repair) while achieving adequate systemic perfusion.

5. Acquired ventricular septal defect

a. Pathophysiology. These patients are desperately ill, with low systemic cardiac output and pulmonary hyperperfusion due to the left-to-right shunt at the ventricular level. This may lead to pulmonary hypertension and biventricular heart failure. Concomitant coronary artery disease in the setting of recent myocardial infarction may be associated with ischemic ventricular dysfunction, which is exacerbated by systemic hypotension and the risk of further myocardial damage.

b. Medical management. The optimal time for attempting repair of this defect remains uncertain, but it appears that "stable" patients (those with no multisystem failure and no worsening of acidosis, hypoxemia, or renal function) are best treated medically for as long as possible to allow recovery from the acute MI. Afterload reduction and augmentation of coronary collateral flow are the two primary principles in ongoing management. An intraaortic balloon pump may assist in stabilization. Any indication that regional perfusion or other body system functions are deteriorating should lead to surgical repair of the VSD.

c. Surgical management. Repair can be a very difficult technical exercise because the tissues surrounding the infarct are friable, leading to poor suture support. Defects near the ventricular apex (LAD occlusion) are the more straightforward of the two common types of defect, and repair is accomplished by debridement followed by primary repair or placement of an apical septal patch of limited size. In cases of posterior VSD (right coronary occlusion), the distortion required for exposure and the often extensive nature of the infarct make surgical repair considerably more difficult. Creative and generous patch reconstruction of the VSD and the ventricular wall is attempted. As with ventricular rupture, weaning from bypass requires attention to afterload reduction to limit intraventricular pressures.

d. Anesthetic considerations. Although the presence of a VSD is a relative contraindication to placement of a PA catheter (due to the risk of paradoxical embolism by air or thrombus), the added information provided by PA monitoring may be extremely valuable in these patients. The balloon should be inflated with carbon dioxide instead of air to ensure rapid dissolution of bubbles should the balloon rupture. Use of a fiberoptic SvO_2 catheter will permit continuous estimation of shunt flow, elevated SvO_2 being associated with a larger left-to-right shunt. Note that thermodilution cardiac output measurements will **not** accurately reflect **systemic** blood flow. The amount of blood shunting across the VSD will be related to the pulmonary/systemic vascular resistance ratio, and factors that lower PVR (such as hypocarbia or marked hyperoxia) can increase shunting to the detriment of systemic perfusion. The development of lactic acidosis implies inadequate systemic perfusion. Maintenance of adequate preload, avoidance of major myocardial depression, keeping $PaCO_2$ equal to 40 mm Hg, and careful titration of LV afterload reduction are general preoperative and anesthetic goals.

6. Papillary muscle rupture

a. Pathophysiology. Rupture of a papillary muscle results in loss of support of portions of both the anterior and posterior mitral leaflets. Acute mitral insufficiency following infarction often leads to pulmonary edema and cardiogenic shock. As opposed to chronic mitral insufficiency (in which a large and compliant left atrium is present), when **acute** regurgitation occurs there is usually a **small, noncompliant left atrium.** Therefore, regurgitation of a given volume of blood into the small atrium produces much higher left atrial and pulmonary artery *pressures* than it does in the chronic situation. Severe biventricular failure is common in these patients.

b. Surgical therapy. The only prudent treatment is mitral valve replacement, which should be performed without delay. Temporizing therapy is of limited benefit, and if mitral valve replacement accomplished swiftly and effectively, the results should be good.

    c. Anesthetic considerations. Afterload reduction, faster heart rate, and maintenance of adequate preload are of primary importance. Slow heart rate, high systemic vascular resistance (SVR), and excessive preload should be avoided because they will increase the regurgitant fraction. Biventricular failure may be present, and PA pressure monitoring is particularly valuable. Hypocapnia and avoidance of nitrous oxide can help to control elevated PA pressures.

D. Postoperative hemorrhage

  1. Pathophysiology

    a. Complications. Continued bleeding following cardiac operations leads to **transfusion** with its attendant risks as well as the potential for cardiac tamponade. **Hypovolemia,** when not treated aggressively, rapidly leads to hypotension and shock with damage to critical organs. If neither pleural space was opened during heart operations, the risk of **cardiac tamponade** is great. If blood within the pleural space is left undrained, there will be late morbidity from **fibrothorax.**

    b. Etiology. All vascular procedures carry an obvious risk of bleeding and reliance on endogenous coagulation mechanisms.

      (1) Bleeding following CPB is not uncommon and is the result of several factors that are incrementally more important as the length of time spent on CPB increases. These factors are:

        (a) Surgical causes of bleeding.

        (b) Many patients have been managed preoperatively with antiplatelet or anticoagulant medications. Platelets are sequestered, and their function is further impaired by bypass.

        (c) Hemodilution and mechanical denaturation of all serum proteins result in decreases in specific serum clotting factors.

        (d) Reversal of the heparin-induced coagulopathy required during bypass is an imperfect science.

      (2) The role of ongoing clotting and fibrolysis locally at the site of suture lines and points of electrocautery is complex, but it appears that such local factors may contribute to continued hemorrhage. Evacuation of clot, therefore, may be construed as important therapy itself.

      (3) Following myocardial revascularization, the internal mammary artery may be a source of added postoperative hemorrhage.

  2. Clinical setting. Chest tubes and mediastinal drains are only moderately effective at removing blood from within the chest. When bleeding continues at hourly rates of more than 300 ml, return to the operating room is prudent simply to stem transfusion requirements. On the other hand, **if the chest tube drainage suddenly ceases,** and clots are or have been present in the drainage, one should suspect that clots within the pericardial space are formidable and that the drainage system is no longer effective. The assumption that the bleeding has stopped is wishful thinking. In this situation, continued hemorrhage will lead to cardiac tamponade, which must be diagnosed by suspicion, hemodynamic measurements, and chest x ray.

  3. Management

    a. Prevention

      (1) In the operating room, before closure of the chest, the surgeon should be certain that no bleeding is further correctable by suture or electrocautery techniques.

      (2) Standard **laboratory tests** of coagulation including platelet count, prothrombin time, partial thromboplastin time, and fibrinogen level should be checked whenever hemostasis is clinically abnormal. A protamine titration test (Hepcon), or, less sensitively, the activated clotting time (ACT) may indicate whether heparin has been fully reversed with protamine and whether additional protamine may be needed.

(3) If bleeding continues from diffuse sites in spite of normal coagulation studies, either platelet function is inadequate or a more complex coagulopathy exists. In this case, **blood component therapy** is indicated. Other adjunctive measures including the use of topical hemostatic agents such as "fibrin glue" and collagen preparations as well as the use of 1-deamino-8-D-arginine vasopressin (DDAVP) or epsilon-aminocaproic acid are of variable and controversial benefit.

b. Postoperative bleeding. Following closure and transport from the OR, ongoing bleeding in excess of 300–400 ml/hr initially or in excess of 1000 ml within the first few postoperative hours should prompt return of the patient to the operating room, particularly if results of coagulation studies are reasonably normal. Obviously, if signs of cardiac tamponade are manifest, urgent reoperation is required. If transport to the OR cannot occur immediately, the inferior aspect of the sternotomy wound can be opened to allow drainage of the pericardium temporarily while formal reexploration is arranged.

c. Anesthetic considerations. Anesthetizing the hypovolemic patient presents particular challenges, especially if the bleeding is so rapid that transfusions cannot restore normovolemia. In this situation, it is critically important to achieve surgical control as rapidly as possible. Scopolamine and muscle relaxants with or without narcotics or ketamine may be the only anesthetics tolerated by a patient in shock until the hemodynamics are improved. Knowledge of the prior filling pressures and other hemodynamic variables are important in guiding fluid resuscitation. All IV fluids should be warmed to avoid hypothermia. CPB rarely is required for surgical management of postoperative bleeding.

E. Massive pulmonary embolism

1. Pathophysiology

a. Vascular occlusion. Massive embolism implies that the normal output of the right heart is compromised by the degree of pulmonary vascular obstruction. Approximately 70% of the pulmonary vascular bed must be occluded to initiate pulmonary hypertension and substantial RV failure.

b. Hypoxemia. Cardiac and cerebral performance are worsened by hypoxemia that results from the intrapulmonary shunting which is typically seen during pulmonary embolism. In addition, the isolated RV failure may elevate RA pressure higher than LA pressure, thereby opening a probe-patent foramen ovale (if present). This right-to-left intracardiac shunt can exacerbate hypoxemia and may allow venous emboli (clot or gas) to reach the left-sided circulation (**paradoxical emboli**), with potentially catastrophic consequences.

c. Etiology

(1) The great majority of emboli arise in the leg veins as deep vein thrombi. If the "internal clot cast" dislodges as one unit, a "saddle" embolus may result, causing significant occlusion of the entire pulmonary circulation. Preexisting heart and lung disease only renders the patient less tolerant of the acute insult.

(2) Air emboli may be caused by opening venous structures during surgery or by disconnected central IV lines.

3. Clinical setting

a. Pulmonary embolism typically results in **clinical findings** of tachycardia, dyspnea, chest pain, and arterial hypoxemia. Sudden severe hypoxemia and cardiovascular collapse are nonspecific signs, but they are the only ones on which to base the decision to initiate extraordinary measures.

b. The **differential diagnosis** includes acute myocardial infarction, pneumothorax, and cardiac tamponade.

c. In the **postoperative** setting, pulmonary embolism must be quickly suspected when other problems are not apparent, or there will not be sufficient time to allow intervention. Certain malignancies are associated with a "hypercoagulable" state, and patients with cancer should be regarded as particularly at risk for this complication.

d. **Rapid diagnosis** can be lifesaving. In the most severe cases, there is no time for perfusion scans or pulmonary angiograms, and this diagnosis is based on suspicion, clinical evaluation, and limited laboratory information.

4. **Management.** Conceptually, the most urgent mission is to reestablish adequate pulmonary and systemic perfusion. Rapid decision making is the first requirement for a successful outcome. **The standard technique of cardiopulmonary resuscitation is of extremely limited value.** External cardiac compression will not significantly augment flow across an obstructed pulmonary vascular bed, and the mechanics of ventilation are not the primary abnormality. There are three methods of treatment for massive pulmonary embolus.

a. Attempted **dissolution of clot** with thrombolytic agents such as streptokinase, urokinase, or tissue plasminogen activator. Such "medical" therapy is reasonable for patients with limited hemodynamic embarrassment. Potential problems relate to the risk of induced bleeding, and thrombolytic agents are contraindicated following recent major surgery. Also, it is unsafe to utilize more aggressive therapy (see sec. **b.** and **c.** below) for at least several hours after a thrombolytic agent has been given.

b. Attempted **removal of clot** with a suction catheter (Greenfield Kim-Ray) through a right femoral vein approach using fluoroscopy. The success of this method depends on the nature of the clot (well-organized or gelatinous) and the extent of vascular obstruction. Transport to the radiology department or catheterization laboratory, pulmonary arteriography, and the suction procedure itself must all be tolerated by the patient. This method may require considerable time and is unsuitable for patients in shock.

c. **"Open" pulmonary embolectomy,** with or without cardiopulmonary bypass. At the present time, optimal care consists of placing the patient on femoral-femoral bypass using percutaneous cannulae and a portable pump-oxygenator, followed by transport to the operating room. The venous cannula is exchanged for inferior and superior vena caval cannulae following sternotomy to allow the heart to be isolated. Then embolic material and clots are removed from the pulmonary artery and its major branches.

d. Placement of a Greenfield **inferior caval filter.** This method is prudent following any major operative procedure for removal of clot.

e. **Anesthetic considerations**

(1) Recording the gradient between arterial and end-tidal PCO_2 reflects the amount of pulmonary dead space. When followed over time at a constant minute ventilation, it provides a relative index of pulmonary blood flow changes during surgery and recovery.

(2) In most cases, management consists primarily of resuscitation with use of tracheal intubation and hyperventilation with oxygen, muscle relaxants, hypnotic drugs (e.g., scopolamine), and inotropic drugs. The goal should be to preserve vital organ function until the establishment of CPB.

(3) In the haste to establish bypass, it is vital to remember to **administer heparin** into a central vein.

(4) Because these patients are in extremis when they arrive in the OR and because survival depends on rapid institution of CPB, it may be necessary to begin surgery with only minimal monitoring (ECG, blood pressure cuff, end-tidal carbon dioxide). After achieving control, the surgeons can pass off a femoral arterial line and RA or LA transthoracic lines.

II. The lung and thorax

A. Pneumothorax

1. Pathophysiology

a. Pneumothorax is the accumulation of air within the pleural (potential) space. Pneumothorax is often categorized as small (less than 20% of pleural space volume), moderate (20–50%), or major (> 50% of pleural space occupied by air). **Tension pneumothorax** refers to progressive accumulation of air, causing positive intrapleural pressure to develop. This process is potentially lethal if it is not promptly recognized. Ventilation becomes progressively less effective, and cardiac venous return is progressively impeded by the positive intrapleural (and intrathoracic) pressure and the mechanical effects of mediastinal shift. Wheezing may occur as a result of extrinsic airway compression.

b. **Etiology.** The most common cause of pneumothorax is iatrogenic puncture of the lung during attempts to place subclavian or internal jugular vein catheters. Vigorous positive-pressure ventilation (by bag or by ventilator) causes barotrauma and will result in alveolar rupture, particularly if underlying disease (blebs or emphysema) is present. Chest trauma is an important cause of pneumothorax (see sec. **IV.** below). Additionally, spontaneous rupture of congenital blebs or emphysematous bullae may occur.

c. During spontaneous ventilation the leakage of air from the lung into the pleural space tends to be progressive because of normal negative intrathoracic pressure. A one-way valve mechanism then exists at the site of the leak, allowing a simple pneumothorax to progress to a tension pneumothorax. Positive-pressure ventilation can seriously exacerbate an ongoing leak as well as the possibility of bleb rupture and thus augment the risk of tension pneumothorax.

2. Clinical setting

a. Diagnosis of pneumothorax can be difficult in the operating room setting but depends in part on adequate monitoring and attention to detail. The classic triad of **hypoxemia, hypotension, and wheezing** should be remembered. Decreasing oxygen saturation should always lead to suspicion of pneumothorax during anesthesia.

b. Access to the chest to listen to breath sounds is often limited during cardiothoracic operations, and the esophageal stethoscope provides limited information owing to its location adjacent to central rather than peripheral airways.

c. Progressive increases in ventilatory pressures (with fixed volumes) signal decreases in **lung compliance,** which can be due to the increasing size of a pneumothorax. Often, however, progression to tension pneumothorax has occurred before impressive difficulties are encountered.

    d. Hypotension, difficulty with ventilation, and clinical findings of right heart failure and shock indicate that tension pneumothorax is the most likely diagnosis. Cardiac tamponade is a much less frequently encountered clinical entity but is the most difficult differential diagnosis, the lack of lung compliance change being the only major distinguishing factor. Acute myocardial infarction with LV failure and pulmonary edema is distinguished by the presence of ECG changes, little or no pulmonary compliance change, and pink, frothy secretions in the tracheal tube.

3. Management

    a. Outside the operating room, an occasional small pneumothorax can be managed expectantly by obtaining serial chest x rays. Because of the high nitrogen content, several days may be required for resolution.

    b. In most cases, however, elimination of intrapleural space air is prudent. Any pneumothorax should be regarded as a threat to life because of its potential for progression to tension pneumothorax. **Tube thoracostomy** is the only reasonable action in operative or preoperative patients. The chest tube should be placed before anesthesia or positive-pressure ventilation is initiated. The precise point of insertion or the position of the chest tube is of much less importance than its presence (Fig. 17-4). Elimination of the air space permits apposition of the pleural surfaces, and resolution of the air leak usually is expedited.

    c. Emergency therapy of tension pneumothorax. Simple placement of a needle (18-gauge or larger) through the appropriate chest wall will relieve the positive intrathoracic pressure and ameliorate the crisis. In the supine patient, insertion at the second or third intercostal space in the midclavicular line will avoid puncture of the internal mammary artery. Be sure to pass the needle close to the **superior surface** of the rib because the intercostal blood vessels lie next to the inferior surface. Subsequent tube thoracostomy then allows control of the process.

    d. Operative treatment of pneumothorax is indicated for prolonged air leaks and for recurrent pneumothoraces. One surgical option is formal posterolateral thoracotomy with stapling or oversewing of blebs and sites of air leakage as well as pleural scarification. An operation of lesser magnitude is the "axillary thoracotomy," by which access to the apex of the chest is gained. This limited exposure may prove adequate for cases of spontaneous rupture of congenital blebs, but it is unsuitable for older patients with complications of emphysema.

    e. Anesthetic considerations. Spontaneous ventilation techniques decrease the risks of forcing additional air into the pleural space compared with positive-pressure ventilation, until the pleural space is vented. Nitrous oxide should be avoided to prevent enlargement of gas in the closed pleural space. At the conclusion of a thoracic operation, the chest tube water seal should always be inspected by the anesthetist before spontaneous ventilation is resumed to prevent room air from being sucked into the pleural space with each breath.

B. Hemorrhage within the airways

  1. Pathophysiology

    a. Massive hemoptysis (>600 ml/24 hr) is cause for immediate investigation and intervention because of the risk of asphyxiation. Ventilatory efforts (spontaneous or controlled) lead to progressive airway occlusion more distally in the involved bronchopulmonary segments, and spillover into other respiratory units is inevitable.

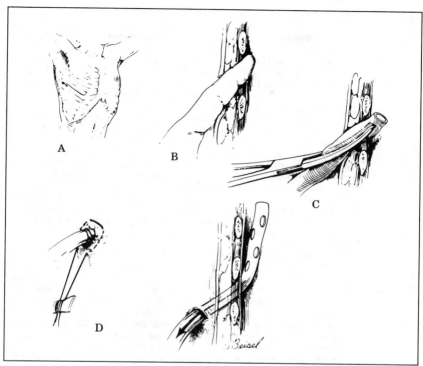

Fig. 17-4. Placement of tube thoracostomy. After applying local anesthesia, a skin incision is made with a knife *(A)*. A finger or a clamp creates a tract *(B)*, then a clamp is used to pass the tube into the pleural space *(C)*. Notice how the tube is tunneled to a different interspace from that of the skin incision (allowing the hole to seal spontaneously when the tube is removed). *D*. Care should be taken to pass the tube near the *superior surface* of the rib (to avoid the intercostal blood vessels). The tube is connected to a water-seal and suction system to evacuate the pleural space and to prevent air from entering the chest cavity with negative-pressure inspiration. (From J.A. Waldhausen and W.S. Pierce. *Johnson's Surgery of the Chest* [5th ed.], Chicago: Year Book, 1985. P. 15. With permission.)

Clotted blood within the airway is "well-rooted" and tenacious, making it difficult for the patient to expectorate and difficult for the endoscopist to remove.

- **b. Hypoxemia.** The blood flow to the nonventilated segments represents shunt flow, which exacerbates the hypoxemia owing to ventilation-perfusion mismatching. The critical nature of the clinical problem is compounded by serious underlying chronic lung disease and other medical problems in many of these patients.
- **c. Etiology**
    - (1) Spontaneous parenchymal bleeding is most frequently **infectious** in etiology and is due to tuberculosis or, increasingly, aspergillosis.
    - (2) **Tumor,** whether primary or metastatic, within the airway causes less severe hemoptysis, but highly vascular lesions may bleed profusely.

(3) **Iatrogenic causes. Endoscopic biopsy** of a bronchial "adenoma" may lead to severe bleeding; **transbronchial biopsy** techniques carry an obvious risk of hemorrhage. Another iatrogenic cause of airway bleeding is related to the use of **pulmonary artery catheters.** Inflation of the balloon when the catheter tip is distally positioned, overinflation of the balloon, and allowing the catheter to remain in a "wedged" position for a prolonged period of time can all lead to rupture of large pulmonary artery branches.

(4) Perhaps the most dread cause of massive hemoptysis is **tracheo-innominate artery fistula,** which is most often a complication of tracheostomy or chronic intubation.

2. **Clinical setting.** Coughing up blood is universally a terrifying experience for patients. Physicians, too, should recognize that "conservative" (expectant) treatment of massive hemoptysis is associated with a 75% mortality. The incidence of rebleeding is also high (80%), so that decisions about definitive treatment should be made early. Selection of patients for operation is based on standard considerations of the medical history and results of spirometry, although spirometry may not be available under emergency circumstances.

3. **Management**

   a. First in priority is confirmation of true hemoptysis followed by efforts to **localize the site** of bleeding. Details of the history will usually differentiate oropharyngeal or upper alimentary bleeding (with regurgitation) from true bleeding within the airway. The patient may also volunteer which side feels abnormal or uncomfortable. A chest x ray will often reveal evidence of underlying disease such as cancer or chronic inflammation. **Bronchoscopy** should be performed promptly in all patients to evaluate the source and nature of the bleeding. Fibrin casts and blood clots within the airway are often very tenacious and difficult to remove simply with suction. Simple lateralization of the source of bleeding to either the left or right lung is information of considerable value. There is wisdom in performing all such bronchoscopies in the operating room, where all opportunities for intervention are available, including selective endobronchial intubation.

   b. **"Simple" hemoptysis.** The capacity to deal with airway bleeding using the flexible bronchoscope is limited by the small size of the working channel and the instruments available, but it is possible to utilize balloon occluders (i.e., Fogarty catheters) through or alongside the bronchoscope. For tumor bleeding in the large airways, the Nd-YAG laser can be extremely effective. Rarely, embolization of pulmonary artery branches or bronchial arteries may be performed (recognizing the risk of neurologic complications), based on the history, bronchoscopic findings, and an assessment of operability.

   c. **Massive hemoptysis.** The initial maneuvers should be designed to protect the patient from asphyxiation. Again, the flexible bronchoscope is of limited value, and the use of a rigid bronchoscope is to be preferred. High-frequency jet ventilation is favored by some centers because accumulation of blood within the instrument is minimized.

   (1) **Isolation of the affected bronchus.** If only limited resources are available, intubation of the **nonbleeding** side with a standard endotracheal tube can also be used to accomplish ventilation. A flexible bronchoscope may assist in optimal placement of the tube. Use of contrast material to inflate the cuff allows confirmation of the tube's position on the chest x ray. Ideal

management involves swift insertion of a **double-lumen endotracheal tube** to provide isolation and selective ventilation of the "normal" lung. The active bleeding from the pathologic side can be accurately quantitated if bleeding continues, and the patient can be transported either to the angiography suite or to the operating room for further intervention. As soon as the tube is secured, the normal side should be cleared of blood and secretions that have spilled over from the bleeding side.

(2) **Surgical management** of hemoptysis generally involves pulmonary resection. Initial control of the bronchus (rather than the vascular structures) is achieved; conservative resections are preferred. As with all resections done with one-lung ventilation, hypoxia due to shunting can be minimized by temporarily occluding the pulmonary artery on the nonventilated side if necessary.

C. Immersion and hypothermia
1. Pathophysiology
a. Body cooling by conduction (immersion) or convection (air exposure) normally induces initial peripheral vasoconstriction and shivering, which generates additional heat.

b. Declining mental status, ataxia, tremulous speech, and hyperreflexia appear as temperature falls to about 32°C, the point at which shivering generally ceases. Below this temperature, stupor progresses and hyporeflexia appears along with muscular rigidity. Early tachypnea is replaced by progressive hypoventilation and respiratory acidosis. Cardiac arrhythmias are common at any reduced temperature, with underlying bradycardias progressing to the fibrillatory threshold at approximately 28°C for patients with normal hearts.

c. Although lowered temperatures are associated with decreased rates of chemical reactions and lowered metabolic demands, a decline in organ perfusion and cerebral blood flow will lead to multisystem organ failure.

2. Clinical setting
a. Prolonged exposure to cold without adequate protection may occur following trauma or in association with central nervous system, psychiatric, or other diseases.

b. Drugs or conditions that interfere with normal cutaneous vasoconstriction or muscle movement can lead to core hypothermia profound enough to induce ventricular fibrillation.

c. Efficient rescue and transport yields the opportunity to provide heroic care for an interesting group of patients, with an occasional spectacular success.

3. Management
a. Core temperature measurements are made by means of rectal or esophageal probes. These sites should provide similar measurements provided the cooling injury proceeded slowly (unlike the situation during CPB). A swift examination is made to determine the existence of other injuries as the available history of the incident is sought.

b. Monitoring should include blood pressure, pulse, ECG, neurologic status, and urine output.

c. Ventilatory control by intubation should be quickly achieved and the airway cleared by suction and bronchoscopy as necessary, because aspiration of vegetable matter is common in drowning victims.

d. The need for cardiopulmonary bypass should be immediately assessed. **Passive rewarming** with hyperthermia blankets and insulation allows rewarming at the rate of 0.5°–1.0°C/hr.

Temperatures below 30°C are best managed by **active rewarming** using cardiopulmonary bypass, which offers the advantage of precise control of temperature, plasma volume, and systemic perfusion. Ventricular fibrillation is an absolute indication for immediate institution of CPB. Femoral vein outflow and femoral artery return will allow flows of at least 2 liters/min, even using percutaneous cannulas. The use of "portable" bypass circuits can expedite and expand this therapy to the emergency room or intensive care unit.

   e. Severe **fresh-water drowning** causes profound hypoosmotic plasma volume expansion as free water is absorbed across the alveolar membrane. Pulmonary edema, congestive heart failure, and hemolysis can result. **Salt-water drowning,** because of its isoosmotic nature, may present less physiologic disturbance.

   f. As warming progresses, arterial blood gas values are monitored to assess the adequacy of ventilation and lactic acidosis. Because pH changes will affect serum K^+ and Ca^{2+} values, serial values of these electrolytes and glucose should be watched.

   g. Toxicology screens for substance abuse and drug level assays (including alcohol, phenophiazines, other psychoactive medications, chronic medications, and thyroid profile) may be important.

III. Chest trauma
A. Blunt trauma to the chest
1. Pathophysiology

   a. Blunt chest trauma can pose a threat to life in three ways:

   (1) The chest wall and/or diaphragm may be sufficiently damaged to interfere with respiratory mechanics.

   (2) Lung parenchymal damage results in bleeding and asphyxiation.

   (3) The heart or large intrathoracic vessels may be injured.

   b. The loss of integrity of the bony framework of the chest results in ineffective ventilation. **"Flail chest"** injuries are those in which a large segment of the chest wall is subject to paradoxical (inward) motion during spontaneous inspiration. The loss of global chest expansion during inspiration results in low tidal volumes and an increased percentage of dead space ventilation. The pneumothorax and pulmonary contusion that frequently coexist compound the inadequacy of spontaneous ventilation.

   c. Open **("sucking") wounds** are those in which an opening in the chest wall permits direct entry of air in and out of the pleural space; the underlying lung injury is always significant. The lung on the affected side will not expand with inspiration owing to lack of negative intrapleural pressure.

   d. **Myocardial contusion** may cause myocardial infarction with ventricular arrhythmias or pericardial tamponade. More severe myocardial injury is most often immediately lethal, but valvular injuries and ventricular septal defects are occasionally diagnosed and successfully repaired.

   e. **Aortic tear.** See Chapter 15 for a discussion of this entity.

2. Management

   a. Supportive management of the patient following blunt chest trauma is the rule rather than operative management. Severe blunt chest trauma is often associated with other injuries, and most of the intrathoracic problems can be managed effectively with control of the airway and the pleural space.

   b. **Endotracheal intubation, mechanical ventilation, and tube thoracostomy** will allow the trauma team to address the other injuries and assess the treatment needs of the patient. Flail chest wall segments should be immobilized, and open (sucking) wounds should be occluded until endotracheal intubation and controlled ventilation ("internal splinting") can be accomplished. It is most unusual for operative fixation of the chest wall to be required, and the only indications for operation center around either intractable bleeding (external, into the pleural space, or into the airway) or a large bronchopleural fistula.

c. Urgent surgical intervention is required for manifestations of **cardiac tamponade** or **tension pneumothorax** (see sec. **I.A.** and **II.A.** above). Urgent diagnosis and surgical intervention is also indicated for **bronchial rupture,** which must be suspected in any patient with posttraumatic hemoptysis, subcutaneous emphysema, or pneumothorax.

d. A brief but attentive **physical examination** and a **chest x ray** are important, searching especially for a widened mediastinum, broken first ribs, or "apical caps." The first job of the trauma team is to keep the patient alive while the patient's assumed multiple injuries are identified. Control of the airway and provision of adequate ventilation take priority over all other initial considerations, followed by assessment of the circulation.

e. In the trauma setting, particularly if there are multiple injuries, any pneumothorax should be treated by **tube thoracostomy.** A large air leak that is not well controlled with a chest tube suggests tracheal or bronchial rupture or an extensive underlying lung injury. **Thoracotomy** is indicated, but **bronchoscopy** and **esophagoscopy** should be carried out initially. The outcome of primary repair of major airway lacerations is far superior to delayed repair. The finding of **mediastinal emphysema** on physical examination or chest x ray should prompt endoscopic evaluation of the airway and esophagus.

f. A chest tube should also be placed to drain fluid or blood in the pleural space **(hemothorax).** Again, on a portable, supine, anteroposterior film significant fluid must be present within the hemithorax to allow any abnormality to be apparent. A patient in extremis with a **total hemothorax** may have an associated major vessel injury. If so, rapid decompression of the chest full of blood will simply exanguinate the patient. The presence of a complete hemothorax is an absolute indication to resuscitate the patient in the operating room. In such a situation, if a chest tube is placed consideration should be given to clamping the tube after a liter of blood is removed. If hypotension occurs, emergency thoracotomy is required.

g. In cases of severe trauma to the lung, the surgeon's primary objective is to control the hilus of the involved lung. The use of a large angled clamp across the entire hilus may allow more precise determination of the extent of the lung injury; this maneuver prevents further blood loss from the lung and internal hemorrhage into the airway and allows optimal ventilation of the opposite lung with minimal transpulmonary shunt. Repair or conservative resection can then be carried out under more stable circumstances.

3. **Anesthetic considerations**

a. In the presence of an unevacuated pneumothorax, **nitrous oxide** must be avoided. In all cases, the anesthesiologist should be attentive to the signs of pneumothorax or cardiac tamponade, which may develop insidiously during nonthoracic surgery. Note that **tension pneumothorax** may develop in the **nonoperative dependent lung** during thoracotomy, with impaired ventilation and circulatory compromise.

      b. Patients with myocardial contusion may develop myocardial ischemia, and appropriate ECG monitoring (i.e., leads II and V_5) should be used.

      c. The use of **regional anesthesia** (epidural or intercostal) may be important for the postoperative management following blunt chest trauma. Pain relief is associated with greater mobility and depth of respirations and improved cough. This may help to reduce secondary pulmonary complications such as atelectasis. Prior to instituting epidural anesthesia, hypovolemia must be ruled out, and pneumothorax must be evacuated prior to beginning an intercostal block.

B. Penetrating trauma to the chest

  1. Pathophysiology. The nature and extent of injury produced by penetrating trauma depends on the weapon or missile involved. The injuries produced by a knife are familiar to all those who work in an operating room. Gunshot wounds, however, are considerably different, for the "zone of injury" produced by high-velocity bullets extends far beyond the tract between entry and exit points.

  2. Clinical setting. Most penetrating chest trauma seen in the emergency room is the result of acts of violence. Penetrating chest trauma is much more likely to be an isolated injury than is blunt chest trauma.

  3. Management. As with blunt trauma, the immediate concerns are the "simple" matters of breathing and circulation. Effective management of the airway includes the ability to provide **selective lung ventilation;** pneumothorax and pericardial tamponade are addressed as previously described.

      a. Adequate **surgical exposure** while maintaining cardiopulmonary control is the key to effective operative treatment of all chest conditions. A variety of incisions, from "classic" posterolateral thoracotomy to sternotomy with extension of the incision into the neck may prove invaluable in providing exposure and control.

      b. The care of patients with **knife wounds** to the chest first requires a decision about whether or not an operation is required. For purposes of decision making these wounds can be separated into three groups by location:

         (1) Median wounds, even of apparently small dimension, may involve the heart.

         (2) Cervicothoracic wounds are always dangerous because of their close proximity to the vital structures in this area, and surgical exploration of such wounds should always be considered.

         (3) Lateral wounds to the lower thorax may have penetrated the diaphragm, with involvement of the spleen, colon, or liver.

      In all these cases, if the knife is still in place it should be left alone and removed only in the operating room, where control of lung and vasculature can be obtained as necessary.

      c. Patients with **bullet injuries** only rarely require removal of the projectile; the injuries caused in or around the path of the missile are the focus of attention. The possibility of internal deflection and fragmentation of the bullet by bony structures also must be recognized. A straight line between entry and exit or between entry and the x-ray location of the bullet is not necessarily the path taken.

      d. The wounding capacity of a bullet is a function of its kinetic energy, which is principally related to its velocity. **Low-velocity** (handgun) bullet injuries are generally rather straightforward to deal with. Aggressive but conservative repair and adequate drainage are the surgeon's goals.

e. High-velocity missiles (hunting and military rifle projectiles) travel at speeds greater than Mach 2 and may be responsible for massive tissue destruction. The bullet itself and the internal shock waves produced within the tissue cause **primary injuries.** Shattered bone fragments may act as multiple **secondary projectiles** and compound the severity of such injuries. All such patients require operating room care. The threat to life is clearly great, and the surgical team is often faced with no option but aggressive resection and debridement.

SUGGESTED READING

Besson, A., and Saegesser, F. *Color Atlas of Chest Trauma and Associated Injuries.* Oradell, NJ: Medical Economics Books, 1983.

Estafanous, F. G. Management of Emergency Revascularization or Cardiac Reoperations. In J. A. Kaplan (ed.), *Cardiac Anesthesia* (2nd ed.). Orlando: Grune & Stratton, 1987. Pp. 833–854.

J. A. Kaplan (ed.). *Thoracic Anesthesia.* New York: Churchill Livingstone, 1983.

Kirklin, J. W., and Barratt-Boyes, B. G. Cardiac Trauma. In J. W. Kirklin and B. G. Barratt-Boyes (eds.), *Cardiac Surgery.* New York: Wiley, 1986. Pp. 1387–1392.

Lake, C. L. Anesthesia and pericardial disease. *Anesth. Analg.* 62:431–443, 1983.

Legler, D. C. Uncommon Diseases and Cardiac Anesthesia. In J. A. Kaplan (ed.), *Cardiac Anesthesia* (2nd ed.). Orlando: Grune & Stratton, 1987. Pp. 785–831.

Lorell, B. H., and Braunwald, E. *Pericardial Disease.* In E. Braunwald (ed.), *Heart Disease.* Philadelphia: Saunders, 1984. Pp. 1470–1527.

Symbas, P. N. *Trauma to the Heart and Great Vessels.* New York: Grune & Stratton, 1978.

J. G. Reves (ed.). *Acute Revascularization of the Infarcted Heart.* Orlando: Grune & Stratton, 1987.

A. J. Roberts (ed.). *Difficult Problems in Adult Cardiac Surgery.* Chicago: Year Book, 1985.

Waldhausen, J. A., and Pierce, W. S. *Johnson's Surgery of the Chest* (5th ed.). Chicago: Year Book, 1985.

Knochel, J. B. Disorders Due to Heat and Cold. In J. B. Wyngaarden and L. H. Smith (eds.), *Cecil Textbook of Medicine.* Philadelphia: Saunders, 1988. Pp. 2382–2385.

Coagulation Management During and After Cardiopulmonary Bypass

Frederick W. Campbell, David R. Jobes, and Norig Ellison

The authors wish to express their gratitude to Renee Whiting for her expert manuscript preparation.

The cardiac anesthesiologist's primary goals during the management of patients undergoing cardiac surgery are (1) the promotion of cardiovascular function and the preservation of other vital organ function, (2) provision of anesthesia, and (3) management of coagulation. The last goal requires the intentional, temporary inhibition of coagulation, thereby permitting cardiopulmonary bypass (CPB), and the restoration of normal hemostasis after cardiac surgery. Proper patient management requires that the anesthesiologist understand the normal hemostatic process, the pharmacology of heparin and protamine, and the effect of cardiac surgery on hemostatic function.

Approximately 10–20% of cardiac surgical patients have abnormal hemostasis requiring transfusion of blood products, and 3% require reoperation for excessive postoperative hemorrhage. The bleeding surgical patient is most effectively managed when the anesthesiologist's knowledge of the hemostatic abnormalities that occur during cardiac surgery permits effective treatment of the bleeding diathesis and minimizes the administration of ineffective or possibly toxic therapies.

I. Physiology of coagulation
A. Mechanism of hemostasis.
Hemostasis is a tripartite function involving blood vessel integrity, platelets, and the coagulation mechanism (Fig. 18-1). Cessation of bleeding requires near normal function in each of these three areas. No matter how meticulous the surgeon at achieving surgical hemostasis, the hemophiliac will continue to bleed until factor VIII levels are raised to acceptable norms. Similarly, no matter how high the factor VIII and platelet count, a slipped arterial ligature will require repair to stop bleeding.

For blood to exist in a liquid form and simultaneously possess the potential to clot at points of injury requires a delicate balance between the procoagulant and anticoagulant components of blood. Thrombin and fibrinogen are necessary to allow clot formation, whereas, antithrombin-III (AT-III) and proteins C and S are inhibitors of the coagulation mechanism. Additionally, there is need for a mechanism to prevent excessive systemic fibrin deposition once coagulation is initiated and to clear blood vessels of the coagulated debris once wound healing is complete. The fibrinolytic system serves this function. Abnormal hemostasis may result from deficiencies in vascular integrity, platelet function, and coagulation as well as abnormalities in the inhibition of coagulation (very rare) and the fibrinolytic systems.

B. Tests of hemostatic function.
Table 18-1 lists commonly used tests of the hemostatic system. These tests may be used to assess a patient's baseline function preoperatively (see sec. **IV.A.**) and to detect abnormalities intraoperatively or postoperatively that predispose to excessive bleeding.

II. Heparin anticoagulation
A. Purpose.
The only nonthrombogenic surface is the endothelial cell, and even then it is nonthrombogenic only in the absence of injury or disease state such as atherosclerosis, both of which expose platelets and procoagulants to activating substances such as subendothelial collagen. Since active metabolic processes are involved, the endothelial cell is unlikely to be duplicated, and current efforts to produce **less** thrombogenic surfaces are not likely to produce a **nonthrombogenic** surface. For that reason inhibition of coagulation is essential during CPB.

Prior to instituting CPB, total hemostatic paralysis must be achieved, and heparin is the only drug used for this purpose.* Heparin

---

*Ancrod, derived from the venom of the Malayan pit viper, has been used experimentally to decrease fibrinogen levels to the range of 40 mg/dl and permits CPB without heparin. The long preparation time, 24 hours, required by this agent to decrease fibrinogen levels prior to surgery and the homologous blood requirements post-CPB make it highly unlikely that Ancrod will ever gain clinical acceptance.

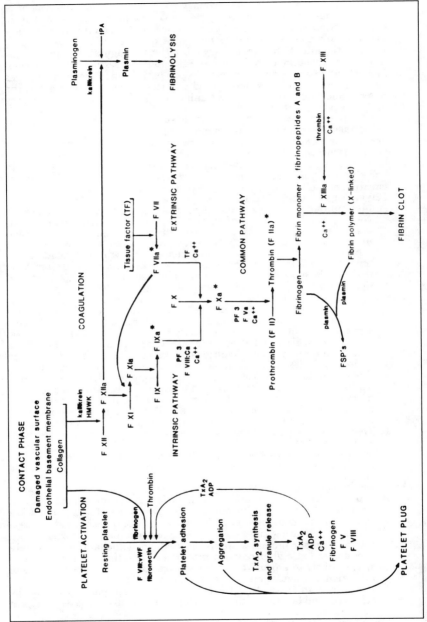

Figure 18-1

Fig. 18-1. Schematic representation of the hemostatic system depicting the vascular, platelet, and coagulation components. The physiologic hemostatic process is initiated on contact of blood with subendothelial basement membrane and collagen in traumatized vessels during the contact phase. Exposure to the vascular subendothelial surface triggers activation of platelet function and production of activated factor XII, Hageman factor (F XII → F XIIa). Synthetic surfaces in the extracorporeal circuitry also induce platelet and factor XII activation. Platelet activation results in a sequence of events beginning with cell adhesion to the subendothelial surface (or extracorporeal circuit). Platelet aggregation to form the hemostatic platelet plug, thromboxane A$_2$ (TxA$_2$) synthesis, and secretion of platelet granule products (ADP, fibrinogen, factor V, calcium) then occur. TxA$_2$ and ADP stimulate continuing platelet aggregation. Fibrinogen is an essential cofactor required for platelet adhesion and aggregation. Fibrinogen and factors V and VIII secreted from the activated platelet and platelet factor 3 (PF 3), a phospholipid in the platelet cell membrane, play important roles in the coagulation cascade. Activated factor XII (F XIIa) initiates the intrinsic pathway of coagulation. Coagulation may also be triggered by means of the extrinsic pathway through the activation of factor VII by a tissue factor (TF). TF is a lipoprotein released into the bloodstream by damaged endothelium and red blood cells. Both pathways lead to the activation of factor X. The common pathway starts with activated factor X (F Xa), which forms a complex with PF 3, factor V, and calcium. This complex converts prothrombin to thrombin. Thrombin is a major regulator of hemostatic function because its many roles include cleaving fibrinogen to fibrin (releasing fibrinopeptides A and B), platelet activation, activation of factors V, VIII:C, and XIII, and activation of the coagulation inhibitor, protein C. Insoluble fibrin, the structural substance of the clot, is formed when fibrin monomers polymerize in the presence of factor XIIIa and calcium. There are two major coagulation inhibitor systems in plasma. In the figure the sites of antithrombin-III inhibition (factors IIa, VIIa, IXa, Xa) are indicated by an asterisk. Also inhibited is factor XIa. Activated protein C, together with its cofactor, protein S, degrades factors Va and VIII:Ca. Fibrinolysis is initiated concurrently with coagulation. The conversion of plasminogen to the active fibrinolytic enzyme plasmin is triggered by factor XIIa and kallikrein formed in the contact phase and by tissue plasminogen activator (t-PA) released from damaged endothelium. The actions of plasmin on the hemostatic system are described in Fig. 18-5. F = coagulation factor, FSPs = fibrin-(ogen) split products, HMWK = high-molecular-weight kallikrein.

Table 18-1. Common clinical tests of hemostatic function

Test	Normal values	Comment
Platelets		
Platelet count	150,000–400,000/μl	
Bleeding time (IVY)	1–8 min	Most widely accepted clinical test of platelet function; inconvenient; arms must be exposed to perform this test.
Coagulation system		
Whole blood coagulation time (WBCT, Lee-White)	2.5–4.25 min	Prolonged by marked deficiencies in intrinsic system or final common pathway; used to monitor heparin therapy; clot can be observed for retraction (platelet function) or dissolution (fibrinolysis); all variables must be controlled for reproducible results.
Activated coagulation time (ACT)	Manual = 90–110 sec Automated = 90–130 sec*	Modified WBCT: commonly performed to monitor heparin in the operating room because of convenience; all variables must be controlled for reproducible results.
Prothrombin time (PT)	12–15 sec; compare to control	Tests extrinsic system and final common pathway; prolonged by clotting factor deficiencies or circulating anticoagulants; used to monitor warfarin anticoagulation.
Activated partial thromboplastin time (aPTT)	35–45 sec; compare to control	Tests intrinsic system and final common pathway; prolonged by clotting factor deficiencies or circulating anticoagulants; used to monitor heparin anticoagulation.
Thrombin time	Less than 17 sec; compare to control	Tests final common pathway; prolonged by heparin, fibrinogen ≤ 90 mg/dl, or an abnormal fibrinogen; increased in fibrinolysis.
Fibrinogen	250–500 mg/dl	Decreased in disseminated intravascular coagulation (DIC).
Fibrinolytic system		
Fibrin(ogen) split products	Less than 12 μg/ml	Increased in primary fibrinolysis and DIC.

*See D.R. Jobes et al. [7]; see also Chapter 6.

is a highly satisfactory anticoagulant because it has few side effects and virtually no limit to duration of use, and an antidote is available. The only contraindication to heparin use in CPB, heparin-induced thrombocytopenia (HIT), has now been successfully managed (see sec. II.E.).

B. Pharmacology. Heparin exerts its anticoagulant property primarily through action with AT-III. Following the binding of heparin with AT-III, the rate of formation of inactive complexes between AT-III and several serine proteases of the coagulation system, including thrombin (factor IIa) and factors VIIa, Xa, IXa, and XIa, is markedly accelerated (Fig. 18-1). In this way one of the three elements required for hemostatic function is inhibited. The degree of inhibition is dose dependent.

   1. Units versus milligrams. Heparin doses should always be described in terms of units rather than weight (i.e., milligrams). Unlike most drugs, heparin is neither chemically nor biologically homogeneous, being composed of chemically related sulfated mucopolysaccharides of varying molecular weights and AT-III binding activity. They share a measurable net anticoagulant activity defined by a very specific in vitro assay. Heparin is prepared, assayed, and dispensed only as units per unit volume (e.g., units/ml), and the exact weight is not identified. Though U.S.P. requires porcine mucosa heparin to have no less than 140 units of activity/mg and beef lung heparin to have no less than 120 units of activity/mg, the actual activity may vary widely between lots of drugs. The continued description of heparin doses in milligrams is not only incorrect but also dangerous because it may lead to underdosing or overdosing the patient.

   2. Heparin administration. Heparin should be administered through a central line with aspiration before and after injection to ensure that the dose is administered to the circulation. This practice may be safely substituted for direct injection into the right atrium by the surgeon. The commonly used dose to initiate anticoagulation for CPB is 300–400 units/kg.

C. Monitoring anticoagulation. It is vital to document **heparin effect** (pharmacodynamic response) following administration of the drug because failure to achieve anticoagulation prior to commencement of CPB will produce intravascular coagulation in the extracorporeal circuit. Clinical testing should be directed toward assessing the in vivo anticoagulant effect rather than the **heparin concentration** (pharmacokinetic response) in blood because it is the effect rather than the heparin blood level that will determine if thrombus formation during CPB is successfully inhibited. Logically, this determination is best accomplished by measuring the actual degree of inhibition of clot formation.

   Assays of heparin concentration, either indirectly by means of protamine titration or, more recently, directly by means of a factor Xa assay, have contributed to a better understanding of heparin pharmacokinetics and permit detection of residual heparin in patients following CPB but do not reliably predict anticoagulant effect.

   1. Activated coagulation time. The activated coagulation time (ACT), first described by Hattersley in 1966, is a modified, accelerated Lee-White whole blood coagulation time. The determination is accelerated by adding diatomaceous earth to the blood sample to decrease the time for contact activation and increase the rate of coagulation. The automated ACT has largely replaced Hattersley's manually performed ACT for reasons of convenience (Table 18-2) and is the most commonly used test of heparin anticoagulant effect in cardiac operating rooms.

   The most widely used automated method (Hemochron*) uti-

*International Technidyne, Edison, New Jersey

Table 18-2. Characteristics of ideal operating room tests of hemostasis

1. Reproducible results obtained with simple maneuvers.
2. Equipment minimal, compact, inexpensive, and quiet.
3. Result available quickly, even with abnormally prolonged time.
4. Whole blood used for test rather than plasma.
5. Test reagents remain stable indefinitely.
6. Does not require prolonged attention away from the operator's primary duties.

lizes glass tubes containing 12 mg of diatomaceous earth and a small cylindrical magnet. A 2-ml blood sample, drawn 3–5 minutes after heparin injection, is added to the tube, which is shaken vigorously and placed in a warmed well where mechanical rotation commences when a timer on the device is started. The magnet remains in close proximity to a detector at the base of the well as long as the blood is liquid. On formation of fibrin strands, the magnet becomes adherent to the test tube wall. Tube rotation displaces the magnet, and a proximity switch trips the timer, recording the time in seconds for coagulation.

A more recently introduced mechanical device (HemoTec*) requires only 0.4 ml of blood and measures the rate of fall of a flag through the blood. As fibrin strands form, the rate of fall is decreased, and this is taken as the end point of coagulation.

2. Safe levels of anticoagulation. Prior to 1975 heparin therapy was based on rigid dose schedules that varied greatly between institutions without any obvious explanation for that variation. In that year two classic articles by Bull et al. demonstrated clearly that there was a wide variation in patient response to heparin therapy both in sensitivity and duration [3,4]. The threefold variation in sensitivity combined with the fourfold variation in duration indicated that there may be as much as a 12-fold variation in individual patient response to the given dose of heparin. Figure 18-2 shows the usual gaussian distribution of heparin dose–ACT responses in which some patients demonstrate a mild insensitivity, which merely represents the lower end of the spectrum of clinical response to heparin. Some patients will, however, demonstrate a lack of response that falls well below the 95% confidence limit, and to these patients the term **heparin resistance** is applied (sec. **II.D..**).

The normal variation in heparin dose-response and the infrequent occurrence of heparin resistance argue strongly that the heparin dose be titrated to achieve the desired anticoagulant effect in the individual patient. The concept of heparin titration was first introduced by Bull, who used a manual ACT. In Bull's system, a patient's response to a subtotal heparin dose is measured, and the specific additional heparin dose required to achieve the desired ACT is determined (Fig. 18-3).

Despite numerous studies during the 35 years that CPB has been in clinical use, absolute criteria for inhibition of coagulation have not been established. In particular, the minimum acceptable ACT remains in question. In his heparin titration, Bull's goal was to maintain the manual ACT between 300 and 480 seconds. Jobes et al. compared the automated ACT to a heparin assay performed by manual protamine titration and concluded that as long as the automated ACT was greater than 300 seconds, anticoagulation was

*HemoTec, Englewood, Colorado

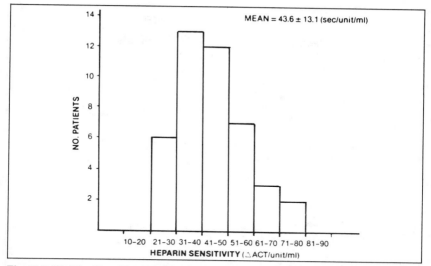

Fig. 18-2. Distribution of heparin resistance or insensitivity demonstrating a typical gaussian distribution. (From R. A. Esposito, A. T. Culliford, S. B. Colvin, et al. The role of the activated clotting time in heparin administration and neutralization for cardiopulmonary bypass. *J. Thorac. Cardiovasc. Surg.* 85:180, 1983. With permission.)

adequate for CPB [8]. Young et al, reported that keeping the automated ACT greater than 400 seconds would prevent microscopic coagulation using as their end point the appearance of fibrin monomer [18].

Empirically, doses that prolong the automated ACT more than 400 seconds are known to be safe. Currently available data do not justify a lower ACT value on a risk-benefit basis. Heparin is a drug whose side effects are minimal, whereas the risk of insufficient heparin dose is possible catastrophic thrombus formation during CPB. In that regard, Bull has emphasized, "The major risk is not too much heparin but too little, with a precipitation of disseminated intravascular coagulation (DIC)."

However, avoidance of heparin underdose does not justify an unwarranted excess. The dose of heparin will dictate the dose of protamine. Protamine's toxic effects are partially dose dependent, and large doses are associated with increased postoperative bleeding (see sec. III.C.).

D. Heparin resistance. In some patients the administration of conventional doses of 300–400 units heparin/kg will produce a negligible effect on coagulation. The response of these patients is well off the usual gaussian distribution of heparin dose–ACT responses. Numerous etiologies separately or in combination have been advanced to explain this phenomenon of heparin resistance (Table 18-3).

Technical reasons (see Table 6-7) must always be considered first in the differential diagnosis of the cause of inadequate ACT elevation after heparin administration. Failure to recognize and correct heparin resistance prior to the onset of CPB may be unlikely to produce catastrophic thrombosis. Rather, low-grade activation of coagulation with the consumption of platelets and procoagulants is likely to occur. Although this can result in microemboli whose effect will vary depending

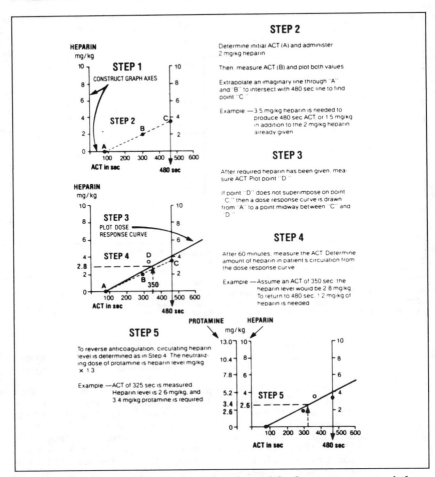

Fig. 18-3. Bull's procedure for construction and use of the dose-response curve in heparin therapy. To accommodate individual patient variation, the concept of heparin titration was introduced by Bull et al. A patient's response to a subtotal dose of heparin is determined and a dose-response curve constructed. Subsequent heparin doses and heparin neutralization may be based on this curve. Bull's goal was to maintain the manual ACT (activated coagulation time) between 300 and 480 seconds. Above 500 seconds, the heparin dose-response curve is nonlinear, and the use of a two-point dose-response curve, therefore, is invalid. As described in the text (sec. II.B.1), the term mg/kg should be replaced by units/kg. (From B. S. Bull, W. M. Huse, F. S. Brauer, et al. Heparin therapy during extracorporeal circulation. II. The use of a dose-response curve to individualize heparin and protamine dosage. *J. Thorac. Cardiovasc. Surg.* 69:686, 1975. With permission.)

on where they lodge, a hemorrhagic diathesis is likely to follow the termination of CPB because of platelet and procoagulant consumption. Heparin resistance is managed by administration of the additional heparin required to produce prolongation of the ACT to values permitting safe CPB. Low AT-III levels, presumably depleted or lowered

Table 18-3. Etiologies of marked heparin resistance

1. Ongoing active coagulation
2. AT-III deficiency, congenital or acquired
3. Previous heparin therapy
4. Drug interaction as with oral contraceptives
5. Presence of other medical conditions such as hypereosinophilia or coronary artery disease
6. Advanced age

secondary to the causes of heparin resistance, can easily be restored by administration of 2 units (in the adult) of fresh-frozen plasma (FFP).

E. **Heparin-induced thrombocytopenia.** Heparin-induced thrombocytopenia (HIT), better termed **heparin-induced platelet activation,** is a complication of heparin therapy that is being diagnosed more frequently. The pathogenesis of HIT is probably immunogenic, involving formation of complement-mediated, heparin-dependent IgG platelet antibody. Antibody-platelet interaction initiates platelet activation and aggregation. The triad of signs seen in HIT usually appears 7–10 days after the initiation of heparin therapy and comprises thrombocytopenia, tachyphylaxis to heparin, and thrombotic complications. The interval between heparin initiation and appearance of signs presumably represents the time necessary for antibody production. The diagnosis is confirmed by the demonstration of heparin-induced in vitro platelet aggregation.

Morbidity and mortality of this syndrome result from vascular thrombosis (involving the coronary, cerebral, splanchnic, and peripheral circulations) and have been reported to be as high as 61% and 20%, respectively. Management of HIT requires discontinuation of heparin. In vitro platelet aggregation to heparin disappears in 4–8 weeks but may persist up to 12 months.

The administration of heparin to sensitized patients will, at the least, decrease the platelet count to dangerously low levels or produce thromboemboli, with serious results depending where they lodge. Cardiac surgery with CPB has been performed in patients with a previous history of HIT after in vitro heparin-induced platelet aggregation is no longer observed [12]. This was done without complication because the duration of heparin exposure during CPB was brief and terminated prior to the formation of platelet antibody.

A dilemma occurs when urgent cardiac surgery is indicated in patients with active HIT or in those recovering from the condition in whom heparin-induced platelet aggregation is demonstrated. Delay of operation until resolution of the platelet aggregation studies may not be practical. Plasmapheresis to remove the heparin-dependent IgG antibody until platelet aggregation studies normalize and inhibition of platelet responsiveness to the antibody with aspirin and dipyridamole have been used to permit CPB with unreliable results. A synthetic analog of prostacycline, iloprost, has been developed that produces effective and reversible (half-life 15–30 minutes) platelet inhibition, in effect desensitizing patients during their reexposure to heparin. Iloprost can be considered the drug of choice for managing HIT patients who require urgent cardiac surgery with CPB [9]. At the University of Pennsylvania, HIT patients are managed successfully by avoiding prolonged exposure to heparin (use of non-heparin-bonded vascular catheters and heparinless flush solution) and titration (to inhibition of in vitro heparin-induced platelet aggregation) of a continuous infusion of iloprost initiated prior to heparinization and maintained through heparin neutralization post-CPB [1]. The drug's effects are dissipated rapidly, permitting platelets to participate in the hemostatic process postoperatively.

III. **Neutralization of heparin.** The neutralization of heparin anticoagulation after the termination of CPB is accomplished by the administration of protamine sulfate. Protamine is the only drug currently available in the United States that is used to neutralize heparin in the clinical setting.

   A. **Protamine pharmacology.** Protamine is commercially prepared from fish sperm and contains low-molecular-weight proteins whose high arginine content makes them strongly cationic.

   Protamine was first used clinically in combination with insulin (e.g., neutral Hagedorn or protamine zinc insulin) to delay absorption and prolong its effect. When an attempt was made to combine protamine with heparin to achieve a similar delay, it was found to inactivate heparin instead. The combination of a strongly cationic substance (protamine) with a strongly anionic substance (heparin) produces a stable complex that is devoid of anticoagulant activity. Heparin–protamine interaction occurs in proportion to the weight rather than the activity of heparin. One milligram of protamine will neutralize 1 mg of heparin regardless of the units of activity per milligram of heparin.

   1. **Protamine dose.** Protamine appears to have the same distribution within the circulatory system as heparin, and the protamine dose required for neutralization, in milligrams, is theoretically equal to the number of milligrams of heparin in the patient's circulation at the time of neutralization. A direct assay of heparin as well as a measurement of plasma volume is required for precise neutralization. These exact values are infrequently obtained in the clinical setting because of time constraints and expense. Thus, virtually all protocols for arriving at an initial dose of protamine are based on approximations of these variables.

      a. **Standard reversal dose.** Most clinicians choose a dose of protamine based on the number of units of heparin administered (milligrams of protamine to units of heparin, assuming that 1 mg of protamine will neutralize 100 units of heparin). Clinical efficacy has been documented using a ratio as low as 0.6 mg protamine to 100 units of heparin administered. Most centers choose a ratio of 1:100. Initial doses using this ratio or the dose-response method (sec **b.** below) result in a mild-to-moderate protamine excess relative to heparin that ensures total neutralization and minimizes the likelihood of subsequent heparin rebound.

      For example, heparin 25,000 units was administered prior to CPB, and no additional heparin was required. The CPB pump prime contained 5000 units. If the entire contents of the pump are returned after bypass to the patient, the ratio of 1:100 would result in 300 mg of protamine as the neutralizing dose. If the pump contents are not returned or if the cells only are returned after washing, the dose would be 250 mg. A ratio of 0.6:100 would result in 180 mg of protamine as the neutralizing dose in the first instance or 150 mg if the pump contents are not reinfused.

      b. **Dose-response curve (method of Bull).** Another method of determining protamine dose is to extrapolate the dose from the heparin dose-response curve previously constructed (Fig. 18-3, step 5). This method determines the existing heparin activity at the time of reversal in units of heparin/kg, and a ratio of protamine (e.g., 1 mg protamine to 100 units heparin) to that number of units would then be administered.

      c. **Protamine titration.** See sec. **B.2.** below.

2. Protamine administration. Protamine is administered at a slow rate of injection (over 5 minutes). The rate of administration is more important than the route of administration in preventing direct adverse hemodynamic effects. Administration may be accomplished manually by using a syringe or by adding the chosen dose of protamine to a small volume of diluent that is dripped from a soluset.

B. Monitoring heparin neutralization

1. ACT. The appropriate step after protamine administration is to test for residual heparin presence. The most common screening test for residual unneutralized heparin is performed by measuring the ACT of a blood sample drawn 5–10 minutes after completion of the protamine injection. If the ACT returns to the patient's baseline (pre-heparin) value ±10%, it is likely that heparin neutralization is complete. An ACT value postprotamine that remains prolonged in relation to the baseline measurement may be due to incomplete heparin neutralization, technical errors, or, less commonly, other hemostatic abnormalities (sec. **V.A.1**).

2. Protamine titration. Protamine titration is a more specific test of heparin neutralization and can (and should be) done if bleeding persists. This test is based on the fact that protamine has anticoagulant properties in vitro and prolongs coagulation of normal blood in test tubes. (Protamine's in vitro anticoagulant potency is approximately one-hundredth of that of heparin.) A qualitative manual titration may be performed with a constant temperature block, clean test tubes, a timer, and a microliter syringe or pipette. Add 1 ml of whole blood to each of two warmed tubes, one empty (control) and the other containing 10 μg of protamine sulfate. Tilt and replace tubes in the block every 0.5 minute noting when the first tube forms a firm clot. If the tube containing protamine clots at the same time or before the control tube, heparin was present and neutralized, permitting the blood to clot before or at the same time as the blood in the tube containing no protamine. This result indicates that neutralization in the patient is incomplete. Conversely, if the blood in the tube containing protamine clots more slowly, no heparin was present, and the protamine exerted an in vitro anticoagulant effect that delayed clot formation. The two commercially available dual-chambered automated ACT devices can be used to simplify the test procedure. A proportional amount of protamine is added to the required blood sample volume in one of the chambers. For example, if a 2-ml sample is required for the Hemochron test, then 20 μg protamine should be added to one tube. If a 0.4-ml sample is required for the HemoTec ACT, 4 μg should be added to one chamber.

The manual protamine titration can be made quantitative by adding protamine to several test tubes in 10-μg increments, usually 0–50 μg/ml, and observing which tube clots first. The neutralizing dose of protamine can be calculated by multiplying the protamine concentration in the test tube or chamber whose blood clots first by the patient's estimated blood volume. For example, when the chamber or tube with protamine at a concentration of 30 μg/ml of blood clots first, a patient whose circulating blood volume is calculated to be 4 liters would require 120 mg protamine. The HemoTec automated protamine titration (see Fig. 9-2) can also be used for this purpose, producing a quantitative assessment of heparin level expressed in micrograms of protamine per milliliter of blood.

C. Adverse effects

1. Hypotension. The most common undesirable effect associated with protamine administration is systemic hypotension, which occurs as an immediate response to drug injection. It is most often seen when the drug is given rapidly or is given to patients who are relatively hypovolemic and vasoconstricted. The effect is possibly mediated by histamine and is characterized by venodilation, reduced cardiac filling, and decreased systemic vascular resistance. A weak negative inotropic action of protamine is debated but probably does not occur. There have been many attempts to modify the hypotensive response (e.g., intraaortic or left atrial administration, protamine pretreatment) with little evidence of predictable success. Only slower rates of intravenous administration (over 5–10 minutes) and simultaneous maintenance of an adequate circulating volume have been shown to be effective in decreasing the incidence of hypotension. Phenylephrine in 100-μg increments (or any short-acting vasopressor) may be used to treat mild-to-moderate hypotension if it occurs.

2. **Thrombocytopenia.** When protamine forms a circulating complex with heparin, a marked increase in complement fractions occurs above that already produced during CPB. Concomitantly, there is a sudden decrease in platelet count. Although these two phenomena seem to be dose related, no immediate observable consequences appear. Platelet function, assessed by in vitro aggregation, is also impaired by the protamine-heparin complex. A number of studies relating protamine dose to postoperative blood loss suggest that lower doses are associated with less bleeding [6,11]. There is enough evidence of undesirable effects to warrant avoiding excessively high doses of protamine.

3. **Idiosyncratic reactions.** Some patients exhibit anaphylactic or anaphylactoid responses to protamine that vary from mild cutaneous flushing and hives to profound vascular collapse. A delayed phenomenon of noncardiogenic pulmonary edema has been identified as well as immediate catastrophic pulmonary vasoconstriction. These are uncommon events and are rarely seen in infants and children. A single exposure to protamine (e.g., at cardiac catheterization) is unlikely to sensitize patients. Diabetic patients taking insulin containing protamine may develop demonstrable antibody to protamine and would appear to be at increased risk. Clinical reactions, however, do not predictably occur in these individuals. Suspected cross sensitivity in cases of fish allergy or autosensitization in males after vasectomy do not seem to put most patients at increased risk.

D. **Management of patients with protamine hypersensitivity.** Clear identification of the patient who will predictably undergo an idiosyncratic life-threatening reaction is not yet possible. However, it seems prudent to take some deliberate measures in patients who have already demonstrated a severe reaction.

Clinically used measures have included antihistamine-steroid prophylaxis, the avoidance of protamine, and the slow infusion of a dilute protamine solution. Other measures, including priming the patient with a small dose of protamine before heparinization or use of alternatives to heparin (Ancrod-induced defibrinogenation) or protamine (hexadimethrine, heparinase) have not been applied or are unavailable to the clinical cardiac surgical patient.

1. **Pharmacologic prophylaxis.** A treatment schedule of steroids (prednisone 50 mg q6h for the preoperative 24 hr with hydrocortisone 200 mg IV during rewarming on CPB) and a histamine receptor blocker (diphenhydramine 50 mg IV during rewarming on CPB) may be given. A 5-mg test dose of protamine has been recommended before the full reversal dose of protamine is given. A similar pretreatment schedule for patients who are sensitive to radiocontrast media reduced the incidence of reactions from 17–35% to 5–7.5%. A few anecdotal reports suggest that benefit occurs in patients sensitive to

protamine, but no conclusive series have been reported. No pretreatment will guarantee protection, and treatment for a severe reaction must be readily available. Furthermore, the immediate catastrophic pulmonary vasoconstriction reaction may not be histamine-mediated and therefore will not be attenuated by antihistamine prophylaxis. This idiosyncratic reaction may be thromboxane mediated [10]. Major responses (severe systemic hypotension, pulmonary hypertension, pulmonary edema, bronchospasm) will require large doses of catecholamines, bronchodilators, volume expansion, or, frequently, reinstitution of cardiopulmonary bypass as a lifesaving measure (see Chapter 6 for a detailed discussion of the management of idiosyncratic reactions). Patients who have survived these catastrophic events with resumption of CPB have been given protamine to neutralize the additional heparin without additional adverse effect.

2. **Withholding protamine.** An alternative is to withhold protamine altogether, permitting the spontaneous decay of heparin activity. Blood losses and replacement have reached 4000–5000 ml in these cases before the heparin effect dissipates. The risk of transfusion-related morbidity must be weighed against the risk of severe reaction in managing patients known to be reactive.

IV. **Hemostatic abnormalities in the cardiac surgical patient.** Abnormalities in hemostasis causing excessive operative and postoperative bleeding may be present preoperatively or acquired during operation.

A. **Preoperative hemostatic screening**

1. **History**

   a. **Medications.** Abnormalities occurring in the preoperative period are commonly the result of administration of medications with primary or incidental anticoagulant effects. It is essential to review current drug therapy, especially anticoagulants and medication containing aspirin or other platelet-inhibiting drugs.

   (1) **Platelet-inhibiting drugs.** Table 18-4 lists the medications that inhibit platelet function or cause thrombocytopenia. Aspirin and other anti-inflammatory drugs are common medications in the adult cardiac surgical population and are potent platelet inhibitors. Although cardiac surgery may be safely performed in patients receiving aspirin, operative blood loss and transfusion requirements have been shown to be increased as a result of the drug's inhibition of platelet function [5]. Medications with antiplatelet actions should be discontinued preoperatively if possible. **The duration of platelet inhibition induced by most drugs is 7–10 days.** This time period may be required for platelet function to normalize and the cardiac procedure to be performed without the risks associated with an increased transfusion requirement. If urgent cardiac surgery does not permit withdrawal of antiplatelet medications, it may be appropriate preoperatively to order the preparation of platelet concentrates for administration **if bleeding is excessive** after CPB. Desmopressin acetate (sec. **IV.D.2**) will reduce the bleeding time resulting from most drug-induced platelet inhibition. However, it is not known whether desmopressin acetate administration will decrease post-CPB blood loss in patients receiving preoperative antiplatelet medications.

   (2) **Warfarin.** Warfarin should be discontinued and prothrombin time (PT) normalized prior to elective operation. Anticoagulant therapy with warfarin depletes the vitamin K-dependent coagulation factors prothrombin (II), VII, IX, and X. Clinically significant anticoagulation due to warfarin usually ceases within 48 hours of the last dose but may last as long as 5 days,

Table 18-4. Medications with antiplatelet effects*

Drugs inhibiting platelet function	Drugs causing thrombocytopenia
Anti-inflammatory drugs	Antibiotics
Aspirin	Cephalothin
Ibuprofen	Gentamycin
Indomethacin	Sulfonamides
Mefenamic acid	Diuretics
Naproxen	Acetazolamide
Phenylbutazone	Chlorothiazide
Sulfinpyrazone	Ethacrynic acid
Antibiotics	Furosemide
Carbenicillin	Cardiovascular drugs
Nafcillin	Heparin
Penicillin G	Protamine
Ticarcillin	Quinidine
Respiratory drugs	Miscellaneous drugs
Aminophylline	Gold salts
Isoproterenol	
Theophylline	
Psychoactive drugs	
Amitryptyline	
Chlorpromazine	
Diazepam	
Doxepin	
Imipramine	
Trifluoperazine	
Anesthetic drugs	
Halothane	
Local anesthetics	
Cardiovascular drugs	
Adenosine	
Diltiazem	
Dipyridamole	
Hydralazine	
Nitroglycerin	
Papaverine	
Propranolol	
Sodium nitroprusside	
Verapamil	
Miscellaneous drugs	
Alcohol	
Caffeine	
Diphenhydramine	

*This list is representative and not all-inclusive. Numerous minor analgesics and over-the-counter preparations contain aspirin.

depending on the commercial preparation used. Intravenous vitamin K can restore coagulation within 6 hours. Two units of fresh-frozen plasma will correct warfarin's effect immediately in adults requiring emergent surgery.

(3) **Thrombolytic therapy.** Streptokinase is administered through intravenous or intracoronary routes for the thrombolytic treatment of acute coronary thrombosis and myocardial infarction.

This drug, by the mechanism of primary fibrinolysis (see sec. **IV.B.4.a.**) depletes the patient of fibrinogen and factors V, VIII:C, IX, and XI for a period of 12–24 hours. Urgent coronary revascularization required within that period of time may be performed safely but is associated with increased bleeding and transfusion requirements. Excessive bleeding not attributable to surgical technique should first be treated with fresh-frozen plasma or cryoprecipitate. Epsilon-aminocaproic acid should be reserved for those cases in which hemorrhage is not controlled by replenishment of depleted procoagulants. The experience with humans suggests that thrombolysis specific to the forming thrombus can be achieved with tissue plasminogen activator (t-PA) without systemic activation of the fibrinolytic system.

    b. Hemorrhagic diathesis. A preexisting hemorrhagic diathesis is best detected by a properly taken history of the patient's bleeding tendency. The most important part of the history is the hemostatic response to any prior surgery, including dental procedures. Any bleeding episode should be characterized by severity, site, duration, and presumed etiology as well as similar episodes, age of onset of symptoms, and family history. Nearly all significant hereditary disorders of coagulation in an adult patient will be identified at this point.

    c. Medical conditions. Renal failure, liver disease, and myeloproliferative disorders are medical conditions associated with acquired hemostatic defects that should be identified preoperatively.

  2. Physical examination. Bruises, purpura, petechiae, telangiectasias, hematomas, hemarthroses, and guaiac-positive stool are physical findings that provide clues to significant coagulation defects.

  3. Laboratory tests. Laboratory tests of hemostatic function should be performed before surgery. The platelet count, Ivy bleeding time, prothrombin time (PT), activated partial thromboplastin time (aPTT), and fibrinogen level or thrombin time (TT) provide a comprehensive quantitative screen of the platelet, coagulation, and fibrinolytic components of the hemostatic system* (Table 18-1). A normal hemostatic profile and negative history support the conclusion that a preexisting hemorrhagic diathesis is not present. Furthermore, the values obtained preoperatively can serve as baseline measurements to which tests obtained during or following surgery can be compared should bleeding problems develop. Observations made on patients undergoing cardiac and major noncardiac surgery suggest that incorporation of a factor VIII: Von Willebrand's factor (factor VIII:vWF) assay into the screening profile may be desirable. In these reports the preoperative level of factor VIII:vWF correlated highly with postoperative blood loss.

B. Abnormalities acquired during cardiac surgery. Abnormalities in the vascular, platelet, coagulation, and fibrinolytic components of the hemostatic system are commonly induced during cardiac surgery.

  1. Loss of vascular integrity. Multiple breaks in the vascular integrity necessitated by the surgical procedure are obviously the most common cause of excessive bleeding. Sources of surgical bleeding include vascular anastomoses, blood vessels in wound edges, and unrecognized vascular perforations in the surgical field (e.g., mammary artery laceration by a sternal wire).

---

*At the Hospital of the University of Pennsylvania, a clinically satisfactory and more economical screening profile is used that consists of a platelet count, PT, and aPTT.

Table 18-5. Factors in cardiac surgery causing quantitative and qualitative platelet deficiencies and their possible mechanisms of antiplatelet action

	Thrombocytopenia	Platelet dysfunction
Precardiopulmonary bypass		
Preoperative antiplatelet therapy	—	i
Pulmonary artery catheters	x?, a?	—
Anesthetic drugs	—	i
Cardiovascular drugs	—	i
Heparin	s, a?	a?
Cardiopulmonary bypass		
Hemodilution	d	—
Hypothermia	s	i
Membrane oxygenators	a	a
Bubble oxygenators	x, a	x, a
Cardiotomy suction	x, a	x, a
Arterial filters	x, a	x, a
Postcardiopulmonary bypass		
Protamine	s, a?	a?
Cell washing	d	—
Transfusion	d	—

Mechanisms: a = platelet activation triggered by interaction with synthetic surface or other agents; d = dilution of circulating platelets; i = direct inhibition of platelet cellular function; s = transient sequestration of platelets from circulation; x = mechanical platelet injury or destruction; — = absence of known platelet effect.

2. **Platelet alterations.** Qualitative (platelet dysfunction) and quantitative (thrombocytopenia) alterations in platelets occur during CPB as the result of interactions between the platelets and synthetic surfaces of the extracorporeal circuit, air-blood interfaces, and other factors (Table 18-5).

   a. **Platelet dysfunction.** Although many hemostatic defects may be observed following CPB, **the most predictable defect resulting from cardiac surgery, after loss of vascular integrity, is platelet dysfunction.** In vitro measurement of platelet function following cardiac surgery with CPB demonstrates that platelets have less affinity for glass beads and diminished ADP and epinephrine-induced aggregation. Bleeding times are prolonged in vivo after cardiac surgery. Sources of platelet dysfunction include:

      (1) **Membrane and bubble oxygenator.** Platelet interaction with the synthetic surfaces of the extracorporeal circuit is the major source of the alterations in platelet function. The largest area of synthetic surface in an extracorporeal circuit is a **membrane oxygenator.** On initiation of extracorporeal circulation, platelets adhere to a layer of fibrinogen deposited on the circuit's synthetic surface. Platelet adhesion, activation, and degranulation are triggered during this surface interaction. The platelet granule contents that are liberated induce platelet aggregate formation. Surface adhesion and platelet-to-platelet aggregation result in a temporary reduction in circulating platelets. Platelets are returned to the circulation following this interaction. Available evidence indicates that a minority of platelets are fully activated, but, more importantly, the majority of platelets circulate with reduced function. The functional defect is not clearly defined but may be due to a reduction of platelet fibrinogen receptors.

During extracorporeal circulation with a **bubble oxygenator,** a direct platelet injury is superimposed on the one that accrues from platelet-surface interaction. Blood-gas interfaces are known to denature plasma proteins, and the mechanical destruction of platelets occurs at the interface. During CPB with a bubble oxygenator, the platelet count declines but more gradually than during CPB with a membrane oxygenator, reflecting the fact that the bubble oxygenator contains less synthetic surface area for synthetic surface-induced platelet adhesion and aggregate formation. In the bubble oxygenator circuit, however, the loss of circulating platelets is progressive, and there is no return of platelets to the circulation, presumably reflecting platelet destruction.

Cardiotomy suction systems and filters in the extracorporeal circuit provide additional sites for platelet activation resulting in cell dysfunction.

(2) **Hypothermia.** Hypothermia contributes to platelet dysfunction after cardiac surgery, the severity of dysfuntion being directly related to the degree of hypothermia. In vitro platelet aggregation is abolished below 33°C. Bleeding times are prolonged when measured at hypothermic skin sites in vivo [16].

(3) **Drugs.** Cardiovascular drug therapy and certain anesthetic agents may also contribute, in part, to platelet dysfunction (Table 18-4). The relative contribution of platelet inhibition by these pharmacologic and anesthetic drugs to the alteration in platelet function that occurs after hypothermic CPB is unknown and is not thought to be a contraindication to the proper use of these agents.

Platelet dysfunction after CPB is usually transient, with normal platelet function returning within 24 hours of surgery. Persistent or severe platelet function abnormalities may occur and may result in excessive postoperative bleeding.

b. **Thrombocytopenia.** Platelet count declines during CPB as a result of hemodilution, platelet interaction at blood-synthetic surface interfaces, and platelet destruction at blood-gas interfaces, in cardiotomy suction systems, and in arterial filters.

(1) **Hemodilution.** Reduction in platelet count results from dilution of the patient's blood volume during CPB by priming solutions consisting of crystalloid fluids or aged homologous blood and by crystalloid cardioplegia solutions. For example, if an adult with a preoperative platelet count of 300,000/µl and blood volume of 6 liters is perfused with an extracorporeal circuit containing a priming volume of 2000 ml and receives 1000 ml of crystalloid cardioplegia solution, the platelet count will be decreased by one-third to 200,000/µl. Hemoconcentration achieved by urinary diuresis will moderate the dilutional reduction in platelet count.

(2) **Bubble oxygenator.** During extracorporeal circulation with a bubble oxygenator, a progressive and permanent loss of circulating platelets results from their destruction at blood-gas interfaces; this destruction occurs in addition to the reduction produced by hemodilution. In contrast, the decrease in platelet count occurring during extracorporeal circulation with a membrane oxygenator is largely due to hemodilution alone.

(3) **Cardiotomy suction.** Cardiotomy suction systems, by returning blood from the operative field to the pump, provide blood-gas and blood-tissue interfaces at which platelet activation,

injury, and destruction occur. The volume of blood aspirated by cardiotomy suction correlates directly with platelet loss.

   (4) Filters. Arterial and cardiotomy filters in the extracorporeal circuit provide additional surfaces for platelet activation and destruction and contribute in part to the loss of functional platelets.

   (5) Drugs and vascular catheters. A transient reduction, by approximately one-third, in circulating platelets occurs when protamine is injected intravenously after CPB. This effect, probably caused by the **protamine-heparin complex,** lasts less than 1 hour and may result from temporary sequestration of platelets in the hepatic circulation. A mild reduction in platelet count may be induced by the administration of other drugs (Table 18-4) and is also associated with intravascular placement of pulmonary artery catheters.

   c. Clinical implications. Although reductions in platelet count occur frequently during cardiac surgery as a result of the factors described above, the platelet count per se is only rarely decreased low enough to explain excessive postoperative bleeding. A large proportion of these platelets, however, circulates with impaired function. Numerous investigations demonstrate that average post-CPB platelet counts exceed the value (50,000–70,000/μl) normally required for hemostasis. Moreover, the occurrence of excessive postoperative hemorrhage does not usually correlate with platelet count. This suggests that **alterations in platelet function are more important than reductions in platelet count in determining the contribution made by platelets to postoperative hemostasis.** Platelet counts generally return to the preoperative level within 1 week of surgery.

   Excessive bleeding due to platelet dysfunction and thrombocytopenia is more likely when CPB is performed with prolonged use of a bubble oxygenator, voluminous cardiotomy suction, deep hypothermia, and inadequate rewarming.

3. Reduction of coagulation factors

   a. Hemodilution. Reductions in coagulation factor activity occur during CPB and parallel the reduction in hematocrit. Thus, the decline in clotting factors, including fibrinogen, is generally the result of hemodilution (Fig. 18-4). Factor V is an exception, decreasing to slightly lower levels than predicted on the basis of hemodilution alone.

   The modest reductions in coagulation factor activities resulting from routine CPB are not great enough to result in a bleeding diathesis. Coagulation guidelines have established that 5–20% is the minimum factor V level and 10–40% is the minimum level for the other coagulation factors necessary for normal hemostasis. Clinically significant coagulation factor deficiencies may occur during cardiac surgery when certain patient-related variables and operative factors are present.

   (1) When **preexisting clotting factor deficiencies** resulting from liver disease, antibiotic-related vitamin K deficiency, warfarin anticoagulation, or thrombolytic therapy are superimposed on the modest decline in coagulation factor levels produced by CPB, clinically significant deficiencies may occur.

   (2) Excessive hemodilution of coagulation factors as well as platelets will result if the patient's blood volume is small in relation to the volume of prime solution in the extracorporeal circuit and the amount of crystalloid cardioplegia solution infused. For example, the blood elements and plasma proteins of

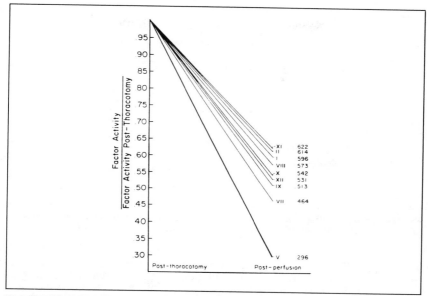

Fig. 18-4. The reduction in clotting factor activity observed after cardiopulmonary by-pass (postperfusion) is expressed as a fraction of the activity measured prior to CPB (postthoracotomy). The magnitude of the proportional decline in clotting factor activities is indicated by the fractions at the right side of the figure, which represent the mean of the declines measured in a series of patients. (From R. D. Kalter, C. M. Saul, L. Wetstein, et al. Cardiopulmonary bypass—associated hemostatic abnormalities. *J. Thorac. Cardiovasc. Surg.* 77:430, 1979. With permission.)

a 3-kg neonate (with a blood volume of 300 ml) undergoing extracorporeal circulation with a circuit primed with 600 ml of crystalloid and aged homologous blood will be diluted to 33% of pre-CPB levels.

b. Cell washing and red blood cell (RBC) transfusion. Coagulation factor losses greater than those expected from hemodilution alone may occur during RBC transfusion therapy (packed cells) for massive blood loss or voluminous cell washing. Cell washing devices, commonly used for the hemoconcentration and salvage of autologous red blood cells during cardiac surgery, effectively cleanse the blood of clotting factors as well as platelets. The relationship between the volume of blood washed and coagulation factor loss is unquantitated to date.

c. Fibrinolysis. Clinically significant reductions in coagulation activities of fibrinogen (I), prothrombin (II), and factors V and VIII may infrequently be caused by excessive fibrinolysis during cardiac surgery.

d. Clinical implications. Replacement of coagulation factors should await documentation of significant laboratory abnormalities **and** clinical evidence of abnormal bleeding because clotting factor levels generally are not reduced during cardiac surgery below those required for coagulation.

4. Fibrinolysis

a. Primary fibrinolysis. Activation of the fibrinolytic system in the absence of active coagulation produces primary fibrin(ogen)olysis.

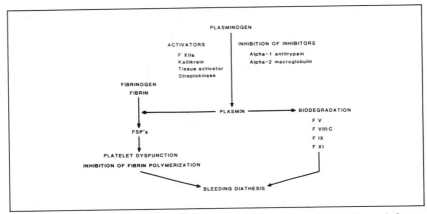

Fig. 18-5. Schematic diagram of the fibrin(ogen)olytic system and the actions of plasmin and fibrin(ogen) split products (FSPs) on hemostatic function. F = factor.

This condition occurs when factors trigger plasminogen activation and increase plasmin-induced lysis of fibrinogen and fibrin (Fig. 18-5). Thrombolytic therapy is a clinical application of primary fibrinolysis in which plasminogen activators (tissue plasminogen activator and streptokinase) are administered to arrest and dissolve intravascular fibrin formation.

b. **Fibrinolytic activity during CPB.** Many investigators have demonstrated increased fibrinolytic activity during CPB. Possible causes include plasminogen activation and inhibition of plasmin inhibitors. Extrinsic (tissue) plasminogen activators are liberated from vascular endothelial and blood cells. Intrinsic plasminogen activity results from factor XII and prekallikrein activation by synthetic surfaces and hypothermia. Decreased activity of the plasmin inhibitors alpha-2 macroglobulin and alpha-1 antitrypsin results from hemodilution during CPB. The resulting lysis of fibrinogen and fibrin generates fibrin(ogen) split products (FSPs). The bleeding diathesis that may be caused by primary fibrinolysis results from several hemostatic defects: lysis of formed fibrin and fibrinogen, coagulation factor degradation, and platelet inhibition (Fig. 18-5).

The incidence of primary fibrinolysis during CPB varies depending on many clinical variables as well as the method used to detect its presence. If elevated FSP titers are the criterion defining the occurrence of fibrinolysis, the incidence ranges from 0–85%. Studies finding modest reductions in plasminogen and fibrinogen levels attributable only to hemodilution and no elevations in FSPs suggest that fibrinolysis is uncommon. In contrast, sensitive clot assay techniques detect the occurrence of increased fibrinolytic activity frequently (in up to 100% of cases) even in the absence of significant plasminogen and fibrinogen reductions or FSP elevations. The measured fibrinolytic activity is shown to increase on initiation of CPB and resolve within minutes of CPB termination.

In summary, it is likely that variable levels of enhanced primary fibrinolytic activity occur during CPB. This activity is commonly of little clinical significance because it decreases to normal levels promptly after CPB and is infrequently associated with hypofibrinogenemia or elevated FSP titers in the post-CPB period. Postoperative hemorrhage related to primary fibrinolysis is possible, however, if plasminogen activation and plasmin generation are excessive during CPB or persist postoperatively.

c. Disseminated intravascular coagulation. Disseminated intravascular coagulation (DIC) is a condition of uncontrolled systemic fibrin deposition and simultaneous fibrinolysis. DIC may be induced when intrinsic or extrinsic coagulation activators are introduced into the circulation, triggering the intrinsic or extrinsic coagulation systems. Fibrinolysis may be triggered simultaneously by intrinsic or extrinsic plasminogen activators introduced into the circulation at the same time or, secondarily, by the excessive production of thrombin and fibrin. A varying combination of thrombosis due to fibrin formation and hemostatic defects due to fibrinolysis may ensue.

d. DIC during cardiac surgery. DIC is an extremely rare occurrence during extracorporeal circulation and cardiac surgery. CPB-related thrombocytopenia, decreases in the levels of fibrinogen and other clotting factors, or the appearance of FSPs have been presumed to reflect the occurrence of DIC in early reports. Borderline or inadequate anticoagulation during CPB may result in low-grade activation of coagulation and may produce secondary fibrinolysis. Reports concerning extensive DIC during CPB were published before the widespread acceptance by the mid-1970s of the concept of heparin titration to a defined end point. The relative lack of reports describing DIC in recent literature may be explained by the existence of uniform adequate anticoagulation that prevents intravascular coagulation and secondary fibrinolysis.

A few clinical circumstances may arise during cardiac surgery that may possibly be associated with DIC: (1) hemolytic transfusion reactions, (2) shock, (3) sepsis, and (4) dissecting aortic aneurysms, which may be the sources of intrinsic and extrinsic coagulation and fibrinolytic activators introduced into the circulation inducing the syndrome. Distinguishing DIC from more common causes of thrombocytopenia, hypofibrinogenemia, and increased FSP titers may be difficult. Demonstration of the formation of fibrin from fibrinogen (elevated fibrinopeptides A and B) distinguishes DIC from primary fibrinolysis.

5. Residual heparin effect. Causes of residual heparin effect after initial neutralization by protamine include the following:

a. Incomplete heparin neutralization resulting from administration of an insufficient protamine dose and heparin rebound are uncommon occurrences in modern practice when excessive heparin is avoided by titrating the dose to measured effect (ACT) prior to CPB and when adequate doses of protamine are administered following CPB.

b. Heparin rebound is the reappearance of heparin effect in blood after complete initial neutralization. It generally occurs within the first 4–6 hours after neutralization. The most likely cause is pharmacokinetic differences between heparin and protamine. On injection, protamine undergoes relatively rapid redistribution, whereas heparin has a longer elimination half-life. Large amounts of heparin present and small doses of protamine increase the likelihood of heparin rebound.

If loss of clot or excessive oozing occurs late in chest closure or postoperatively, the patient's blood should again be checked for heparin effect. Reappearance of heparin can be quickly and easily

Table 18-6. Hemostatic defects associated with cardiac surgery

Loss of vascular integrity
Platelet dysfunction
Primary fibrin(ogen)olysis
Thrombocytopenia
Clotting factor deficiencies
Residual heparin effect
Disseminated intravascular coagulation

Note: Defects are listed in probable order of decreasing prevalence.

tested using manual or automated methods to perform a protamine titration.

  c. **Residual heparin in anticoagulated pump blood** transfused post-CPB is effectively treated by administration of 25–50 mg of additional protamine following each unit (500 ml) of unwashed blood.

  6. **Summary.** Vascular, platelet, coagulation, and fibrinolytic defects are unavoidable consequences of cardiac surgery and extracorporeal circulation. The specific hemostatic defects observed following hypothermic CPB are listed in probable order of decreasing prevalence in Table 18-6.

  The acquired hemostatic deficiencies are generally transient in duration and variable and unpredictable in degree. **The demonstration of one or more of these acute acquired hemostatic defects does not predict that excessive bleeding is likely to occur.** Platelet dysfunction, for example, can be measured in all patients undergoing CPB, but only a small fraction have excessive hemorrhage after surgery.

  Likewise, levels of thrombocytopenia and FSP titer elevations observed after CPB do not generally correlate with blood loss. Knowledge of the frequency and hemostatic significance of the coagulation abnormalities that occur during cardiac surgery should, however, aid the physician managing **the bleeding patient** by guiding the selection of diagnostic tests and available therapies.

C. **Prevention of acquired abnormalities**

  1. **Surgical technique.** Skilled surgical dissection and meticulous control of bleeding sites prior to closure will reduce the likelihood of postoperative hemorrhage resulting from the primary cause of bleeding, inadequate surgical hemostasis. Particular attention should be paid when attending to vascular anastomoses and suture lines as well as to sternal wires prior to closure of the chest.

  2. **Cardiotomy suction.** Controlled cardiotomy suction may reduce platelet injury and destruction, liberation of plasminogen activators, and denaturation of plasma proteins that occur as a result of the interaction of blood with air and tissue in these devices. Tips of suction cannulae should be immersed in blood, if possible, rather than permitted to aspirate a turbulent air-blood froth. During intracardiac repairs, lowering the flows of CPB perfusion within acceptable levels will reduce blood return to the heart and decrease the volume of blood aspirated by cardiotomy suction.

  3. **Choice of oxygenator.** The use of membrane oxygenators for CPB durations exceeding 120–180 minutes rather than bubble types will minimize the progressive destruction of platelets and plasma proteins that occurs at air-blood interfaces. Platelet dysfunction and thrombocytopenia occurring after CPB employing a bubble oxygen-

ator may be less than that following use of a membrane oxygenator when the duration of extracorporeal circulation is very brief. This results from the comparatively smaller degree of platelet adhesion and activation that occurs in an oxygenator with a smaller synthetic surface area.

4. **Rewarming.** Adequate rewarming following hypothermic CPB and the prevention of post-CPB hypothermia will reduce temperature-related platelet dysfunction.

5. **Heparin and protamine dose.** Administration of heparin in a dose titrated to anticoagulation effect for each patient and heparin neutralization with an adequate dose of protamine that is confirmed by ACT or protamine titration will prevent residual anticoagulation.

D. **Prophylactic therapy**

1. **Prophylactic FFP, platelets. There is little justification for the routine administration of FFP or platelets during cardiac surgery in the absence of excessive bleeding because the presence of any of the predictably occurring acquired coagulation abnormalities resulting from hypothermic CPB is not correlated with and does not predict postoperative hemorrhage.** Numerous studies have demonstrated no clinical benefit from prophylactic FFP or platelet transfusion following CPB.

2. **Desmopressin acetate.** 1-Deamino-8-D-arginine vasopressin (desmopressin acetate, DDAVP) produces increases in the circulating levels of coagulation factors VIII:C and VIII:vWF by an unknown mechanism. Factor VIII: vWF plays a major role in platelet function by serving as a bridge for the adhesion of platelets to vascular subendothelium or to other platelets. Desmopressin acetate is known to normalize the bleeding time in cases of platelet dysfunction from many causes, presumably because it promotes platelet-to-platelet and platelet-to-subendothelium interaction.

   The effect of desmopressin acetate (0.3 µg/kg) administration following CPB on platelet dysfunction, **prevention** of blood loss, and reduction of transfusion requirements in cardiac surgical patients has been studied by only a few investigators [13,14]. The results are contradictory and may not support the routine use of the agent to prevent excessive bleeding from cardiac surgery. The use of this drug in the **treatment** of a bleeding diathesis following cardiac surgery has not been evaluated. Currently, the only absolutely acceptable indication for desmopressin acetate use in cardiac surgery occurs in patients who are deficient in factor VIII:vWF.

   Possible hazards of desmopressin acetate administration are hypotension due to vasodilation, antidiuresis, plasminogen activation causing fibrinolysis, and tachyphylaxis to repeated doses.

3. **Epsilon-aminocaproic acid (EACA) and tranexamic acid.** EACA (Amicar) and tranexamic acid inhibit plasminogen activation and fibrinolysis. The prophylactic administration of EACA after CPB has not been shown consistently to produce a clinically significant reduction in postoperative blood loss [17]. The effect of tranexamic acid administration during and after CPB on fibrinolytic activity and postoperative bleeding is under study. These drugs should not be administered to patients in whom DIC with secondary fibrinolysis is suspected.

V. **Management of post-CPB bleeding.** Despite pre-anesthetic screening and appropriately conducted CPB, cases of excessive bleeding will be encountered. An algorithm for the management of the patient bleeding after cardiac surgery is suggested in Figure 18-6.

A. **Evaluation of hemostatic function.** Empiric or "shotgun" approaches to the treatment of bleeding are not prudent in view of the risks of

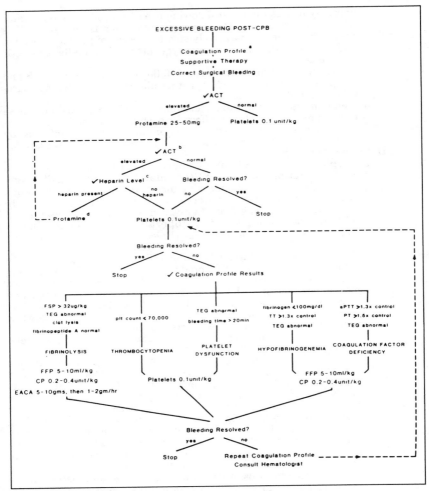

**Fig. 18-6. An algorithm for the treatment of patients bleeding excessively after CPB.
a. Commonly includes platelet count, PT, aPTT, TT, fibrinogen level, FSPs. Template
bleeding time or TEG is desirable if available and feasible. b. Heparin level may be
checked at this step. c. Most commonly by in vitro whole blood protamine titration
(manual or automated); alternatively, by protamine corrected TT. d. Protamine dose
determined by measured heparin level. Disseminated intravascular coagulation (DIC)
is a rare cause of post-CPB hemorrhage and therefore is not included in the outline of
coagulation profile results and treatment of post-CPB hemostatic abnormalities shown
in the lower portion of the figure. It would be suspected on the occurrence of hypofibrinogenemia, thrombocytopenia, and elevated fibrinopeptides in association with increased FSPs, clot lysis, or a TEG characteristic of fibrinolysis. The treatment of DIC
includes identification and arrest of the inciting cause and coagulant replacement
with FFP, CP, and platelets. EACA should not be administered to the patient with
DIC and secondary fibrinolysis because of the risk of intravascular thrombosis. ACT
= activated coagulation time, aPTT = activated partial thromboplastin time, CP =
cryoprecipitate, EACA = epsilon-aminocaproic acid, FFP = fresh frozen plasma, FSP
= fibrin(ogen) split products, plt count = platelet count, PT = prothrombin time, TEG
= thromboelastogram, TT = thrombin time.**

Table 18-7. Causes of ACT prolongation after cardiopulmonary bypass

Technical errors
  Contamination of blood sample by heparin flush
  Excessive sample volume in tube or cuvette
  Inadequate agitation of sample and activator
  Unwarmed tube or cuvette
  Unwarmed detection well
  Failure of tube rotation (Hemochron)
  Separation of flag from detector (HemoTec)
  Machine failure
Hemostatic abnormalities
  Circulating anticoagulant (heparin, warfarin)
  Severe thrombocytopenia ($\leq 50,000/\mu l$)
  Severe procoagulant deficiencies

debilitating and life-threatening viral infection acquired through unnecessary or excessive transfusion of blood products. Selection of therapy for post-CPB hemorrhage must be based on an understanding of the hemostatic abnormalities that occur in the cardiac surgical patient and their relative prevalence (Table 18-6).

Knowledge of the individual patient and the hemostatic consequences of the specific operative and perfusion techniques employed may point to likely etiologies. Specific diagnosis-directed therapy is preferable and possible if blood specimens for coagulation testing are drawn promptly on clinical diagnosis of excessive bleeding and processed by a coagulation laboratory responsive to the need for rapid results in the cardiac OR and ICU.

1. ACT and coagulation profile

  a. Blood sampling. When excessive bleeding occurs, the ACT should be repeated and a coagulation profile obtained: platelet count, PT, aPTT, fibrinogen, and FSP (Table 18-1). Blood specimens may be obtained through indwelling arterial or central venous catheters. It is mandatory to employ careful technique to prevent contamination of the specimen by the heparin flush solution used to maintain line patency. An adequate aliquot must be aspirated before a sample is collected. For example, in an arterial line with a dead space of 2 ml between patient and sampling port, withdrawing 4 ml into one syringe before collecting the sample into a second syringe will eliminate the chance of heparin contamination. If a venopuncture is performed to collect the blood specimen, it must be accurate and atraumatic to avoid introducing tissue fluid. One way to ensure this is to use a two-syringe technique in which the first syringe is discarded after collection of 0.2 ml and a second syringe is attached to the indwelling needle to collect the sample.

  b. ACT interpretation. An elevated ACT after heparin neutralization strongly suggests the presence of residual heparin effect, another circulating anticoagulant, or changes in the operator's technique (Table 18-7). Although marked deficiencies in the intrinsic coagulation system or severe thrombocytopenia (due to insufficient platelet factor 3) may theoretically prolong the ACT, the test is generally not sensitive enough to detect the degrees of hemostatic deficiencies encountered after cardiac surgery. Platelet dysfunction does not cause ACT prolongation.

  c. Coagulation profile interpretation. The results of laboratory coagulation tests must be interpreted with caution in the patient following cardiac surgery. In one series, 80% of 512 patients had elevations of PT after cardiac surgery, yet only 4% had clinically significant bleeding, and all patients had 70–80% levels of factors II, V, VII, and X [2]. In another series, excessive bleeding was observed in only 51% of patients with abnormalities in a post-CPB laboratory coagulation profile consisting of platelet count, PT, aPTT, and fibrinogen level [15]. In a third report, post-CPB bleeding occurred in only 5 of 40 cardiac surgical patients, each of whom had one or more abnormal laboratory coagulation test values [11]. The extreme sensitivity of these coagulation tests to post-CPB alterations in hemostatic function that are variable in clinical significance dictates that the anesthesiologist should **treat the patient, not the patient's numbers!** If a patient is not bleeding excessively despite abnormal laboratory coagulation values, any therapy offers only risks and no clinical benefit. In a **bleeding** patient, however, the abnormalities in the coagulation profile may serve as a basis for the selection of therapy.

Platelet function may be evaluated by the measurement of a template bleeding time. However, the precision required in the performance of the test and lack of correlation of abnormal results with clinically significant hemorrhage are reasons this test has not been popular in the cardiac surgery setting.

2. **Protamine titration.** Performing a protamine titration, either by manual or automated methods, permits one to make or exclude a diagnosis of residual heparin effect. It is particularly useful when ACT prolongation persists or increases despite additional protamine administration.

3. **Thromboelastography and Sonoclot.** Thromboelastography (TEG) is a qualitative measure of viscoelastic clot strength that has been widely used in the comprehensive hemostatic evaluation of the patient undergoing hepatic transplantation and has recently been introduced to the field of cardiac surgery. The TEG measures and displays the shear elasticity of a sample of whole blood through the sequence of initial fibrin formation, fibrin cross-linking, and clot retraction. Abnormalities in platelet, coagulation, and fibrinolytic components of the hemostatic process result in alterations in the viscoelastic qualities of forming clot and therefore may be observed by TEG. The characteristic TEG tracing and the measurements commonly derived from it are depicted in Figure 18-7.

The Sonoclot is another viscoelastic measure of whole blood clotting. This test may be a sensitive indicator of variations in platelet function; however, the effects of other coagulation abnormalities on Sonoclot-measured whole blood clotting are not well documented. Like the TEG, there is little published experience documenting the application and usefulness of this test in cardiac surgery.

B. **Supportive therapy.** As soon as excessive bleeding is apparent, several supportive management steps should be taken to control hemorrhage and prevent secondary coagulation derangements. These actions may be carried out while tests of coagulation are performed, the likely causes(s) of the bleeding is (are) identified, and specific therapy is prepared.

1. **Volume repletion.** Adequate quantities of volume expanders, crystalloid or colloid, must be available for infusion to maintain normal intravascular volume and cardiac output. Shock and circulatory failure must be prevented to avoid complications that include DIC.

2. **Maintain normothermia.** Patient normothermia must be achieved and maintained to avoid hypothermic-related platelet dysfunction.

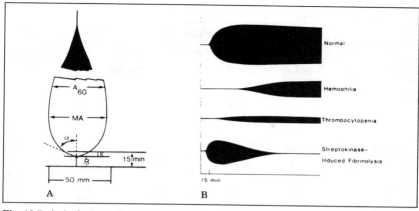

Fig. 18-7. *A.* A characteristic thromboelastogram (TEG) tracing and standard R, K, α°, MA, and A$_{60}$ measurements. The R value (reaction time) is measured from the time of sample placement in the TEG machine until the tracing amplitude reaches 1 mm. This value represents the time required for initial fibrin formation (normal R = 7.5–15 min). Prolongation of the R value may be due to heparin administration, clotting factor deficiencies, or severe hypofibrinogenemia. The K value (coagulation time) is measured from the R value to the point where the amplitude of the tracing measures 20 mm (normal K = 3–6 min). The α° is the angle formed by the upslope of the TEG tracing from the R value (normal α° = 45°–50°). Both the K and the α° represent the rate of clot formation, fibrin cross-linking, and platelet-fibrin interaction. Decreased values may occur with hypofibrinogenemia, thrombocytopenia, or thrombocytopathy. The maximum amplitude (MA) value represents maximum clot strength (normal MA = 50–60 mm). Depression of this parameter occurs for the same reasons as depression of K and α° angle values. The A$_{60}$ is the amplitude of the tracing measured 60 minutes after the MA and is a measure of clot retraction or lysis (normal A$_{60}$ = MA − 5 mm). The A$_{60}$ may be very small in cases of primary fibrin(ogen)olysis and DIC. (Modified from International Anesthesia Research Society, K. J. Tuman, B. D. Spiess, R. J. McCarthy, et al. Effects of progressive blood loss on coagulation as measured by thromboelastography. *Anesth. Analg.* 66:857, 1987. With permission.) *B.* Characteristic qualitative abnormalities in TEG tracing resulting from specific coagulopathies are illustrated in these horizontally arranged representative examples. (From B. D. Spiess and A. D. Ivankovich. Thromboelastography: A Coagulation-monitoring Technique Applied to Cardiopulmonary Bypass. In N. Ellison and D. R. Jobes [eds.], *Effective Hemostasis in Cardiac Surgery.* Philadelphia: Saunders, 1988. P. 165. With permission.)

3. **Prevent hypertension.** Mild reductions in blood pressure and, in particular, avoidance of hypertension are important strategies to control blood loss during and after cardiac surgery. Hypertension may be prevented by adequate levels of anesthesia intraoperatively, analgesia and sedation postoperatively, avoiding overtransfusion, and, if necessary, infusion of antihypertensive drugs.

4. **Positive end-expiratory pressure.** Positive end-expiratory pressure (PEEP) during controlled ventilation after chest closure is used by some to 'tamponade' mediastinal bleeders and reduce hemorrhage. Controlled studies evaluating the efficacy of PEEP in this regard have yielded contradictory results.

C. **Correction of surgical bleeding.** The first specific therapeutic action should consist of a vigorous effort to identify and correct surgical bleeding sites. "Medical bleeding" due to systemic coagulopathy may be distinguished from "surgical bleeding" on the basis of generalized oozing from previously dry wound edges, vascular cannulation sites, and epistaxis or hematuria. When blood loss is confined to the surgical

Table 18-8. Chest drainage criteria for reoperation

Preoperative weight (kg)	Hourly amount (ml/hr)			Total amount (ml)	
	No. of successive hours[a]			Hour no.[b]	
	1	2	3	4	5
5	70	60	50	120	130
6	70	60	50	130	155
7	70	60	50	150	180
8	90	70	50	175	200
9	90	80	60	195	230
10	100	90	65	220	260
12	130	100	80	260	300
14	150	120	90	300	360
16	170	140	100	350	400
18	195	150	120	390	460
20	200	175	130	450	520
25	270	220	160	540	650
30	325	260	195	650	770
35	380	300	230	760	900
40	430	350	260	800	1035
45	500	400	300	975	1150
50[c]	500	400	300	1000	1200

[a]Reoperation is advisable if the patient has bled the amount indicated in any 1 hour (column 1), the lesser amount in column 2 during each of any 2 successive hours, or the still smaller amount (column 3) in each of any 3 successive hours.

[b]Reoperation is advisable if the patient has bled in total the amount indicated by the end of the fourth or fifth postoperative hour.

[c]Chest drainage criteria for reoperation in *adult patients larger than 50 kg* based on ml of blood/kg values extrapolated from those for the patient with a 50 kg preoperative weight are as follows: Reoperation is advisable if the patient has bled 10 ml/kg/hr in any 1 hour, or 8 ml/hr/kg during each of any 2 successive hours, or 6 ml/kg/hr in each of any 3 successive hours. Reoperation is also advisable if the patient has bled in total 20 ml/kg by the end of the fourth postoperative hour.

Source: From J. W. Kirklin and B. G. Barratt-Boyes, *Cardiac Surgery*. New York: Wiley, 1986. P. 159. With permission.

wound in the absence of generalized oozing, surgical bleeding is likely. **No amount of blood or blood components will stop bleeding resulting from inadequate surgical hemostasis!** Prior to chest closure, all vascular anastomoses and suture lines should be examined, the wound inspected thoroughly, and the sternal wire sites noted for bleeding.

Postoperatively, if residual heparin effect is excluded by protamine titration, a repeat coagulation profile is normal, and bleeding time or TEG demonstrates normal platelet function in spite of continued bleeding, reexploration of the chest should be performed with the expectation of finding a surgical bleeder. Rapid hemorrhage may require reoperation prior to completion of diagnostic tests. Criteria based on blood loss per hour used by Kirklin and Barratt-Boyes as indications for reexploration are listed in Table 18-8.

D. Management of post-CPB hemostatic abnormalities. When meticulous surgical hemostasis has been performed and hemorrhage persists, bleeding resulting from acquired hemostatic abnormalities is considered. The order in which the anesthesiologist acts on the possible hemostatic deficiencies related to cardiac surgery and extracorporeal circulation may be determined by (1) the relative speed and accuracy with which specific causes can be identified or excluded, and (2) a risk-benefit analysis of the administration of the available therapeutic options. A recommendable scheme (Fig. 18-6) for the management of post-CPB hemorrhage is based on the limited capacity of clinical coagulation laboratories to provide rapid diagnostic information about a patient's hemostatic system and an estimation of achievable benefits founded upon knowledge of the coagulation abnormalities occurring in the cardiac surgical patient.

In this scheme (Fig. 18-6):

1. After the collection of blood for a laboratory coagulation profile, institution of supportive treatment measures, and efforts to achieve surgical hemostasis, assessment is made for **residual heparin effect.** Although it is generally an uncommon cause of excessive hemorrhage, residual anticoagulation is readily detected using methods (manual or automated protamine titration) that can be performed at the OR or ICU bedside. Furthermore, the risks of injection of a small additional dose of **protamine** to neutralize suspected or confirmed residual heparin are minimal.

2. Once residual heparin anticoagulation is corrected or excluded and **if bleeding continues,** therapy is next directed at the commonly observed **platelet dysfunction** unless knowledge of patient, operative, or perfusion-related factors suggests strongly that another cause is more likely. Until additional research demonstrates the common occurrence of clinically significant hemostatic derangements resulting from other etiologies, it is prudent to direct initial treatment at platelet function. The transfusion of **platelet concentrates** will predictably restore platelet function. Increasing levels of factor VIII activity achieved by the administration of desmopressin acetate, FFP, and cryoprecipitate have led to improved platelet function in several nonsurgical conditions (e.g., uremia, von Willebrand's disease). Although, these agents avoid or reduce the risk or infection acquired from a blood product pooled from multiple donors (i.e., platelet concentrate), their efficacy in the treatment of platelet dysfunction in the patient bleeding after cardiac surgery is uncertain.

3. If bleeding persists following administration of platelet concentrates, **results of the initial coagulation profile or TEG** (now likely to be available from the laboratory) **are analyzed** to determine the presence of the other, variably occurring, etiologies of post-CPB hemorrhage. **Specific drugs or blood products** (Table 18-9) are then selected.

4. Treatment is followed by observation of the rate of hemorrhage and **repeat coagulation tests** to determine whether continued therapy is needed or additional coagulation abnormalities have occurred.

5. If a specific cause for post-CPB bleeding cannot be identified, administration of appropriate fluids and blood products in adequate volumes may be necessary for many hours to achieve a favorable outcome. Through **persistent attention** to volume replacement, correction of anemia, and support of normal hemodynamic function, the rate of bleeding will often decrease and eventually stop without a specific diagnosis being made.

Table 18-9. Blood products and drugs used in the treatment of excessive bleeding after cardiac surgery

Blood product/drug	Constituents	Indications	Dose	Comment
Whole blood	Hct 35% Plasma deficient in factors V, VIII No functional platelets Approx. vol. 500 ml/unit	Hemorrhage	Titrated to measures of hemoglobin and blood volume	35-day-old blood: K^+ 17–26 mEq/L, pH 6.7, lactate 200 mg/dl
Fresh whole blood (<6 hr)	Hct 35% Plasma contains all clotting factors Functional platelets Approx. vol. 500 ml/unit	Hemorrhage and coagulopathy related to clotting factor or platelet deficiencies	See whole blood	Fresh blood: K^+ 3.5–5.5 mEq/L, pH 7.2, lactate 20 mg/dl
Red blood cells	Hct 70% Approx. vol. 250 ml/unit	Anemia	See whole blood	
Fresh frozen plasma	All clotting factors No platelets Approx. vol. 200–250 ml/unit	Bleeding diathesis with: PT>1.5 × control, aPTT>1.3 × control, TT>1.3 × control, fibrinogen <100 mg/dl or abnormal TEG	5–10 ml/kg	
Cryoprecipitate	Fibrinogen Factors VIII, XIII Approx. vol. 10–20 ml/unit	Bleeding diathesis with: TT>1.3 × control, fibrinogen <100 mg/dl, or known factor VIII deficiency	0.2–0.4 unit/kg	Risk of disease transmission correlates with number of donors (units) to which recipient is exposed

Platelet concentrate	≥5.5 × 10¹⁰ platelets/ unit Plasma	Bleeding diathesis with thrombocytopenia (<70,000/μl) or platelet dysfunction (bleeding time >20 min, abnormal TEG)	0.1–0.2 unit/kg	See cryoprecipitate
Protamine sulfate	Ampules contain 50 or 250 mg lypholized drug, or 1% solution	Bleeding diathesis with residual heparin documented by protamine titration	Determined by protamine titration; 1 mg/100 units measured heparin activity	Possible side effects: hypotension, thrombocytopenia, idiosyncratic reactions
Desmopressin acetate	Each 1 ml vial contains 4 μg desmopressin acetate	Bleeding diathesis with factor VIII deficiency and platelet dysfunction (bleeding time >20 min, abnormal TEG)	0.3 μg/kg, administer in 50 ml diluent over 15 min	Possible side effects: hypotension, tachyphylaxis to repeated doses, antidiuresis, fibrinolysis
Epsilon-amino-caproic acid	Each 20 ml vial contains 5 g EACA	Bleeding diathesis with primary fibrinolysis (FSPs >32 μl/ml, abnormal TEG, fibrinopeptide A normal)	Loading dose: 5 g IV over 1 hr Maintenance dose: 1 g/hr IV	Possible side effects: hypotension, arrhythmias, catastrophic intravascular thrombosis may result if administered during secondary fibrinolysis (i.e., DIC)

Hct = hematocrit, K⁺ = potassium, PT = prothrombin time, aPTT = activated partial thromboplastin time, TT = thrombin time, TEG = thromboelastography, EACA = epsilon-aminocaproic acid, FSPs = fibrin(ogen) split products, DIC = disseminated intravascular coagulation.

REFERENCES

1. Addonizio, V. P., Fisher, C. A., Kappa, J. R., et al. Prevention of heparin-induced thrombocytopenia during open heart surgery with iloprost (ZK 36374). *Surgery* 102:796–807, 1987.
2. Bachmann, F., McKenna, R., Cole, E. R., et al. The hemostatic mechanism after open-heart surgery. I. Studies on plasma coagulation factors and fibrinolysis in 512 patients after extracorporeal circulation. *J. Thorac. Cardiovasc. Surg.* 70:76–85, 1975.
3. Bull, B. S., Korpman, R. A., Huse, W. M., et al. Heparin therapy during extracorporeal circulation. I. Problems inherent in existing heparin protocols. *J. Thorac. Cardiovasc. Surg.* 69:674–684, 1975.
4. Bull, B. S., Huse, W. M., Brauer, F. S, et al. Heparin therapy during extracorporeal circulation. II. The use of a dose-response curve to individualize heparin and protamine dosage. *J. Thorac. Cardiovasc. Surg.* 69:685–689, 1975.
5. Ferraris, V. A., Ferraris, S. P., Lough, F. C., et al. Preoperative aspirin ingestion increases operative blood loss after coronary artery bypass grafting. *Ann. Thorac. Surg.* 45:71–74, 1988.
6. Guffin, A. V., Dunbar, R. W., Kaplan, J. A., et al. Successful use of a reduced dose of protamine after cardiopulmonary bypass. *Anesth. Analg.* 55:110–113, 1976.
7. Jobes, D. R., Campbell, F. W., Ellison N: Limit(ation)s for the ACT. *Anesth. Analg.,* In press 1989.
8. Jobes, D. R., Schwartz, A. J., Ellison, N., et al. Monitoring heparin anticoagulation and its neutralization. *Ann. Thorac. Surg.* 31:161–166, 1981.
9. Kappa, J. R., Horn, M. K., III, Fisher, C. A., et al. Efficacy of Iloprost (ZK 36374) versus aspirin in preventing heparin-induced platelet activation during cardiac operations. *J. Thorac. Cardiovasc. Surg.* 94:405–413, 1987.
10. Morel, D. R., Zapol, W. M., Thomas, S. J., et al. Ca5 and thromboxane generation associated with pulmonary vaso- and broncho-constriction during protamine reversal of heparin. *Anesthesiology* 66:597–604, 1987.
11. Moriau, M., Masure, R., Hurlet, A., et al. Haemostasis disorders in open heart surgery with extracorporeal circulation. *Vox Sang.* 32:41–51, 1977.
12. Olinger, G. N., Hussey, C. V., Olive, J. A., et al. Cardiopulmonary bypass for patients with previously documented heparin-induced platelet aggregation. *J. Thorac. Cardiovasc. Surg.* 87:673–677, 1984.
13. Rocha, E., Llorens, R., Paramo, J. A., et al. Does desmopressin acetate reduce blood loss after surgery in patients on cardiopulmonary bypass? *Circulation* 77:1319–1323, 1988.
14. Salzman, E. W., Weinstein, M. J., Weintraub, R. M., et al. Treatment with desmopressin acetate to reduce blood loss after cardiac surgery: A double-blind randomized trial. *N. Engl. J. Med.* 314:1402–1406, 1986.
15. Spiess, B. D., Tuman, K. J., McCarthy, R. J., et al. Thromboelastography as an indicator of post-cardiopulmonary bypass coagulopathies. *J. Clin. Monit.* 3:25–30, 1987.
16. Valeri, C. R., Cassidy, G., Khuri, S., et al. Hypothermia-induced reversible platelet dysfunction. *Ann. Surg.* 205:175–181, 1987.
17. Vander Salm, T. J., Ansell, J. E., Okike, O. N., et al. The role of epsilon-aminocaproic acid in reducing bleeding after cardiac operation: A double-blind randomized study. *J. Thorac. Cardiovasc. Surg.* 95:538–540, 1988.
18 Young, J. A., Kisker, C. T., and Doty, D. B. Adequate anticoagulation during cardiopulmonary bypass determined by activated clotting time and the appearance of fibrin monomer. *Ann. Thorac. Surg.* 26:231–240, 1978.

SUGGESTED READING

Addonizio, V. P., and Colman, R. W. Platelets and extracorporeal circulation. *Biomaterials* 3:9–15, 1982.

Bick, R. L. Hemostasis defects associated with cardiac surgery, prosthetic devices, and other extracorporeal circuits. *Semin. Thromb. Hemost.* 11:249–280, 1985.

Edmunds, L. H., Ellison, N., Colman, R. W., et al. Platelet function during cardiac operation. Comparison of membrane and bubble oxygenators. *J. Thorac. Cardiovasc. Surg.* 83:805–812, 1982.

Ellison, N., and Jobes, D. R., (eds.). *Effective Hemostasis in Cardiac Surgery.* Philadelphia: Saunders, 1988.

Harker, L. A., Malpass, T. W., Branson, H. E., et al. Mechanism of abnormal bleeding in patients undergoing cardiopulmonary bypass: Acquired Transient platelet dysfunction associated with selective αgranule release. *Blood* 56:824–834, 1980.

Horrow, J. C. Protamine allergy. *J. Cardiothorac. Anesth.* 2:225–242, 1988.

Lee, K. F., Mandell, J., Rankin, J. S., et al. Immediate versus delayed coronary grafting after streptokinase treatment. Postoperative blood loss and clinical results. *J. Thorac. Cardiovasc. Surg.* 95:216–222, 1988.

Mammen, E. F., Koets, M. H., Washington, B. C., et al. Hemostasis changes during cardiopulmonary bypass surgery. *Semin. Thromb. Hemost.* 11:281–292, 1985.

Mantia, A. M., Lolley, D. M., Stullken, E. H., et al. Coronary artery bypass grafting within 24 hours after intracoronary streptokinase thrombolysis. *J. Cardiothorac. Anesth.* 1:392–400, 1987.

Marder, V. J., and Sherry, S. Thrombolytic Therapy: Current status. *N. Engl. J. Med.* 318:1512–1520, 1585–1595, 1988.

van den Dungen, J. J. A. M., Karliczek, G. F., Brenken, U., et al. Clinical study of blood trauma during perfusion with membrane and bubble oxygenators. *J. Thorac. Cardiovasc. Surg.* 83:108–116, 1982.

Mechanical Support of
the Circulation

Cardiopulmonary Bypass Circuits and Design

Kane M. High, Dennis R. Williams, and Mark Kurusz

The authors would like to sincerely thank Ms. Kathy Seiple for her help in the preparation of this chapter.

Modern cardiopulmonary bypass (CPB) has evolved during the past century with the development of the individual elements of the CPB circuit. The first of the essential elements of CPB to be developed were film and bubble oxygenators. Prototypes were made as early as the 1880s and were used primarily for physiology experiments. The discovery of heparin in 1916 by McLean [10] made possible extended contact of blood with foreign surfaces without clotting, and the use of roller pumps by DeBakey [3] in the 1930s provided a reliable and simple pumping system. The clinical use of bubble oxygenators became feasible with the development of adequate blood defoaming in the early 1950s. Finally, in 1953 Gibbon [6] performed the first successful human CPB for cardiac surgery. In the past 35 years, CPB devices and techniques have been refined, permitting safe CPB to be routinely performed on more than 250,000 patients in the USA annually.

This chapter will describe the current components of the CPB circuit as well as many of the safety features that have been developed. Medical management of the patient on CPB is discussed in Chapter 7 and the specific pathophysiologic effects of CPB are discussed in Chapter 20.

I. **Goals of Cardiopulmonary bypass.** The essential goals of CPB are to provide a stilled bloodless heart with blood flow temporarily diverted to an extracorporeal circuit that functionally replaces the heart and lungs. The goals of CPB may then be classified as:
   A. **Respiration**
      1. **Ventilation. Adequate and controllable carbon dioxide elimination in accordance with carbon dioxide production to maintain PCO_2 in a desired range for the temperature of the blood.** As temperature decreases, carbon dioxide production is decreased and requires less "ventilation" through the oxygenator by decreasing the gas flow into the oxygenator. The choice of the desired $PaCO_2$ depends on the particular management scheme (alpha-stat versus pH-stat) and is discussed in Chapter 20.
      2. **Oxygenation. Provide oxygen transport to blood matching body oxygen consumption.** The large surface area (either bubble surface or membrane) of the oxygenator provides for adequate oxygen transport. Under normal operating conditions, much higher PaO_2 values are maintained (PaO_2 = 200–400 mm Hg), particularly with a bubble oxygenator, than are normally maintained during mechanical ventilation. Although it is possible to maintain PaO_2 in a more physiologic range, lack of demonstrable ill effects has led most teams to accept these elevated values, which provide an additional small margin of safety.
   B. **Circulation. It is necessary to maintain a desired perfusion pressure and flow while minimizing trauma to the formed elements of the blood.** Some hemolysis during CPB is inevitable owing to abnormal pressures and shear stresses in the CPB flow, but elevations in free plasma hemoglobin are only slight and transient except during prolonged CPB or excessive use of the cardiotomy suction.
   C. **Temperature regulation**
      1. **Decreased body metabolism with hypothermia**
         a. **Hypothermia permits the use of lower blood flows, thereby decreasing blood trauma and permitting a longer safe CPB period.** Also, less blood returning to the heart at a lower flow rate provides a drier operative field. Typical blood temperature ranges for hypothermia are given in Table 19-1. Today virtually all institutions routinely employ hypothermia during CPB.
         b. **With reduction in body temperature to profound hypothermic levels it is possible to reduce metabolism to the point**

Table 19-1. Typical temperature ranges for hypothermia

Mild	28–34°C
Routine	20–28°C
Profound	<20°C

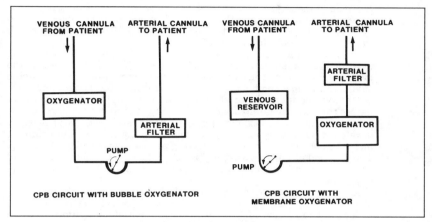

Fig. 19-1. Schematic of the CPB circuit for bubble and membrane oxygenators: *A.* CPB circuit with bubble oxygenator: oxygenator placed before pump head. *B.* CPB circuit with membrane oxygenator: oxygenator placed after pump head.

where the body tolerates total circulatory arrest for extended periods of time without demonstrable cellular destruction. Usually temperatures in the range of 16°–20°C are employed. With this degree of hypothermia, it is generally agreed that circulatory arrest periods of up to 45 minutes can be safely undertaken [7].

2. **Provide hypothermic myocardial preservation. Intravascular and topical cooling are excellent adjuncts to flaccid hyperkalemic myocardial arrest used in myocardial preservation.** The heart is actively chilled by cold cardioplegic solution and by ice slurry applied to the surface of the heart by the surgeon. Also, to minimize warming of myocardium by surrounding tissue (and to avoid cold injury to the phrenic nerve) an insulating pad is applied to the posterior surface of the heart in the pericardial well to prevent direct heat transfer between warmer tissues and the heart. Cardioplegia typically decreases the myocardial temperature to approximately 10°C. When a single right atrial–inferior vena cava cannula is used to provide venous return, myocardial temperatures need to be carefully monitored because venous blood returning to the right atrium is 20–28°C. Two cannulae, one in the inferior vena cava (IVC) and another in the superior vena cava (SVC), can be used to keep venous blood from entering the heart and warming the heart.

II. The cardiopulmonary bypass circuit

A. **Circuit design.** The essential elements of the CPB machine remain the same despite different manufacturers and different machine designs. Figure 19-1 shows a schematic of the essential elements of CPB. Tracing the path of blood flow in this diagram, desaturated blood exits the patient's vena cava through the venous cannula(e) and is **drained by gravity** through large-bore polyvinyl chloride (PVC) tubing into a reservoir that is either an integral part of the oxygenator (as in bubble oxygenators) or a separate element (in membrane oxygenators). Newer membrane oxygenators may have an integral venous reservoir. When a bubble oxygenator is used, the blood flows by gravity through the oxygenator and then is pumped to the systemic circulation through a smaller-bore PVC tube. If a membrane oxygenator is used, the blood is drawn from the venous reservoir by the pump and then passes through the oxygenator. In both systems the blood then flows through an arterial filter and back through the arterial cannula to the aorta.

There is a fundamental design reason for the difference in the location of the membrane and bubble oxygenators, which relates to the pressure drop across the oxygenator. The pressure drop across a bubble oxygenator is low and blood easily passes through the oxygenator without active pumping. In most membrane oxygenators, the blood first passes through the pump because of the much higher resistance to flow across the membrane oxygenator. One membrane oxygenator recently developed has a pressure drop low enough to permit gravity drainage and does not require the higher driving pressure provided by the pump. The detailed circuit drawing in Fig. 19-2 shows the bypass circuit and the other pump heads typically used during CPB with a bubble oxygenator.

B. **The pumps: roller and centrifugal.** There are currently two types of blood pumps used in the CPB circuit. They are the nonocclusive roller pump and the constrained vortex, or centrifugal, pump. Of these two, the most commonly used is the roller pump.

1. **Roller pump**
   a. **Principles of operation.** The roller, or peristaltic, pump was first patented by Porter and Bradley in 1855, and modifications were made by DeBakey in 1934. The roller pump causes blood to flow by compressing plastic tubing between the roller and the horseshoe-shaped backing plate as the roller turns in the raceway (Fig. 19-3). Each pump has two roller heads placed 180 degrees apart to maintain continuous roller head contact with the tubing.
   b. **Adjustment of occlusion**
      (1) To minimize hemolysis, the occlusion, or separation between the rollers and the raceway, must be properly set. In essence, this provides a mechanism for setting the resistance to backflow past the roller head. The occlusion is set by adjusting the distance between the raceway and each of the roller heads, which control the cross-sectional area inside the tubing at the point of compression by the roller head. The occlusion adjusting nut (Fig. 19-3) at the top of the pump head is used to set the occlusion with the head at two different positions on the raceway.

      Total occlusion is not used because increased hemolysis and excessive tubing wear will result. A problem with hemolysis can also develop, though, if too large an area is left between the pump head and the backing plate. In this case, a rapid backflow causing large velocity gradients and excessive shear stresses on red cells can occur, in turn causing hemolysis. Too little occlusion can also lead to decreased forward flow to the patient.

      The usual **method for setting occlusion** involves holding the arterial line, which is primed with clear fluid, vertically so that the top of the fluid column is approximately 30 inches above the pump. The occlusion is adjusted until the fluid level

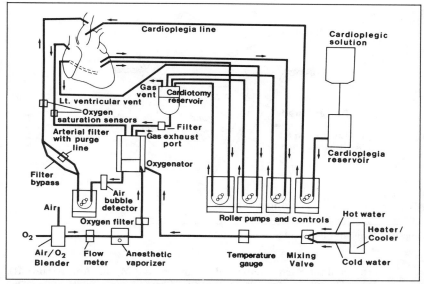

Fig. 19-2. Detailed diagram of CPB circuit. The main CPB circuit is located in the left corner of the figure and shows the roller pump, oxygenator, and arterial line with filter returning to the patient. The heat exchanger is usually included as an integral part of the oxygenator. An arterial line pressure monitor (not shown) is usually connected distal to the arterial filter to measure pressure in the arterial line between the roller pump and the patient. The other roller pumps are used for suction, ventricular venting, and providing a supply of cold cardioplegic solution. Normally, a clamp is applied to the arterial filter bypass line. When bubble oxygenators are employed the blender is set to deliver 100% O_2 or not used at all. (Modified from C. C. Reed and T. B. Stafford. *Cardiopulmonary Bypass* [2nd ed.]. Houston: Medical Press, 1985. P. 270-A. With permission.)

falls at a rate of 1 cm/min based on studies of roller pump hemolysis [1].

(2) Although not totally occlusive, roller pumps are not significantly affected by arterial pressure. When occlusion is properly set, the pump flow rate does not significantly decrease as the afterload (arterial pressure) increases. High pressures can occur in the arterial line if the arterial cannula is blocked as a result of either tube kinking or a tubing clamp. Pressures high enough to cause line separation or rupture can occur. Also, if the roller head pump inlet tube is restricted, it is physically possible for a roller pump to create a negative pressure, pulling gas out of solution. However, this does not usually occur because the tubing entering the roller pump is short and is connected directly to a reservoir that contains enough blood to preclude any significant negative pressure from developing.

c. **Pulsatile flow.** Newer roller pumps generate pulsatile flow by varying the instantaneous rate of rotation of the pump head. The use of pulsatile perfusion during CPB remains controversial (see Chap. 20).

2. **Constrained vortex pumps (centrifugal pumps)**

a. Currently there are only two manufacturers of **centrifugal pumps used for CPB:** the Bio-Pump (BioMedicus, Eden Prairie, MN)

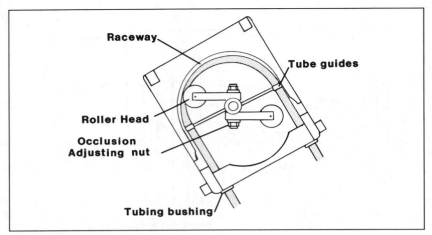

Fig. 19-3. Typical roller head pump with tubing.

and the Sarns/Centrimed Pump (Sarns/3-M, Inc, Ann Arbor, MI). The constrained vortex Bio-Pump (see Fig. 22-3) consists of a series of vaneless rotor cones mounted in a clear plastic housing that spin, causing circular motion of the blood and generating flow and pressure by centrifugal force. The cones spin by means of a magnetic connection to a drive shaft. The two outer cones are attached at a few points to each other and to the innermost cone. Blood enters along the axis of the pump and exits at the other end of the pump at the periphery.

   b. This type of **pump is nonocclusive** and flow is dependent on the pressure change created by the spinning cones in the pump. The flow rate is affected by the size of the cannula, length of the tubing, diameter of the tubing, restrictions in the tubing, and changes in the patient's SVR. That is, as the pressure distal to the pump increases, the flow decreases. Such decreases in flow can be partially prevented by increasing the pump speed. A flow meter is requisite when a centrifugal pump is used and is placed in the arterial line between the patient and the pump to determine accurately the actual flow rate.

   Earlier claims were made that centrifugal pumps could not pump air (thereby making them safer than roller pumps) and that the patient need not be heparinized to use this type of pump [4]. Certainly centrifugal pumps cannot pump if they become filled with air because they rely on centrifugal force to generate pressure. However, centrifugal pumps can easily pump bubbles into the bloodstream without difficulty if they are present in the blood. A summary of the advantages and disadvantages of centrifugal and roller pumps is given in Table 19-2.

C. Oxygenators. "Oxygenators" provide an environment for carbon dioxide and oxygen exchange similar to that in the alveolar-pulmonary capillary unit. In the design of an oxygenator, it is desirable that ventilation (i.e., carbon dioxide elimination) be separable from oxygenation so that ventilation and oxygenation can be controlled without affecting each other.

   1. General principles of design and operation

Table 19-2. Comparison of roller head and centrifugal pumps

	Advantages	Disadvantages
Roller head	Predictable pump flow based on pump speed	Can pump **large** quantities of air
	Capable of pulsatile flow	Can overpressurize lines causing them to burst
Centrifugal	Cannot pump **large** quantities of air	Output not necessarily indicated by pump speed
	Cannot overpressurize lines	Not capable of pulsatile flow

    a. Optimize gas transport by (1) minimizing the gas transport distance in the blood, (2) maximizing the effective area for gas diffusion, and (3) increasing the blood transit time in the oxygenator.

    b. Minimize formed element trauma by minimizing shear stresses and provide smooth blood-contacting surfaces.

    c. The priming volume should be as small as possible.

    d. The reservoir should be of large capacity and permit easy viewing of the blood levels at all times.

2. Bubble oxygenators. The first disposable bubble oxygenator was used successfully by DeWall and Lillehei in Minneapolis in 1956 [9]. The safe use of a disposable oxygenator allowed for the explosive development of cardiovascular surgery. Until this time oxygenators were large, bulky, and difficult to clean, limiting the number of cases which could be performed. Today many types of "bubblers" are available, but the design and principles are similar. There are three main compartments in the bubble oxygenator: the oxygenation section, the defoamer, and the arterial reservoir, as shown in Figure 19-4.

    a. Compartments of bubble oxygenator

        (1) The oxygenation section. This type of oxygenator employs the "fish tank" principle in which oxygen is bubbled through venous blood, which drains by gravity through the oxygenation chamber with a direct blood-gas interface. Oxygenation and carbon dioxide elimination are determined by the size and number of bubbles. The number of bubbles is determined by both the rate of gas flow and bubble size. Bubble size is determined by the size of the screen through which the oxygen flows. Large bubbles create less surface area, whereas small bubbles (at the same gas flow rate) increase surface area for greater exposure of blood to gas, thereby improving oxygenation. However, if bubbles of 100% oxygen are too small, they are completely absorbed very quickly, thus limiting carbon dioxide elimination. Carbon dioxide removal is increased with increased gas flow, which can also cause excessively high PaO_2 levels. It is preferable to use 100% oxygen in bubble oxygenators because nitrogen flowing through the oxygenator is far less soluble and more dangerous if it gains access to the arterial cannula.

        (2) The defoamer. The arterialized blood and foam enter the "defoaming" compartment, where they pass through a polyurethane mesh sponge coated with an antifoam agent, silicone Antifoam-A. A large portion of actual gas exchange occurs while the blood is passing through the defoamer. **The oxygenator must be able to "defoam" the blood quickly**

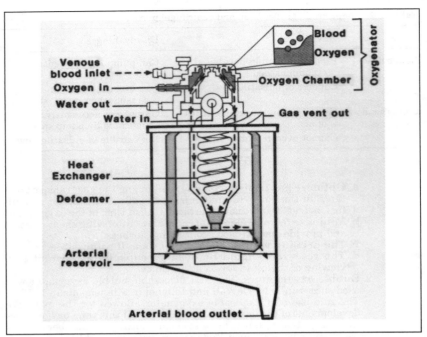

Fig. 19-4. Typical bubble oxygenation section, with its compartments: oxygenator, heat exchanger, defoamer, and arterial reservoir. (Modified from American Bentley. Irvine, CA. 1978. With permission.)

enough to maintain the rated blood flow of the oxygenator without spillage of bubbles into the arterial line port. All bubble oxygenators have a maximum flow rate that is determined by the manufacturer. Defoaming is completed in the arterial reservoir, where the buoyancy of the residual foam causes it to rise to the top of the arterial reservoir.

(3) **The arterial reservoir.** From the defoamer the blood falls into the arterial reservoir or collecting chamber and then is pumped out to the patient. Flow through the reservoir must be smooth, not turbulent, to avoid creating more bubbles. Adequate volume in the reservoir allows time for gaseous microemboli to be absorbed or to float away from the arterial outlet located at the bottom of the reservoir. Also, a greater volume increases the reaction time needed by a perfusionist to prevent accidental emptying of the reservoir and pumping of air. All manufacturers state the minimum volume levels required for various blood flow rates, and it is a common safety practice to maintain sufficient volume to have a 15-second reaction time. Therefore, at a flow rate of 4 liters/min, a minimum volume of 1 liter of blood should be maintained in the arterial reservoir.

b. **Considerations for operation.** The bubbler is an efficient, inexpensive oxygenator that is easy to prime and use for most short-term cardiac surgical procedures. However, a few limitations still remain. Because of the desirability of using 100% oxygen, it is usually more difficult to control oxygen and carbon dioxide exchange independently. In longer CPB cases, bubble oxygenators may tend to cause hemolysis and disrupt the clotting mechanisms to a greater degree than do membrane oxygenators. Generally, if the CPB time is expected to exceed 3 hours a membrane oxygenator should be used.

3. **Membrane oxygenators.** The membrane lung more closely imitates the natural pulmonary anatomy by interposing a thin membrane between the blood and gas. This creates a definite blood space and gas space within the oxygenator. The first membrane oxygenator was developed by Kolff and used by Effler [5] and Clowes [2] in 1956. This oxygenator, although used clinically in 100 cases, was bulky, required an extremely large priming volume, and was prone to leaking and difficult to set up. However, it proved to be a prototype for further development. -

Problems of design included developing membranes that were sufficiently permeable to exchange both oxygen and carbon dioxide while providing a barrier to bulk gas and blood movement. Compactness was another problem owing to the large surface area required for adequate gas exchange for the volume of blood flow required for adult perfusion.

Current membrane oxygenators have a large surface area, approximately 2–4 m², which is either fan-folded, coiled, or shaped into capillary tubes. The blood passes through the oxygenator as a thin film, minimizing the diffusion distance for gases in the blood and thus maximizing gas exchange.

a. **Types of membrane oxygenators.** The membrane materials commonly used are very thin sheets of polypropylene, Teflon, or silicone rubber and "hollow fiber" capillary membranes of microporous polypropylene. The sheets of silicone rubber are nonporous and rely entirely on gas diffusion through the silicone for gas exchange. In contrast, the polypropylene sheets and fibers have pores that are potential physical connections between the gas and blood space.

(2) **Hollow fiber (microporous) membranes.** The microporous fibers are packed together in a parallel fashion as shown in Fig. 19-5. Either the blood flows through the capillaries surrounded by gas, or the gas flows through the capillaries with blood around them. Models in which the blood passes through the capillaries do have problems with plugging of the tubes, leading to decreased gas transfer secondary decreased blood transit times through the remaining patent fibers.

There is some question whether hollow fiber membranes should be regarded as "true membranes" because of the presence of pores in the membrane responsible for gas exchange. As mentioned, at the onset of bypass there is a direct blood/gas interface at these pores that is present until a thin protein layer covers the hollow fibers to form a molecular membrane. These hollow fiber membranes are not suitable for extended long-term extracorporeal membrane oxygenation (ECMO) perfusion owing to protein leakage that eventually clogs the pores. Only the coiled silicone membrane of the **Sci-Med** oxygenator, developed by Kolobow and Bowman [8] in 1963 has proved adequate for long-term perfusion such as that used in ECMO.

(2) **True (nonporous) membrane oxygenators.** "True" membrane oxygenators are manufactured by coiling silicone rubber sheets in a cylindrical fashion. Blood is kept on one side of the membrane and gas on the other. Gas transfer through the membrane is dependent on the permeability of the membrane,

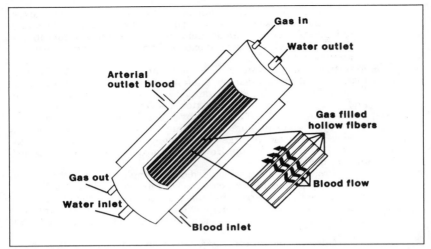

Fig. 19-5. Typical membrane oxygenator with exploded view of hollow fibers and blood flow.

the diffusion distance of the gas in blood, and the driving pressure of gas on either side of the membrane. Membranes must be 20–30 times more permeable to carbon dioxide than to oxygen due to the lower driving pressure of carbon dioxide.

(3) **Characteristics of operation.** Because of the high resistance to blood flow through most membrane oxygenators, blood must be actively pumped through the oxygenator by the roller pump or centrifugal pump. Excessive pressure through the membrane can cause rupture, creating either a blood leak or air embolism.

A major advantage of membrane oxygenators is the capability of exerting independent control of gas exchange. Because all gas present in the blood phase is in solution, an air-oxygen blender can be used to control the PaO_2. The gas flow can be controlled independently to remove carbon dioxide, allowing better control of blood gases on bypass.

Except at the onset of bypass with use of a hollow fiber membrane there is no direct blood-gas interface. This lack of blood-gas interface allows more gentle handling of blood with a lower rate of hemolysis during longer bypass runs.

D. Arterial and venous cannulae

1. **Venous cannulae.** Venous blood returning to the right heart is drained by gravity to the oxygenator or venous reservoir through either two venous cannulae inserted into both the IVC and SVC or one venous cannula inserted into the right atrial appendage. If both the IVC and SVC are cannulated with heavy ligatures (commonly referred to as caval tapes) around the cavae and cannulae, all the blood returning through the venae cava is diverted to the oxygenator. There is no ejection of blood from the left ventricle and therefore no arterial pulsations. This is "total bypass" (see Fig. 6-3). This type of cannulation is used to create a bloodless operative field and to prevent rewarming of the heart by venous blood. If a single atrial cannula is used, it most often is a **single** "two-stage" cannula in which

blood is drained from the right atrium and the IVC by this single tube with concentric flow channels. Representative venous cannulae are shown in Fig. 6-5. When using a two-stage cannula or bicaval cannulation without caval tapes, some blood may pass into the right atrium, through the right heart, and into the pulmonary circulation. The amount of blood passing into the right atrium can be controlled by restricting venous return to the bypass circuit. Restriction of blood return to the CPB machine causes blood to pass through the pulmonary circulation, and some arterial pulsation occurs; this condition is called partial bypass.

Several factors affect venous return to the pump. The driving pressure for blood flow in the venous cannulae is the hydrostatic pressure head from the right atrium to the venous reservoir less any pressure drop incurred in the venous system of the CPB circuit. **Remedies to consider when venous return is less than desired include:**

a. **Relieve inflow obstruction** caused by caval wall obstruction of the cannula(e) inlet or too deep insertion of the IVC cannula (e.g., into the portal vein).

b. **Undo kinking** of the cannula(e), particularly as it passes over the sternal retractor.

c. **Increase the height difference** (elevate the operating room table or drop the oxygenator reservoir) between the cavae and the venous reservoir-oxygenator (i.e., increase the hydrostatic pressure head).

d. **Remove all clamps** from the venous line at the pump.

e. **Use larger venous cannula(e)** because they have less flow resistance and allow greater flows at the same pressure drop.

Single venous cannulae for individual cannulation of the IVC and SVC range in size from 16–46 Fr. Selection is based on the patient's weight and anticipated flow requirements. The **single** two-stage cannulae range from small (40 × 32 Fr [outside cannula by inside cannula]) to large (51 × 36 Fr) and are chosen also by the patient's weight and flow requirements.

2. **Arterial cannulae.** Arterialized blood is returned to the patient from the CPB circuit through an arterial cannula placed either in the ascending aorta or the femoral artery. Size of the cannula is chosen to minimize the pressure drop across the cannula at the patient's calculated flow rate. A standard cardiac index of 2.4 liters $\cdot$ $min^{-1} \cdot m^{-2}$ for adults and 2.6 liters $\cdot min^{-1} \cdot m^{-2}$ for pediatric patients is used to determine the calculated flow rate required at normothermia. Representative cannulae are shown in Fig. 6-4.

Pump flow must be high enough to prevent the occurrence of metabolic acidosis, which usually requires maintaining a mixed venous PaO_2 of 25–30 (at blood temperature). Flows used at the University Hospital, Penn State University are shown in Table 19-3. These flows are typical of those used around the country and are based on the oxygen consumption curves discussed in Chapter 20.

As a general rule, the pressure drop across the cannula should not exceed 100 mm Hg. Size is then determined by the smallest cannula that can provide calculated flow with a gradient of less than 100 mm Hg. Pressure gradients are determined by manufacturers, and pressure drop-flow charts come with cannula packages. Gradients can also be determined by allowing fluid to flow through the pump circuit and the cannula and measuring the pressure. Newer "high-flow" cannulae are thin-walled and allow a greater flow with a smaller outside diameter.

E. **Ancillary equipment**

Table 19-3. Typical cardiac indexes with hypothermia

Temperature (C)	Cardiac index ($liters \cdot min^{-1} \cdot m^{-2}$)
34–37	2.4
30–34	2.0
25–30	1.8
20–18	1.5
<18	1.0

1. **Blood filters**
   a. **Filter types.** There are two primary types of filters used for blood filtration during CPB, depth filters and screen filters. A depth filter is composed of packed fibers of Dacron. They filter by absorption on their large wetted surface areas. **With depth filters, particulate removal depends on:**
      (1) The amount of wetted surface area.
      (2) The chemical structure of the particles and filter material.
      (3) The diameter of blood flow pathways.
         Screen filters are made of a woven mesh of polyester fibers with specific pore sizes in the mesh. Particulate material is trapped in this filter because the particles are larger than the pores. Pore size must be more than 20 μ for adequate blood flow without causing excessive back pressure. Both types of filters make effective bubble traps as well.
   b. **Filter location.** Most filters in the arterial line are screen filters. A bypass line (Fig. 19-2) around the arterial line filter is recommended should the filter become obstructed. The pressure drop across the filter should be measured to monitor obstruction of the filter. The bypass line around the arterial filter is normally occluded by a clamp that can be readily released in the event of filter obstruction.
         Because the cardiotomy reservoirs receive blood that contains a large quantity of debris, they contain an integral filter that utilizes a combination of both depth and screen type filters.
2. **Blood suctioning.** Suction is used during CPB to remove blood and cardioplegic solution from the operative field as well as to drain cardiac chambers or great vessels. When the fluid drained is primarily cardioplegic solution, the hospital suction system is used, and this fluid does not enter the CPB circuit. However, when the fluid is primarily blood, the pump suction lines are used to return the fluid to the circuit and the patient.
      The pump suction lines are powered by use of a roller pump to draw a vacuum (Fig. 19-2). Generally, two pump heads are dedicated to this purpose. Blood from the pump suction lines is pumped into the cardiotomy reservoir and returned to the patient. Usually these roller pumps are activated only when needed by the surgeon. **Leaving these roller pumps turning continuously is a major source of hemolysis and should be avoided.** Indiscriminate use of suction pumps also causes aspiration of room air, which is less easily removed by the cardiotomy filters and defoamers and can increase the risk of gaseous microemboli.
3. **Arterial line pressure monitor.** Electronic strain gauge pressure transducers are used to monitor the pressure in the arterial line.

These are usually connected to the circuit at a port on the arterial filter. This monitor is extremely important for detecting restrictions to flow in the arterial line caused by an inadvertent clamp or kinking of the line.

4. **Heat exchangers.** Heat exchangers usually are an integral part of the CPB oxygenator. Either hot or cold water is circulated through the heat exchanger and provides a temperature gradient to warm or cool the blood. Management of rewarming during CPB is discussed in Chapter 7.

5. **Temperature sensors.** The temperature of the blood in the venous and arterial lines is continuously monitored during CPB to determine the temperature gradient during warming and cooling. The temperature is measured by either thermocouple or thermistor and is displayed on the CPB machine.

6. **Anesthesia vaporizer.** An anesthesia vaporizer is placed in the fresh gas line to the CPB oxygenator. This vaporizer is the same as the vaporizers found on anesthesia machines. Isoflurane is the agent usually utilized because of its low blood solubility and its prominent vasodilating effect. The vaporizer should not be located directly above the oxygenator because anesthetic liquid spilled onto the oxygenator during filling of the vaporizer can cause damage or cracking of the oxygenator.

7. **Ultrafiltration.** Occasionally during CPB it is necessary to remove excess water (with electrolytes) to increase the patient's hematocrit. This process is easily accomplished on CPB by the use of ultrafiltration. In comparison with diuretics ultrafiltrators are readily controllable and do not cause excessive losses of potassium.

Ultrafiltrators usually consist of hollow fiber membranes that allow the separation of water and electrolytes from formed elements and larger molecules (i.e., proteins) in the blood. Blood is either pumped from a reservoir through the ultrafiltrator by an auxiliary roller pump or shunted from the arterial line. Pressure is created by the resistance to flow within the ultrafiltrator and occasionally by a downstream clamp that partially occludes the return line. This hydrostatic pressure forces water out of the blood and across the membrane, concentrating the remaining blood. Up to 45 ml/min of effluent can be removed from the blood in this fashion.

III. **Priming the cardiopulmonary bypass circuit.** Prior to the early 1960s it was thought that large volumes of donor blood were needed to prime the CPB circuit. This practice was associated with many postoperative complications including fluid overload and capillary sludging, resulting in poor tissue perfusion with renal failure, seizures, stroke, and the "pump lung" syndrome.

Due to advances in the understanding of concepts of hemodilution and hypothermia plus new concerns about transmission of blood-borne diseases, the use of a total nonblood prime is now standard CPB procedure in adults and large children. Patients weighing less then 35 kg, however, usually must still receive blood in the CPB prime because of their small blood volume relative to the prime volume. Moderate hypothermia to 25°–28°C is usually employed to allow improved myocardial and cerebral preservation during CPB. However, the viscosity of the blood is increased during hypothermia. The use of hemodilution, in contrast, decreases the viscosity of the blood and causes increased tissue perfusion at lower flow rates. Therefore, there is a decrease in red cell trauma, improved renal function postoperatively, and less need for banked blood when hemodilution to a hematocrit of 21–24% is employed during CPB.

A. **Priming solution.** Four major factors must be considered when priming the bypass circuit.

Table 19-4. Standard adult CPB primes used at the University of Texas and Pennsylvania State University

University of Texas		Pennsylvania State University	
Plasma-Lyte A	1300 ml	Plasma-Lyte A	1500 ml
Heparin	5000 units	Heparin	5000 units
Sodium bicarbonate	25 mEq	Sodium bicarbonate	45 mEq
25% albumin	250 ml	Mannitol	25 g
D/W 5% with 0.45% normal saline solution	650 ml		

1. **Osmolality.** The fluid should be isotonic or slightly hypertonic to preserve the interstitial-intravascular fluid balance.
2. **Electrolytes.** Normal electrolyte balance must be maintained to avoid electrolyte depletion postbypass.
3. **Volume.** Adequate volume of priming solution must be utilized to fill the circuit and oxygenator to a safe level and provide adequate bypass flow rates. The total volume of fluid needed to prime the circuit is determined by the volume of the circuit tubing and the volume required to prime the components of the circuit such as the cardiotomy and venous reservoir, oxygenator, and arterial line filter. The total volume used must be enough to allow initiation of CPB with adequate blood flow rates but not too much to cause excessive hemodilution and volume overload to the patient.
4. **Hemodilution.** It is undesirable to reduce the hematocrit to less than 18% with the initiation of bypass. The initial bypass hematocrit can be estimated using the following equation:

$$Hct_{int} = (Hct \times EBV)/(EBV + \text{volume of prime} + \text{prebypass IV fluids})$$

where EBV = estimated blood volume of patient
Hct_{int} = initial hematocrit on CPB
Hct = preoperative hematocrit

Solutions used for priming vary from institution to institution. Adult primes at University Hospital, Pennsylvania State University and the John Sealy Hospital, University of Texas, Galveston are compared in Table 19-4. Generally, an isotonic, balanced electrolyte solution such as Ringer's lactate or Plasma-Lyte is used. Sodium bicarbonate is employed as a buffer. Osmotic agents such as mannitol are often added to improve renal function, and a colloid solution such as albumin or hetastarch can be utilized to maintain oncotic pressure and to coat the foreign surfaces of a membrane oxygenator. The prime should be heparinized to prevent dilution of the heparin dose given prebypass.

B. **Method of priming.** The goal of priming is to wet and debubble the bypass circuit completely. The actual methods employed to accomplish this vary greatly among perfusionists. Generally, a carbon dioxide flush of the filter and oxygenator for several minutes is used to remove all room air from the circuit. Carbon dioxide is used to purge the dry circuit because of its high water solubility. This is followed by recirculation of priming solution through the circuit (with the venous and arterial lines connected together). All circuit elements and stopcocks must also be primed. Any carbon dioxide bubbles that are not washed from the circuit are quickly absorbed into the prime.

The prime should then be recirculated at a maximum calculated flow rate to test the circuit and monitor for excessive line pressure. Recirculation with gas flow also allows excessive carbon dioxide to be removed from the circuit before commencing bypass. An attempt should be made to approach a physiologic acid-base status prior to initiating CPB.

IV. Malfunctions during cardiopulmonary bypass and their correction. Mechanical malfunction of equipment and components can occur during CPB. These problems require quick thinking on the part of the perfusionist and members of the surgical team. Each problem must be determined rapidly, evaluated, and corrective measures instituted. Specific protocols to deal with problems can save valuable time when dealing with emergencies during CPB.

A. Malfunctions of the arterial roller pump

1. **Electrical failure** of the pump due to a power interruption in the OR does occur. In this instance perfusion is maintained by using the manual crank or battery back-up to maintain circulation. The crank should always be available and should be stored on the CPB machine. When needed, it is applied to the axle of the pump head and turned. Newer hand cranks are ratcheted so that they will operate in only one direction to prevent accidental reversal of flow. A battery-operated light source must be readily available so that perfusionist can observe the level in the oxygenator reservoir. Even with manual operation it is possible for an air embolus to occur if the reservoir is drained.

2. The **pump motor controller can fail** and the arterial pump head turn at its maximum speed, a condition referred to as **runaway arterial pump head.** In this instance the pump's electrical plug must be immediately pulled out and the arterial line clamped. The arterial line is then changed to another pump head.

3. **"Pump creep"** is a phenomenon noticed when the arterial pump continues to rotate very slowly after pump rotation has been stopped with the control knob. The danger in pump creep lies in the possibility that air will be inadvertently pumped into the arterial system or the arterial line will be overpressurized. For this reason it is a safe practice to activate the off switch and clamp the arterial line when no pumping is desired.

B. Oxygenator failure. Hypoxemia of blood leaving the oxygenator may result from either **oxygen supply failure** or **failure of the oxygenator** itself. Failure to oxygenate the blood can be detected either by observing the color of the arterial blood or by an inline oxygen monitor. If failure of oxygenation is noticed at the onset of bypass and is due to the oxygenator itself, it may be possible to take the patient off bypass and change the oxygenator. If the problem becomes apparent later during bypass the oxygenator must be changed during circulatory arrest.

Loss of oxygen supply can occur owing to loss of wall oxygen pressure or leaks in the oxygen supply line in the room; the constant presence of a reserve oxygen supply in close proximity to the pump is required. Also, the tubing and connectors that supply oxygen to the oxygenator may develop leaks or cracks, leading to an oxygenator failure.

C. Occlusion malfunction. There have been reported instances of occlusion malfunction of the arterial pump head. This can result in the roller head becoming totally occlusive to the point where it cannot move. Total occlusion may cause the circuit breaker for that roller head to trip and the roller head to stop. If it cannot be easily corrected, the tubing must be changed to another pump head.

The opposite problem in occlusion malfunction can occur if the roller head becomes totally nonocclusive. This will result in inadequate flows to the patient and may cause hemolysis and tearing or shredding of the arterial pump tubing in the roller head. The pump must be stopped and the occlusion properly set.

D. Inadequate anticoagulation. The causes and management of inadequate anticoagulation are discussed in Chapters 6 and 7. If clots appear in the oxygenator, a dose of heparin equal to that initially administered prior to CPB should be given again, preferably drawn from a different bottle of heparin. If the arterial filter becomes obstructed it is necessary to open the filter bypass line.

E. Switching of arterial and venous lines. There have been case reports of inadvertent switching of the arterial and venous lines, resulting in blood draining from the aorta and pumping into the venous circulation, leading to excessive venous pressure and possible damage to the vena cava. This can be immediately noticed by a **widening of the pulse pressure** (rather than the usual decrease in pulse pressure) and distention of the vena cava on institution of CPB.

The arterial line is smaller than the venous line, and this mistake should not occur. If it does occur it should be readily appreciated. Patency of the arterial cannula and line should be verified prior to beginning CPB by the presence of a pulsatile aortic pressure in the arterial line that correlates with the systemic blood pressure. If switching of the lines does occur, CPB must be stopped and the connections corrected.

E. Inadvertent air infusion. As previously mentioned, both roller head and centrifugal pumps can deliver air to the arterial circulation. One of the primary functions of the perfusionist is to ensure that during the course of CPB the reservoir from which the pump draws blood does not become empty and allow air to enter the arterial cannula. Air can be entrained into the arterial line even if the reservoir has not become completely empty in the form of bubbles that have been mixed into the blood (vortexing). Should air be detected entering the aorta, CPB should be immediately discontinued and treatment begun according to the protocol outlined in Table 7-3.

V. Safety devices

A. Devices to detect and prevent air embolism. Besides the most important safety device, a vigilant perfusionist, many mechanical and electronic safety devices are available that are designed primarily to detect and prevent air embolism.

1. **Low-level alarm.** Blood level alarms (both high and low) were used on early disk oxygenators in the 1950s and 1960s. With the advent of hard shell disposable bubble oxygenators the low-level alarm became a standard accessory on the CPB console. A photoelectric sensor is attached to the side of the blood reservoir at a user-determined level. When the blood level is above the sensor no alarm sounds, but if the blood level drops below the sensor an alarm sounds and a light flashes. Low-level alarms also can be engaged to shut off the arterial pump automatically or simply warn of a low-level condition (manual mode). Newer low-level alarms rely on capacitance or infrared sensors instead of visible light.

2. **Air bubble detector.** The air bubble detector has many years of use in the hemodialysis field and has become available for CPB in the last 10 years. A sensor head clamps onto the arterial tubing and an infrared signal detects bubbles greater than 0.5–1.0 cc in size. Pump shut-off is automatic unless the air bubble detector is turned off. Discrete bubbles are necessary to trip the detector, and **the detector can fail to detect foam** (microbubbles) passing through the arterial line.

3. **Arterial line filter or bubble trap.** Both these devices can be placed in the arterial line between the pump and the patient. They capture gross air emboli physically. Arterial screen filters also are effective in retaining gaseous microemboli. Both should be operated with an open purge line to allow air to escape to maximize their effectiveness.

4. **Purge line.** The purge line itself is a very important safety device. It originates from the top of the arterial line filter or bubble trap and connects to the manifold for blood sampling and then to the venous reservoir. By allowing a continuous flow of approximately 40 ml/min to drain the top of the arterial filter, it serves as an air purge to prevent air embolism. Also, this flow prevents the accidental injection of air into the arterial circuit that might otherwise occur during blood sampling or drug injection.

5. **Oxygenator weight arm.** This device is available on only one manufacturer's CPB console. It detects decreases in blood volume in the oxygenator by sensing the presence of less weight exerted on the preset weight arm. The arm mechanism is servoregulated to the arterial pump. When less weight is detected the pump slows; conversely, with increased venous return and more weight, the arterial pump will speed up.

6. **In-line ball-check valve.** This invasive device is similar to a ball-in-cage cardiac valvular prosthesis. It is placed just below the arterial reservoir in the arterial line and before the pump head. As long as blood fills the tubing the hollow ball remains unrestrictive to blood flow. If air enters the arterial line, the ball drops down and seals the arterial line, thus preventing transmission of air. One disadvantage of this device is that the roller pump will continue to operate, creating excessive vacuum and cavitation in the blood line between the ball valve and the pump. The ball-check valve also reportedly does not work with centrifugal pumps.

7. **One-way vent valves.** These valves can be designed to prevent air from being pumped through a suction or vent line in the wrong direction if either the pump is operated in reverse or the tubing is loaded into the pump head incorrectly at the time of assembly.

B. **Devices to monitor blood oxygenation, ventilation, and acid-base status on CPB.** Until recently the only monitor of oxygenation and ventilation on CPB was the intermittent drawing of blood samples for blood gas analysis. This has the advantage of accurate results but the disadvantage of being intermittent and subject to delay while results are being determined in the blood gas laboratory.

Recently, continuous in-line monitoring of blood gas parameters and electrolytes has become available. Thus continuous measurement of arterial and venous blood gases is now available. The advantage of these systems is rapid detection of changes in patient and CPB perfusion status.

C. **Devices to monitor coagulation status.** Prior to the mid-1970s coagulation was not closely monitored. With closer monitoring of coagulation with the activated clotting time (ACT) in recent years, the incidence of disseminated intravascular coagulation during CPB has decreased. Since patient response to heparin solutions varies greatly depending on factors including levels of anti-thrombin III, previous doses of heparin, and the potency of the heparin administered, it is imperative to monitor the degree of anticoagulation.

The standard in the OR for measurement of coagulation is currently the ACT. CPB is not initiated until the ACT is greater than 300 seconds. During the course of CPB the ACT is checked every 15–30 minutes and maintained at greater than 400 seconds. Measurement of the ACT is discussed in Chapters 6 and 18.

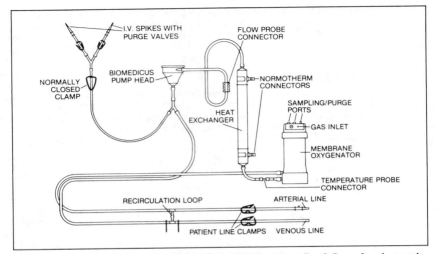

Fig. 19-6. Diagram of emergency CPB circuit of CPS system, Bard, Inc., showing position of centrifugal pump, heat exchanger, oxygenator, and arterial and venous cannulae. (From BARD CPS System Instruction Manual, Catalog H-4300. Billerica, MA: C.R. Bard, 1988. P. 2. With permission.)

VI. **Emergency cardiopulmonary bypass.** Occasionally patients with coronary or valvular disease **that are amenable to surgery** undergo acute cardiovascular decompensation outside the OR, in the intensive care unit, hospital floor, or the cardiac catheterization laboratory. The condition of these patients remains viable only if adequate perfusion can be maintained to vital organs such as the heart, brain, liver, and kidneys. A marked improvement in perfusion compared with closed chest massage can be obtained with the use of a portable cardiopulmonary bypass circuit. The patient can be placed on CPB, stabilized on CPB, and then transferred to the OR in an orderly manner. These patients need not be intubated, although they often are in the early course of their resuscitation. Although this system in principle might improve outcome, survival rates in published studies are low, presumably because of the time required to identify the patients' need for CPB and then transport the equipment. To be effective, this technique requires the preoperative coordination of a surgical team including surgeon, perfusionist, anesthesiologist, and surgical nurse.

A. **Equipment and circuit.** The equipment used for emergency bypass must be easily stored and quickly assembled and primed with fluid ready for use. C.R. Bard, Inc. has developed the system shown schematically in Fig. 19-6. It consists of one BioMedicus Bio-Pump, Bard oxygenator, heat exchanger, PVC tubing and connectors, hospital cart, and battery. Similar systems can be assembled from existing CPB hardware.

Once assembled, it must be readily primed and purged. Figure 19-6 demonstrates how this system is quickly purged of air. After an initial infusion of crystalloid into the circuit, the lines are purged to the clamps. Then the circuit is recirculated, and further purging is done from the top of the oxygenator by withdrawing any air that collects there.

CPB is established percutaneously through the femoral vein and artery because of their accessibility and the need for only local anesthesia in patients who remain alert. Once CPB has begun chest compressions may not be necessary if the aortic valve is competent, but concern for ventricular distention in the fibrillating heart requires at least slow chest compressions in patients with aortic insufficiency. The patient is then transported to the OR for definitive treatment. After induction of anesthesia, the chest is prepared and opened, and conventional CPB is performed with cannulation through the ascending aorta and caval drainage. CPB then proceeds in the usual manner. While in the OR the femoral cannulae are removed and their insertion sites surgically closed.

  B. System storage. All the equipment necessary to assemble, prime, and institute emergency CPB must be available on an easily transported cart so that it can be taken rapidly to the patient. It is imperative that the equipment be in "ready to travel" condition and that it not be used for any other purpose.

VII. Summary. CPB has evolved into a safe but sophisticated system of hardware that requires intensive training to operate. It is the function of certified perfusionists to maintain and operate this equipment during CPB. However, it is the responsibility of the anesthesiologists and surgeons caring for patients undergoing CPB to understand this equipment and its function in order to manage these patients properly.

REFERENCES

1. Bernstein, E. F., and Gleason, L. R. Factors influencing hemolysis with roller pumps. *Surgery,* 61:432–442, 1967.
2. Clowes, G. H. A., Jr., Hopkins, A. L., and Neville, W. E. An artificial lung dependent upon diffusion of oxygen and carbon dioxide through plastic membranes. *J. Thorac. Surg.* 32:630–637, 1956.
3. DeBakey, M. E. A simple continuous-flow blood transfusion instrument. *N. Orleans Med. Surg. J.* 87:386, 1934.
4. Dixon, C. M., and Magovern, G. J. Evaluation of the Bio-pump for long-term cardiac support without heparinization. *J. Extra-Corpor. Technol.* 14:331, 1982.
5. Effler, D. B., Kolff, W. J., Groves, L. K., et al. Disposable membrane oxygenator (heart-lung machine) and its use in experimental surgery. *J. Thorac. Surg.* 32:620–629, 1956.
6. Gibbon, J. H., Jr. Application of a mechanical heart and lung apparatus to cardiac surgery. *Minn. Med.* 37:171, 1954.
7. Kirklin, J. W., and Barratt-Boyes, B. G. Hypothermia, Circulatory Arrest, and Cardiopulmonary Bypass. In J. W. Kirklin, and B. G. Barratt-Boyes (eds.), *Cardiac Surgery.* New York: Wiley, 1985. P. 29.
8. Kolobow, T., and Bowman, R. L. Construction and evaluation of an alveolar membrane artificial heart-lung. *Trans. Am. Soc. Artif. Int. Org.* 9:238–243, 1963.
9. Lillehei, C. W., Warden, H. E., DeWall, R. A., et al. Cardiopulmonary bypass in surgical treatment of congenital or acquired cardiac disease. *Arch. Surg.* 75:928–945, 1957.
10. McLean, J. The thromboplastic action of cephalin. *Am. J. Physiol.* 41:250–257, 1916.

SUGGESTED READING

Reed, C. C., and Stafford, T. B. *Cardiopulmonary Bypass* (2nd ed.). Houston: Texas Medical Press, 1985.

Taylor, K. M. (ed.). *Cardiopulmonary Bypass, Principles and Management.* London: Chapman and Hill, 1986.

Reed, C. C., Kurusz, M., and Lawrence, A. E., Jr. *Safety and Techniques in Perfusion.* Stafford, TX: Quali-Med., 1988.

Pathophysiology of Cardiopulmonary Bypass

Peter G. Hild

Cardiopulmonary bypass (CPB) is often regarded as a routine procedure by laymen and medical personnel alike and as such is frequently taken for granted. This attitude is perhaps due to the large number of cases performed and the relatively low incidence of morbidity and mortality associated with CPB.

It should be remembered that CPB technology is relatively new and has improved rapidly during the past 25–30 years. Improvements in oxygenator design, addition of various filters and defoaming devices, improved monitoring of anticoagulation, and greater understanding of blood damage by high flow rates and shear stresses have contributed to the relative safety of CPB. However, the low frequency of complications associated with CPB is due more to the human organism's ability to adapt to physiologic insults than to any inherent safety of CPB techniques.

The three major physiologic aberrations introduced by CPB are (1) alterations of pulsatility and blood flow patterns, (2) exposure of blood to nonphysiologic surfaces and shear stresses, and (3) exaggerated stress responses. In addition, modern CPB usually involves varying degrees of hypothermia and hypotension and their attendant physiologic changes.

I. Cardiopulmonary bypass as a perfusion system
A. Normal circulatory homeostasis.
In the normal situation, the maintenance of adequate cardiac output, oxygen delivery, and metabolic waste elimination is governed by metabolic needs of the body. Heart rate, ventricular filling pressures, myocardial contractility, and systemic vascular resistance are modulated by autonomic nervous system tone and circulating catecholamine levels.

Autonomic nervous system activity is modulated by the various baroreceptors and chemoreceptors in the central nervous system (CNS) and periphery in response to changes in blood pressure, pH, PO_2, and PCO_2 which are in turn directly related to tissue metabolism. As metabolic requirements increase, sympathetic tone is increased. Consequently, cardiac output and oxygen delivery are increased.

B. Circulatory control during CPB.
The maintenance of circulation during CPB is no longer dependent on the above homeostatic mechanisms. "Cardiac output" on CPB is the pump flow rate and can be set at any level desired. Systemic and venous blood pressures are partially dependent on the patient's autonomic tone but are easily manipulated by increasing or decreasing venous drainage and by administering vasopressors or vasodilators. Thus circulatory parameters during CPB are controlled in large part by the perfusionist and the anesthesiologist.

C. Circulatory changes during CPB
1. Changes at onset of CPB.
At commencement of CPB, there is usually a fall in systemic blood pressure due to several factors. Blood pressure is determined by cardiac output and systemic resistance, and the decreased blood pressure must be due to a fall in one or both of these parameters.

a. Usually pump flow rates are comparable to cardiac output prior to initiating CPB, and decreases in blood pressure due to decreased "cardiac output" are unusual.

b. The major cause of decreased blood pressure at the initiation of CPB is a dramatic decrease in systemic vascular resistance (SVR). This phenomenon is due to

(1) Decreased blood viscosity secondary to hemodilution by the pump priming fluid.

(2) Decreased vascular tone secondary to

(a) Dilution of circulating catecholamines.

(b) Temporary hypoxemia. Hypoxemia due to initial circulation of pump priming fluid has also been postulated as a cause of decreased SVR.

2. Circulatory status during hypothermic CPB

a. Increased SVR. There may be considerable patient-to-patient variations in SVR response during CPB. However, as CPB progresses, there will generally be a steady increase in systemic pressure due to increasing SVR if flow rates are kept constant. However, SVR rarely exceeds the values that are present prior to initiation of CPB. The observed increase in SVR during the course of CPB is probably due to several factors:

(1) Actual decreases in vascular cross-sectional area due to closure of portions of the microvasculature.

(2) Constriction of vascular tree due to
   (a) Hypothermia.
   (b) Increasing levels of circulating catecholamines.

(3) Increase in blood viscosity secondary to hypothermia, increased urine output, or translocation of fluid into the interstitial compartment (variable effects).

Patients undergoing coronary artery bypass grafting (CABG) have a higher SVR prior to and during CPB compared to patients undergoing repair of valvular lesions.

b. Decreased SVR. Transient decreases in SVR and systemic pressure may be observed shortly after infusion of cardioplegic solutions, especially if these solutions contain nitroglycerin.

c. Flow rate. Cardiac output or pump flow rates are completely under external control and can be manipulated at will. Pump flow rates are usually expressed as ml/kg or, more frequently as liters $\cdot$ min$^{-1} \cdot$ m^{-2}. In awake patients, it is generally accepted that a cardiac index less than 2.0–2.2 liters $\cdot$ min$^{-1} \cdot$ m^{-2} is not sufficient to provide tissues with an adequate oxygen supply. This also appears to be the lower limit of sufficient cardiac output during **normothermic** CPB. With increasing degrees of hypothermia, the patient's oxygen demand decreases, and consequently **pump flow rates may be reduced significantly.** Kirklin has calculated curves relating oxygen consumption to pump flow rates at differing temperatures (Fig. 20-1). These hyperbolic curves are mathematically expressed by the equation

$$\dot{V}O_2 = 0.4437(Q - 62.7) + 71.6$$

and describe "best fit" lines for measured $\dot{V}O_2$ at varying flow rates (using nonpulsatile flow) from several animal studies. The small x's on each curve represent clinically used flow rates at each temperature at the University of Alabama. Pump flow rates greater than 2.2 liters $\cdot$ min$^{-1} \cdot$ m^{-2} at normothermia do not result in greater tissue oxygen consumption and expose blood to greater damage from higher shear rates. The significance of oxygen consumption will be discussed later in sec. 4.c.

d. Arterial blood pressure. Although acceptable flow rates are fairly well established, there is considerably more controversy about acceptable arterial pressures during CPB. At any given flow rate, there is marked variability in arterial pressure from patient to patient. The overriding concern with low arterial pressures is adequacy of organ perfusion. The brain and kidney are the organs at greatest risk. Short periods of hypotension with a mean arterial pressure (MAP) of less than 30 mm Hg are certainly well tolerated.

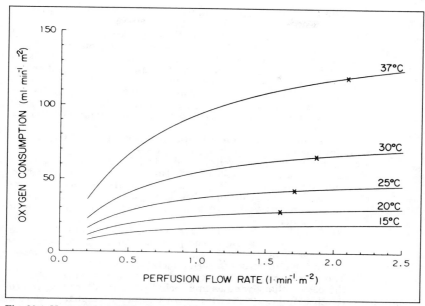

Fig. 20-1. Nomogram relating oxygen consumption ($\dot{V}O_2$) to perfusion flow rate ($\dot{Q}$) and temperature (T). (From J. W. Kirklin and B. G. Barratt-Boyes. Hypothermia, Circulatory Arrest, and Cardiopulmonary Bypass. In J. W. Kirklin and B. G. Barratt-Boyes [eds.], *Cardiac Surgery.* New York: Churchill Livingstone, 1986. P. 35. With permission.)

Fox and others have demonstrated that cerebral autoregulation is fairly well preserved during moderately hypothermic CPB [2]. Govier et al. demonstrated that cerebral blood flow was relatively constant down to a MAP of about 30 mm Hg in patients who were normotensive preoperatively and in whom alpha-stat blood gas management was employed during hypothermic CPB [3]. In this study, flow rates were held constant and low arterial pressure represented low systemic vascular resistance. Despite these findings, many anesthesiologists use vasopressors and vasodilators to keep mean arterial pressure between arbitrarily set limits of 50 and 100 mm Hg during CPB. Some institutions, notably the Stanford group, routinely use lower flow rates and lower perfusion pressures than those described above with no greater reported incidence of mortality. [4]

The disadvantages of higher arterial pressures during CPB are more rapid rewarming of the ischemic heart secondary to greater flow through noncoronary collaterals and possibly greater risk of cerebral hemorrhage in anticoagulated patients. In addition, pump tubing disconnections are more likely with higher line pressure and patient pressures.

3. **Circulatory changes during the rewarming phase of cardiopulmonary bypass**
   a. As the perfusate temperature is increased to rewarm the patient, variable circulatory responses are observed depending on the anesthetics used, patient hematocrit, underlying disease, and other factors. Frequently SVR and MAP increase during rewarming

from 25°C to 32°C. Occasionally, as temperature increases above 32°C, SVR and MAP will decrease.

    b. A more consistent decrease in SVR and MAP usually occurs with release of the aortic cross-clamp and reperfusion of the heart. Despite cardioplegia and hypothermia, there is some degree of ongoing metabolic activity and utilization of myocardial energy stores during cardiac arrest. When the heart is reperfused, accumulated metabolites are washed out of the heart into the general circulation. Some of these metabolites, most notably **adenosine,** are potent vasodilators that induce a marked decrease in SVR.

4. Changes in the microcirculation and adequacy of tissue perfusion during cardiopulmonary bypass

    a. During CPB, cardiac output and arterial pressure can be easily maintained at "normal" values. However, several observations suggest that tissue perfusion and oxygen delivery can be impaired to varying degrees during CPB. These factors are

        (1) Postoperative organ dysfunction, both temporary and permanent.

        (2) Variable decreases in oxygen consumption during normothermic CPB at flows and pressures that are comparable to pre-CPB values.

        (3) Variable increases in serum lactate levels.

    b. The microcirculation lies between the precapillary arterioles and the postcapillary venules and includes the capillary bed, the interstitial fluid space, and the microcirculatory lymphatics. Normal microcirculatory physiology is poorly understood and requires further clarification. However, it is clear that microcirculatory function during CPB may be impaired by

        (1) Constriction of precapillary arteriolar sphincters with or without formation of arteriolar-venular shunts.

        (2) Increased interstitial fluid volume (edema).

        (3) Decreased lymphatic drainage.

        (4) Loss of pulsatile flow.

        (5) Inefficient flow or "sludging" in the capillaries.

            Attempts to optimize microcirculatory function during CPB may include use of vasodilators to inhibit arteriolar constriction, addition of mannitol to the pump priming fluid to inhibit interstitial fluid accumulation, use of pulsatile perfusion techniques, and hemodilution to a hematocrit between 25% and 30% to optimize capillary flow.

    c. Monitoring adequacy of tissue perfusion. The best indicator of adequacy of perfusion during CPB is the absence of any significant postoperative organ dysfunction. Ideally, however, one would prefer some means of ensuring adequacy of perfusion during CPB rather than waiting to see if the patient exhibits any organ dysfunction postoperatively. The most precise indicator of adequate perfusion would be the measurement of actual tissue PO_2. However, this cannot be done easily in the clinical setting. Therefore, other, less precise measures of adequacy of perfusion are employed.

        (1) Global measures of adequacy of perfusion. In anesthetized patients who are not on CPB, microcirculatory function is assumed to be normal, and tissue oxygen consumption is assumed to be constant. In these patients oxygen delivery to tissues can be assumed to be adequate if cardiac output and arterial oxygen content are normal. Arterial oxygen content is easily monitored by determination of hematocrit and analysis of arterial blood gases. Cardiac output can be monitored grossly by measurement of blood pressure, palpation of peripheral pulses, or observation of capillary refill. More precise information about cardiac output can be obtained with thermodilution techniques utilizing pulmonary artery catheters. Also, if arterial oxygen content is stable, oxygen consumption or mixed venous oxygen content (or mixed venous PO_2 or oxygen saturation) can be used as indicators of cardiac output and tissue oxygen levels.

(a) The usefulness of $C\bar{v}O_2$ **and** oxygen consumption as indicators of cardiac output and tissue perfusion during CPB is based on the Fick equation, which relates cardiac output ($\dot{Q}$) to oxygen consumption ($\dot{v}O_2$) and the difference between arterial and mixed venous oxygen content ($CaO_2 - C\bar{v}O_2$)

$$VO_2 = Q(CaO_2 - C\bar{v}O_2)$$

Under normal physiologic circumstances, oxygen consumption and CaO_2 are relatively constant and are independent of perfusion. Under these conditions, $C\bar{v}O_2$ varies directly with changes in cardiac output and is a useful index of perfusion.

$$C\bar{v}O_2 = CaO_2 - \frac{VO_2}{Q}$$

During CPB, however, $C\bar{v}O_2$, represented by the partial pressure of oxygen in mixed venous blood ($P\bar{v}O_2$), varies with changing temperatures, and cardiac output is under the control of the perfusionist. Further, one can no longer assume that microcirculatory function is normal during CPB. When arterial blood is shunted past closed portions of the microvasculature, $C\bar{v}O_2$ will increase despite reduced tissue perfusion. Therefore:

(i) $C\bar{v}O_2$ alone can be a deceptive indicator of tissue perfusion, an abnormally high $C\bar{v}O_2$ indicating either excess cardiac output or hypoperfusion with closed microvasculature and shunting of arterial blood.

(ii) Oxygen consumption, because it considers both cardiac output and $C\bar{v}O_2$, provides a somewhat better index of perfusion. A normal oxygen consumption for any given temperature usually indicates **at least** adequate tissue perfusion. The difficulty arises, however, in determining what is the **normal** $\dot{V}O_2$ for a given patient at a given temperature. Based on the absence of significant organ dysfunction following CPB during which $\dot{V}O_2$ values were determined, Fox et al. have suggested that a measured $\dot{V}O_2$ of 85% of the maximum predicted value for a given temperature will ensure adequate tissue perfusion and oxygen delivery (see Fig. 20-1).

(iii) If the "normal" relationships between $C\bar{v}O_2$, or $P\bar{v}O_2$, cardiac output, and temperature were determined, as has been done for oxygen consumption, then measured values of $P\bar{v}O_2$ would become a more sensitive indicator of perfusion.

(b) **Lactate levels.** Theoretically, if tissue perfusion is inadequate, serum lactate levels should increase secondary to increased anaerobic metabolism. With closure of or shunting past the microcirculation, lactate buildup from ischemic tissue may not be washed out into the venous blood until reestablishment of normal microcirculatory flow. Often high levels of lactate reflected in large base deficits occur with reinstitution of bypass after a prolonged period of circulatory arrest.

Unfortunately, increases in serum lactate levels are variable and have not proven to be useful moment-to-moment indicators of tissue perfusion.

   (2) Monitoring specific organ function during CPB as a means of ensuring adequate tissue perfusion
   (a) Cerebral function. In awake patients cerebral perfusion is assumed to be adequate if the patient is conscious and mentating normally. Because patients on CPB are anesthetized, paralyzed, and hypothermic, the level of consciousness and appropriate mentation cannot be used as signs of cerebral perfusion. Electroencephalography (EEG), evoked responses, and cerebral blood flow monitors may be used, but effects of anesthetic medication and hypothermia also limit their usefulness as cerebral function monitors.
   (b) Renal function. Urine output is the simplest measure of renal function. However, different blood flow patterns, varying perfusion pressures, effects of hypothermia, and the presence or absence of diuretics in the pump priming fluid may affect urine output and render it an inaccurate indicator of overall tissue perfusion.

5. Pulsatile versus nonpulsatile flow during cardiopulmonary bypass. One of the major physiologic derangements introduced by CPB is loss of pulsatility of flow. Intuitively, it would be desirable to reproduce normal flow patterns as closely as possible while patients are undergoing CPB. However, there is considerable controversy about the merits of pulsatile perfusion compared with conventional nonpulsatile perfusion.
   a. How to produce pulsatile flow. Several methods are commonly employed to maintain arterial pulsations during CPB.
   (1) If partial CPB is being used, variable amounts of blood may be left in the patient to produce some cardiac ejection.
   (2) If an intraaortic balloon is in place, it may be used to impart pulsatility to the flow.
   (3) Pulsations may also be produced by roller pumps designed to rotate at varying speeds.
   b. Damping effects of the aortic cannula. The first two methods of producing pulsations are much more effective because they generate the pulse in the aorta itself. Though many pumps produce effective pulsations in the pump outflow, they are limited by the damping effects on the amplitude of the pulsations caused by the narrow aortic cannula.
   c. Nature of pulse waveform. The energy and dynamics of the normal arterial pressure waveform are very complex. It is becoming increasingly evident that more significant differences between pulsatile and nonpulsatile perfusions are manifest when the pulse contour more closely resembles the normal arterial pulse. Many early studies that found no significant differences between the two techniques employed pulse contours that were nearly sine wave in nature, in contrast to those using the rapid systolic upstroke and slower diastolic runoff characteristic of the normal arterial pulse.

Table 20-1. Advantages of pulsatile perfusion

Parameter studied	Purported advantage of pulsatile flow
Renal function	
Isolated kidney preparations	Greater renal venous return at any given flow rate
	Less pooling of blood in kidney
	Less microscopic evidence of ischemia
	Less tissue hypoxia or metabolic acidosis
	Greater maintenance of cortical blood flow
	More rapid resumption of function in transplanted homografts preserved with pulsatile perfusion
Whole animal experiments	Greater urine output
	Greater creatinine clearance
Edema formation, lymph flow	More rapid clearance of dye injected into interstitial space
	Greater capillary flow
	Less capillary sludging
	Less microscopically observed perivascular edema
Oxygen consumption	Greater oxygen consumption at any given flow rate
	Less accumulation of lactic acid
Mean arterial pressure, total peripheral resistance	Both parameters increase less during pulsatile perfusion

    d. Microvascular effects of pulsatile flow. Approximately twice as much energy is required to produce pulsatile as nonpulsatile flow. This additional energy may be transferred to the microvasculature where it may
      (1) Hold open capillary beds.
      (2) Enhance diffusion of oxygen and other substrates secondary to "vascular shocks" or "jiggling" of perivascular interstitial fluid.
      (3) Enhance lymph formation and flow secondary to the "pumping" action of arterial pulsation, reducing edema formation.
    e. Advantages of pulsatile flow. The table above is a summary of the claimed advantages of pulsatile perfusions compared with conventional nonpulsatile perfusions (Table 20-1). For every study supporting these advantages there is at least one other study concluding that there are no differences between pulsatile and nonpulsatile flow. Most clinical studies involving patients on CPB have failed to show any significant differences between pulsatile and nonpulsatile flow. Difficulties encountered in demonstrating any differences between the two techniques may be attributable to the adaptive and compensatory responses of patients. In any event, the controversy over pulsatile versus nonpulsatile flow needs further clarification and is likely to continue for some time.
II. Cardiopulmonary bypass as an oxygen delivery system
    A. Oxygenator function. The details of oxygenator design and the efficiency of those designs are discussed in detail in Chap. 19. The oxygenator serves the function of the lungs—namely, oxygenation of, and elimination of carbon dioxide from, the venous blood. During CPB the intricacies of pulmonary physiology are eliminated, and gas exchange occurs merely by bringing blood and gas into direct contact (bubble

oxygenators) or close proximity (membrane oxygenators). The resulting PaO_2 and $PaCO_2$ are determined by the FiO_2 of the gas mixture and the rate at which the gas mixture flows through the oxygenator. Varying amounts of carbon dioxide may be added to the gas mixture flowing through the oxygenator (see sec. **III.4.a.**)

B. **Blood gas monitoring during cardiopulmonary bypass.** Modern oxygenators are very efficient gas exchangers, and arterial blood gas tensions are easily and precisely controlled by the perfusionist. Frequent blood gas determinations are becoming less necessary with the advent of in-line blood gas monitors in the CPB circuit. During normothermic CPB arterial blood gases are maintained near conventional values: pH 7.40, $PaCO_2$ 35–45, and PaO_2 more than 100.

III. **Hypothermia and cardiopulmonary bypass**

A. **Effects of hypothermia on biochemical reactions.** The Q_{10} for chemical reactions is a measure of changes in rate of reaction for a change in temperature of 10°C. For human tissues, the Q_{10} is approximately 2. That is, for each 10° decrease in body temperature, the rate of reaction (i.e., metabolic rate or oxygen consumption) is roughly halved.

B. **Effects of hypothermia on blood viscosity.** Hypothermia increases blood viscosity. In the early history of CPB, hemodilution was not performed, and the high morbidity and mortality were probably secondary to this hyperviscous state (i.e., stroke, organ infarcts). Today, all patients are hemodiluted to hematocrits of 20–30% during CPB. Although oxygen-carrying capacity is decreased secondary to hemodilution, oxygen delivery is improved because the decreased viscosity provides improved microcirculatory flow.

C. **Changes in blood gases associated with hypothermia**

1. **Changes in oxygen-hemoglobin dissociation curve.** As temperature decreases, the affinity or strength of binding between oxygen and hemoglobin is increased. A lower partial pressure of oxygen is required to force a given amount of oxygen onto the hemoglobin molecule. The oxygen-hemoglobin dissociation curve is shifted to the left. Release of oxygen from hemoglobin at the tissue level is less efficient.

2. **Changes in solubility of oxygen and carbon dioxide.** As temperature decreases, gases become more soluble in liquid. For a given amount of oxygen or carbon dioxide, more gas will be dissolved in the plasma, and the partial pressure of the gas will decrease. This is much more significant for carbon dioxide because it is very soluble in plasma at any given temperature.

3. **Changes in arterial blood gases of poikilotherms and hibernators, and behavior of in vitro blood samples, with varying temperatures**

a. **In vitro blood samples.** If a sample of normal arterial blood with pH of 7.40, $PaCO_2$ 40, and PaO_2 90–100 is placed in a gas-free, blood-filled, airtight container, the pH and $PaCO_2$ will vary predictably with changes in temperature. The carbon dioxide content of the blood remains constant. As the blood cools, more carbon dioxide goes into solution, and the $PaCO_2$ decreases.* Concomitantly, the pH increases. For each degree Celsius decrease in temperature, the pH increases 0.0147 units:

$$\Delta pH/°C = 0.0147$$

*The molecular interaction of water and carbon dioxide is decreased with hypothermia and therefore formulation of H^+ is minimal.

b. Poikilotherms. Observations of poikilothermic animals indicate that arterial blood gases vary with temperature, as described above. Poikilotherms behave as if they were closed systems with a constant carbon dioxide content. In reality, they are open systems in which carbon dioxide content is held relatively stable by the balance between carbon dioxide production in the tissues and carbon dioxide elimination by the lungs.

c. Hibernating animals. In contrast to poikilotherms, hibernators appear to maintain blood pH close to 7.4 (measured at their actual temperature) as their temperature decreases. To do this, they must increase the carbon dioxide content of their blood. They seem to have evolved a different but equally effective means of dealing with hypothermia.

4. Differing strategies of blood gas analysis and interpretation in hypothermic human subjects. There has been considerable controversy about appropriate blood gas values for hypothermic humans. The question is whether hypothermic patients should be treated as if they were poikilothermic or hibernating animals. The two strategies have become known, respectively, as the alpha stat and pH stat methods of blood gas interpretation.

a. pH stat method. This strategy of blood gas management aims at keeping arterial pH at or close to 7.4 at any given temperature (i.e., the patient is treated as if he were a hibernating animal). Usually the maintenance of pH at 7.4 requires the addition of carbon dioxide to the oxygenator gas mixture. Because most blood gas machines measure every blood sample at 37°C, complex formulas are used to calculate the derived blood gas values for a hypothermic patient at his actual body temperature. If the patient's pH at 28°C is 7.4, when the blood is warmed to 37°C in the machine, it will have a measured pH of 7.26.

b. Alpha stat method. The alpha stat strategy of blood gas interpretations is based on the premise that the pH of blood is regulated to keep the stage of dissociation of the imidazole moiety (i.e., the alpha of imidazole) constant. Histidine, which contains the imidazole moiety, is an integral part of the active site of many enzyme systems. Enzyme function has been shown to be optimal in an environment in which the ratio of $OH^-:H^+$ ions is about 16:1. As we shall see, this ratio represents different pH values at different temperatures.

(1) Using the alpha stat technique, one simply draws an arterial blood sample from the patient and analyzes it at 37°C. If the values are appropriate at 37°C, they are assumed to be appropriate for the hypothermic patient regardless of his actual temperature (i.e., the patient is treated as if he were a poikilotherm).

(2) Observations that support the alpha stat technique are as follows:

(a) **Neutrality of water.** Neutral water is water in which the $[H^+]$ is equal to the $[OH^-]$. At 37°C the pH of neutral water is 6.8. At 25°C the pH of neutral water is 7.4. As temperature decreases, the pH at which water is "neutral" changes in a linear fashion. The neutral pH increases 0.017 units for each degree Celsius decrease in temperature.

$$\Delta pH/°C = 0.017$$

(b) **Constancy of $OH^-:H^+$ ratio.** Clearly human blood is not neutral. That is, $[OH^-]$ is not equal to $[H^+]$. Instead, the observed ratio is approximately 16:1, resulting in a pH of

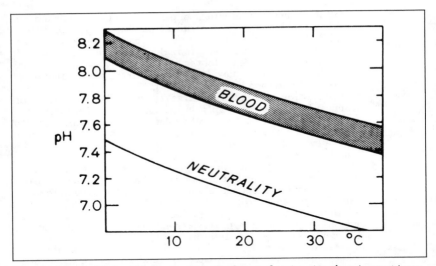

Fig. 20-2. Blood pH of poikilotherms and pH of neutral water at various temperatures (values at actual temperatures). (Modified from H. Rahn, R.B. Reeves, and B.J. Howell. Hydrogen ion regulation, temperature, and evolution. The 1975 J. Burns Amberson Lecture. *Am. Rev. Respir. Dis.* 112:167, 1975. With permission.)

7.4 instead of 6.8 at 37°C. In poikilothermic animals and in vitro human blood samples this 16:1 ratio is maintained as the temperature varies. Consequently, the pH of blood is maintained about 0.6 units more alkaline than the neutral pH of water at any given temperature, but both curves parallel one another (Fig. 20-2). It is hypothesized that this constancy of OH^-:H^+ ions maintains a state of dissociation of the imidazole of histidine that results in optimal enzyme function despite varying temperatures.

(c) **Buffer systems.** Albery and Lloyd proposed that the in vitro behavior of blood requires a buffer system with a pK value near 7.0 [1]. Reeves demonstrated that the imidazole of the peptide-histidine buffer system satisfies this requirement. Aqueous solutions of carbonic acid, bicarbonate, and imidazole in concentrations resembling those in blood produce a pH versus temperature curve that has a slope similar to the one characteristic of the in vitro behavior of blood [6].

c. Which strategy of blood gas management is more appropriate?
(1) Studies contrasting alpha stat and pH stat indicate that myocardial function during hypothermic CPB is better preserved when the alpha stat method is employed. When pH was held at 7.4 by addition of carbon dioxide, myocardial lactate extraction decreased, indicating the presence of either myocardial ischemia or, more likely, depression of cellular function due to a relatively acidotic condition. Also, during pH stat perfusions contractility, myocardial oxygen consumption, and coronary blood flow have been shown to decrease. These observations are believed to indicate depressed cellular function in the acidotic environment produced by maintaining the actual body temperature pH at 7.4 during hypothermia. Similar

depression of cellular function may occur in other organs as well.

    (2) Maintenance of cerebral blood flow autoregulation appears to remain intact with alpha stat management, whereas flow becomes pressure passive with pH stat management [5].

    (3) Based on the preceding findings most centers now use alpha stat management of arterial blood gases during hypothermic CPB. However, outcome studies to date have failed to demonstrate the superiority of one method over the other.

IV. Systemic effects of the bypass environment

A. Hematology

    1. Coagulation. Changes in the coagulation cascade, platelets, and fibrinolytic cascade are discussed in Chapter 10.

    2. Changes in formed elements

      a. Red blood cells (RCBs)

        (1) During CPB red cells become stiffer and less distensible. This change may interfere with microcirculatory blood flow. Stiffer RBCs are also more susceptible to hemolysis.

        (2) Hemolysis and free hemoglobin. During CPB, RBCs are exposed to nonphysiologic surfaces and shear stresses. The degree of hemolysis is increased by both higher flow rates and the accompanying increase in rate of shear, and by a greater gas-filled interface in the CPB apparatus. As red cells are lysed, the free hemoglobin produced is bound to haptoglobin. When the amount of free hemoglobin generated exceeds the binding capacity of haptoglobin, serum hemoglobin concentrations increase, and hemoglobin begins to be filtered by the kidney, resulting in hemoglobinuria.

      b. Leukocytes. CPB affects primarily neutrophils (polymorphonuclear leukocytes, PMNs) and to a lesser degree monocytes. Shortly after the onset of CPB there is a marked decrease in circulating PMNs (Fig. 20-3). Neutrophil counts decrease to a greater extent and remain decreased longer when membrane oxygenators are used. The reason for this difference is unknown. The observed neutropenia is due to both margination of neutrophils along vessel walls and aggregation of neutrophils. Examination of biopsy specimens indicates that neutrophils are sequestered primarily in the pulmonary circulation. However, margination, diapedesis, and both intravascular and extravascular accumulation of PMNs has also been demonstrated in the microcirculation of heart and skeletal muscle. Blockage of vessels by PMNs or microcirculatory derangements induced by substances released from PMNs may contribute to organ dysfunction after CPB.

        As CPB progresses, a rebound neutrophilia becomes evident and is more pronounced in patients treated with corticosteroids. The neutrophilia is less dramatic during hypothermia, but circulating PMN levels increase dramatically on rewarming. Both neutrophils released from the pulmonary circulation and younger cells released from the bone marrow contribute to the observed neutrophilia.

        Effects of CPB on host defense functions of PMNs are controversial. Studies demonstrating decreased responsiveness of PMNs to chemotactic and aggregating stimuli indicate impaired defense mechanisms. However, other studies indicate that the bacteriocidal activity of PMNs is increased for up to 3 days following CPB.

    3. Changes in plasma proteins. Proteins are globular molecules with very specific structures. Generally, polar, hydrophilic groups are ori-

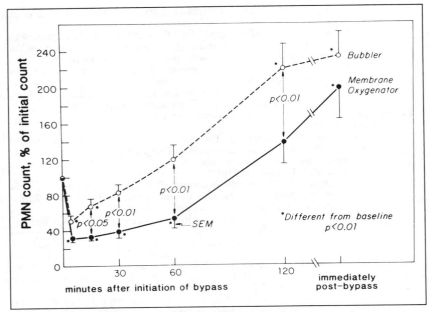

Fig. 20-3. Neutrophil counts during cardiopulmonary bypass, expressed as percentage of prebypass values. (From D. E. Hammerschmidt, D. F. Stroncek, T. K. Bowers, et al. Complement activation and neutropenia occurring during cardiopulmonary bypass. *J. Thorac. Cardiovasc. Surg.* 81:372, 1981. With permission.)

ented toward the outside of the molecule, and nonpolar, hydrophobic groups are located internally. When proteins approach a gas-liquid interface, strong electrostatic forces at that interface result in varying degrees of unfolding of these molecules by disrupting the internal sulfhydryl and hydrogen bonds.

a. Consequences of protein denaturation

    (1) **Altered enzymatic function.** Denatured proteins lose some or all of their function. This may be one mechanism by which coagulation becomes impaired during and after CPB.

    (2) **Aggregation of proteins.** Denatured proteins have a tendency to aggregate and may produce precipitates. IgM aggregates are strong activators of the complement cascade.

    (3) **Altered solubility characteristics.** Denatured proteins are less soluble in plasma and cause increased blood viscosity.

    (4) **Release of lipids.** Denaturation of lipoproteins and the protein fractions of chylomicrons results in chylomicron aggregates and free lipid globules in the circulation. These lipid emboli may become large enough to occlude small vessels.

    (5) **Absorption of denatured proteins onto cell membranes.** RBCs may become "sticky." Resulting red cell aggregates promote capillary sludging and may contribute to microcirculatory dysfunction.

b. Membrane oxygenators may induce less protein denaturation by virtue of the absence of a direct gas-fluid interface.

4. Activation of humoral cascade systems

a. **Coagulation and fibrinolytic cascade systems.** See Chapter 18.
b. **Complement system.** Stimulation of PMNs to aggregate and adhere to vessel walls is probably mediated by activated components of the complement cascade. The complement system consists of about 20 proteins that play an integral part in host defense. Activation of the complement cascade facilitates the inflammatory reaction, resulting in opsonization of bacteria, increased capillary permeability, and activation of leukocytes. Intense and excessive activation can result in membrane damage, organ dysfunction, and activation of other humoral cascades.

   During CPB, activated complement component C3a and C5a increase. Conversely, there is depletion of inactive complement precursors as demonstrated by significant depression of CH_{50}.

   The complement cascade may be activated by antibody molecules through the classic pathway after reaction with a specific antigen or following minor denaturation of antibodies. The cascade can also be activated through an alternate pathway by many macromolecular structures such as endotoxin, zymogen, thrombin, and plasmin. Both pathways probably play a roll in complement activation during CPB.
c. **Kallikrein-kinin cascade.** Activation of this cascade elaborates bradykinin and other substances that may contribute to increased vascular permeability during CPB.
B. **Fluid balance and interstitial fluid accumulation during CPB**
   1. Starling's law of transcapillary fluid movement describes fluid fluxes at the microcirculatory level. Alteration in the determinants of fluid flow during CPB favors interstitial fluid accumulation. The following table lists the factors in the Starling equation that are altered by CPB and measures that may be used to counteract these CPB-induced derangements (Table 20-2).
C. **Central nervous system changes.** Most patients who have undergone CPB sustain no major permanent neurologic dysfunction despite the vulnerability of the central nervous system (CNS) to ischemic or anoxic insults. CNS damage may be caused by decreased perfusion of the brain secondary to low blood flows or embolic occlusion of vessels or to adequate perfusion with a hypoxic perfusate. The latter scenario is rare and easily preventable. Embolic phenomena and changes in CNS perfusion are more likely to occur during CPB.
   1. **Changes in cerebral autoregulation.** Normally, autoregulation holds cerebral blood flow fairly constant between mean arterial pressures of 50–100 mmHg. Establishment of CPB itself does little to affect autoregulation. However, some anesthetic drugs are known to inhibit autoregulation to varying degrees. As hypothermia is introduced, cerebral blood flow decreases in proportion to decreases in cerebral metabolic rate. Although flow rates or arterial pressure may decrease, autoregulatory functions keep CBF relatively constant over a wide range of flows and pressures provided alpha stat blood gas management is maintained.
   2. **Adequate perfusion pressure.** Flow-pressure relationships and adequacy of perfusion have been discussed previously. In awake hypertensive patients the autoregulatory curve is shifted to the right. Although no comparable shift has been demonstrated in hypertensive patients on CPB, it may be wise to keep perfusion pressures higher than those seen in normotensive patients. Likewise, patients with occlusive cerebrovascular disease may benefit from higher pressures during CPB.

Table 20-2. Starling equation: tissue fluid accumulation = $K[(P_C - P_{IF}) - \sigma(\pi_C - \pi_{IF})] - Q_{LYMPH}$

Parameter of Starling equation		CPB-induced derangement	Possible countermeasures
K	= Permeability coefficient of capillary membrane	↑ By complement activation	Administer corticosteroids?
		↑ by vasoactive substances released from neutrophils or platelets	Administer corticosteroids or prostaglandin inhibitors?
P_c	= Mean intracapillary hydrostatic pressure	↑ Venous pressure	Ensure adequate venous drainage
		↑ Arterial pressure	Administer vasodilators
			Ensure adequate anesthesia
P_{IF}	= Mean interstitial hydrostatic pressure	Unchanged	None
σ	= Reflection coefficient of macromolecules	Unchanged	None
π_c	= Intracapillary oncotic pressure	↓ By hemodilution	Add albumin or mannitol to pump prime
π_{IF}	= Interstitial oncotic pressure	Unchanged	None
Q_{LYMPH}	= Lymph flow	↓ By microcirculatory dysfunction or loss of pulsatility of flow	Use pulsatile flow?

3. **Embolic phenomena.** Most neurologic morbidity that results during CPB is due to emboli of various types. Air embolization is a significant risk during CPB for any procedure but is more likely during procedures involving opening of cardiac chambers. Emboli may also consist of preexisting thrombi, platelet and leukocyte aggregates, fat globules, or foreign substances from the CPB apparatus.

4. **Impact of blood glucose levels on postischemic neurologic sequelae.** Recent studies of anoxic brain damage suggest that injury is greater when preischemic blood glucose levels are high. One theory to explain this finding is that metabolism, and the subsequent generation of oxygen-free radicals and other metabolites, is greater when the preischemic glucose is high, resulting in more cellular damage. It may be prudent to keep blood glucose levels between 100 and 200 mg/dl during CPB. If glucose-free solutions are utilized, blood sugar levels should be determined to rule out hypoglycemia (usually unlikely, especially after institution of CPB).

D. **Renal function**

1. **Significance of urine output during CPB.** Urine output is a crude indicator of renal function. There is no correlation between the amount of urine output during CPB and the incidence of postoperative renal failure. Urine output is greater when mean arterial pressure is higher, when pulsatile perfusion is employed, and when mannitol is added to pump priming fluids.

2. **Decreased tubular function.** Tubular function is depressed by hypothermia alone. During CPB tubular function is further depressed, resulting in reductions in urine output.

3. **Renal blood flow.** Global renal blood flow usually decreases during CPB secondary to diminished flow rates and pressures or loss of pulsatility. As in other low-flow or shocklike states, there is a redistribution of renal blood flow from the cortex to the outer medulla. This redistribution of blood flow appears to be less severe during pulsatile perfusion.

4. **Hemoglobinuria.** Intravascular hemolysis resulting in hemoglobinuria can cause acute tubular necrosis. It is not clear whether the mechanism is precipitation of pigment in the renal tubules and subsequent blockage of tubular flow or glomerular-tubular injuries caused by red cell stroma and other substances liberated from lysed RBCs.

5. **Renal failure.** Renal failure following CPB is a persistent cause of morbidity and mortality in cardiac surgical patients. Its incidence is reported to be less than 1% in adult patients but may be as high as 2–10% in infants undergoing open intracardiac operations. Development of renal failure depends more on the preoperative and postoperative hemodynamic state than on various manipulations used to maintain urine output during CPB.

E. **Hepatic function**

1. **Jaundice** may occur in up to 23% of patients following surgery employing CPB, but severe jaundice (bilirubin levels $\geq$ 6 mg/dl) occurs in only 6% of patients. As with renal failure, hepatic dysfunction is more dependent on hemodynamic status before and after CPB than on any direct effect of CPB. The probability of postoperative jaundice is high when right atrial pressures are elevated, when there is significant hypoxia during operation, when there is persistent hypotension following CPB, or when large amounts of blood are transfused. If hemodynamics and nutritional status are kept normal postoperatively, hepatic function will gradually improve.

F. **Pulmonary function**

1. **Complete versus partial CPB.** Complete CPB implies that all systemic venous blood is drained into the oxygenator, and there is ab-

solutely no blood flow to the right heart or pulmonary circulation. Complete CPB employs two venous cannulae with tapes around them to prevent blood from entering the right atrium. Partial CPB employs a single venous cannula or two venous cannulae without tapes. During partial CPB variable amounts of blood can flow into the right atrium and ventricle, through the lungs, and eventually reach the left heart. During partial CPB some anesthesiologists maintain minimal ventilation of the lungs to avoid delivery of hypoxic blood to the left heart. Also, flow of relatively warm blood through the pulmonary circuit can contribute to early rewarming of the heart.

2. **Pulmonary dead space, ventilation-perfusion ($\dot{V}/\dot{Q}$) mismatching after CPB.** Variable degrees of pulmonary dysfunction are seen after CPB. There is an almost inevitable increase in extravascular lung water during CPB. Development of intrapulmonary shunts and increased dead space ventilation result in less efficient matching of ventilation to perfusion. Increased dead space is reflected in greater end tidal-arterial carbon dioxide gradients after CPB in the majority of patients. $\dot{V}/\dot{Q}$ mismatching results in increased alveolar-arterial oxygen gradients and decreased PaO_2, and these are the most consistent abnormalities noted following CPB.

3. **Pulmonary sequestration of neutrophils and release of vasoactive compounds.** PMNs sequestered in the lung during CPB or dialysis may undergo release reactions causing localized, intense vasoconstriction or membrane damage with subsequent edema formation, resulting in increased dead space ventilation and $\dot{V}/\dot{Q}$ mismatching.

4. **Metabolic functions of the lung**
   a. **Inactivation of catecholamines.** Under normal circumstances the lung is a major site of inactivation of norepinephrine. During CPB the lungs are bypassed, and lack of degradation may contribute to the increasing levels of catecholamines seen during CPB. Following CPB and reinstitution of pulmonary blood flow, inactivation of catecholamines resumes. However, decreasing catecholamine levels during this time are primarily due to decreased production of catecholamines.
   b. The lung also plays a role in the renin-angiotensin system and in the metabolism of prostaglandins and serotonin. The physiologic impact of CPB on these functions is not well understood and merits further investigation.

5. **Sequestration of narcotics in the lungs.** This phenomenon has been described with fentanyl, which is widely used in cardiac anesthesia. The lungs have a high affinity for fentanyl. During CPB, plasma levels of fentanyl steadily decrease. On reperfusion of the lungs there is an increase in the plasma fentanyl concentration due to release of sequestered fentanyl and a further slow decline as fentanyl is metabolized.

6. **Changes in pulmonary vascular resistance and hypoxic pulmonary vasoconstriction**
   a. **Pulmonary vascular resistance (PVR).** Numerous factors influence pulmonary vascular tone following CPB. Many congenital cardiac lesions are associated with increased pulmonary resistance. Efforts to limit increases in PVR and maintain pulmonary blood flow include hyperventilation and administration of $NA^+HCO^-_3$ to maintain an alkaline pH, and maintenance of adequate oxygenation. Increased catecholamine levels during and after CPB may contribute to increased PVR. Likewise, catecholamine infusions can induce pulmonary vasoconstriction. Notable

exceptions are isoproterenol and dobutamine. Effects of CPB on increased PVR associated with underlying disease are unclear.

b. Hypoxic pulmonary vasoconstriction (HPV). Direct effects of CPB and hypothermia on HPV are poorly understood. However, use of volatile anesthetics and vasodilators after CPB may interfere with HPV, leading to $\dot{V}/\dot{Q}$ mismatching and decreasing PaO_2.

7. Postpump pulmonary dysfunction. Pulmonary dysfunction following CPB may range from mild decreases in PaO_2 to full-blown respiratory failure resembling the adult respiratory distress syndrome. Most patients exhibit some decrease in PaO_2 immediately postoperatively, and it is difficult to predict which patients will develop more serious pulmonary insufficiency.

Those patients who develop greater respiratory insufficiency exhibit further increases in $A\text{-}aDO_2$ and decreases in PaO_2 during the second postoperative day. Mild hyperventilation is noted. The chest x ray reveals patchy infiltrates and small areas of consolidation. During the next 36–48 hours $\dot{V}/\dot{Q}$ mismatching worsens, with shunt fractions reaching 20–40% of cardiac output. Pulmonary compliance decreases, resulting in further increases in respiratory rate. Chest x ray shows increasing pulmonary edema and confluence of pulmonary infiltrates. By the third or fourth postoperative day the full-blown picture of respiratory failure has developed. Arterial hypoxemia is severe with shunt fractions reaching more than 40%. The lungs are extremely noncompliant, requiring 50–80 cm H_2O of airway pressure to maintain ventilation. The chest x ray reveals the classic "white out" or complete opacification of all lung fields.

Although full-blown respiratory failure following CPB is relatively rare, its incidence is directly related to preoperative pulmonary dysfunction, duration of CPB, and postoperative hemodynamic status. Events during CPB which may contribute to development of pulmonary dysfunction include:

a. Decreased pulmonary blood flow due to
  (1) Emboli of various composition leading to localized areas of $\dot{V}/\dot{Q}$ mismatching and edema formation
  (2) Localized vasoconstriction due to elevated endogenous catecholamines, catecholamine infusions, or substances released from PMNs trapped in the pulmonary capillaries.

b. Edema formation enhanced by membrane damage due to
  (1) Complement activation. Activated complement components increase membrane permeability.
  (2) Vasoactive compounds released from PMNs. These enhance capillary permeability and may lead to localized areas of interstitial edema.
  (3) Oxygen free radicals. Direct cellular toxins can lead to altered permeability at the capillary level.

c. Edema formation secondary to increased pulmonary hydrostatic pressure, which is due to
  (1) Inadequate left ventricular venting.
  (2) Increased bronchial blood flow.

G. Stress or neuroendocrine response to CPB

1. Serum catecholamine levels. During CPB and aortic cross-clamping, circulating levels of both epinephrine and norepinephrine increase significantly (Fig. 20-4). Epinephrine levels increase more dramatically, indicating that the response is primarily adrenomedullary in nature. It has been suggested that catecholamine release may be triggered through reflexes initiated by baroreceptors and chemoreceptors in the heart and lung when those organs are excluded from the circulation.

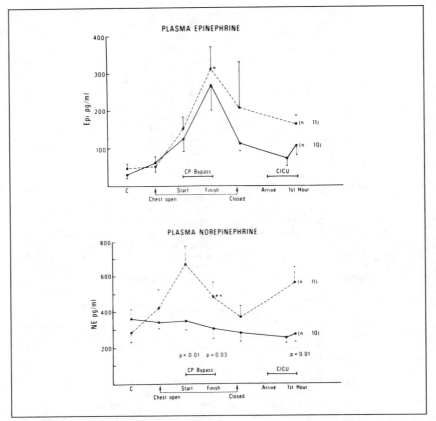

Fig. 20-4. *Top.* Changes in plasma epinephrine during and after CABG surgery in patients with *(dashed line)* and without *(solid line)* postoperative hypertension. *Bottom.* Changes in plasma norepinephrine during and after CABG surgery in patients with *(dashed line)* and without *(solid line)* postoperative hypertension. (From R. Wallach, R. B. Karp, J. G. Reves, et al. Pathogenesis of paroxysmal hypertension developing during and after coronary bypass surgery: A study of hemodynamic and humoral factors. *Am. J. Cardiol.* 46:562-563, 1980. With permission.)

    a. **Hypertensive versus normotensive patients.** Serum norepinephrine levels rise to higher levels and remain elevated for longer periods in patients known to be hypertensive prior to surgery and in patients exhibiting hypertension after CPB, regardless of the presence or absence of preoperative hypertension.

    b. **Significance of increased catecholamines.** Elevated catecholamine levels may have adverse effects on regional and organ blood flow patterns. Also, catecholamines increase myocardial oxygen consumption. Reperfusion of the heart with blood containing high concentrations of catecholamines may adversely affect the balance between myocardial oxygen supply and demand during this critical time.

2. **Other "stress hormones."** As does any major stress, CPB causes increases in antidiuretic hormone, cortisol, glucagon, and growth

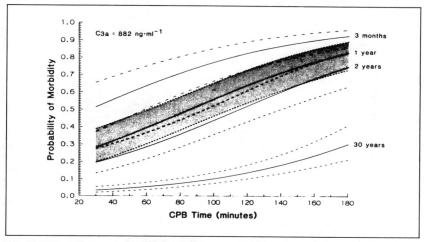

Fig. 20-5. Probability of morbidity related to duration of cardiopulmonary bypass in pediatric patients of different ages. Mean C3a level of 882 mg·ml⁻¹ at conclusion of CPB. (From J. K. Kirklin, S. Westaby, E. H. Blackstone, et al. Complement and the damaging effects of cardiopulmonary bypass. *J. Thorac. Cardiovasc. Surg.* 86:853, 1983. With permission.)

hormone. The effect of these substances is to increase catabolic reactions, leading to consumption of energy, tissue breakdown, and possible impairment of wound healing. Glycogenolysis and gluconeogenesis are enhanced, and the effects of insulin on glucose metabolism are inhibited. Patients undergoing CPB are relatively resistant to the effects of exogenously administered insulin.

VI. Summary. This chapter has focused primarily on the aberrations of normal physiology imposed by the bypass environment, with only secondary emphasis on specific organ dysfunction. Certainly not all of the pathophysiology described is seen in every patient undergoing CPB. Many patients appear to suffer no ill effects at all. Indeed, the absence of significant organ dysfunction is probably the best indicator of successful CPB. Post-CPB organ dysfunction constitutes a spectrum ranging from mild dysfunction in one or more organ systems to death resulting from irreparable damage to one or more organ systems. The probability of significant morbidity increases with duration of CPB and decreasing age of the patient within the pediatric age group (Fig. 20-5). Morbidity has also been correlated with C3a levels measured 3 hours following CPB (Fig. 20-6).

The impact of preexisting organ dysfunction on post-CPB morbidity is not well defined, but it seems likely that poor overall condition prior to CPB results in greater morbidity after CPB.

Finally, it should be emphasized that placing a patient on CPB is a physiologic trespass against that patient. Absence of significant damage caused by CPB depends primarily on a particular patient's ability to compensate for the derangements introduced by that trespass.

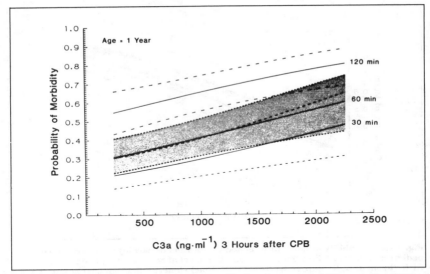

Fig. 20-6. Probability of morbidity related to C3a levels measured 3 hours after CPB for three different time periods on CPB. (From J. K. Kirklin, S. Westaby, E. H. Blackstone, et al. Complement and the damaging effects of cardiopulmonary bypass. *J. Thorac. Cardiovasc. Surg.* 86:853, 1983. With permission.)

REFERENCES

1. Albery, W. J., and Lloyd, B. B. Variation of Chemical Potential with Temperature. In A. V. de Reuck and R. Porter (eds.), *Development of the Lung.* Boston: Little, Brown, 1967. Pp. 30–33.
2. Fox, L. S., Blackstone, E. H., Kirklin, J. W., et al. Relationship of brain blood flow and oxygen consumption to perfusion flow rate during profoundly hypothermic cardiopulmonary bypass. *J. Thorac. Cardiovasc. Surg.* 87:658–664, 1984.
3. Govier, A. V., Reves, J. G., McKay, R. D., et al. Factors and their influence on regional cerebral blood flow during nonpulsatile cardiopulmonary bypass. *Ann. Thorac. Surg.* 38:592–600, 1984.
4. Kolkka, R., and Hilberman, M. Neurologic dysfunction following cardiac operation with low-flow, low-pressure cardiopulmonary bypass. *J. Thorac. Cardiovasc. Surg.* 79:432–473, 1980.
5. Murkin, J. M., Farrar, J. K., Tweed, W. A., et al. Cerebral autoregulation and flow/metabolism coupling during cardiopulmonary bypass: The influence of $PaCO_2$. *Anesth. Analg.* 66:825–832, 1987.
6. Reeves, R. B. An imidazole alphastat hypothesis for vertebrate acid-base regulation: Tissue carbon dioxide content and body temperature in bullfrogs. *Resp. Phys.* 14:219–236, 1972.

SUGGESTED READINGS

Kirklin, J. K., Westaby, S., Blackstone, E. H., et al. Complement and the damaging effects of cardiopulmonary bypass. *J. Thorac. Cardiovasc. Surg.* 86:845–857, 1983.
Kirklin, J. W., and Barratt-Boyes, B. G. Hypothermia, Circulatory Arrest, and Cardiopulmonary Bypass In J. W. Kirklin, and B. G. Barratt-Boyes (eds.), *Cardiac Surgery.* New York: Wiley, 1986. P. 29.

Mavroudis, C. To pulse or not to pulse. *Ann. Thorac. Surg.* 25:259–271, 1978.

Ratliff, N. B., Young, W. G., Hackel, D. B., et al. Pulmonary injury secondary to extracorporeal circulation. *J. Thorac. Cardiovasc. Surg.* 65:425–432, 1973.

Reves, J. G., Karp, R. B., Buttner, E. E., et al. Neuronal and adrenomedullary catecholamine release in response to cardiopulmonary bypass in man. *Circulation* 66:49–55, 1982.

Rudy, L. W., Heymann, M. A., and Edmunds, L. H. Distribution of systemic blood flow during cardiopulmonary bypass. *J. Appl. Physiol.* 34:194–200, 1973.

Solen, K. A., Whiffen, J. D., and Lightfoot, E. N. The effect of shear, specific surface and air interface on the development of blood emboli and hemolysis. *J. Biomed. Mater. Res.* 12:381–399, 1978.

White, F. N. A comparative physiologic approach to hypothermia. *J. Thorac. Cardiovasc. Surg.* 82:821–831, 1981.

Myocardial Preservation During Cardiopulmonary Bypass

Craig B. Wisman, Christopher J. Peterson, and Frederick A. Hensley, Jr.

I. Introduction

A. Goals. For all forms of intracardiac surgery two goals must be met.

  1. A motionless, bloodless heart.
  2. A heart that has not been significantly structurally or functionally impaired by the lack of adequate oxygen or metabolic substrates.

B. Historical perspectives

  1. Inflow occlusion and profound hypothermia (1950s)

   a. Early cardiac surgeons employed simple inflow occlusion combined with aortic cross-clamping to provide a bloodless but not motionless field.

   b. Moderate hypothermia (32°C) was employed, primarily to protect the brain, but allowed only about 10 minutes of effective operating time.

   c. The use of extracorporeal circulation with profound hypothermia (15°C) and aortic cross-clamping provided a motionless and relatively bloodless field that was safe for up to 1 hour [4].

  2. Elective cardiac arrest (1960s). Gerbode, Melrose and others popularized "elective cardiac arrest" [5]. They injected a solution of 2.5% potassium citrate into the aortic root after applying a cross-clamp. This provided a flaccid empty heart. Other clinicians modified the technique and developed other "cocktails" based on potassium, magnesium, neostigmine, and other agents.

   a. The technique did work and was at least technically easier in many patients than profound hypothermia.

   b. Impairment of postarrest myocardial function was reported by Waldhausen [10]. and others, and fatal myocardial necrosis was linked to the use of potassium citrate-induced cardiac arrest [7].

   c. The clinical use of elective cardiac arrest virtually disappeared by the mid 1960s.

  3. Continuous coronary perfusion (1960s–1970s). Because of the technical limitations of profound hypothermia and the apparent difficulties attributed to elective cardiac arrest, surgeons turned to what appeared to be the most natural of methods, continuous coronary perfusion.

   a. At normothermia or slight hypothermia the coronary arteries were perfused through the aortic root or individually with special perfusion catheters.

   b. Elective ventricular fibrillation with coronary perfusion was used to produce less cardiac motion.

   c. Subendocardial necrosis was still observed, especially in hypertrophied hearts. Buckberg was able to relate subendocardial necrosis to disordered distribution of coronary flow associated with poor coronary perfusion and ventricular fibrillation [1].

   d. Technical problems associated with cannulation of individual coronary arteries such as dissection and late stenosis were also reported.

  4. Normothermic ischemia (1970s). Although coronary perfusion was popular, the cumbersome cannulae and the occasional disasters resulting from direct coronary perfusion prompted some to advocate simple normothermic aortic cross-clamping.

   a. This technique never achieved great popularity but is still practiced today by some cardiac surgeons.

  5. The return of elective cardiac arrest (1970s)

   a. The cardiac necrosis that occurred with earlier potassium citrate arrest solutions was attributed to a high potassium concentration. Subsequently, solutions with lower concentrations of potassium were found to be safe and effective means of arresting myocardial activity.

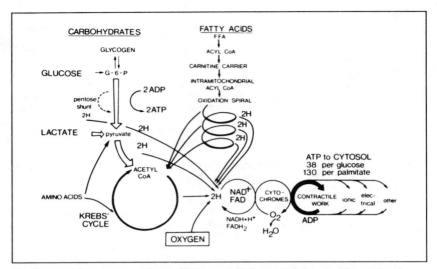

Fig. 21-1. The major myocardial fuels are carbohydrates (glucose and lactate) and non-esterified free fatty acids (FFA). Ultimately, all fuels are broken down to acetyl coenzyme A (CoA), which produces hydrogen atoms (H) by various dehydrogenases to form reduced nicotinamide adenine dinucleotide (NADH$_2$ or NADH + H$^+$), which in turn interacts with the cytochrome chain to produce adenosine triphosphate (ATP). Fatty acids also produce reduced flavin adenine dinucleotide (FADH$_2$) from the oxidation spiral, which likewise enters the cytochrome chain. One molecule of glucose undergoing complete oxidation produces 36 molecules of ATP. In the absence of oxygen, glucose undergoing aerobic glycolysis provides a net of only two ATP molecules that can be used for cardiac work. G-6-P = glucose 6-phosphate; ADP = adenosine diphosphate. (From L. H. Opie. Fuels. In L. H. Opie [ed.], *The Heart.* New York: Grune & Stratton, 1984. P. 111. With permission. Figure copyright by L. H. Opie.)

    b. The combination of a biochemical contractile "arrest" with cardiac hypothermia seemed to meet most of the needs of the surgeon and the patient. Using the cardioplegic solution to cool the heart as well as to arrest it was conceptually and mechanistically elegant.

C. General principles of myocardial metabolism. To appreciate existing techniques of myocardial protection and to develop new and rational methods of preservation, the metabolic basis of ischemia must be understood.

    1. Overview of metabolism (Fig. 21-1).

        a. Each of the metabolic pathways shown in Fig. 21-1 are available in the myocardium for production of high-energy phosphates (adenosine triphosphate [ATP] and creatine phosphate [CrP], which provide the energy for contraction and all cellular functions) given the availability of the substrates (glucose, lactate, free fatty acids [FFA], ketone bodies and amino acids) and oxygen.

        b. In the absence of oxygen essentially all pathways are shut down except anaerobic glycolysis.

    2. Control of myocardial metabolism. Regulation of energy production by metabolic pathways is controlled by

        a. Substrate availability

            (1) The myocardium can use almost any available substrate to produce energy (this was originally shown by Bing in the 1800s using coronary sinus sampling).

(2) In a fasted individual (NPO past midnight) who has high levels of circulating FFAs, FFAs are the primary substrate utilized (70%).

(3) In a patient receiving a glucose and insulin infusion, glucose would be the major substrate.

(4) A high plasma level of lactic acid, such as occurs after rigorous exercise, seizures, or sepsis, would promote lactate utilization by the heart.

b. Enzyme levels. Myocardium is the classic "red" muscle.

(1) It maintains a high activity of oxidative enzymes and is efficient during continuous activity in the presence of oxygen.

(2) Thirty-five percent of the total volume of heart muscle is composed of mitochondria.

(3) The heart functions poorly under hypoxic conditions because of the low activity of glycolytic enzymes and the low energy yield per substrate molecule under anaerobic conditions (2 molecules of ATP under anaerobic conditions versus 36 ATP molecules produced under aerobic conditions for each molecule of glucose utilized).

c. Modification of enzymes. Enzyme modification occurs under normal conditions and with hypoxia and ischemia. Enzymes are either inhibited or stimulated to determine which pathways will be primarily utilized for energy production (Fig. 21-2).

(1) Normal state

(a) Seventy percent of energy utilized comes from free fatty acids.

(b) In the presence of oxygen, free fatty acid utilization yields high citrate and ATP levels, which by feedback mechanisms **inhibit glycolysis** at phosphofructokinase (PFK).

(2) Hypoxia or anoxia

(a) The presence of a low arterial oxygen tension (with preserved flow) stimulates glycolysis. This is the Pasteur effect.

(b) Without oxygen, oxidative metabolism ceases, and ATP and citrate levels decrease, adenosine monophosphate, adenosine diphosphate, and phosphate increase. These changes stimulate glycolysis at PFK.

(c) Glycogen breakdown is also stimulated, and glucose transport into the cell is increased tenfold.

(d) Even with accelerated glycolysis, the hypoxic heart generates only 5–7% of the ATP produced in well-oxygenated hearts.

(3) Ischemia

(a) Inadequate arterial blood flow results in limited substrate supply, decreased oxygen delivery, and, perhaps most important, decreased removal of the products of anaerobic metabolism.

(b) There is decreased oxidative metabolism with decreased ATP and CrP; also, lactate, hydrogen ions, and reduced nicotinamide adenine dinucleotide ($NADH_2$) accumulate because flow is inadequate to remove those products from the tissues or metabolize them.

(c) These end products inhibit glycolysis at PFK and glyceraldehyde-3-P-dehydrogenase and probably play a role in the irreversible damage seen with prolonged myocardial ischemia.

(d) High lactate levels, not low ATP and CrP, have been correlated with poor recovery of ventricular function in ischemic hearts [8]. This finding supports the use of multiple

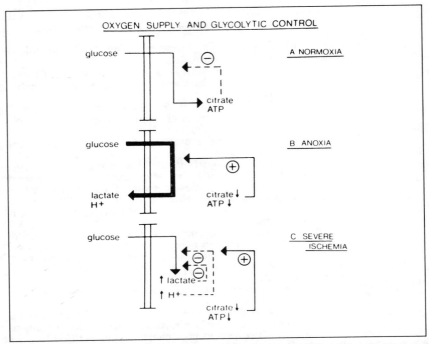

Fig. 21-2. Oxygen supply and glycolytic control. *A.* In the normally oxygenated heart, tissue citrate and adenosine triphosphate (ATP) levels are high, thereby inhibiting glycolysis and using minimal glucose. *B.* When oxygen is removed (because of hypoxia or anoxia) but the coronary flow rate is allowed to increase, glycolysis is stimulated, and glucose becomes the primary fuel. *C.* In severe ischemia (deprivation of both oxygen and coronary flow) the accumulation of lactate and protons inhibits glycolysis, shutting off the only method of myocardial production of ATP. (From L. H. Opie. Fuels. In L. H. Opie [ed.], *The Heart.* New York: Grune & Stratton, 1984. P. 112. With permission. Figure copyright by L. H. Opie.)

dose cardioplegia to wash out hydrogen ions, lactate, and other toxic metabolites (see sec. **III.B.**).

II. **Myocardial preservation during the initiation of cardiopulmonary bypass before cardioplegic arrest.** In the beating heart on cardiopulmonary bypass (CPB) prior to cross-clamping of the aorta, there are many factors that may adversely affect myocardial oxygen supply-to-demand ratio and lead to myocardial energy depletion and ischemia. Many of the same concerns of oxygen supply and demand presented here apply to both the aortic cross-clamp period (i.e., fibrillation and distention) and the period after the aortic cross-clamp is removed and coronary flow is reestablished. The problem of reperfusion injury is an additional concern in the time period after the cross-clamp is removed.

A. **Factors leading to decreased myocardial oxygen supply**

1. **A decreased hematocrit** of the CPB perfusate occurs when bypass is initiated. The hemodilution is most marked with a crystalloid prime.

2. **Air, debris,** and **emboli** may all lead to obstruction of coronary blood flow. The source of this material may be either atherosclerotic

plaque subsequent to cannulation or foreign material from the cardiopulmonary bypass circuit.

3. **Ventricular distention** may result from numerous causes. The most common cause is inadequate venous drainage. Inadequate drainage will lead to an increased left ventricular end-diastolic pressure and a subsequent decrease in subendocardial perfusion.

4. **Hypothermia** may reduce subendocardial blood flow, necessitating higher perfusion pressures [2].

5. Ventricular **fibrillation** may limit subendocardial blood flow with time secondary to a progressive increase in subendocardial vascular resistance. This increase in subendocardial vascular resistance may be the result of evolving myocardial edema.

6. **Tachycardia** minimizes diastolic filling time and flow to the subendocardium. Because the cold perfusate on initiation of cardiopulmonary bypass usually induces bradycardia, this is usually not a problem.

7. **Very low perfusion pressures** may limit coronary blood flow. A mean arterial pressure minus left ventricular end-diastolic pressure gradient of greater than 50–70 mm Hg is usually adequate.

8. The presence of **atherosclerotic coronary obstructions** may potentiate myocardial ischemia if low perfusion pressures and flows are present distal to the coronary stenoses. Measurements have been made of coronary artery pressures distal to coronary artery stenoses. In severe lesions there may be up to a 60 mm Hg difference between the distally measured pressure and the pressure in the proximal aorta. This suggests that collateral flow may not compensate for the pressure drop across the coronary lesion in severe coronary artery disease.

9. **Left ventricular hypertrophy** (LVH) further decreases the subendocardial blood flow, and the effects of fibrillation on oxygen supply are further enhanced in the presence of left ventricular hypertrophy [6] (Fig. 21-3).

B. **Factors leading to an increased myocardial oxygen demand.** Myocardial oxygen demand is decreased with initiation of bypass secondary to a decrease in preload and stroke work. This decrease in work load occurs even during partial bypass when the heart is still ejecting. However, because the heart still beats, energy demands are a function of contractility and heart rate.

1. An increased heart rate directly increases contractility (Bowditch effect). With initiation of hypothermic bypass, however, lower heart rates usually ensue. Studies with empty beating hearts show that oxygen consumption per minute decreases with the decrease in temperature primarily because of a decrease in heart rate. However, **oxygen consumption per beat increases** with a decrease in temperature, probably because of an increase in inotropic state, as shown by a greater intraventricular systolic pressure development at a given left ventricular end-diastolic volume [2].

2. Inadequate venous drainage to the CPB pump can increase ventricular preload to both the right and left ventricles, causing an increase in wall stress and a secondary increase in oxygen demand and a decrease in subendocardial blood supply.

3. On complete bypass afterload is not a concern because no ventricular ejection is occurring. However, if the heart is on partial bypass (partial heart ejection), theoretically afterload could increase myocardial oxygen demand.

4. **Fibrillation** in a **normal** nonhypertrophied, vented, normothermic, and spontaneously fibrillating heart creates a greater oxygen demand than when the same heart is spontaneously beating. However,

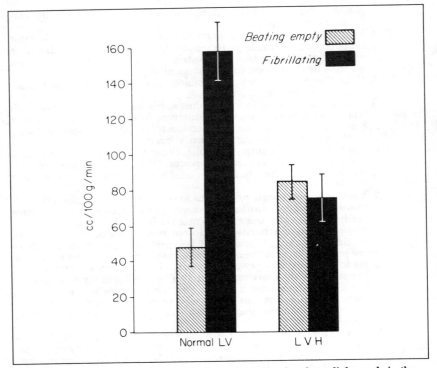

Fig. 21-3. Blood flow through dog left ventricular (LV) subendocardial muscle in the normal and hypertrophied heart (LVH) when the hearts are beating and nonworking and after 60 minutes of spontaneous ventricular fibrillation at normothermia. Mean arterial pressure was maintained at 100 mmHg by regulating pump flow. Note the approximately 300% increase in subendocardial flow during fibrillation in normal hearts. Conversely, coronary flow to the subendocardial muscle does not increase during fibrillation in hypertrophied hearts. (From C. E. Hottenrott, B. Towers, H. J. Kurkji, et al. The hazard of ventricular fibrillation in hypertrophied ventricles during cardiopulmonary bypass. *J. Thorac. Cardiovasc. Surg.* 66:746, 1973. With permission.)

blood flow to the inner shell of the left ventricle is increased to meet the increased demands. Coronary vascular resistance may increase with prolonged fibrillation and limit blood flow and oxygen supply.

In patients with **coronary artery disease** or **left ventricular hypertrophy** blood supply can **fail** to meet the increased demands even when the ventricle is collapsed and fibrillating spontaneously, thus jeopardizing oxygen supply-demand balance (Fig. 21-3).

5. **Distention** of the **left ventricle** in combination with fibrillation greatly increases oxygen demand and limits subendocardial blood supply. Decompression, usually by venting (see sec. **III.D.**) restores a more favorable supply-demand ratio and limits the amount of myocardial ischemia and damage.

6. **Cooling** a fibrillating heart increases the compliance of the ventricle, [2] which is opposite to the situation seen in the beating heart. In spite of this, wall tension is higher in the fibrillating heart than in the beating heart during diastole at the same temperature.

7. Electrical fibrillation is sometimes used in a perfused heart to allow repair of simple defects such as atrial septal defects. The current applied with electrical fibrillation is greater than the current generated during spontaneous fibrillation. As the frequency and voltage of electrical stimulation is increased there is:

  a. An increase in intramural tension.

  b. An increase in intraventricular pressure.

  c. An increase in oxygen needs.

  d. Decreased blood flow to the subendocardium.

  The rise in intraventricular pressure that occurs with electrical stimulation makes ventricular decompression mandatory to decrease oxygen consumption and increase subendocardial blood flow.

C. Management of oxygen supply and demand of the beating myocardium on CPB. Prior to application of the aortic cross-clamp:

  1. A hemoglobin concentration of between 7 and 10 gm/dl is probably adequate when on bypass to meet oxygen demands. Higher hemoglobin levels were associated with thrombotic and embolic complications in the early history of CPB. These were related to the increased viscosity of cold blood with a high hematocrit.

  2. Prevention of arterial emboli by proper bypass management includes the use of arterial line filters, avoiding the manipulation of vein grafts, and careful surgical technique.

  3. A perfusion pressure gradient greater than 50 mm Hg is probably adequate in patients **without** left ventricular hypertrophy or severe coronary artery disease.

  4. Tachycardia and increased contractility lead to increased oxygen demand at the initiation of bypass. Therefore, recommendations include discontinuing pacing at rapid rates and discontinuing inotropes if they were utilized in the prebypass period.

  5. Utilizing proper venting methods and ensuring adequate venous return to the pump helps to avoid ventricular distention. Raising the operating table also enhances venous drainage. Monitoring of left atrial and pulmonary artery pressures and palpation by the surgeon of the left ventricle should be performed to ensure that ventricular distention is not occurring.

D. Strategies for cooling the myocardium by the bypass circuit on initiation of bypass. There are essentially two accepted ways to cool the myocardium from the time of initiation of bypass until the aortic cross-clamp is applied. Both techniques have advantages and disadvantages, and no definitive studies have proved or disproved completely the overall benefit of one technique over the other.

  1. Gradual cooling. This technique involves a gradual cooling of the CPB perfusate by the heat exchanger of the CPB circuit. The cooled perfusate supplies the coronary blood and reduces myocardial oxygen demand. The cross-clamp is applied when ventricular fibrillation occurs.

   a. Theoretical advantages

     (1) More uniform cooling of the myocardium in a beating heart as long as possible.

     (2) Low myocardial oxygen demand with potential energy repletion (continuous oxygenated blood flow) prior to the further ischemia associated with aortic cross-clamping.

   b. Disadvantage. The technique may require a longer period on bypass. Lidocaine 1–2 mg/kg may be administered to prevent ventricular tachycardia and fibrillation during cooling with this technique.

    2. Rapid cooling. Rapid onset of profound cooling of the perfusate results in early ventricular fibrillation, and the aortic cross-clamp is then applied.

      a. Advantage. Shorter bypass time.

      b. Theoretical disadvantage. Patchy cooling of the myocardium, especially when severe coronary lesions are present.

E. Management suggestions for specific cardiac pathologies

    1. Coronary artery disease and severe left ventricular hypertrophy. The **mean arterial pressure** should be maintained at **greater than 70 mm Hg** in the presence of severe coronary disease or left ventricular hypertrophy prior to cross-clamp placement. Premature ventricular fibrillation may occur if there is a low perfusion pressure at the onset of bypass in the setting of left ventricular hypertrophy or coronary disease. If the rapid cooling procedure described above is utilized, the cross-clamp is immediately applied, and cardioplegic solution is administered. Therefore, when this cooling technique is utilized, maintenance of perfusion pressure in this higher range limit is probably not as important as it is during the longer gradual cooling procedure.

    2. Severe aortic regurgitation. Management should be aimed at keeping the mean perfusion pressure of the heart on bypass at less than 50 mm Hg prior to aortic cross-clamp placement. This is done to **prevent distention** of the left ventricle (LV) due to regurgitant flow of blood into the LV secondary to the incompetent valve. Therefore, vasopressors such as phenylephrine should not be utilized during this time. Often a left ventricular vent is placed prior to initiation of bypass to prevent ventricular distention.

III. Current technique of intraoperative myocardial preservation during aortic cross-clamping (cardioplegic arrest)

A. Key components of the cardioplegic arrest technique. There are two key components to successful myocardial preservation:

    1. Hypothermia reduces oxygen consumption and high-energy phosphate utilization of the heart and other organs. The rate of enzymatic reactions is roughly halved for each 10°C decrease in temperature.

    2. Electromechanical arrest prevents **rapid** depletion of energy stores because most of the heart's energy is used to fuel myocardial contraction.

B. Clinical application of cardioplegic arrest

    1. The technique of **multiple dose** cardioplegia serves three primary goals:

      a. To maintain the myocardium at an optimum temperature.

      b. To deliver agents needed to maintain the arrested state, which may have been depleted through metabolism or diffusion, or washed out by collateral blood flow.

      c. To wash out metabolic products that inhibit anaerobic metabolism and cause irreversible ischemic damage and decrease myocardial performance (see sec. **I.C.**).

C. Hypothermia. Present cardioplegic techniques rely heavily on the cooling capacity of the cardioplegic infusate, which is generally delivered at between 4 and 12°C. However, virtually all surgeons also employ some form of supplemental external cooling technique to aid the initial induction of hypothermia and to maintain hypothermia during the operative procedure.

    1. Protective effects. Hypothermia will maintain electromechanical silence as the initial chemical cardioplegic agent is washed out by noncoronary collateral circulation. In addition to its use in reducing basal energy utilization, hypothermia may provide additive protective effects on intracellular membranes. Stabilization of membranes by hypothermia-induced lipid phase transitions may reduce calcium- or oxygen-mediated reperfusion injury.

2. **Disadvantages.** Hypothermia is not without drawbacks. Cold injury can occur because inhibition of the sodium-potassium transmembrane pump can lead to intracellular ion redistribution and subsequent cellular edema.

3. **Technique—initial cooling by infusion of the cardioplegic solution.**
   a. The infusion of cold cardioplegic solution (4–12°C) into the aortic root provides rapid and direct myocardial cooling.
   b. Occlusive coronary artery disease can cause uneven distribution of cardioplegic cooling. Regional variations and significant epicardial and endocardial differences have been demonstrated.
   c. Monitoring of myocardial temperature during the initial infusion of cardioplegia, especially if it is monitored in multiple regions, may demonstrate areas of inadequate preservation.

4. **External cooling**
   a. One of the simplest techniques is irrigation of the pericardium with saline or lactated Ringer's solution at 4°C. Variations on the technique involve continuous versus intermittent irrigation and drainage methods.
   b. Ice is commonly added to the pericardial wall.
      (1) **Advantages**
         (a) Ice stabilizes temperature and reduces or eliminates the need for continuous irrigation.
         (b) Ice can achieve colder intrapericardial temperatures.
      (2) **Disadvantages.** Ice can cause phrenic nerve injury (temporary or permanent). Because of this, its routine use is declining [9].
   c. Other techniques such as wrap-around jackets with circulating cold water or cold gel-filled bags exist, but all are cumbersome and have limited utility, especially when work is being done on the posterior aspect of the heart.

5. **Cardiac rewarming.** Despite external cooling, the myocardium will rewarm after the initial infusion of cold cardioplegia. The major causes of rewarming are
   a. **Warm venous return blood.** The blood temperature is almost always about 20°C, and venous return to the right atrium will rewarm it and the atrial septum. If bicaval cannulae are employed, especially with caval snares (i.e., complete bypass), this effect is lessened or eliminated.
   b. **Conductive transfer from warmer pericardial tissues.** The surrounding tissues of the mediastinum are, at best, at the arterial perfusion temperature, which is 20°C or greater. Direct contact, especially with the posterior LV, allows conductive heat transfer. Continuous pericardial irrigation, cooling pads or jackets, and foam insulation pads reduce this effect.
   c. **Noncoronary collateral circulation.** Myocardial blood flow derived from noncoronary arterial sources is a small fraction of total myocardial flow, but it can be increased in patients with long-standing ischemic coronary occlusive disease or after previous cardiac surgery (mediastinal adhesions). This flow cannot be readily controlled by physical maneuvers on the operative field. Maintaining low systemic arterial temperatures and minimizing systemic perfusion pressure are the only effective remedies.
   d. **Heat transfer** to the heart from the environment is difficult to quantify, but it seems reasonable to keep the room temperature low during the ischemic period.

Table 21-1. Cardioplegia additives

Constituent	Rationale
Blood	Provide oxygen
KCl	Maintain arrest
THAM	Buffer
Histidine	Buffer
Sodium bicarbonate	Buffer
Aspartate	Substrate enhancement
Glutamate	Substrate enhancement
Glucose	Substrate enhancement
Mannitol	Prevent edema
Coenzyme Q	Oxygen radical scavenging
Procaine, lidocaine	Abolish vasoconstriction
Nitroglycerin	Abolish vasoconstriction
Calcium channel antagonists	Limit calcium entry
	Abolish vasoconstriction

6. **The ideal temperature.** The ideal temperature to be maintained during ischemia is not known, and clinical and experimental "ideal temperatures" may not be the same. Practical use dictates that myocardial temperatures be maintained between 8° and 15°C.

D. **Biochemical cardiac arrest**
1. **Hyperkalemia.** The second component of modern cardioplegia is electromechanical arrest. Hyperkalemic solutions infused into the coronary arteries cause rapid cessation of electrical and mechanical activity, the major energy consumers of the heart. By rapidly stopping the major energy demands, depletion of high-energy phosphates during the period of cooling is reduced.

   a. **The mechanism of hyperkalemic diastolic arrest.** Hyperkalemia induces diastolic arrest by producing depolarization of the membrane and inhibiting membrane repolarization. Depolarization caused by increased extracellular K^+ ($[K^+]_o$) lowers the resting membrane potential (causing it to become less negative) toward the threshold potential and depolarizes the cell. Intracellular calcium (Ca^{2+}) rises, and contraction occurs. Ca^{2+} is then sequestered in intracellular sites, and the myocardium relaxes, but the cell membrane remains depolarized, and repolarization is prevented. The value of the resting membrane potential in ventricular myocardium is about -84 mV at a $[K^+]_o$ of 5.4 mEq/liter and -60 mV at $[K^+]_o$ of 16.2 mEq/liter. At this level the fibers are inexcitable to ordinary stimuli.

   b. Historically, potassium citrate was utilized first, however, magnesium, acetylcholine, neostigmine, and local anesthetics such as procaine have all been employed clinically to arrest the heart electively.

   c. Most modern cardioplegic solutions are based on potassium chloride, with potassium concentrations generally ranging between 15 and 30 mEq/liter.

2. **Other cardioplegic components** (Table 21-1)
   a. Osmolality is adjusted with albumin or mannitol. Most solutions are iso-osmolar or slightly hyperosmolar.

b. Calcium is present at least in small amounts to avoid the "calcium paradox" on reperfusion (see sec. **III.G.6.**).

c. Other additives may include vasodilators (nitroglycerin, calcium channel blockers), glucose and insulin, and lidocaine. Compelling data supporting the use of each agent are not available.

3. Blood versus crystalloid cardioplegia. There is controversy at present about whether cardioplegic solutions based on dilute blood solutions provide better myocardial protection than asanguinous crystalloid-based solutions. The hematocrit of blood cardioplegia varies from 10–25% depending on the clinical technique. Many clinical experimental studies purport to compare these two techniques. Comparisons are difficult because varying clinical and experimental techniques are used.

  a. Theoretical advantages of blood-based cardioplegia
    (1) Blood can carry much more oxygen than asanguinous solutions.
    (2) It has superior buffering capacity.
    (3) Plasma proteins provide important osmotic balance.

  b. Theoretical disadvantages of blood-based cardioplegia
    (1) Mixing and delivery systems are more complex.
    (2) Osmotic regulation does not require plasma proteins.
    (3) Hemoglobin cannot transfer much oxygen at hypothermic delivery temperatures.
    (4) Myocardial oxygen requirements may be satisfied with oxygenated crystalloid solutions (oxygen bubbled through crystalloid cardioplegia prior to administration).

  c. Some surgeons recommend a period of warm induction cardioplegia in patients with significant preoperative cardiac dysfunction. In this technique, warm hyperkalemic blood-based cardioplegic solution (often with "substrate enhancement") is infused after the cross-clamp is applied. Theoretically, this allows the myocytes to replenish depleted high-energy phosphates prior to global ischemia.

E. Technical aspects of cardioplegia infusion

  1. Pressure. The cardioplegia solution is generally infused into the coronary arteries at a pressure approximating the normal mean aortic pressure (80–100 mm Hg). Excessive pressure results in myocardial edema, and low infusion pressure can result in maldistribution of cardioplegia solution.

  2. Temperature. Most crystalloid solutions are infused at 4–10°C, and most blood-based solutions are infused at 10–12°C (to avoid potential red cell aggregation).

  3. Reinfusion. Most surgeons reinfuse cardioplegia periodically during the ischemic period, intervals between infusions being determined by time or myocardial temperature. Some surgeons infuse only one dose of cardioplegic solution initially and rely on external cooling to maintain myocardial preservation. In this situation the end products of metabolism are not washed out, and one of the key benefits of multiple-dose cardioplegia is lost.

  4. Retrograde cardioplegia. In most cardioplegia techniques the cardioplegic solution is infused antegrade into the aortic root or into the coronary arteries directly. As previously mentioned (see sec. **3b**) in the case of obstructive coronary lesions, maldistribution of the cardioplegia can occur. Experimental and limited clinical use of retrograde cardioplegia techniques (infusion into the coronary veins through the coronary sinus) shows promise as a means of improving delivery of cardioplegia solution. Current techniques are technically more difficult than routine antegrade methods but are undergoing further development.

F. Venting. Mechanical aspects of the conduct of cardiopulmonary bypass also affect myocardial preservation. Routine left ventricular venting of the heart is infrequent in the current practice of cardiac surgery when the cardiac chambers are not opened. The salutary effects of this technique warrant familiarity with it. Preload and ventricular distention can be minimized by venting.

1. Decompression of the ventricle can be accomplished in many cardiac procedures by good venous drainage through the venous return cannula(e) and an aortic root vent (usually incorporated as part of the cardioplegic administration apparatus).

2. Monitoring of left atrial pressure (LAP) or pulmonary artery pressure (PAP) is beneficial in patients who are not vented or minimally vented (aortic root vent) and is important for determining the need for ventricular decompression. In vented hearts this may help determine the efficiency of venting. Concern should arise if the PAP or LAP is more than 15 mm Hg.

3. In the unvented heart, decompression should be provided if ventricular distention is detected. Decompression can be achieved by
   a. Changing the surgical traction on the heart.
   b. Rearranging the venous cannula(e).
   c. Correcting mechanical obstruction to blood flow extrinsic to the heart.
   d. Decreasing the bypass flow rate or increasing the level of venous gravity drainage.
   e. If the above measures are unsuccessful a form of left ventricular venting should be considered, usually in addition to the aortic root vent (Fig. 21-4).

4. **Advantages of venting**
   a. A dry surgical field is created, which is especially important during distal graft anastomoses in a myocardial revascularization operation. Usually an aortic root vent is adequate for this purpose.
   b. Oxygen consumption is reduced by decreasing myocardial wall tension.
   c. Impedance to subendocardial blood flow is reduced by lowering wall tension.
   d. Rewarming resulting from return of warm blood is decreased.
   e. Distribution of cardioplegic solution, especially to the subendocardium, is improved.
   f. Evacuation of intracardiac air before the patient is taken off CPB (especially after open cardiac procedures) can be performed through appropriate vents.

5. **Disadvantages of venting**
   a. Operative time may be prolonged for placement or removal of a vent or repair of a vent site.
   b. Air may be entrained into the heart, especially if beating occurs.
   c. Technical problems may arise including bleeding.
   d. Damage to the ventricle may result when vents are inserted through the ventricular tissue.
   e. Venting by pulmonary artery decompression does not ensure left ventricular decompression, and a pressure gradient may exist between the atrium and the ventricle.

6. Venting of the left ventricle during cardiac procedures has been an area of clinical controversy. Much of the data supporting the use of venting was acquired before the current use of cold cardioplegic arrest and was generated in hearts undergoing prolonged periods of ventricular fibrillation. Most recent studies suggest that venting

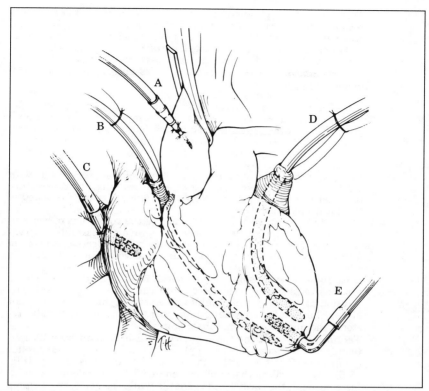

Fig. 21-4. Drawing of the sites for venting the left heart. _A._ A Texas Heart Institute aspirating needle in the ascending aorta proximal to the cross-clamp. _B._ Cannulation of the area between the superior vena cava and the aorta with the cannula extending down into the left ventricle. _C._ Cannulation of the right superior pulmonary vein with the cannula in the left atrium. If a longer cannula is used, it may be threaded into the left ventricle (this is a very common approach used to perform left ventricular venting). _D._ Cannulation of the left atrial appendage with the cannula positioned in the left ventricle. _E._ Cannulation of the ventricular apex. (From C. C. Reed and T. B. Stafford. Cannulation. In C. C. Reed and T. B. Stafford [eds.], _Cardiopulmonary Bypass_ [2nd ed.]. Houston: Texas Medical Press, 1985. P. 277. With permission.)

during cardiac surgery using cold cardioplegic arrest may improve postarrest myocardial function.

7. With cold cardioplegic arrest, venting is more important during the early postischemic reperfusion period, when elevated intraventricular pressure may reduce subendocardial perfusion and increase metabolic needs of the heart.

G. **Reperfusion injury.** Reperfusion injury is a term used to describe damages, both functional and ultrastructural, that become apparent during the reestablishment of flow following a period of ischemia. In addition to relieving ischemia, restoring perfusion may result in a number of deleterious effects, including

1. Necrosis of irreversibly injured myocytes.
2. Marked increases in cell swelling (myocardial edema).
3. Nonuniform return of blood flow to all portions of the myocardium.

This is termed the **"no reflow" phenomenon** and is the failure to reestablish microcirculatory flow despite the reestablishment of macrocirculatory flow. This is the result of the vicious circle of vascular endothelial edema, reduced local perfusion, more damage, more edema, and so on. Its incidence and severity may be reduced by maintaining modest reperfusion pressures and adding oncotic supplements to the reperfusate.

4. Conversion of ischemia to a hemorrhagic infarct, resulting in extension of myocardial necrosis and decreased compliance of the ventricle.

5. Oxygen-derived free radicals that disrupt membranes through lipid peroxidation. Free-radical scavengers such as superoxide dismutase, catalase, and mannitol have theoretical and experimental support for their use during reperfusion, but none, other than mannitol, is currently routinely used clinically.

6. If perfused with a calcium-free cardioplegic solution, reperfusion with calcium will cause membrane damage, cell swelling, and contracture (the "calcium paradox"). Hence, a small amount of Ca^{2+} is added to the cardioplegic solution.

H. **Controlled reperfusion.** Efforts to modify the conditions of reperfusion have been proposed in an effort to improve myocardial preservation. Controlled reperfusion has been used for selective control of myocardial perfusate flow, temperature, and composition before the aortic cross-clamp is removed [3].

1. **Rationale.** The infusion into the aortic root, while the cross-clamp remains in place, of oxygenated blood cardioplegic (hyperkalemic) solution at normothermia maintains electromechanical silence but allows the cellular enzymatic processes to proceed and rapidly restores the high-energy phosphate stores.

2. **Technique.** Separating the coronary perfusion circuit from the systemic perfusion circuit is accomplished by using an auxiliary roller pump to perfuse the aortic root proximal to the cross-clamp. (Fig. 21-5). Warm (normothermic) oxygenated blood cardioplegia is infused through the cardioplegia cannula while the aortic cross-clamp is still applied. This allows the surgeon to control completely the pressure and temperature of the coronary perfusion during the critical initial reperfusion period. After an initial period of reperfusion with warm blood cardioplegia (usually about 5 minutes), reperfusion is continued with normothermic blood from the oxygenator for an additional 10–15 minutes or until vigorous cardiac activity is present. Aortic root perfusion pressure is maintained at 50 mm Hg for the first minute and then at 70–80 mm Hg thereafter. Rapid increases in the resistance of the coronary vascular bed can be easily detected and treated immediately with coronary vasodilators (typically nitroglycerin) injected directly into the aortic root (Fig. 21-5). Rapid increases in coronary vascular resistance, if they occur, are most common in the first 10–20 minutes after reperfusion is initiated[3].

3. These specialized techniques appear to be most useful when the myocardium has been compromised significantly prior to the period of ischemia, such as in patients with markedly reduced ejection fraction or in those who are in cardiogenic shock due to an acute event.

4. Venting the heart is an important part of all controlled reperfusion techniques.

IV. **The right ventricle: special concerns.** As improved techniques of myocardial preservation allowed patients to survive extended periods of ischemia with satisfactory left ventricular function, occasional episodes of severe right ventricular dysfunction have called attention to the unique needs of the right ventricle.

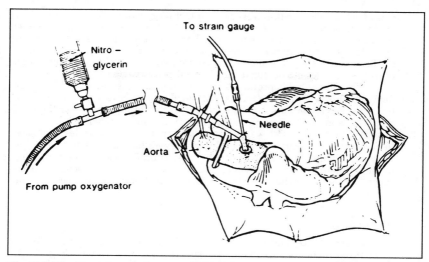

Fig. 21-5. The arrangements for controlled aortic root reperfusion. The aortic arterial cannula (not shown) is in place distal to the aortic cross-clamp in the position indicated by the purse-string suture. A 14Fr trimmed hepatic artery catheter with a thin-wall pressure recording needle incorporated within it has been inserted into the ascending aorta just after cardiopulmonary bypass has been established. The catheter is connected to an auxillary pump and the cardioplegia reservoir by tubing. In this tubing is incorporated a tap through which boluses of nitroglycerin can be injected. The cross-clamp is placed, and the cold cardioplegic infusion is given. After the repair and with the cross-clamp still in place, the warm and initially hyperkalemic reperfusion is begun, followed without interruption by normokalemic reperfusion. The aortic cross-clamp is left in place, and the normokalemic controlled aortic root reperfusion is continued until the heart is beating vigorously in a steady sinus rhythm. (From W. A. Lell, J. W. Kirklin, and B. A. Freeman. Case conference. *J. Cardiothorac. Anesth.* 2:561, 1988. With permission.)

1. **Rewarming.** The right ventricle is exposed anteriorly during most cardiac procedures. It is readily rewarmed by the operating theater lights. It is frequently not immersed in the cold pericardial irrigant. Noncoronary collateral return to the right atrium through the coronary sinus serves to rewarm the right heart. The typical practice of cardiac surgery rarely utilizes bicaval cannulation with caval snares for myocardial revascularization or aortic valve replacement. Incomplete removal of venous return tends to rewarm the right atrium and the right ventricle as well.

2. **Cardioplegia maldistribution.** The right coronary artery is frequently involved with occlusive disease. Collaterals are frequently poorly developed.

3. Right ventricular impairment is manifest by the need for high central venous pressures to achieve modest left-sided filling pressures. It may be manifest by severe ventricular arrhythmias. Right heart failure, when severe, can be more difficult to treat because of the lack of routinely available mechanical support devices suitable for right-sided support.

4. More frequent use of **bicaval cannulation** and increased use of **topical cooling** directed at the right heart may improve right heart preservation.

V. Conclusion. Myocardial preservation techniques have developed rapidly during the last 25 years. Periods of ischemia, feared 15 years ago, are now routinely tolerated. It is very clear, however, that no one technique or formulation is the ultimate answer. Attention to the management of myocardial oxygen supply and demand before and after global ischemia is an important aspect of successful myocardial preservation.

The future holds promise for extending the safe ischemic time even further. This will further reduce the incidence of severe postarrest dysfunction. Developments can be expected in two broad areas, cardioplegic additives and maneuvers to modify the conditions of reperfusion.

Our original goal was to provide a motionless, bloodless surgical field without causing unacceptable or irreversible damage to the heart. This is reliably achievable at the present time for operations requiring up to 2–3 hours of ischemic time. The basic principles of myocardial preservation remain biochemical arrest of the electromechanical processes and hypothermia.

REFERENCES

1. Buckberg, G. D., and Hottenrott, C. E. Ventricular fibrillation: Its effect on myocardial flow, distribution and performance. *Ann. Thorac. Surg.* 20:76–85, 1975.
2. Buckberg, G. D., Brazier, J. R., Nelson, R. L., et al. Studies of the effects of hypothermia on regional myocardial blood flow and metabolism during cardiopulmonary bypass. *J. Thorac. Cardiovasc. Surg.* 73:87–109, 1977.
3. Digerness, S. B., Kirklin, J. W., Naftel, D. C., et al. Coronary and systemic vascular resistance during reperfusion after global myocardial ischemia. *Ann. Thorac. Surg.* 46:447–454, 1988.
4. Drew, C. E., and Anderson, I. M. Profound hypothermia in cardiac surgery: Report of three cases. *Lancet* I:748–750, 1959.
5. Gerbode, F., and Melrose, D. The use of potassium arrest in open cardiac surgery. *Am. J. Surg.* 96:221–227, 1958.
6. Hottenrott, C. E., Towers, B., Kurkji, H. J., et al. The hazard of ventricular fibrillation in hypertrophied ventricles during cardiopulmonary bypass. *J. Thorac. Cardiovasc. Surg.* 66:742–753, 1973.
7. McFarland, J. A., Thomas, L. B., Gilbert, J. W., et al. Myocardial necrosis following elective cardiac arrest induced with potassium citrate. *J. Thorac. Cardiovasc. Surg.* 40:200–208, 1960.
8. Neely, J. R., and Grotyohann, L. W. Role of glycolytic products in damage to ischemic myocardium: Dissociation of adenosine triphosphate levels and recovery of function of reperfused ischemic hearts. *Circ. Res.* 55:816–824, 1984.
9. Rousou, J. A., Parker, T., Engelman, R. M., et al. Phrenic nerve paresis associated with the use of iced slush and the cooling jacket for topical hypothermia. *J. Thorac. Cardiovasc. Surg.* 89:921–925, 1985.
10. Waldhausen, J. A., Braunwald, N. S., Bloodwell, R. D., et al. Left ventricular function following elective cardiac arrest. *J. Thorac. Cardiovas. Surg.* 39:799–807, 1960.

SUGGESTED READING

Buckberg, G. D. Recent Progress in Myocardial Protection During Cardiac Operations. In D. C. McGoon (ed.), *Cardiac Surgery* (2nd ed.). Philadelphia: F. A. Davis, 1987 Pp. 291–319.

Chitwood, W. R., Jr. *State of the Art Reviews,* Vol. 2, No. 2. Philadelphia: Hanley and Belfus, 1988.

Hearse, D. J., Brambridge, M. V., and Jynge, P. *Protection of the Ischemic Myocardium: Cardioplegia.* New York: Raven Press, 1981.

Roberts, A. J. *Myocardial Protection in Cardiac Surgery.* New York: Marcel Dekker, 1987.

Circulatory Assist Devices

Kane M. High, William S. Pierce, and Thomas M. Skeehan

The perioperative use of circulatory assist devices has become increasingly common in clinical practice. It is vital that anesthesiologists caring for patients who require these devices thoroughly understand their mechanical and physiologic functions.

Circulatory assist devices have undergone a substantial transformation from preliminary laboratory tools to conventional medical therapy [1]. Twenty-five years ago intraaortic balloon pumps were used only for patients **in extremis.** Today balloon pumps are used commonly, and ventricular assist devices are used for the sickest patients in major research centers. The total artificial heart is used today in only a very few centers for patients who are candidates for heart transplantation, have exhausted conventional therapies, and will not survive without further intervention. It seems certain that the use of these devices will increase as they are improved and their utility is further documented.

I. **Indications for mechanical support of the circulation.** Prior to discussing the indications for particular mechanical devices to assist the failing ventricle, it is necessary to define ventricular failure. Common criteria for failure of each ventricle are listed in Table 22-1.

Mechanical support of the circulation is indicated if these criteria are met in spite of maximal inotropic support of the circulation. An **approximation** of maximum inotropic support would be any combination of **two or more** of the following:

1. > 10 µg/kg/min of dobutamine
2. > 10 µg/kg/min of dopamine
3. > 0.2 µg/kg/min of epinephrine
4. > 10 µg/kg/min of amrinone

Higher levels of inotropic support can be expected to be of little further benefit to the patient and are likely to have prohibitive toxicity.

II. **Selection of mechanical assist devices.** The type of assist device utilized depends on the extent of ventricular failure that is present. The intraaortic balloon pump (IABP) is the first mechanical device that is employed to support the failing left ventricle. For patients with more profound left ventricular failure the ventricular assist device (VAD) should be considered if no medical contraindications exist. Either left or right heart failure or both may precipitate the need for ventricular assistance [4]. If a single VAD (usually on the left side) is not sufficient, then biventricular assist should be undertaken. Currently, the total artificial heart (TAH) is reserved at **most** centers only for cardiac transplant candidates suffering transplant rejection (who will be difficult to cross match and may have a prolonged wait for a compatible donor) and those with nonrepairable acquired ventricular septal defect (VSD) or ventricular rupture.

Special clinical indications for each modality of mechanical support of the circulation are as follows:

A. **Postcardiopulmonary bypass.** At the completion of cardiopulmonary bypass (CPB), some patients will meet the criteria for ventricular failure despite maximal pharmacologic support, and these should then be considered for circulatory assist devices. Occasionally there are factors that can predict the need for mechanical support prior to the time the need arises.

   1. **Preoperative predictors of the need for circulatory assistance**
      a. Preoperative ventricular dysfunction (ejection fraction < 0.30).
      b. Severe valvular disease with end-stage myocardial impairment.
      c. Coronary artery disease that is only partially amenable to bypass grafting with associated poor ventricular function.
      d. An anticipated long time on CPB.

Table 22-1. Criteria for ventricular failure

	Left ventricle	Right ventricle
Cardiac index (liters·min^{-1}·m^{-2})	<1.7	<1.7
Systolic blood pressure (mm Hg)	<100	N/A*
Vascular resistance (dynes·sec·cm^{-5})	<1200 (SVR)	<200 (PVR)
Mean atrial pressure (mm Hg)	>20	>20
Ionized Ca^{2+}	Normal	Normal
Heart rate (beats/min)	>80	>80

SVR = systemic vascular resistance, PVR = pulmonary vascular resistance
*Right ventricular failure can occur with or without pulmonary hypertension. The work performed by the right ventricle is related to the difference between the right atrial and pulmonary artery mean pressure. As this difference approaches zero, pulmonary blood flow is passive and right ventricular failure is present.

If such preoperative predictors exist, additional leads for synchronizing the IABP with the electrocardiogram (ECG) should be placed preoperatively so that they are available if needed. Also, at least one groin should be prepared in the surgical field for ready access. Consideration should be given to placing a femoral arterial line after induction of anesthesia to facilitate percutaneous IABP placement if it is required to separate the patient from CPB.

2. **Intraoperative predictors**
   a. Pre-CPB ischemia
   b. Prolonged CPB
   c. Incomplete repair or bypass
   d. Air or particulate embolus in the coronary artery
   e. Large ventriculotomy or ventricular aneurysm resection

B. **Ventricular failure after myocardial infarction.** Treatment of ventricular failure after myocardial infarction is initiated with inotropes and afterload reduction. Usually the use of inotropes is limited as much as possible after myocardial infarction because of the risk of extension of the infarction. Treatment with the IABP [11] is initiated earlier in this setting to reduce afterload and increase coronary perfusion.

The use of VADs in the setting of acute myocardial ischemia or infarction has not been evaluated. There has been no evidence to date that the use of VADs affects the course or outcome of these patients as does the IABP. It is conceivable that the VAD could be used to salvage selected patients who would be candidates for transplantation following an acute myocardial infarction.

C. **Bridge to cardiac transplantation.** Any patient that is a candidate for heart transplantation and becomes hemodynamically unstable due to ventricular failure should be considered for mechanical support. The first form of therapy in these patients is the IABP. For those with severe ventricular failure, a VAD is the next line of therapy. For those with severe biventricular failure, a total artificial heart or biventricular assist pump may be used. [3,8] Current worldwide results indicate similar hospital discharge rates for patients "bridged" with unilateral, biventricular, or TAH support [6].

III. **Intraaortic balloon counterpulsation**

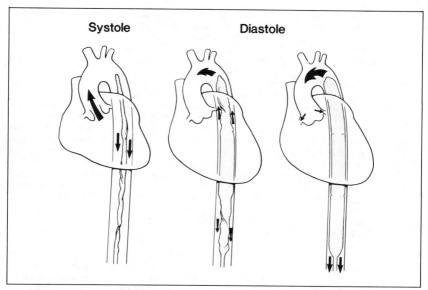

Systole   **Diastole**

Fig. 22-1. Placement of intraaortic balloon pump (IABP) in aorta. The IABP is shown in the descending aorta with the tip at the distal aortic arch. During systole the balloon is deflated to enhance ventricular ejection. During diastole the balloon inflates, forcing blood from the proximal aorta into the coronary and peripheral vessels.

A. **Functional design of the IABP.** The intraaortic balloon is a long, narrow balloon placed in the thoracic aorta, usually percutaneously from the groin (Fig. 22-1). The balloon is inflated during diastole, displacing blood from the thoracic aorta and increasing the aortic pressure. Balloon inflation increases the coronary perfusion pressure and coronary blood flow and thus is beneficial during periods of myocardial ischemia. During systole the balloon is deflated, giving the left ventricle a lower afterload into which to eject. This reduces myocardial wall tension and thus decreases myocardial oxygen consumption. The reduced afterload may also cause increased forward flow.

The IABP drive console consists of a pressurized gas reservoir that is connected to the balloon supply line through a solenoid valve that is electronically controlled. The gas used to inflate the balloon is either carbon dioxide or helium. The advantage of carbon dioxide is its increased blood solubility. It dissolves in blood more rapidly, thereby reducing the consequences of balloon rupture with gas embolization. The advantage of helium is its decreased density, which thereby decreases the Reynolds number and allows the same flow through a smaller drive line. A tube with a smaller diameter decreases the injury to the artery from the puncture and also decreases the risk of infection and arterial thrombosis.

B. **Placement of the IABP**
1. Insertion of the IABP is usually accomplished through either percutaneous or surgical cutdown into the femoral artery utilizing the Seldinger technique for placement of a large-diameter introducer. If the femoral approach is technically difficult and the chest is open, then transthoracic placement is an option.
2. The balloon-drive line unit is then passed through the introducer.

3. The balloon is ideally positioned so that its tip is at the junction of the descending aorta and the aortic arch as shown in Fig. 22-1. This promotes the removal of blood from the proximal aorta and minimizes the risk of renal artery occlusion by the balloon.

C. **Control of the IABP.** Several parameters are important during the setup and operation of an IABP.

   1. **Synchronization of the IABP.** Synchronization of the IABP with the cardiac rhythm is accomplished by using either the largest electrical deflection of the ECG signal (usually the QRS complex) or the arterial pressure waveform. If there is a natural pulse pressure (> 40 mm Hg), use of the arterial waveform for synchronization is preferred in the operating room because the electrical artifact produced by using the electrocautery inhibits most IABP control units. Some monitoring systems have suppression circuitry that eliminates the problem of electrical noise during electrocautery and improves IABP performance during ECG synchronization. Also, pacemakers can cause difficulties in obtaining synchronization when the ECG mode is used because the IABP senses the pacer spikes instead of or in addition to the R wave and triggers balloon inflation prematurely.

   2. **Timing of balloon inflation and deflation.** When setting the timing of inflation and deflation (Fig. 22-2), it is important to time the onset of the pressure rise caused by balloon inflation at the dicrotic notch of the arterial waveform. If inflation begins sooner, the IABP will impinge on ventricular ejection. If it begins later, the effectiveness of the balloon in augmenting coronary perfusion and reducing afterload will be limited.

      Deflation should be timed so that the arterial pressure just reaches its minimum level at the onset of the next ventricular pulse. If it deflates too soon, time during the cycle is wasted, and the aorta is not maximally evacuated before ventricular contraction. Coronary perfusion is also reduced during this time. If the balloon deflates too late, it provides an extra impedance to ventricular ejection.

   3. **Ratio of native ventricle pulsations to IABP pulsation.** Pumping is begun usually at a beat ratio of 1:2 (one IABP beat for every two cardiac beats). The 1:2 ratio is chosen so that an easy comparison can be made between natural ventricular beats and augmented beats to determine IABP timing.

   4. **Stroke volume of the balloon.** The volume of gas used to inflate the balloon is determined by the balloon used and the patient's size and is generally not adjusted once it has been set at the beginning of pumping. Increasing the volume of gas over that for which the balloon was designed risks balloon rupture with gas embolization.

   5. **Balloon filling.** The time required for the balloon to fill and empty is determined by the density of the gas used, gas pressure, the length and diameter of the gas line, and balloon volume. These values are usually constant for any particular balloon. At high heart rates, the time required for balloon filling may limit the balloon stroke volume.

D. **Weaning from the IABP.** Weaning the patient from the IABP is done primarily by gradually decreasing the ratio of balloon-augmented to natural heart beats (from 1:1 to 1:2 to 1:4 to 1:8) while monitoring cardiac output to ensure that it remains acceptable. Once the patient is weaned to a ratio of 1:8 the balloon pump is removed. The balloon is never turned off while it remains in the aorta except when the patient is fully anticoagulated during CPB because of the risk of thrombus formation on the balloon.

   A comparison of native ventricular pulsations to balloon pulsations during the course of operation of the balloon can serve as an indicator of ventricular performance. As the ventricular performance

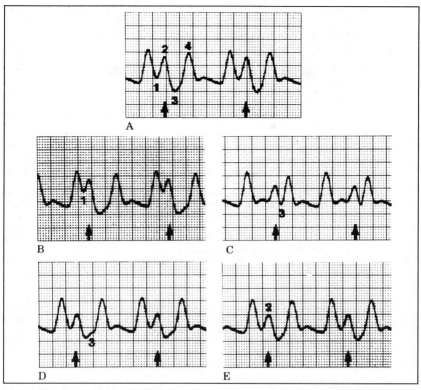

Fig. 22-2. Manipulation of the timing of inflation and deflation of intraaortic balloon pump. Tracings illustrate 1:2 support for the sake of clarity. *A.* Normal tracing. Augmentation commences after the dicrotic notch (1) augments diastolic pressure (2) and reaches its nadir just before the next contraction (3). Peak systolic pressure in the next beat is decreased (4). *B.* Early inflation. Augmentation commences before aortic valve closure (1), thereby increasing afterload and possibly inducing aortic regurgitation. *C.* Late inflation. Diastolic augmentation is inadequate, and end-diastolic pressure is no different from that in the unassisted cycle (3).
D. Early deflation. Diastolic augmentation and afterload reduction are impaired. *E.* Inadequate filling time. Timing is satisfactory, but diastolic augmentation is impaired. (From R. N. Sladen. Management of the Adult Cardiac Patient in the Intensive Care Unit. In A. K. Ream and R. P. Fogdall [eds.], *Acute Cardiovascular Management in Anesthesia and Intensive Care.* Philadelphia: Lippincott, 1982. P. 509. With permission.)

improves, the magnitude of the natural pulse will increase relative to the balloon pulse. By comparing the magnitude of these two pulses over time, one can obtain a qualitative assessment of ventricular performance.

E. Management of anticoagulation during IABP. During extended IABP use of some type of anticoagulation is advisable. In the immediate post-CPB period, anticoagulants are not used until drainage from the chest tubes is acceptable (< 100–150 ml/hr). Although low-molecular-weight dextran (LMD) is generally useful in preventing thrombosis in patients with IABP, it is not readily reversible. Heparin is useful in preventing thrombosis and is readily reversed with protamine, a very desirable feature in patients preoperatively and postoperatively. In any patient who has an IABP in place and is being considered for surgery, heparin should be employed in preference to LMD.

E. **Complications.** The incidence of complications from the use of the IABP has decreased significantly as experience with the device has increased. Complications include:

1. Infection, primarily at the groin site of the transcutaneous introducer.
2. Coagulopathies (thrombocytopenia).
3. Vascular occlusion (primarily of the renal or femoral artery from the pump itself or from emboli).
4. Vascular injury (arterial dissection or tear).
5. Balloon rupture with gas embolus. When this occurs blood is usually seen in the gas drive line, and the arterial pressure deflection caused by the IABP is lost. Most pumps have an alarm that indicates low balloon pressure.
6. Air embolism from the pressure monitoring line. Air embolism to the brain is a larger risk from the IABP than from a radial artery line because the monitoring port is located at the tip of the balloon, which is located in a very proximal position in the aorta. **Blood gases should be drawn through the IABP pressure monitoring line only if no other locations are available.**

G. **Limitations.** The ability of the IABP to augment cardiac output and unload the left ventricle (LV) is limited. If the LV is in severe failure, the IABP will not provide sufficient flow to sustain the circulation. When the LV cannot eject blood into the aorta, the IABP will simply cause pulsations in the arterial waveform without resulting in significant increases in blood flow. In this situation a more effective assist device such as a VAD must be considered.

Balloon pumps are not very effective in irregular and rapid cardiac rhythms. Balloon control devices have difficulty in tracking these rhythms and hence are unable to create properly timed balloon inflations and deflations. The IABPs are ineffective pumps at fast rates because there is insufficient time for the gas to fill and empty the balloon.

H. **Contraindications**

1. **Aortic insufficiency.** Use of the IABP is relatively contraindicated in patients with aortic valve insufficiency because the incompetent aortic valve allows the ventricle to distend during diastole (balloon inflation), thus potentially decreasing coronary perfusion pressure.
2. **Sepsis.** Bacteremia should be treated prior to placement of an IABP. Infections are very difficult to treat if prosthetic surfaces become seeded with bacteria.
3. **Severe vascular disease.** Placement of IABP may be technically very difficult or impossible in arteriosclerotic vessels. Such vessels are much more prone to arterial thrombosis during use of an IABP. Patients with abdominal aortic aneurysms are at increased risk of rupture, although balloons have been successfully passed and employed in such patients.

I. **Pulmonary artery balloon pumping.** Balloon pumps are also used in the pulmonary artery at some centers to assist the failing right ventricle. Although not commonly used, they do provide some augmentation of right ventricular output and may be useful, particularly at the end of CPB for management of right ventricular failure. They are limited in stroke volume (i.e., balloon volume) because the short length of the pulmonary artery limits the length and hence the volume of the balloon. However, a vascular graft may be attached by means of an end-to-side anastomosis to the side of the pulmonary artery to increase the effective pulmonary artery length and accommodate a larger balloon. An IABP is inserted through the other end of the graft and remains inside the graft during operation.

IV. Ventricular assist devices

A. **Types of assist devices.** Various types of pulsatile and nonpulsatile blood pumps (Fig. 22-3) have been developed to augment the function of the human left and right ventricles. Functionally, they all pump blood against an afterload at physiologic flow rates. The assist pumps used today are placed either outside the chest wall or upper abdomen or implanted in the abdomen.

1. **Pulsatile pumps.** These pumps function as blood sacs to which external pressure is applied during ejection to force blood into the arterial tree. The direction of blood flow is controlled by prosthetic valves, which operate as they would in a natural ventricle. The blood sac is compressed externally by gas (the pneumatic pumps) or pusher plate (electric motor pumps).

   a. **Pneumatic pumps.** During systole the blood sac is squeezed by increased gas pressure within the pump case. During diastole the pump case is maintained at a negative gauge pressure, causing blood to be drawn into the pump.

   The pressures that drive the pumps are generated by a drive unit that is connected to the ventricles by air lines or "drive lines." The drive unit contains positive pressure (systolic) and negative pressure (diastolic) drive tanks, which are alternately connected to the drive lines through a solenoid valve. The systolic and diastolic tanks are maintained in the pressure ranges shown in Table 22-2.

   The most commonly used pneumatic assist pumps currently available are versions of the **Pierce-Donachy** pump commercially produced by Sarns-3M, Inc. (Ann Arbor, MI) and Thoratec Laboratories Corporation (Berkeley, CA). The maximum stroke volume of the Pierce-Donachy pump is 70 ml.

   b. **Pusher plate pump.** The pusher plate pump uses plates rather than gas to compress the blood bag. Solenoid valves control beam springs that transfer energy from the two solenoids to the pusher plates. The **Novacor Left Ventricular Assist Device (LVAD)** [10] is a pusher plate pump manufactured by Novacor, Inc. (Oakland, CA). Unlike the pneumatically driven pump, this pump is synchronized with the native ventricle and fills passively during native ventricular ejection, reducing left ventricular afterload.

2. **Nonpulsatile (centrifugal) pumps.** [2,7] This type of pump causes a rotational acceleration of the blood by means of a spinning impeller powered by an electric motor. Several important differences between this type of pump and the pulsatile pump exist. The centrifugal pump has:

   a. **Nonpulsatile flow.** Because the pump creates flow by the turning of an impeller at a constant rate, the resultant pressure produced is not pulsatile. Although there is debate about the physiologic consequences, several long-term studies of metabolic and biochemical parameters have shown that this type of perfusion probably does not cause any deleterious sequelae.

   b. **Nonocclusive venous inflow.** Whether the centrifugal pump is used for left- or right heart assist, the inflow to the pump is maintained by the vacuum created by the pump. There are no check valves in this type of pump because the pump maintains continuous forward flow.

   c. **A role as a temporary nonimplantable device only.** To date, several problems still exist with centrifugal pumps that limit their

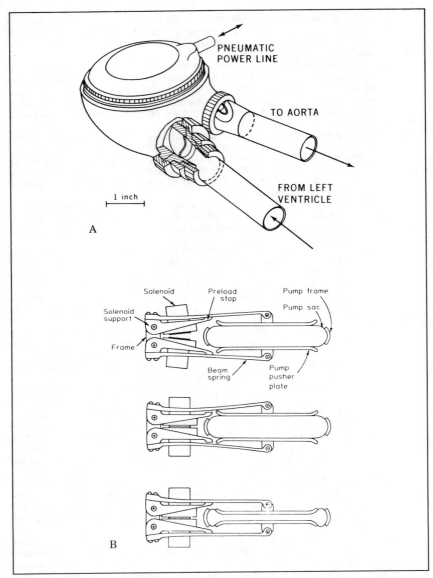

Fig. 22-3. Types of assist pumps: pneumatic, pusher plate, and centrifugal. *A.* Pierce/Donachy pneumatic assist pump. This pump is a flexible sac inside a rigid case. Drive line attachment allows air to squeeze the bag, causing ejection out of the pump. Diastolic vacuum causes the bag to reexpand with blood entering through the inlet valve. *B.* Novacor pusher plate pump. A metal plate squeezes the bag causing ejection. The pump is shown in the end-diastolic position *(top),* at onset of systole *(middle),* and in the end-systolic position *(bottom).* (From P. M. Portner, P. E. Oyer, J. S. Jassawalla, et al. A Totally Implantable Ventricular Assist Device for End-Stage Heart Disease. In F. Unger [ed.], *Assisted Circulation* [2nd ed.]. Heidelberg: Springer-Verlag, 1984. P. 122. With permission.)

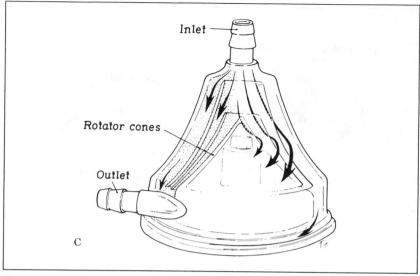

Fig. 22-3 (continued) *C.* BioMedicus centrifugal pump. A spinning impeller causes the centrifugal acceleration of blood. Blood enters near the axis of the pump and exits at the periphery. (From C. C. Reed and T. B. Stafford. *Cardiopulmonary Bypass* [2nd ed.]. Houston: Texas Medical Press, 1985. P. 378. With permission.)

Table 22-2. Standard drive tank pressures (mm Hg gauge)

	Diastolic	Systolic
Left heart	0 to -50	200–300
Right heart	0 to -50	100–200

long-term use. The major one is the heat produced in the bearing housing, which predisposes to thrombus formation in this area. Until this problem is overcome, the centrifugal pump will remain an important form of **temporary** ventricular support.

Currently there are two manufacturers of centrifugal pumps: Sarns/Centrimed and BioMedicus. The Bio-Pump produced by BioMedicus is currently also used as a part of a portable assist system (CPS, by Bard) employed for support after acute cardiac decompensation (see Chap. 19).

3. **Roller pumps.** The standard roller head pump (discussed in Chap. 19) is used at some institutions as a VAD. This has the advantage of being familiar to personnel, simple to set up, and simple to operate. Blood is drained from the left atrium and is returned to the ascending aorta through a single silicone tube that runs through the roller head. No venous reservoir is usually used. The pump is manually controlled in the standard manner for roller pumps. The setting of the roller head occlusion is discussed in Chapter 19. Flow rates of up to 4 liters/min can be obtained and are adjusted according to left atrial pressure.

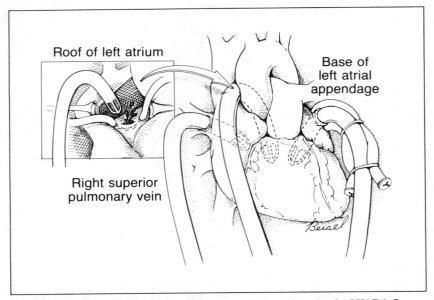

Fig. 22-4. Positions of LVAD inflow cannula. Possible positions for the LVAD inflow cannula. This cannula draws pulmonary venous blood into the assist pump that is then returned to the ascending aorta. Placement of the cannula in the left ventricle, though used under some circumstances, is not shown here.

B. **Placement of assist devices.** Outflow cannulas of LV assist pumps are generally placed in the ascending aorta through a median sternotomy incision. Inflow cannula placement is more variable and depends on accessibility (Fig. 22-4) and the intended function of the assist. In patients in whom significant recovery of ventricular function is anticipated, the left atrium should be used. When the pump is used as a bridge to transplantation or a Novacor pump is used, the inflow cannula can be placed in the left ventricle. Most VAD have both VAD cannulae that traverse the chest wall at the level of the diaphragm as shown in Fig. 22-5. For centrifugal pumps, the cannulae are somewhat longer, and the pump is fixed to the patient's bed. The cannulae for Novacor LVAD traverse the diaphragm to connect to the pump, which is located in the abdomen. The outflow cannula of a right ventricular assist device (RVAD) is connected to the pulmonary artery, and the inflow cannula is connected to the right atrium. They function in a manner analogous to that of the LVAD. Before any of these pumps are activated, meticulous de-airing of the cannulae and pump is performed.

C. **Control and operation of assist pumps.** Table 22-3 provides an overview of the currently used assist pumps and a description of their control and operation. Details of operation are discussed below.

1. **Pulsatile**

   a. **Pierce-Donachy pump.** Initially, pumping is controlled by changing the pumping rate and driving pressures on the drive unit by hand (manual mode). In the manual mode, a pump rate is set, and the pump may or may not be filling and emptying completely. Once the patient has been weaned from CPB and is stable, usually the pump rate is controlled automatically. In the

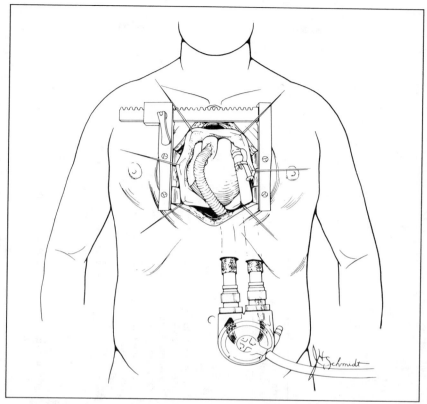

Fig. 22-5. Positioning of pneumatic LVAD. The typical positions of an LVAD as oriented to the patient and patient's heart. The inlet and outlet cannulae traverse the diaphragm and pass through the skin in the upper abdomen.

automatic mode, the Pierce-Donachy VAD varies its beat rate to maintain a **full to empty** ventricle. This mode of operation provides good washing of the blood sac and inhibits the formation of thrombus. Ventricular filling and emptying are determined by monitoring of the drive line pressure trace and determination of "full and empty flags" as shown in Fig. 22-6 [5]. These "flags" represent periods when gas flow into and out of the VAD has stopped and the pneumatic drive line pressure has come into equilibrium with the drive unit pressure tanks.

The systolic and diastolic driving pressures can also be adjusted to improve pump performance. They are adjusted to provide full to empty pumping while maintaining the desired pump output. The systolic duration can also be adjusted to vary filling and emptying.

b. Novacor pump. The Novacor pumps are usually synchronized to the cardiac cycle and pump during the diastolic portion of the cardiac cycle. This synchronization is accomplished by one of two methods: either by detecting the R wave of the ECG or by detecting the end of the native ventricular ejection into the pump. End of

Table 22-3. Comparison of operation and control of assist pumps

Pump	Mode of operation	Pump-controlled variables	Response to increased preload	Response to increased afterload
Pulsatile pumps Pierce-Donachy Thoratec-VAD 3-M Sarns				
Manual	Variable filling to full to empty	Rate, systolic, and diastolic drive pressures, systolic duration	Increased output if increased stroke volume	Little
Automatic	Full to empty	Systolic and diastolic drive pressures, systolic duration	Increased rate, thus increased output	Little
Novacor	Variable filling synchronized with cardiac cycle	None	Increased filling thus stroke volume and increased output	Little
Centrifugal pumps BioMedicus Medtronic Sarns/Centrimed	Continuous rotation	Speed of rotation	Increased output	Moderate decrease in output

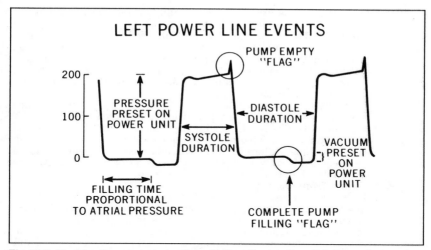

Fig. 22-6. Air drive line pressure tracing—"full and empty flags." At the end of pneumatic pump systole there can occur a short time in which there is no pump ejection. During this time there is no volume change in the gas in the rigid pump case, and the pressure in the case and the drive line equilibrate with the pressure in the systolic drive tank in the drive unit. This causes a sharp rise in pressure called an "empty flag" because it signals emptying of the pump. Similarly, during pump diastole, after the pump fills the gas pressures come into equilibrium, and a "full flag" occurs. Vertical axis is drive line pressure; horizontal axis is time.

ejection of the native ventricle is detected by a halt in the motion of the pusher plate. Thus, this pump does not necessarily fill and empty during each stroke; the stroke volume varies depending on the rate of filling and emptying. Because of its control mode, the inlet cannula must be placed in the left ventricle.

2. **Nonpulsatile (centrifugal) pumps.** The pump rate is manually adjusted so that the pump maintains adequate pressure on its outflow side while effecting adequate decompression on its inflow or venous side. Thus, for left heart assist, the left atrial pressure would need to be kept below an acceptable maximum value, whereas the mean arterial pressure would be maintained at an acceptable minimum value. For right heart assist, the central venous pressure would be kept below a safe maximum, whereas the mean pulmonary pressure or left atrial pressure would be kept at a reasonable minimum value. This is accomplished by adjusting the pump speed and blood volume. However, unlike most pulsatile pumps, centrifugal pump output can be reduced because of elevated systemic afterload. Therefore, continuous monitoring of pump output is critical.

D. **Anticoagulation and antiplatelet drugs during assist pumping.** The use of anticoagulants during assist pumping is still not a totally resolved issue. The risk of bleeding must be weighed against the risk of thrombus formation. As a general rule, it is helpful to maintain regular native ventricular contractions in addition to the use of anticoagulants to help reduce the risk of clot formation within the native ventricle.

1. **Pulsatile pumps.** Currently, some form of anticoagulation or antiplatelet therapy is generally used for patients with an intact coagulation system. Full heparinization does not need to be employed

since the pumps are designed to inhibit thrombus formation, although it occasionally is used to elevate the activated clotting time (ACT) to 1.5 times normal. Low molecular-weight dextran has fallen from use when any further surgery is planned because its prolonged half-life may cause a long-term coagulopathy. During weaning from pulsatile assist pumps, when the pump flow becomes less than 2 liters/min, the ACT is usually increased to 250–350 seconds by increasing the infusion of heparin.

2. **Nonpulsatile pumps.** Studies have been done using these pumps with and without systemic heparinization. In these studies, the ACT was maintained at levels ranging from normal control (100 seconds) to approximately 200 seconds, using heparin in small doses as needed. However, the data are inconclusive, and medical judgment should be used. If bleeding is minimal, some level of anticoagulation is advisable when centrifugal pumps are used.

E. **Weaning from assist pumps**
1. **Pulsatile pumps.** Fortunately, the presence of the inflow and outflow cannulae does not impair the native circulation. With pneumatic assist pumps, usually the first step in weaning these patients is to reduce the diastolic vacuum. This causes a reduction in flow into the pump and a decrease in pumping. The atrial pressure increases, and the native heart should begin to fill and eject, providing an opportunity to observe the native ventricle's performance. The pump output is kept at about 2 liters/min for 24 hours to increase the native ventricle workload. To test the native ventricle, VAD pumping may be temporarily stopped and the cannulae clamped (the "clamp test"). This is done for only short periods (usually 1–2 minutes) every 6 hours because of the increased risk of thrombus formation secondary to stagnation inside the pump.

Use of the Novacor pump has been reported only as a "bridging device" that has not been weaned. However, it may be weaned by decreasing its beat ratio relative to the native ventricle.

2. **Nonpulsatile pumps.** Weaning from centrifugal pumps is performed by decreasing the pump speed and observing the function of the native ventricle. However, at pump flows of less than 2 liters/min, the pump rotor is more prone to thrombus formation, and care must be taken to make sure that adequate anticoagulation is maintained during the weaning period.

F. **Complications and limitations**
1. **Right ventricular failure.** Many patients who have been supported until transplantation with an LVAD have marginal right ventricular function. Sometimes when an LVAD is applied right heart failure is observed; this can sometimes be corrected by concomitant use of inotropes and vasodilators. A second assist device may be needed for simultaneous right ventricular support.
2. **Danger of diastolic vacuum.**
   a. **Probe patent foramen ovale.** This condition occurs in approximately 25% of the general population and can cause severe intracardiac shunting if left atrial pressure is reduced below right atrial pressure (with the aid of a diastolic vacuum). Accordingly, the foramen should **always** be checked and surgically closed at the time of insertion of the left ventricle assist cannulae.
   b. **Open chest.** Diastolic vacuum may draw air into the circulation prior to closure of the chest. Similarly, the negative inflow pressure generated by centrifugal pumps has the potential to draw air into the circulation at suture lines or central venous catheters.
3. **Infection.** Two large-diameter tubes passing transcutaneously through the abdominal wall present a serious risk of infection. De-

spite vigorous efforts to maintain sterility at the cannula sites and the use of velour sleeves to allow tissue ingrowth, the risk of infection persists throughout the time an assist pump is used. Prophylactic antibiotics are usually used.

Once infection is present in these devices, it is very difficult to eradicate. Cardiac transplantation in an infected patient also carries considerable risk because of the use of immunosuppressive agents. However, successful outcomes have been reported under these circumstances.

4. **Coagulation.** The risk of thrombus formation or excessive bleeding is present whenever assist devices are used. The particular risk in any one patient depends on the amount of anticoagulants used. Although thrombi are unusual, they can occur and present a constant risk to the patient. During the perioperative period the risk of hemorrhage is ever present, particularly along the suture lines that attach the pump to the patient.

5. **Inflow occlusion.** Obstruction to flow into assist pumps continues to be a concern. Either thrombus formation inside the cannula or extrinsic compression of the cannula or atrium by clot or tissue can prevent adequate flow of blood into the pump.

6. **Pulsatile versus nonpulsatile pump.** There appear to be no complications that are specific to the use of pulsatile or centrifugal pumps for ventricular assist. The possible disadvantage of nonpulsatile flow has not been substantiated. If some form of pulsatile flow is desired with a centrifugal pump, the centrifugal pump can be combined with IABP to establish a pulse pressure.

G. **Contraindications.** Active sepsis would preclude the insertion of an assist device. In addition, there must be some anticipated improvement in ventricular performance or the prospect of cardiac transplantation. The VAD will perform in any patient but is warranted only in those judged capable of receiving some long-term benefit.

V. Total artificial hearts: bridge to transplantation

A. **Types of artificial hearts.** Two types of pulsatile artificial hearts have been developed to date. These are the pneumatic driven pumps and the electric motor driven pump.

1. **Pneumatic pumps.** Of the pneumatic pumps, the Jarvik pump designed at the University of Utah and the heart designed at The Penn State University have received the most attention and clinical use. These devices are fairly similar in design and function. Both consist of two pumps similar to pneumatic assist pumps, the major difference occurring in the angulation of the inflow and outflow ports and in control of their operation.

2. **Electric pumps.** Electric motor pumps are still in the animal testing stage and have not been used clinically. These pumps have either a reciprocating shaft and pusher plates to squeeze two blood bags, as in the pump currently under development at Penn State, or a fluid pump that passes a liquid from one pumping chamber to another with the fluid squeezing the blood bags (University of Utah design).

B. **Placement of the total artificial heart.** Surgical implantation of these TAHs are similar, connecting cannulas (quick connects) being applied to both atria and both great arteries prior to connection of the ventricles as depicted in Fig. 22-7. The suture lines are pressure tested before they are applied to the ventricles. After a meticulous de-airing of the left ventricle, the ventricle is allowed to begin pumping slowly, while the right ventricle is attached and de-aired. This slow pumping prevents elevated left atrial pressure.

C. **Operation and control of the TAH**

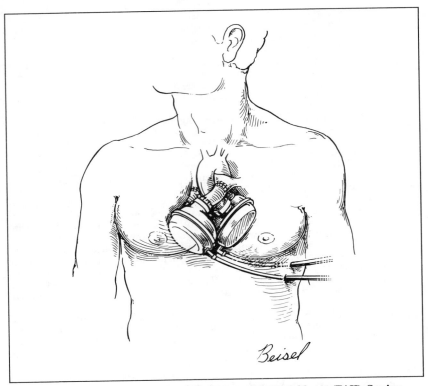

Beisel

Fig. 22-7. Surgical placement of the Penn State total artificial heart (TAH). Sewing rings are sutured to the atrial cuffs that were created when the recipient heart was excised. Dacron grafts are attached to the pulmonary artery and aorta. These four connectors are attached to the appropriate ports on the two pumps.

1. **Pneumatic pumps.** Differing schemes have been developed at The Penn State University and the University of Utah to control their TAH. The Penn State University pump is usually run in the "full to empty" automatic mode on both left and right pumps, so that cardiac output is determined by the left pump beat rate.* Alternatively, negative feedback loops can be used that result in a decreased left or right pump rate in response to elevated aortic or left atrial pressures, respectively. The aortic pressure is inferred from the end-systolic drive line pressure, and the left atrial pressure is inferred from the time it takes to fill the left heart based on the fill flag. Thus the two ventricles operate independently and usually have different pumping rates.

   The right heart often has a significantly slower rate because flow through the pump during diastole is limited only by the small difference between the central venous pressure and the pulmonary artery pressure. Thus the right heart does not have to beat as often to match the left heart output. Also, there is more backflow (regur-

*The stroke volume is known to be 70 ml for the standard adult pump; this volume multiplied by the beat rate, gives the cardiac output.

gitant flow) through the valves of the left pump because of the higher pressures to which they are exposed.

At the University of Utah, the driving pressures and heart rate are kept relatively constant, and the cardiac output is adjusted intrinsically by increased diastolic filling. This operation is referred to as the "fill limited" mode of operation.

2. Electric motor pumps. The control logic for electric motor artificial hearts is continuing to be developed. It entails an electronic system that counts the rotations of the motor armature to determine the position of the pusher plate and hence the volume of the pumping chamber. Generally, a full to empty mode of pumping is employed.

Also, the afterload can be inferred from the amount of current required by the pump to move the pusher plate. As the afterload increases the current required to move the pusher plate increases. The ability to infer the afterload can then also be used to control pumping without the need for a pressure transducer.

D. Anticoagulation and the TAH. The problems of thrombus formation and bleeding continue to be balanced against each other to provide the proper coagulation milieu. Most centers are currently using a combination of antiplatelet drugs and warfarin. Warfarin has the dual advantages of inhibiting the coagulation system as well as the formation of calcium deposits on the blood-contacting surfaces [9]. These therapies are begun postoperatively after the surgical bleeding has subsided.

E. Complications and limitations. The complications of the TAH are essentially the same as those associated with the VAD.

1. Hemorrhage or thrombosis. Perioperative bleeding should not be more than that seen in patients undergoing CPB with great vessel surgery. Late thromboembolism continues to occur in patients with a TAH and is probably related to prosthetic valves, foreign surfaces, and the numerous interfaces present.

2. Infection. Infection is a constant threat for patients who have transcutaneous lines in place. Generally, though, the risk seems to be small with current nursing care and the velour-covered lines that allow tissue ingrowth. Sepsis, once present, is extremely difficult to treat effectively.

VI. Anesthetic management of patients with circulatory assist devices

A. Monitoring of the circulation

1. Adequacy of perfusion is determined by the usual methods including:

a. Skin color and temperature

b. Urine output

c. Acid-base status

d. Mixed venous oxygen saturation

2. Cardiac output

a. IABP. For patients supported with an IABP, a Swan-Ganz catheter can still be used to measure cardiac output accurately. The altered arterial pressure wave will not affect the output calculation.

b. LVAD. The cardiac output is the total of the output of the natural ventricle plus that of the assist device. It may be calculated as the assist pump output alone if the arterial waveform does not have native ventricular pulsations. For pulsatile pumps, cardiac output is calculated by multiplying the VAD pump rate by the stroke volume (known if the device is pumping in a full to empty mode). If the arterial waveform does show native ventricular pulses, thermodilution cardiac outputs are valid measures of combined native ventricle and pump output.

Centrifugal pumps use flow meters on the outflow line to measure pump output either in line or as an attachment to the line. Either electromagnetic flow meters or Doppler flow meters are used for this purpose.

   c. RVAD. Thermodilution cardiac outputs cannot be reliably used in patients with an RVAD because of the differing transit times of blood through the RVAD and the native right ventricle. Estimates of RVAD output can be made if the stroke volume of RVAD (full to empty mode) and rate are known. Again, this will be the total cardiac output if the native ventricle is not ejecting. If the native right ventricle is ejecting, the cardiac output can be determined by the standard dilutional method using indocyanine green dye. Dye is injected into the pulmonary artery or left atrium, and its concentration is measured in a peripheral artery.

   d. TAH. The output of a TAH can be determined from the stroke volume of the left pump (full to empty) and rate of pumping with the Penn State TAH. The Jarvik pump utilizes a unique system called the COMDU (Cardiac Output Monitoring and Diagnostic Unit). This system utilizes a pneumotachograph in the drive line to measure the gas flow, from which the pump output is inferred. In lieu of this device, the cardiac output can be determined with the dilutional method using green dye. Thermodilution cardiac outputs are unavailable because a Swan-Ganz catheter should not be placed through the prosthetic valves.

3. Other monitors. All standard anesthesia monitors (esophageal stethoscope, pulse oximeter, end-tidal CO_2 monitors) are appropriate in these patients. In addition to an arterial catheter, a central venous pressure (CVP) catheter or Swan-Ganz catheter (if an RVAD is not used) is useful for drug infusion and monitoring cardiac function. A left atrial line is also very important in monitoring left heart filling pressures.

B. Induction of anesthesia and discontinuation of CPB with an assist device in place. Proper anesthetic management requires an understanding of pump design, function, and control of the unit employed. In addition, it is necessary to consider the right ventricle and the pulmonary circulation separately from the left ventricle and the systemic circulation. If a device is employed to assist or replace the LV (IABP or VAD), the effects of anesthetics on the right ventricle become paramount. In patients with assist devices:

1. Adequate preload must be maintained.

   a. Anesthetics often cause vasodilation, reducing central blood volume and therefore limiting the ability of the assist device to fill.

   b. In patients with a pulsatile VAD **it is desirable not to use vacuum during diastole while the chest is open** to reduce the risk of air entrainment. Therefore, it is necessary to maintain adequate blood volume to permit the VAD to fill. At the same time, it is necessary not to overload the patient, precipitating ventricular failure in the unassisted ventricle.

2. Inotropes are often required for the ventricle that does not have an assist device. In addition, vasodilating drugs may be helpful to enhance the output from the unassisted ventricle. The effects of any drug must be considered, particularly the effects on both the pulmonary and systemic vasculature and the unassisted ventricle.

3. Effects of ventilation. In a patient with an LVAD in place, mechanical ventilation needs to be managed according to its effects on pulmonary vascular resistance (PVR). On one hand, high airway pressure may increase PVR. On the other hand, hyperventilation may reduce reactive PVR.

4. It is necessary to **maintain good communication** with the individual controlling the assist device to ensure that it is functioning appropriately and to help optimize its functioning.

VII. Summary. Various forms of mechanical assist devices are currently available to assist the failing ventricle. The clinical conditions used to select an assist device have been discussed. The basic functioning of these devices and the control systems for these devices were discussed. It is very important to all physicians caring for patients with assist devices to have a fundamental understanding of these devices so that appropriate decisions regarding their use can be made.

On the horizon is the use of the TAH. Initially this will be used as a bridge to cardiac transplantation, but with the experience thus gained as well as continued development of these pumps, implantation for permanent circulatory support will begin.

REFERENCES

1. Birtwell, W. C., Clauss, R. H., Dennis, C., et al. The evolution of counterpulsation techniques. *Medical Instrumentation* 10:217–223, 1976.
2. Golding, L. A. R. Centrifugal Pumps. In F. Unger (ed.), *Assisted Circulation 2.* New York: Springer-Verlag, 1984. Pp. 142–152.
3. Hill, J. D., Farrar, D. J., Hershon, J. J., et al. Use of a prosthetic ventricle as a bridge to cardiac transplantation for postinfarction cardiogenic shock. *N. Engl. J. Med.* 314:626–628, 1986.
4. Jorge, E., Pae, W. E., and Pierce, W. S. Left Heart and Biventricular Assist. In D. Bergman (ed.), *Critical Care Clinics: New Techniques in Mechanical Support* 2(2):267–275, April 1986.
5. Landis, D. L., Pierce, W. S., Rosenberg, G., et al. Long-term in vivo automatic electronic control of the artificial heart. *Trans. Am. Soc. Artif. Intern. Organs* 23:519–525, 1977.
6. Pae, W. E., and Pierce, W. S. Combined registry for the clinical use of mechanical assist pumps and the total artificial heart: Second official report—1987. *J. Heart Transplant.*, in press.
7. Pennington, D. G., Merjavy, J. P., Swartz, T., et al. Clinical experience with a centrifugal pump ventricular assist device. *Trans. Am. Soc. Artif. Intern. Organs* 28:93–98, 1982.
8. Pennock, J. L., Pierce, W. S., Campbell, D. B., et al. Mechanical support of the circulation followed by cardiac transplantation. *J. Thorac. Cardiovasc. Surg.* 92:994–1004, 1986.
9. Pierce, W. S., Donachy, J. H., and Rosenberg, G. Calcification inside artificial hearts: Inhibition by warfarin-sodium. *Science* 208:601–603, 1980.
10. Portner, P. M., Jassawalla, J. A., Chen, H., et al. A new dual pusher-plate left heart assist blood pump. Proc. 2nd Meeting of the International Society for Artificial Organs. *Artif. Organs [Suppl.]* 3:361–365, 1979.
11. Sturm, J. T., McGee, M. G., Fuhrman, T. M., et al. Treatment of postoperative low output syndrome with intraaortic balloon pumping: Experience with 419 patients. *Am. J. Cardiol.* 45:1033–1036, 1980.

SUGGESTED READING

Unger, F. (ed.). *Assisted Circulation 2.* Berlin: Springer-Verlag, 1984.
Bergman, D. (ed.). *Critical Care Clinics: New Techniques in Mechanical Cardiac Support* 2(2), April, 1986.

Extracorporeal Membrane Oxygenation

Michael T. Snider, Kane M. High, David B. Campbell, and Dennis R. Williams

I. Introduction. Severe adult respiratory distress syndrome (ARDS) can result in a mortality approaching 100%. Death is due primarily to the natural course of lung injury and secondarily to further lung trauma induced by the high concentrations of inspired oxygen (FIO_2) and airway pressures required for adequate arterial oxygenation during mechanical ventilation. Extracorporeal membrane oxygenation (ECMO) with artificial lungs can supplement the pulmonary gas exchange of the damaged natural lung and can minimize the secondary injuries of oxygen toxicity and barotrauma.

This chapter is written to aid the cautious and deter the flippant. Here we briefly review prior attempts to use ECMO and give practical details for using veno-venous (V-V) perfusion to supplement pulmonary gas exchange in those few selected patients with severe ARDS who may be aided by its use. When appropriate, contrasts will be made with the use of veno-arterial (V-A) perfusion to treat neonatal respiratory distress syndromes (NRDS). Our recommendations are based on our recent experience with V-V ECMO at Penn State, the senior author's prior experience at the Massachusetts General Hospital, and his 25 years of laboratory experiments [5,7,8].

A. Early attempts. Unsuccessful attempts to use ECMO for the treatment of neonatal disease were described first by White in 1971. Hill reported the first successful use of long-term ECMO utilizing a membrane oxygenator in ARDS in 1972. Since then many patients have survived NRDS and ARDS by means of gas exchange support with ECMO.

B. Major adult series

  1. National Heart, Lung and Blood Institute (NHLBI) ECMO Study. Between 1974 and 1977, 90 patients were studied in nine medical centers during the prospective, randomized study of V-A ECMO sponsored by the NHLBI [7]. Patients between the ages of 12 and 65 years with the diagnosis of ARDS and an illness of less than 3 weeks in duration were eligible for the study if sustained severe hypoxemia was present without evidence of left ventricular failure. They were randomized to either a control group that continued to receive mechanical ventilation with positive end-expiratory pressure (PEEP) or a treatment group that received V-A ECMO in addition to mechanical ventilation with PEEP. Although the FIO_2 was lowered to 0.65 and airway pressures were decreased in the ECMO group, both groups had the same low survival rate of 9%. ECMO produced no demonstrable improvement in survival. Based on this study, ECMO is no longer performed for ARDS at many centers.

  2. The Milan experience. Recently, Gattinoni and coworkers reported a survival rate of 47% in 55 patients with ARDS who were treated with V-V perfusion [4]. They used low extracorporeal blood flows and high extracorporeal gas flows through membrane lungs mounted in series. Hyperventilation of the blood passing through the extracorporeal circuit transferred most of the patients' carbon dioxide production but provided only small amounts of extracorporeal oxygen transfer. Barotrauma was minimized because the diminished need for carbon dioxide removal by the injured natural lung permitted the use of less vigorous mechanical ventilation. Specifically, they used intermittent mandatory ventilation with small tidal volumes, very low ventilator frequencies, an inverse inspiratory to expiratory time (I-E) ratio and an FIO_2 of 0.6. Since this technique provides only small amounts of membrane oxygenation, it has been termed extracorporeal carbon dioxide removal ($ECCO_2R$). No randomized comparison was made with patients treated solely with mechanical ventilation.

3. The Penn State experience. Recently, we reported the treatment of patients with severe ARDS with high-flow V-V perfusion [5]. This technique provided 80–90% of a patient's oxygen and carbon dioxide exchange while enabling the FIO_2 to be reduced from 1.0 to between 0.2 and 0.3. Three of seven patients survived and returned to their previous level of activity. Airway pressures were only slightly lowered. No randomized comparison was made with patients treated solely with mechanical ventilation. Our experience forms the basis for the practical techniques given in this chapter.

4. Why the widely differing survival rates? The reason for the improvement in survival among the patients in the NHLBI ECMO study, the $ECCO_2R$ series, and our recent experience is unclear. The patients in all series appear to have the same degree of arterial hypoxemia prior to perfusion. Gattinoni has attributed the improvement in survival obtained with $ECCO_2R$ mainly to the lower airway pressures generated during the less vigorous mechanical ventilation [4]. On the other hand, a greater lowering of the FIO_2 in our series may have aided in the resolution and repair of damage from pulmonary oxygen toxicity. Another important difference is the route of extracorporeal pumping. V-V pumping may be more beneficial to the lung in patients with ARDS than V-A pumping. Although the patients in all series may have had similar diagnoses and degrees of hypoxemia, the reversibility of the lung injury at the initiation of perfusion may have been different.

5. Lack of general acceptance. These improved results with $ECCO_2R$ and high blood flow V-V ECMO have not had a major widespread effect on the current practice of treating ARDS. This lack of general application of ECMO in ARDS may have resulted from (1) ignorance on the part of the critical care physicians of these newer and more encouraging results, (2) general lack of knowledge of how and when to apply these techniques, (3) lack of agreement on what constitutes maximal medical therapy prior to the initiation of ECMO, and (4) disbelief because no classic randomized, prospective study has compared $ECCO_2R$ or high blood flow V-V ECMO against mechanical ventilation techniques.

Currently, $ECCO_2R$ is being compared with mechanical ventilation in a randomized prospective study by Alan Morris at the Latter Day Saints Hospital in Salt Lake City, Utah, using rigorous protocols for medical management before and during perfusion [3]. Without randomized prospective comparisons, **one may legitimately ask whether patients with ARDS survive because of ECMO or despite ECMO.** We believe a small number of adults need ECMO to survive ARDS and will present arguments to this point. **ECMO should not be withheld from these selected patients with ARDS while awaiting the outcome of randomized studies.**

C. Major neonatal series. ECMO has provided an excellent alternative treatment to positive pressure mechanical ventilation for patients with several neonatal pulmonary and cardiovascular diseases that produce NRDS. At the present time, approximately 500 neonatal ECMO perfusion attempts are performed yearly at more than 15 centers in the United States. The survival rate during the treatment of severe NRDS by V-A ECMO is currently 79% [2]. Retrospective studies suggest that these neonatal patients would have had a survival rate of only 20% if ECMO had not been used. Despite the lack of a classic randomized study comparing equal numbers of patients in ECMO and non-ECMO groups, V-A ECMO is now the accepted therapy for infants with severe NRDS that is unresponsive to conventional ventilator and pharmacologic therapies. In contrast, V-V ECMO has not been used as successfully in neonates.

Why is the survival rate higher in neonatal ECMO as compared with adult ECMO? Four factors may be responsible. First, the technology and personnel training for neonatal ECMO is uniform throughout treatment centers. Most efforts have closely duplicated the pioneering program of Robert Bartlett at the University of Michigan. Second, the number of neonatal diseases causing NRDS is small, and large numbers of salvageable patients with uniform pathophysiology exist in each disease. Third, the techniques of neonatal mechanical ventilation may not be as highly developed as those used in adults and may be a less competitive therapy to ECMO. Last, NRDS resolves not only by repair and scarring but also by further maturation and development of the neonatal lung. Regardless of the cause of the difference in survival rates, the success of neonatal ECMO has stimulated and encouraged further efforts to treat ARDS with ECMO.

II. Current indications

A. Neonatal respiratory distress syndrome. NRDS is defined by the presence of hypoxemia in the neonate that is accompanied by persistent panlobar infiltrates on chest film. These patients often require prolonged mechanical ventilation with high airway pressures and elevated FIO_2. V-A ECMO is indicated in severe NRDS due to hyaline membrane disease, persistent fetal circulation, pulmonary hypertension either as a primary disease or secondary to meconium aspiration, and congenital diaphragmatic hernia.

To identify those neonates who would profit from invasive ECMO techniques, a major emphasis has been placed on defining quantitative criteria for the severity of NRDS that would predict survival or death if standard mechanical ventilation were continued. These criteria are based on the level of positive inspiratory pressure and duration for which a large alveolar-arterial oxygen gradient is required for support. Such survival criteria work well at individual institutions but often fail to predict mortality accurately elsewhere because of local differences in overall patient management. Information from the Neonatal ECMO Central Registry shows that the most common reason for the institution of ECMO is worsening of the patient's condition despite maximal medical management.

B. Total pulmonary lavage in adults. ECMO has been used infrequently to support gas exchange during simultaneous lavage of both lungs for the treatment of severe alveolar proteinosis. However, most of these patients can be successfully treated without severe hypoxemia by using a double-lumen tube that allows lavage of one lung at a time. Few patients require ECMO for this reason.

C. Cardiopulmonary support. V-A ECMO can provide temporary left ventricular or biventricular cardiac support to a few patients who suffer from heart failure with severe, intractable hypoxemia or intractable cardiopulmonary arrest.

1. Biventricular failure and severe hypoxemia. Most patients with left ventricular failure or biventricular failure can be treated successfully with inotropes and vasodilators. Mild hypoxemia due to pulmonary edema can usually be treated with supplemental inspired oxygen by mask or, if necessary, by endotracheal intubation and mechanical ventilation. Those who fail to respond to pharmacologic therapy but are still salvageable can be supported by an intraaortic balloon pump or ventricular assist device coupled with mechanical ventilation. See Chapter 22 for details. The rare, salvageable patient who requires higher levels of both cardiac and pulmonary support may profit from short-term, high-flow V-A pumping with ECMO.

2. Intractable cardiopulmonary arrest. Some centers now use portable ECMO devices to institute rapid support of the circulation and gas exchange with intractable cardiopulmonary arrest caused by either myocardial infarction or pulmonary embolus. Full cardiopulmonary bypass is instituted using peripheral cannulation.

D. Adult respiratory distress syndrome. ARDS is defined as the progressive development of hypoxemia in adults with the appearance of panlobar infiltrates without evidence of left ventricular dysfunction or failure. This condition is often accompanied by a decreased lung compliance, hypercapnia, thrombocytopenia, and pulmonary artery hypertension. Sometimes a presumptive diagnosis of systemic sepsis, pulmonary contusion, fat embolus, aspiration pneumonitis, or bacterial pneumonia can be made. Usually a definitive cause for the lung injury cannot be established. All patients who undergo positive pressure ventilation, but especially those with ARDS, are at risk for pulmonary barotrauma due to high airway pressures and oxygen toxicity due to prolonged exposure to high FIO_2.

1. Barotrauma. The usual manifestations of barotrauma include pneumothorax, pneumomediastinum, pneumopericardium, and subcutaneous emphysema. This risk is increased during ARDS because the decrease in lung compliance causes an increase in airway pressures during positive pressure ventilation. Thus, for any given tidal volume the peak airway pressure will be higher than normal and will predispose the patient to barotrauma. Also, increased levels of PEEP, used in an attempt to correct the arterial hypoxemia, may further increase the working ventilating pressures. Animal data suggest that barotrauma itself can cause ARDS. Finally, patients with ARDS tend to develop subpleural pulmonary infarcts that have less mechanical strength than the normal pulmonary parenchyma. These may rupture and cause pneumothoraces.

2. Oxygen toxicity. These patients also are exposed to increased FIO_2 in an attempt to correct their hypoxemia. Prolonged exposure to a higher FIO_2 can itself cause ARDS, with progressive, further impairment of pulmonary gas exchange. The longer the duration of the exposure and the higher the FIO_2, the greater the damage. Sensitivity to pulmonary oxygen toxicity varies widely. Coughing and substernal distress can begin in healthy volunteers after as short an exposure as 12–24 hours to 100% oxygen at sea level. Unfortunately, at present there is no simple battery of specific tests that indicates whether a given FIO_2 is safe for a specific patient. Clearly, prolonged exposure of lungs to a high FIO_2 can be detrimental, and the lower the FIO_2 the better for the patient.

3. Who with ARDS requires ECMO to survive? The most important decision is to determine which few of the many adult patients with ARDS will profit from the additional expense and manpower required to institute and maintain ECMO. The usual justification for using ECMO in patients with ARDS is that the chance of survival is so low with the use of mechanical ventilation alone that the additional risk of ECMO is acceptable. Quantitative survival criteria have been used or suggested as indications for ECMO in the major reported series. These relate the survival rate from ARDS during mechanical ventilation to the severity of ARDS as judged by the FIO_2 and PEEP required to maintain a given arterial partial pressure of oxygen (PaO_2), the duration of mechanical ventilator support, and the duration of the disease process.

To aid in making this paramount decision of who should receive ECMO, a summary of survival rates of patients with ARDS of increasing severity who were treated only by mechanical ventilation

Table 23-1. Survival rates in ARDS with conventional ventilation criteria based on PaO_2 and level of ventilator support

Survival rate (%)	Level of ventilator support			Reference
	FIO_2	PEEP (cm Hg)	PaO_2 (mm Hg)	
61	≥0.5	5	>75	[1]
31			<75	[1]
9	≥0.6	≥5	≤50	[7]
8	1.0	≥5	≤50	[7]
0	1.0	≥5	≤45	[7]
0	1.0	≥5	≤35	[7]

Note: See Appendix for duration of mechanical ventilation, names of criteria, and number of measurements required.

is given in Table 23-1. By comparing a given patient's observed PaO_2 with the level and duration of ventilator support in this table, the chances of survival without ECMO can be estimated. The basis of this table and the theoretical limitations of these criteria are detailed in the Appendix to this chapter (sec. **XIII**).

4. **Practical limitations of current survival criteria.** Table 23-1 shows the estimated survival rates at a few **specified levels or bounds of FIO_2 and PEEP.** Unfortunately, **no interpolation is available** that allows the clinician to assess the survival rates of patients at intermediate levels of support. It is likely that the ventilator settings, chosen on clinical grounds for a given patient, will be different from those defined by these criteria. Thus, if one wants to assess the survival rate of a given patient, the ventilator settings must be manipulated to criteria values, and additional blood gas determinations must be made that are not immediately relevant to clinical care. This may be a potential hazard. At the criteria ventilator settings, the patient will usually have a significantly lower PaO_2 than at the immediately previous ventilator settings that were chosen on clinical grounds to avoid hypoxia. **If prudent, gradual adjustments are made in FIO_2 and PEEP while monitoring arterial saturation with a pulse oximeter, these criteria can be applied to a patient without undo risk.**

5. **Who with ARDS receives ECMO at Penn State?** We employ V-V ECMO only in patients with ARDS who meet all the following conditions. They must have:

   a. A lung injury of less than 21 days' duration.

   b. A lung injury that has the potential to reverse during 1–2 weeks of ECMO.

   c. No other irreversible, life-threatening disease process.

   d. Been receiving maximal medical therapy.

   e. A PaO_2 of less than 50 mm Hg on measurements made hourly during a 2-hour interval. At the times of measurement the ventilator settings must have been maintained at a FIO_2 of 1.0 and a PEEP of at least 5 cm H_2O for at least 15 minutes. [Between criteria measurements, any combination of FIO_2 and PEEP settings are permitted.]

   f. Extreme barotrauma causing life-threatening impairment of ventilation or oxygenation.

g. Not been exposed to FiO_2 of 1.0 for more than 4 days.

Patients meeting these criteria have less than a 9% chance of surviving on mechanical ventilation (see Table 23-1). Using these criteria we have achieved a survival of three of seven patients using V-V ECMO. It is important to note that approximately **only 1% of all patients with ARDS in our 24–27 bed surgical-medical intensive care unit (ICU) during the last 8 years have met these criteria.**

III. Contraindications

A. Irreversible primary disease. Any panlobar viral pneumonia except varicella pneumonitis is felt to be an absolute contraindication by the authors.

B. Lung injury for more than 3 weeks. Pulmonary fibrosis becomes more likely as the duration of the pulmonary disease increases. Also, longer acting disease processes are believed to require longer repair periods. Three weeks was the arbitrary limit chosen in the NHLBI ECMO study. Any use of data from this study to predict survivors must consider this fact.

C. Active hemorrhage. Hemorrhagic diathesis and cerebral hemorrhage can be devastating during the systemic heparinization required for ECMO.

D. Sepsis. Infection is a common problem that may be either the primary disease or a secondary complication of ARDS. In general, sources of infection should be diligently sought and treated prior to ECMO to avoid contaminating the artificial surfaces that contact the blood. Active bacteremia and sepsis can make the maintenance of ECMO impossible.

E. Severe multiple organ failure. Severe organ dysfunction of the kidney, liver, heart, or brain is considered a relative contraindication to ECMO because of the lower overall physiologic reserve possessed by such patients. Prolonged multiple organ failure heralds a hopeless situation and should be considered an absolute contraindication to ECMO.

F. Old age. Although old age is not an absolute contraindication to ECMO, the decrease in physiologic reserves with age and the residual lung damage seen in survivors suggests that this expensive therapeutic option should be reserved only for younger adults, children, and neonates. There is no absolute age limit, but we would hesitate to perfuse patients older than 50 years.

G. Concomitant lethal disease. Patients with diagnosed diseases that are known to be lethal within 5–10 years are poor candidates. Patients with concomitant severe brain injury who have little chance of functional recovery are not candidates.

IV. Sequence of medical management and ventilator support of ARDS patients prior to ECMO at Penn State. The management of all adult surgical patients in our ICU is supervised by a team of anesthesiologists and surgeons trained in intensive care management. This team approach results in a continuous and more uniform sequence of escalation of the level of ventilator support and medical therapy in patients who develop ARDS. The following approximates the usual management of the patient with ARDS at our institution.

A. Cardiopulmonary monitoring. Variables to be monitored on-line in patients with ARDS include breath-by-breath end-tidal carbon dioxide levels, systemic arterial pressure (SAP), pulmonary artery pressures, pulmonary capillary wedge pressure (PCWP), central venous pressure (CVP), arterial oxygen saturation (SaO_2) by pulse oximetry, and mixed venous oxygen saturation ($S\bar{v}O_2$) by Optimetrix fiber optic pulmonary artery catheter (Abbott Critical Care, Mount View, CA). The right femoral vein and right internal jugular vein may be needed for future cutdowns to insert ECMO cannulae. If these sites must be used for percutaneous catheters early in the patient's management, these catheters should be removed and the sites rested prior to ECMO cannulation.

B. **Initial level of ventilator support and medical therapy.** After intubation of a hypoxic patient with respiratory failure, we attempt to maintain a PaO_2 of more than 70 mm Hg. Our initial settings during an intermittent mandatory mode of mechanical ventilation with a volume ventilator are usually:
1. **$FIO_2 = 0.60$**
2. **PEEP = 5 cm H_2O**
3. **Tidal volume 10–15 ml/kg body weight**
4. **I/E ratio of 1:2**
5. **A ventilator rate that keeps the arterial partial pressure of carbon dioxide ($PaCO_2$) between 35 and 45 mm Hg**
6. **A patient respiratory rate between 2 and 30 breaths/minute**

    In patients who have a diagnosed lung injury that has the potential to reverse during 1–5 weeks and who also have no other irreversible life-threatening disease process, we recommend that the criteria for survival from ARDS be applied systematically to determine as early as possible which of those few patients might profit from ECMO. The first criteria measurements should be made soon after stable mechanical ventilation has been achieved. At this time ventilator settings should be chosen to evaluate the criteria for survival from severe rapidly developing ARDS (see Appendix and Table 23-1).

    As soon as possible we institute vigorous chest physiotherapy including percussion, vibration, postural drainage, and endotracheal suctioning. In general, steroids and empiric antibiotic therapy have no proved benefit and are avoided. If the platelet count is less than $40,000/\mu l$ or the prothrombin time and partial thromboplastin time are prolonged, platelet concentrates or fresh-frozen plasma are administered.

C. **Escalation of the level of ventilator support and medical therapy.** If, following the initial ventilator settings, a PaO_2 of less than 70 mm Hg is seen, the FIO_2 is raised to 0.80 in 0.05 increments during the next few hours. If the PaO_2 still remains less than 70 mm Hg, the PEEP is slowly raised to 20 cm H_2O in 2.5-cm H_2O increments in an attempt to reach a PaO_2 of 70 mm Hg.

    Fiberoptic bronchoscopy and rocker beds are used to maximize pulmonary toilet. Furosemide is given to promote free water diuresis in order to raise the serum sodium level to the range of 145–155 mEq/liter. This total body dehydration tends to draw water from injured areas of the lung and improve gas exchange.

D. **Ongoing search for a treatable diagnosis.** Sometimes a presumptive diagnosis of systemic sepsis, pulmonary contusion, fat embolus, aspiration pneumonitis, or bacterial pneumonia can be made. Most of the time, a definitive cause for the lung injury cannot be established. Sustained fever and leukocytosis imply infection. Identification of the source and organism requires the frequent taking of Gram stains with cultures of blood, sputum, urine, and wounds. If meningeal signs are present, lumbar puncture may be needed to obtain cerebrospinal fluid for culture.

    Open lung biopsy sometimes can yield valuable information. Bacterial cultures from the biopsy may be positive even when repeated blood cultures are negative. This can occur because airway closure may trap infected mucous, which then cannot be mobilized and drained by chest physiotherapy. Intracellular inclusion bodies characteristic of viral pneumonitis may be seen. The extent of fibrosis and its reversibility is difficult to judge because only 20–40 g of lung tissue is sampled.

Open lung biopsy is probably not needed if one is relatively sure of the nature of the lung injury causing ARDS. If one is unsure and suspects a viral pneumonia, the information obtained may indicate that ECMO should be withheld. Often no clinically useful information is found. Open lung biopsy is accompanied by significant risks including hemorrhage, tension pneumothorax, and development of a bronchopleural fistula. Hemorrhage may become a major problem after systemic heparinization for ECMO. Transport to and from the operating room (OR) is complicated by the need to ventilate a patient on high FIO_2 and PEEP with a large dead space and venous admixture. Under all circumstances, transthoracic and transbronchial biopsies should be avoided because the amount of tissue sampled is too small and the risk of pneumothorax too high.

E. **Maximal ventilator support with maximal medical therapy.** If the PaO_2 still remains less than 70 mm Hg, the patient is sedated with morphine or fentanyl and chemically paralyzed with pancuronium or vecuronium using continuous intravenous infusions. If the PaO_2 continues at less than 70 mm Hg, one or all of the following are attempted:

1. **Increase the FIO_2 up to 1.0.**
2. **Raise the PEEP further.**
3. **Induce mild hypothermia by surface cooling (34–35°C) to reduce oxygen consumption and carbon dioxide production.**
4. **Attempt reverse I/E ratio ventilation.**
5. **Accept a PaO_2 less than 70 mm Hg.**

At these ventilator settings, barotrauma and oxygen toxicity are very likely to further injure the lung already damaged by ARDS. Therefore, ventilator settings should be chosen as often as practical to evaluate the **criteria for survival from severe, rapidly developing ARDS** to determine whether a given patient could profit from V-V ECMO. However, all the conditions in sec. **II.D.5** must be met prior to the institution of V-V ECMO. We have saved some patients who met the **criteria for lethal ARDS** using V-V ECMO (see Appendix and Table 23-1).

V. **Methods**
   A. **Comparison of ECMO with cardiopulmonary bypass for cardiac surgery**
   1. It is helpful to consider the major differences between conventional cardiopulmonary bypass (CPB) for cardiac surgery and the three possible extracorporeal pumping routes used for ECMO. These differences are summarized in Table 23-2.
   2. The goal of standard CPB is to provide total cardiac support while providing total oxygen and carbon dioxide transport for the patient. The closest comparison to CPB is V-A ECMO, which is prolonged partial CPB. In V-A ECMO, some pulmonary blood flow remains, and the heart and lungs function partially. With V-V ECMO pulmonary and systemic blood flows are equal, and the heart assumes the total workload.
   3. Generally, the activated clotting time (ACT) is kept much lower on ECMO than with standard CPB. To avoid the destruction of platelets in the already thrombocytopenic patient with ARDS, bubble traps and blood filters are not used in the extracorporeal circuit.
   4. In CPB, thoracotomy is usually required for central cannulation of the great vessels. Cardiotomy suction and venting of the left ventricle are needed to provide a bloodless surgical field and to decompress the left ventricle. None of these maneuvers are needed during ECMO for ARDS.

B. **Pumping routes and their cardiopulmonary consequences.** Regardless of the cannulation sites used, extracorporeal gas exchange

Table 23-2. Comparison of standard cardiopulmonary bypass with most common ECMO routes

	Cardiopulmonary bypass	ECMO routes		
		Veno-arterial	Veno-venous	Arteriovenous
Synonyms	Total heart-lung bypass	Partial heart-lung bypass		
Extracorporeal flow	Total cardiac output	30–80% of total cardiac output	30–90% of total cardiac output	20–30% of total cardiac output
Cardiac effect	Full support	Partial support	None	Extra load
Pulmonary blood flow	Very low	Low	Normal	High
Blood drainage sites	Inferior and superior vena cava	Inferior vena cava	Inferior vena cava	Umbilical, radial artery
Blood infusion sites	Aortic root	Axillary, carotid or femoral artery	Superior vena cava	Superior vena cava
Duration	30 min to 5 hour	1–21 days	1–21 days	1–5 days
Usual ACT range	>400 sec	150–250 sec	150–250 sec	150–250 sec
% O_2 consumption transported extracorporeally	100%	20–90%	20–90%	20%
% CO_2 production transported extracorporeally	100%	20–90%	20–90%	50%
Pulmonary arterial saturation	?	Low	Normal to high	Normal to high

provided by all ECMO pumping routes keeps the patient's oxygen consumption and carbon dioxide production approximately constant at the preperfusion level. However, during ECMO the patient's preperfusion gas exchange, which was previously carried out solely by the natural lung, is now divided between the membrane lung and the natural lung. Specific differences among pumping routes are outlined below.

1. **Veno-arterial (V-A) pumping. At the present time V-A pumping is the most commonly used route for ECMO in neonates.** Venous blood is drained by gravity from a large-bore cannula inserted in either the right internal jugular or femoral vein and advanced so that its tip is near the right atrium. Blood is pumped through the membrane lung, where it is arterialized and then returned to the patient through a cannula placed in a systemic artery. A ligated carotid artery has served as the return site in most neonatal perfusions to date. In adults either the axillary artery or the femoral artery has been used.

   a. **Nonuniform arterial blood gases are likely.** Regardless of where the tip of the return cannula lies, V-A ECMO will more or less disrupt the usually uniform oxygen saturation (SO_2) and partial pressure or carbon dioxide (PCO_2) of the arterial tree and will produce three regions where the saturation varies widely [6] (Fig. 23-1). Thus, this perfusion route produces a similar but inverse problem to that seen in the right-to-left shunt of a patient with a patent ductus arteriosus. Regions near the flow stream at the tip of the return cannula receive well-oxygenated and decarbonated blood from the ECMO circuit. Regions away from the tip receive the hypoxic and hypercapnic blood from the injured natural lung as it exists in the left ventricular outflow. Vascular beds between the left ventricular outflow and the cannula stream receive blood with an oxygen content and carbon dioxide content that is a flow-weighted average of the oxygen and carbon dioxide contents of the blood exiting from the artificial lung and the injured natural lung. The closer the tip of the return cannula to the aortic root or the higher the extracorporeal flow rate, the more uniform the oxygen saturation and PCO_2 of the blood in the arterial tree. Regardless of the site of cannula insertion, one can guarantee that normoxic arterial blood will perfuse the brain only if the tip of the return cannula lies between the aortic arch and the aortic root. Similarly, normoxic arterial blood will be provided to the coronary bed only if the tip of the return cannula is placed in the aortic root. The possibility of nonuniformity of blood gases in the arterial tree must be considered in choosing sites for inserting arterial monitoring lines and in interpreting "arterial" PO_2, PCO_2, and pH on subsequent blood samples. Similarly, the site of placement of a cutaneous pulse oximetry probe may make interpretation difficult. That is, **"arterial" blood gases and pulse oximetry may fail to reflect either improvement in the functioning of the injured natural lung or the oxygenation of blood flowing to vital organs.**

   b. **Cardiac assistance is given, but pulmonary blood flow and S̄vO are low.** During V-A ECMO the total peripheral flow equals the sum of the left ventricular cardiac output and the extracorporeal return flow. Both right and left ventricular cardiac outputs decrease as the extracorporeal flow increases, so that total peripheral blood flow remains almost constant. This can be a potent method of cardiac assistance if the natural heart begins to fail. With optimal selection and placement of cannulas, up to 90% of the pre-ECMO cardiac output can be diverted to the extracorporeal

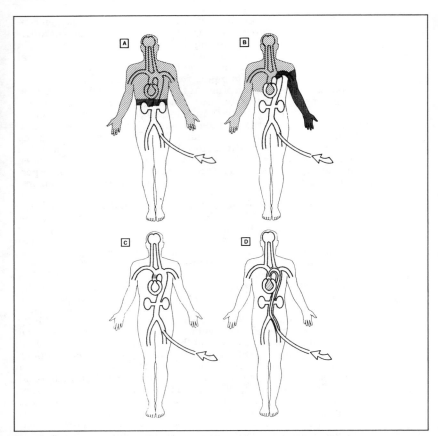

Fig. 23-1. During V-A ECMO the distribution of well-arterialized blood in the aorta depends on both the site of the tip of the return cannula and the magnitude of the extracorporeal blood flow. Depicted are *(A)* low and *(B)* moderate return flows delivered to the femoral artery. Also shown are high return flows to the *(C)* femoral artery and *(D)* the aortic root. Open areas = well-oxygenated blood from the extracorporeal stream, hatched areas = poorly oxygenated blood from the injured natural lung, dotted areas = a mixture of the latter two streams.

circuit. Then cardiac output decreases to 10% of the prebypass value. Only the coronary sinus venous return fails to be drained into the extracorporeal circuit. This coronary venous flow can become the major fraction of the right ventricular cardiac output that is pumped into the pulmonary artery. Thus, the pulmonary circulation is perfused by blood at a low flow rate and with extremely low SO_2 (10–20%). This combined ischemic and hypoxic condition may further damage the lung already injured by ARDS. On the other hand, pulmonary artery pressures are often lowered from their ARDS values of 40–50 mm Hg to normal values because of the low cardiac output. Since injured pulmonary arteries have a higher closing pressure, pulmonary decompression during V-A ECMO tends to close off flow to injured areas and match perfusion and ventilation in less damaged portions of the lung. Paradoxically, the calculated venous admixture decreases and the PO_2 of the left ventricular outflow increases, but the lung injury has not resolved and may be worse.

c. **Erroneous cardiac output determinations are likely.** Cardiac output determinations by obtained thermodilution with superior vena caval or right atrial injection may be falsely high [6]. Portions of the injectate are stolen by the extracorporeal drain. This keeps the total amount of thermal indicator from following its usual course through the right ventricle and then past the sensing thermistor in the pulmonary artery. Thus, a lower temperature change is sensed, and cardiac output will be read as falsely high. This problem can be avoided by injecting the thermal indicator through the right ventricular port of the pulmonary artery catheter designed for ventricular pacing. This allows the tricuspid valve to shield the injectate from steal by the drainage cannula and yields accurate values of cardiac output. Cardiac output determinations by injection of green dye into the pulmonary artery and sampling of systemic arterial blood are usually inaccurate because the left ventricular outflow usually mixes with the returning extracorporeal flow in an undefined way.

2. **Veno-venous (V-V) pumping. At the present time V-V pumping is the most commonly used route for adult ECMO.** Blood is drained by gravity from a wide-bore cannula inserted in the femoral vein and advanced so that its tip lies just below the diaphragm in the inferior vena cava. Blood is pumped through the membrane lung, where it is arterialized and then returned to the patient through a cannula inserted in the right internal jugular vein and advanced so that its tip lies just above the right atrium.

a. **Uniform arterial blood gases.** Unlike V-A pumping, V-V pumping maintains uniform blood gas values throughout all systemic arteries because extracorporeal return and the venous blood from the peripheral tissues are well mixed by passage through four cardiac valves before entering the systemic arterial tree. Simultaneous sampling of systemic and pulmonary arterial blood gases allows the venous admixture of the injured lung to be calculated easily and accurately.

b. **Efficiency of extracorporeal gas exchange depends on venous cannula positions.** To transfer all of the patient's gas exchange from his injured natural lung to the membrane lung while maintaining normal arterial blood gas values, the entire venous return from the patient's peripheral tissues must be drained into the extracorporeal circuit while the entire output of the extracorporeal circuit is directed into the right ventricle without mixing these two streams. Drainage of the coronary venous return and complete separation of these streams are impossible when cannulas are lying in the vena cava. In approaching this goal, the relative placement of the tips of the drainage and reinfusion cannula becomes crucial (Fig. 23-2). To maximize stream separation, the tip of the drainage cannula should lie in the inferior cava a few centimeters below the diaphragm, and the return cannula should lie in the superior vena cava with its tip a few centimeters above the tricuspid valve.

c. **No direct hemodynamic effects occur, but no cardiac assistance either.** Except for alleviating the cardiovascular effects of hypoxemia and hypercarbia, V-V ECMO has no effect on hemodynamics. Because increasing extracorporeal blood flow does not

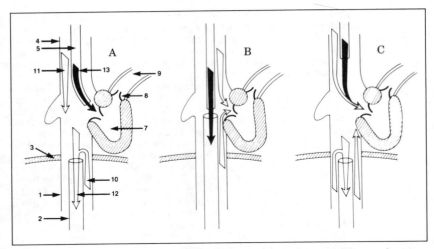

Fig. 23-2. Effects of the locations of the tips of the extracorporeal drainage and return cannulae on the efficiency of extracorporeal gas exchange during V-V ECMO. *A.* The best possible cannula positioning in which the extracorporeal return stream is directed toward the tricuspid valve and shows little mixing with the systemic venous return, which passes into the extracorporeal drainage cannula. *B.* The worst possible cannula positioning in which close end-to-end placement shunts the extracorporeal return immediately back to the extracorporeal drain without any mixing with the systemic venous return. *C.* A mediocre cannula positioning in which the return cannula is placed too high in the superior vena cava, resulting in excessive mixing of the extracorporeal return and venous blood draining upper body. (1) inferior vena cava, (2) ECMO drainage cannula, (3) diaphragm, (4) superior vena cava, (5) ECMO return cannula, (6) tricuspid valve, (7) right ventricular cavity, (8) pulmonic valve, (9) pulmonary artery, (10) venous return stream from lower body, (11) venous return stream from upper body, (12) extracorporeal drain stream, (13) extracorporeal return stream.

change the cardiac output or peripheral arterial blood flow to the tissues, it cannot assist the heart.

    d. Pulmonary blood flow and $S\bar{v}O_2$ remain normal. Because the cardiac output remains constant, there is no decompression of the pulmonary circulation and no direct lowering of the pulmonary artery pressures. Because the $S\bar{v}O_2$ and the partial pressure of oxygen in the mixed venous blood ($P\bar{v}O_2$) rise to normal or above normal levels, pulmonary hypertension may be lowered indirectly because pulmonary vasoconstriction is relieved by correcting mixed venous hypoxemia and hypercapnia. Healing may be enhanced because the pulmonary capillary bed is perfused at a normal blood flow with normal PO_2 and PCO_2.

    e. Erroneous cardiac output determinations are possible. Cardiac outputs measured by thermodilution may be elevated falsely during V-V pumping owing to loss of the thermal indicator into the drainage cannula in the same way as occurs in V-A pumping. This problem can be avoided by injecting the indicator into the right ventricle. Because the entire arterial tree is perfused with blood leaving the left ventricle with uniform PO_2 and PCO_2, cardiac output measurements can be performed by injecting cardiac green dye into the pulmonary artery and sampling the dye washout from any systemic arterial site. With V-V ECMO the systemic blood flow is equal to the cardiac output.

3. **Arteriovenous (A-V) pumping. At the present time, A-V pumping is the most commonly used route for dialysis and hemultra-filtration in adults, but it is not used for ECMO.** In the past, neonates with NRDS were treated unsuccessfully by using the natural heart to propel blood through a membrane lung by means of an A-V fistula.

   a. **Flow load on heart.** Following the opening of an A-V fistula, the cardiac output increases by the amount of the blood flow rate passing through the fistula. A large-bore A-V fistula can double the cardiac output and eventually cause high-output cardiac failure. The blood flow through a membrane lung mounted in an A-V fistula is largely limited by the hydraulic resistance of the blood phase of the membrane lung. Thus, extracorporeal flows are constrained to be less than 1000 ml/min in a pumpless system. During A-V pumping, the peripheral blood flow equals the cardiac output.

   b. **Low oxygen transfer rate expected.** Because of the low blood flow, the maximal oxygen transfer rate of the membrane lungs in a pumpless system is less than 30 ml/min. Membrane lungs with lower hydraulic resistances might double the oxygen exchange.

   c. **Moderate carbon dioxide transfer rate possible.** Hemodialysis through an artificial kidney in a pumpless A-V fistula can remove large quantities of carbon dioxide from the blood. A carbon dioxide transfer rate of about 100 ml/min can be obtained with a blood flow of 1000 ml/min. Carbon dioxide in the form of bicarbonate anions passes from the blood into the dialysate and is replaced by acetate anions. To maintain a steady state, the acetate must be continuously metabolized to regenerate bicarbonate. No prolonged application of this type has been made in man. Because many membrane lungs can be hyperventilated by high extracorporeal gas flows, significant $ECCO_2R$ might be possible in the future using a pumpless A-V system.

C. **Extracorporeal V-V circuit used at Penn State.** In our V-V circuit (Fig. 23-3), blood from the patient drains from the inferior cava through a 28F cannula (see [A] in Fig. 23-3) which was inserted through the right femoral vein and advanced to the level of the hepatic veins. Because the inferior vena caval cannula occludes the lumen of the common femoral vein at the site of its insertion, the distal vein must be drained by an 18F cannula [B] to avoid veno-occlusive edema. The blood streams from the two cannulae are combined and then drained by gravity through a ½-inch inside diameter (id) polyvinyl chloride (PVC) tubing [C] into the venous reservoir bag [F], which has a 2000-ml volume. A heparin solution [D] is added by continuous infusion through port [E]. Blood is pumped out of the reservoir bag by three roller pumps. The major portion passes through the two pumps [G1 and G2], which are fitted with ⅜-inch id PVC tubing and mounted in parallel. Note the extra lengths of tubing that are needed to alternate the segments that are compressed by the rollers and prevent tubing rupture. The output of the two pumps is joined, subsequently redivided, and then propelled into two 3.5 m² Sci-Med Spiral Coil Membrane Lungs (Sci-Med Life Systems, Inc., Minneapolis, MN) [H1 and H2] which are mounted in parallel. After undergoing oxygenation and decarbonation in the membrane lungs, the blood is joined as a single stream and returned to the patient through ⅜-inch id PVC tubing [I]. The processed blood is delivered just above the tricuspid valve by a 22F cannula inserted through the right internal jugular vein [J]. A minor portion of the blood in the reservoir bag is drawn by a third roller pump [G3] fitted with ¼-inch id PVC tubing and propelled through a D30 Diafilter hemultrafilter (Amicon Division, WR Grace & Co., Danvers, MA) [H3] and then re-

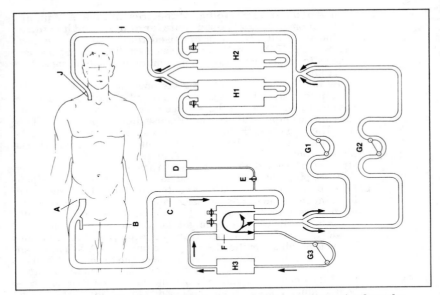

Fig. 23-3. Schematic display of a patient with cannulation apparatus in place; the equipment has been connected to the extracorporeal circuit for V-V ECMO. The path of the extracorporeal return line has been positioned at the head of patient for clarity. A common key to the extracorporeal components is used in Figs. 23-3, 23-4 and 23-7. See text.

turned to the reservoir bag [F]. **The entire perfusion apparatus must be compactly mounted so that it can be placed conveniently at the foot of a patient's bed in the intensive care unit.** Our circuit is mounted on a 36- × 24-inch wood platform with wheels and a pipe scaffolding for mounting the reservoir bag, membrane lungs, and intravenous pumps for medication, as shown in Fig. 23-4.

D. Extracorporeal circuit components

1. Membrane lungs. Prolonged extracorporeal gas transfer requires gentle handling of the blood to avoid accelerated destruction of the formed elements of the blood and plasma proteins. High surface forces are avoided by separating the blood and gas phases by a thin permselective membrane (for further details see Chapter 19).

Currently, the only true membrane lung available commercially in the United States is the Sci-Med Spiral Coil membrane lung, which was designed by Kolobow in 1963. Its basic design features are unchanged since that time except for the addition of an integral heat exchanger. Externally, the Sci-Med has the appearance of a large cylindrical spool (Fig. 23-5). Note that the external and internal features in Fig. 23-5 and 23-6 share the same set of identifying numbers indicated in the text by brackets. Some numbers appear only in one figure.

a. Blood flow path. The incoming blood is directed to a ⅜-inch id inlet connector mounted at the center on the top of the membrane lung [1]. The blood flow then passes through 19 silicone coated, stainless steel tubes that are 3/16 inches id and 16 inches long. These tubes are mounted in parallel [2] and are contained within a plastic cylinder [3], which lies inside the center of the spool.

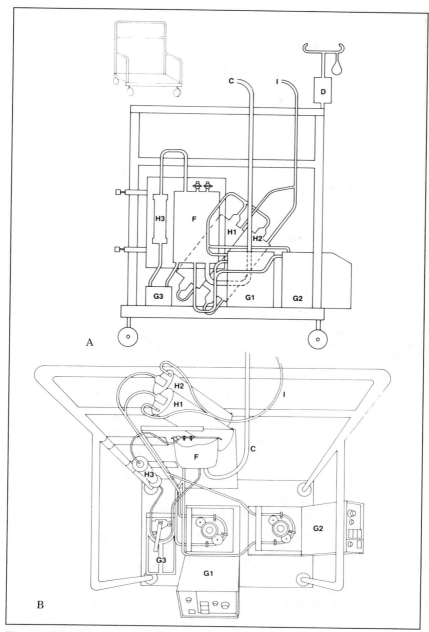

Fig. 23-4. Pictorial display of assembled extracorporeal circuit mounted compactly on mobile cart. *A.* Front view. *B.* Top view. See text for key to components.

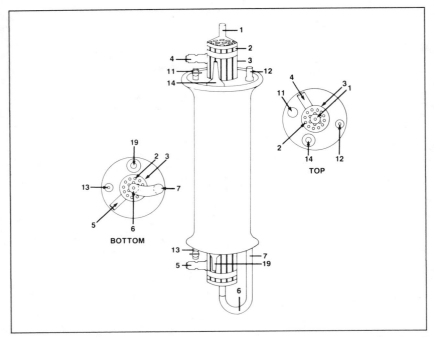

Fig. 23-5. External appearance of the Sci-Med 3.5 m² membrane oxygenator. See text for key to component parts.

Simultaneously, water, which has been heated or cooled by an external unit, enters the plastic cylinder through a ½-inch id plastic connector [4]. After bathing the outer surfaces of the stainless steel bundle [2], the water exits through a similar connector on the bottom of the machine [5] and is recirculated to the external unit. Thus, the blood and water streams are separated physically, and countercurrent heat exchange occurs by conduction across the walls of the steel tubes. The thermally equilibrated blood exits from the inside of the tubing bundle, passes through a ⅜-inch id short PVC tube that has a 180-degree turn [6], and is delivered back through a ⅜-inch id connector [7] mounted on the lower face of the spool. Internally the blood flows out from the later ⅜-inch connector into the dispersal manifold [8] and then passes upward between the adjacent membrane envelope layers [9], which are wrapped into a tight spiral. Decarbonation and oxygenation occur while the blood passes upward through this space. Carbon dioxide and oxygen diffuse across the silicone membrane separating the blood and gas compartments. The arterialized blood continues to flow upward into the collecting manifold [10], which lies above the membrane envelope. The collected blood passes externally through a ⅜-inch id connector mounted on the top of the spool [11]. Stopcock ports on the top [12] and bottom [13] allow sampling of inlet and outlet blood.

b. **Gas flow path.** Inlet gas for ventilating the lung enters through a ¼-inch id connector on the upper surface of the spool [14] and flows into four silicone rubber tubes [15] that are ¹/₁₆ inch id. These

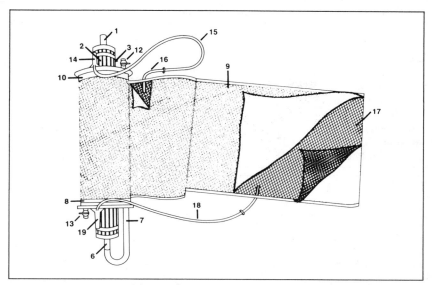

Fig. 23-6. Internal structure of the Sci-Med 3.5 m² membrane oxygenator in which the spiral membrane bundle has been unwound. See text for key to component parts. Note the pulling back of the membrane and screen to show the inside of the membrane envelope. Only one of the four gas delivery tubes (15) and one of the gas collection tubes (18) are shown. These have been lengthened to indicate the gas flow path.

convey the gas through the blood of the outlet collector header into the four equally spaced sites [16] on the top rim of the sealed membrane envelope. This envelope [9] has sides made of fiberglass-reinforced silicone rubber and is wrapped into a tight spiral. The gas flows downward around the mesh of a PVC screen [17], which is sandwiched like a letter between the two membranes (stippled area in Fig. 23-6). Thus, the blood and gas streams flow in countercurrent directions. The gas leaves the bottom rim of the sealed membrane envelope through four equally spaced silicone tubes that are ¹⁄₁₆ inch id [18]. These convey the gas through the blood of the outlet dispersal manifold and into a ¼-inch id outlet gas connector mounted on the bottom surface of the spool [19].

c. **Dimensions.** The dimensions of the components of the membrane envelope give some insight into the functional characteristics of this membrane lung. Within a single Sci-Med membrane lung of 3.5 m² surface area, the width of the envelope is 26 cm and its length is 6.7 m. Thus, each of the two sides of the envelope has a surface area of of 1.75 m². The length of the blood path traversed by the erythrocyte and the length of the gas flow path during gas exchange are both 26 cm. The screen strut forming the gas phase is made from a rectangular mesh 15 × 18 fibers per inch and is 0.76 mm thick. Thus, the gas phase width is 0.76 mm. Mathematical modeling of pressure-flow data in the blood phase and geometrical calculations imply a blood film thickness of 200 μm. The membrane thickness is 0.2 mm. These dimensions are summarized in Table 23-3 and contrasted with those of the healthy natural lung. The thick blood film of the membrane lung provides

Table 23-3. Comparison of natural lung and Sci-Med membrane lungs

	Sci-Med lung	Natural lung
Surface area (m^2)	3.5	70
Blood path length (mm)	250	1
Blood path thickness (μm)	200	6
Membrane thickness (μm)	200	0.3
Gas space size (μm)	750	100
Maximum CO_2 transfer (ml/min)	200	2500
Maximum O_2 transfer (ml/min)	200	2500
Number of function units	1	400,000,000

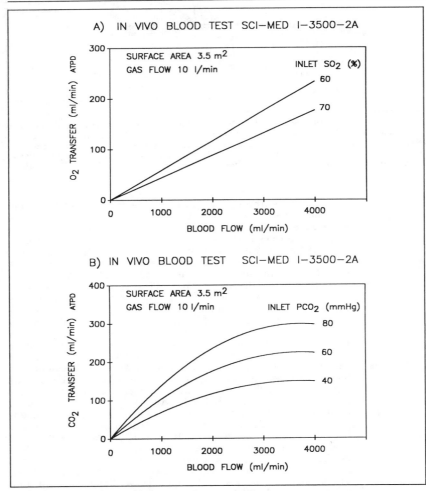

Fig. 23-7. Operating performance curves for the Sci-Med 3.5 m^2 membrane oxygenator.
A. Oxygen transfer as a function of blood flow and inlet blood oxygen saturation.
B. Carbon dioxide transfer as a function of blood flow and inlet blood PCO_2.

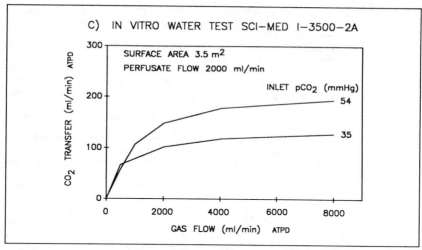

C. Carbon dioxide transfer as a function of gas flow and mock blood flow. (*A* and *B* after Friedman, Richardson and Galletti; *C* from unpublished data of senior author.)

a major resistance to gas diffusion. Thus, a long blood path length is needed for equilibration of diffusion.

d. Operating performance curves. The expected oxygen and carbon dioxide transfer rate from the Sci-Med Spiral Coil membrane lung are summarized by operating performance curves. These curves are based on in vivo animal perfusions or in vitro water perfusions and plot the membrane lung gas transfer versus blood flow rate, gas flow rate, and inlet blood gas concentrations. Oxygen transfer rate is a direct linear function of blood flow rate and an inverse function of inlet blood SO_2 (Fig. 23-7A). At even higher blood flow rates than those shown in Fig. 23-7A, the oxygen transfer rate approaches a plateau value limited by the rate of diffusion in the blood phase. The oxygen transfer rate also drops with decreases in hematocrit, the concentration of oxygen in the inlet gas, and the inlet gas flow rate. Carbon dioxide transfer rate increases with blood and gas flow but becomes increasingly diffusion limited by the membrane at higher flow rates (Figs. 23-7B and C). Carbon dioxide transfer rate is also a strong linear function of inlet blood PCO_2 (Fig. 23-7C). Hematocrit and the concentration of carbon dioxide in the inlet gas also influence carbon dioxide exchange. To determine the total extracorporeal gas transfer when membrane lungs are mounted in parallel, one sums the exchanges of individual units. If one allows for variations in blood and gas inlet conditions, significant variations of observed gas transfers from these curves during a clinical perfusion imply early membrane lung dysfunction.

2. Pumps (see Chapter 19 for a detailed discussion)
  a. Roller pumps. Roller pumps with precisely adjusted occlusion are the most inexpensive and effective way of propelling blood through the extracorporeal circuit. If a proper maintenance schedule is maintained on the drive bearings and moving motor parts, failure of the pump itself is rare during prolonged extracorporeal use. However, one must always perform preventive maintenance

at the end of a prolonged trial of ECMO. The wear on the pump for one 14-day ECMO treatment represents the cumulative wear of approximately 50–80 runs for total CPB in the operating room. Cumulative wear on the segment of plastic tubing that lies beneath the rotating roller heads is the most frequent cause of failure. Regardless of the cause, a failed pump must be replaced. For greater safety we now mount two pumps in parallel and alternate the low and high speeds of each pump. Hence, wear is distributed, and the tubing under one roller head or the entire roller pump can be replaced without lowering the extracorporeal blood flow rate.

    b. Centrifugal pumps. Although not used for ECMO at Penn State, centrifugal pumps offer several advantages. The Bio-med pump (BioMedicus, Minneapolis, MN) allows blood propulsion without concern about the disastrous effects of undetected, inadvertent outflow or inflow occlusion of the pump. Safety is achieved because the centrifugal pump stalls without generating high suction or outflow pressures whenever occlusion occurs. The initial cost of purchase is high ($13,000) and a new disposable pump head must be installed every 48 hours to avoid the buildup of fibrinous deposits in the blood phase (cost per unit, $250). Pump heads with ¼ inch id blood inflow and outflow connectors are available for neonatal use, and pump heads with ⅜ inch connectors are available for adult use. Propelling blood by such a device is simpler and places significantly less demand on personnel than use of roller pumps. Hemolysis and other damage to formed blood elements is similar to that encountered with roller pumps.

3. Tubing and connectors. Medical grade PVC tubing is the most frequently used conduit material for passing blood to, from, and within the extracorporeal circuit. Although silicone rubber tubing has been advocated in the past, its extra expense does not appear to be warranted. Currently, the interconnections of tubing segments and circuit components are made of polycarbonate connectors. These are inexpensive and usually trouble free.

4. Cannulae. The cardiovascular surgeon performing the cannulation will select the cannulae to be used in conjunction with the perfusionist. One should strive to use the cannula with the thinnest wall and with the largest bore possible that can pass through the veins without tearing them. This provides a maximum radius for the drainage and reinfusion of blood at low hydraulic resistances. Catheters whose walls are reinforced with spiral wound wire avoid kinking and have a low hydraulic resistance. Most commonly used infusion catheters have a rounded tip that is perforated with multiple end holes. Most commonly used drainage cannulae also have multiple side holes. A normal sized adult will usually require a 28F drainage cannula and a 22F reinfusion cannula.

5. Hemultrafilters. Ultrafiltration by hollow capillary fiber devices can be used to remove plasma water and electrolytes from blood continuously during ECMO. The Diafilter-30 Hemultrafilter is constructed as a cylindrical cartridge. Blood enters a dispersal manifold at the bottom of the cartridge and is distributed to vertically mounted hollow fibers. During ascent through the fibers, ultrafiltration of molecules with a molecular weight of less than 17,000 daltons takes place. After exiting the fibers, the concentrated blood is collected in the outflow manifold and is returned to the reservoir bag. The ultrafiltered plasma water and electrolytes are collected in the cylindrical space surrounding the fibers and exit at the top of the cartridge for quantitation and subsequent disposal. The transmembrane pressure gradient between the blood in the capillary and the surrounding ultrafiltrate determines the ultrafiltration rate. This gradient can be lowered by partially occluding the ultrafiltrate outlet or raised by increasing the blood flow through the device. Up to 80 ml/min of plasma water and electrolytes can be removed from the blood. A minimal blood flow of 100 ml/min must be maintained through the device to avoid thrombosis. A newer design, the Hemocor Plus hemoconcentrator (Minntech Corp., Minneapolis, MN), no longer requires the washout of glycerin from the fibers prior to use.

6. **Pump occlusion monitors and servo control.** In our extracorporeal circuit the perfusionist visually monitors the blood inflow to the pump and manually lowers the shaft speed of the roller pump if the volume of the reservoir bag drops suddenly. Boredom and sensory monotony can lead to inattention and slower response. To improve human performance, other groups have used automatic servos for this purpose. Simple on or off control has been provided by using a lever arm tangent to the full reservoir bag, which is attached to the pivot of a micro switch. The electric current driving the roller pump passes through the closed micro switch when the bag is full. As the bag empties the lever drops, the micro switch pivots open and stops the pump until the bag refills. An audible alarm sounds whenever the pump stops to warn the perfusionist.

Automatic signaling of pump outflow occlusion and its servo correction are more difficult problems. Their solution is complicated by the short time interval between occlusion and blowout of the connectors or rupture of the membrane lung.

7. **Blood flow meters.** Extracorporeal blood flow is usually estimated as the product of the roller pump shift speed and the volume of blood displaced from the tubing under the pump rollers during a single rotation of the shaft. This assumes that the pump rollers occlude the tubing and displace the blood in a forward direction during shaft rotation. During prolonged ECMO the tubing under the pump roller can become deformed, or the mechanical linkage that holds the rollers at a fixed distance from the tubing track can slip. This may cause blood to regurgitate under the pump rollers because the pump is no longer occlusive. The blood flow estimated from the shaft rotational speed will be more than the real value. This error will go undetected unless there is an independent flow meter monitoring the pump outflow. Electromagnetic and ultrasonic flow meter probes have been used for this purpose. (For details on operation see Chapter 19.) Pump occlusion can be readjusted by tightening the mechanical linkage until the blood flow indicated by the meter matches the pump setting.

E. **Architectural requirements in the intensive care unit.** Choice of a large enough room at the right location in the ICU is important. Once ECMO is begun, it is difficult to move the patient to an alternate site. Up to ten intravenous pump controllers may be required for administering drips. To accommodate the routine and special equipment, a room at least 16 feet by 15 feet in floor area with at least thirty 110 volt AC outlets is required. Communication errors are minimized if the room is equipped with a dedicated telephone line. The choice of a room located away from the main traffic flow can control the access of curious visitors and may lessen the risks of infection.

VI. **Medical management during V-V ECMO at Penn State.** The medical management of patients on ECMO is directed optimally by a team of physicians trained in intensive care management and consisting of both anesthesiologists and surgeons. Time from the decision to use ECMO to its initiation should take no more than 3 hours. Throughout the perfusions, a physician familiar with perfusion and respiratory care together with a perfusionist and nurse should be in constant attendance.

A. **Circuit priming.** Circuit components in this section are keyed to the labels in Fig. 23-3. Prior to priming, the drainage line [C] and the reinfusion line [I] are joined with a ⅜- × ½-inch polycarbonate straight connector fitted with a stopcock. The hemultrafilter is not yet mounted, and its inlet and outlet lines are also joined. The circuit is flushed first for 5 minutes with filtered carbon dioxide, which enters the reservoir bag [F] and exits through the stopcock at the junction of the drainage and reinfusion lines. During the flush the roller pumps [G1, G2, and G3] are run at low speed. Then the perfusion circuit is isolated by closing the stopcocks at the reservoir bag and the junction of the drainage and reinfusion lines. A solution of heparinized (2 units/ml) lactated Ringer's is infused into the reservoir bag. This crystalloid prime slowly fills the entire circuit by serving as an eager solvent for the carbon dioxide. If done correctly, no bubbles will remain in the circuit. If any are present, these can be displaced to the reservoir bag by running the roller pumps G1 and G2 at high speed. The accumulated air at the top of the bag can be drawn off through one of the stopcocks. The hemultrafilter [H3] is then flushed with 2000 ml of normal saline and placed in the circuit. After the crystalloid is emptied from the reservoir bag, 2000 ml of citrated fresh whole blood is heparinized (2 units/ml) and slowly added to the circuit. Roller pumps G1 and G2 are run at 1000 ml/min to recirculate the prime. The gas ventilating the membrane lung is set at a concentration of 100% oxygen and a flow of 1000 ml/min. This avoids excessive hyperventilation of the blood in the prime and normalizes the PCO_2. During the next 2 hours, most of the initial crystalloid in the prime is ultrafiltered by running G3 at a blood flow of 300 ml/min and partially occluding the ultrafiltrate outflow. An extracorporeal prime is produced with a hematocrit of 25–30%. Calcium chloride and sodium bicarbonate are added to correct the base deficit and the ionized calcium levels. The integral heat exchanger maintains the extracorporeal blood temperature at 37°C prior to the initiation of bypass.

B. **Cannulation.** While the extracorporeal circuit is being assembled and primed, peripheral cannulations of the right internal jugular vein and right common femoral vein are performed either in the operating room or the intensive care unit under general anesthesia. Use of the former will maintain better infection control but requires transport of a severely hypoxic patient requiring high FIO_2 and PEEP on a battery-powered portable ventilator accompanied by mobile oxygen cylinders.

We usually employ high-dose fentanyl (50 μg/kg) and pancuronium (0.1 mg/kg) for muscle relaxation. The antimuscarinic effect of pancuronium minimizes the bradycardia seen when the endotracheal tube of the ARDS patient is disconnected from the ventilator for suctioning. Potent inhalation drugs often produce hypoxemia by blunting vasoconstriction of the injured pulmonary circulation and are best avoided. Small doses of scopolamine ensure amnesia.

A pulmonary artery catheter must be in place prior to cannulation. It is very difficult to thread one in later around the large-bore drainage cannula in the superior vena cava. After performing cutdowns on the right iliac and internal jugular veins with meticulous hemostasis, the patient is given heparin to achieve an activated clotting time (ACT) of 300–400 seconds. This typically requires more than 5000 units of heparin. The cannulae are inserted and occluded. Then the patient is transported back to the ICU.

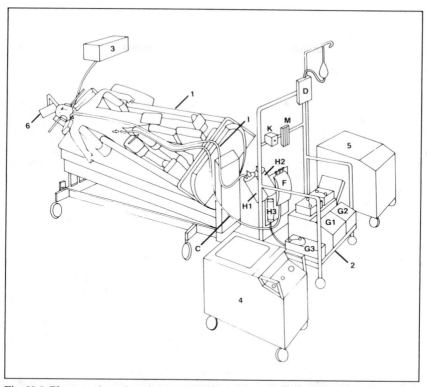

Fig. 23-8. Blow-up view of equipment in patient's room during ECMO. Note extracorporeal circuit mounted on the mobile cart (2) at the foot of rocker bed (1). Pressure transducers are kept at a constant level at the axis of the rotation of the bed (6). The adjacent mechanical ventilator (3), hot or cold water source for heat exchanger (4), and mass spectrometer (5) require a room with floor dimensions of at least 16 feet by 15 feet. See text for key to circuit components.

C. **Cardiopulmonary monitoring.** On arrival in the ICU from the OR, the patient is placed on a rocker bed that rotates up to 70 degrees each way around a longitudinal axis (Fig. 23-8). Cardiopulmonary monitoring is then reestablished. Pressure transducers must be positioned at the axis of the rocker bed to prevent periodic shifts in the zero level during bed rotation. Cardiac outputs can be measured by injecting cardiac green dye into the pulmonary artery or by thermal dilution with injection of room temperature saline into the right ventricular pacing port of the pulmonary artery catheter.

D. **Startup of V-V ECMO.** The number of personnel in the room must be kept at a minimum to avoid confusion and subsequent errors at the startup of perfusion.

1. **Connection of patient to ECMO circuit.** After cardiopulmonary monitoring is established, the cart containing the ECMO circuit is placed at the foot of the patient's bed (Fig. 23-8). The connector joining the blood drainage and infusion lines is removed sterilely. The occlusion of roller pumps G1 and G2 is set to have a leak of 1

cm/min against an outflow blood column 30 inches high. The drainage and reinfusion lines are primed sterilely with heparinized saline and connected to the appropriate cannulae. By allowing the drainage and infusion lines to leave the bed at the longitudinal axis at the foot of the bed, postural drainage can be accomplished without danger of obstructing the inlet or outflow of the extracorporeal blood flow.

2. **Initiation of pumping and its special dangers.** Fatal disasters can occur rapidly at the startup of ECMO. While watching the systemic arterial, central venous, and pulmonary arterial pressures, ECMO is started slowly. The initial turns of roller pumps are made manually without using a pump crank while the drainage line is occluded with a tubing clamp. Then the electric motor of the pump is started. The occlusion of the drainage line is slowly released and the shaft rotational speed gradually increased until blood flow of 1250 ml/m^2/min is obtained. Simultaneously, by adjusting the gas blender and rotameter, 100% oxygen is delivered to the membrane lung gas inlet at a flow equal to twice the blood flow rate. **This slow startup of pump speed during ECMO is in stark contrast to the usual quick beginning of total CPB during cardiac surgery.** Specific dangers that may be avoided, detected, or easily eliminated by a slow startup include:

   a. **Outflow occlusion of the roller pump.** An inadvertently placed or forgotten tubing clamp placed distal to the roller pump outflow as well as a kinked extracorporeal return line can cause the ECMO circuit to blow out within seconds at high flows. Acute overflow occlusion is most likely to occur at the start of ECMO because of the hurried efforts to alleviate the patient's severe hypoxemia. Outflow occlusion can be felt as an extreme resistance to roller rotation if the roller is moved manually without a crank handle. If present, the site must be found and eliminated before increasing the pump flow.

   b. **Acute circulatory collapse.** Marked systemic arterial hypotension can occur soon after the start of ECMO. Differential diagnosis of the causes of circulatory collapse and their possible treatments include the following:

      (1) **"Bleeding" into the reservoir bag.** The most common cause of hypotension at the start of ECMO is the rapid displacement of large volumes of blood from the patient's veins to the reservoir bag in the extracorporeal circuit. If the reservoir bag volume is low, blood may drain rapidly from the patient's central veins by gravity and into the extracorporeal circuit to fill it. This sudden hypovolemia is reflected by a low CVP and PWCP. Stable hemodynamics can be restored quickly by clamping the drainage line and returning blood back to the patient with the roller pump. A lower extracorporeal blood flow rate and a partial clamping of the drain line may be needed until more blood or colloid has been transfused into the patient's venous system. High extracorporeal blood flows will be possible only when the total blood volume of the central veins and reservoir bag is large enough to be partitioned to provide both an adequate CVP and an adequate reservoir bag pressure.

      (2) **Overdistention of the right ventricle.** Occasionally the reservoir bag may be overfilled during the priming, or the reservoir may be squeezed between two transparent compression plates to reduce its compliance. Because the compliance of the reservoir bag is always nonlinear and decreases with increasing filling, the elastic recoil of the overfilled bag will produce a very high blood pressure in the reservoir. Opening the clamp

on the extracorporeal drainage line at the start of perfusion displaces blood quickly from the reservoir bag into the patient's venous system. This rapid transfusion can raise the CVP quickly, overstretch the right ventricle, and cause severe lethal heart failure. Treatment must be rapid. Any compression plate must be removed from the reservoir bag. A small amount of decompression can be obtained immediately by increasing the ECMO flow. This has a limited effect because the blood is recirculated wholly in the veins during V-V pumping. Rapidly raising the bed and increasing the hemultrafiltration to maximum will remove 400–800 ml of circulating volume from the central vein in 5–10 minutes. Venodilation with nitroglycerin or removal of blood from the extracorporeal circuit into blood donor bags may be necessary.

(3) **Delivery of hyperventilated blood from the circuit prime.** The blood leaving the membrane lung at the start of ECMO tends to be hypocapnic and alkalotic ($PCO_2 < 10$ mm Hg and pH > 7.85). While waiting for the completion of cannulation, extremely prolonged hyperventilation of the extracorporeal prime can occur during recirculation. The transient effect of this initial bolus of hyperventilated blood on the patient's cardiovascular system depends on the ECMO pumping route. If V-V ECMO is started at low extracorporeal blood flows, the venous return dilutes the low PCO_2 and high PO_2 of the extracorporeal return, and there are no adverse effects on the pulmonary or systemic circulations. In contrast, a rapid startup of V-A ECMO with aortic root return can deliver this hyperventilated blood directly to the coronary arteries, which may result in disastrous ventricular dysrhythmias. The best way to eliminate this problem is to ventilate the membrane lung after priming with a gas mixture of 5% carbon dioxide and 40% oxygen in a balance of nitrogen. The gas ventilating the membrane lung must be changed to 100% oxygen before starting perfusion.

(4) **Transfusion reaction.** In rare instances, circulatory collapse at the startup of ECMO may be due to a transfusion reaction initiated by the homocorporeal blood in the extracorporeal prime. A slow startup allows gradual mixing of the prime with the patient's blood and may allow treatment of hypotension prior to total collapse with mannitol, vasopressors, and steroids. Increasing the extracorporeal blood flow rate during V-V ECMO while clamping the drainage line will have little if any effect on blood pressure. Removal of the current ECMO circuit with its offending blood may not be feasible.

If these maneuvers do not reverse the circulatory collapse, one must remember that there is no means of partial cardiac support with V-V pumping. With V-A pumping, however, nearly full cardiac support may be available.

c. **Inadequate venous drainage.** If necessary, the rocker bed can be raised to provide a greater pressure head for better drainage of the patient's venous blood into the reservoir. Two designs of rocker beds have been used. The Rotorest Bed (Mediscus Products, Inc., Buena Park, CA) requires slow elevation by manual jacks for placement of blocks. The Keane Mobility Bed (Ethos Medical Ltd., Athlone, Ireland) is driven by electrical motors that allow rapid vertical elevations of up to 2 feet.

    d. Shivering and movement. Prior to the startup of ECMO, the patient must be well paralyzed and sedated. The drop in blood drug levels at the start of ECMO, because of dilution by the extracorporeal prime, may result in a resumption of a hypermetabolic state with shivering and movement. A large increase in the patient's oxygen consumption may cause a worsening of PaO_2 and SaO_2.

E. Anticoagulation. The ACT is monitored every 30 minutes for the first 4 hours of perfusion and is maintained between 160 and 240 seconds by adjusting the rate of continuous heparin infusion into the reservoir bag from 0–3000 units/hr. Thereafter, the ACT is checked every hour, and the heparin infusion rate is adjusted accordingly. Care must be taken when administering platelet concentrates, fresh-frozen plasma, and cryoprecipitate because these may rapidly lower the ACT to dangerous levels when such low-dose heparin infusions are deployed. Thrombosis of blood in the extracorporeal circuit may ensue rapidly. Heparin boluses of 1000–5000 units may be needed to restore the ACT to an appropriate value.

F. Monitoring natural and extracorporeal lung gas exchange. Oxygen and carbon dioxide transport by the injured natural lung can be calculated using the Fick principle with the Haldane correction for steady state nitrogen excretion. This requires that the concentrations of oxygen (FIO_2), carbon dioxide ($FICO_2$), and nitrogen (FIN_2) in the inspired gas are monitored online by mass spectrometry while the expired gas is collected in a 120-liter Douglas bag. After the collected expired gas has mixed by diffusion, its composition is similarly measured off line for mixed expired oxygen concentration ($F\bar{E}O_2$), mixed expired carbon dioxide ($F\bar{E}CO_2$), and mixed expired nitrogen ($F\bar{E}N_2$). During the sampling time, the expired minute volume ($\dot{V}_E$) is measured by the bag and box system within the Engstrom Erica or the flow meter in the Servo 900C mechanical ventilators. Natural lung oxygen transfer ($\dot{V}O_2$) and the natural lung carbon dioxide transfer ($\dot{V}CO_2$) are calculated by the following equations (Eqn. 1 and 2).

$$\dot{V}O_2 = \dot{V}_E \cdot [FIO_2 \cdot (F\bar{E}N_1/FIN_2) - F\bar{E}O_2] \tag{1}$$

$$\dot{V}CO_2 = \dot{V}_E \cdot [F\bar{E}CO_2 - FICO_2 \cdot (F\bar{E}N_2/FIN_2)] \tag{2}$$

Determination of gas exchange in the membrane lung requires precise measurement of gas inflow ($\dot{v}I$) to the membrane lung and sequential determination of inlet concentrations of oxygen, carbon dioxide, and nitrogen (FIO_2, FIO_2, and FIN_2) and exit concentrations of oxygen, carbon dioxide, and nitrogen (FEO_2, $FECO_2$, and FEN_2) by mass spectrometry (Fig. 23-9). Membrane lung oxygen transfer ($\dot{v}O_2$) and membrane lung carbon dioxide transfer ($\dot{v}O_2$) are calculated by the following equations using the Fick principle with the Haldane correction (Eqn. 3 and 4 respectively).

$$\dot{v}O_2 = \dot{V}I \cdot [FIO_2 - (FIN_2/FEN_2) \cdot FEO_2] \tag{3}$$

$$\dot{v}CO_2 = \dot{V}I \cdot [(FIN_2/FEN_2) \cdot FECO_2 - FICO_2] \tag{4}$$

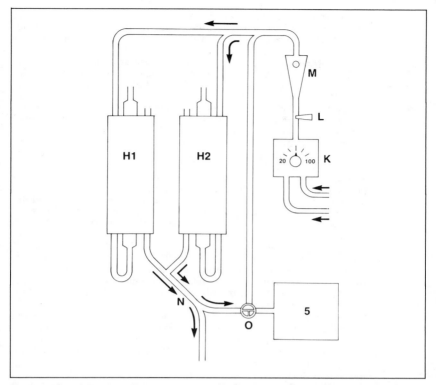

Fig. 23-9. Gas delivery and measurement system for membrane lungs. Compressed oxygen and air are mixed in the blender (K), which allows the oxygen and nitrogen concentrations of the inlet gas to the membrane lung to be selected. The needle valve (L) mounted in series with a rotameter (M) controls and indicates the inlet gas flow rate. The gas stream is divided to pass through the two 3.5 m² Sci-Med membrane lungs mounted in parallel (H1 and H2). Gas streams exiting from the membrane lungs are combined and mixed (N). A stopcock (O) permits either the inlet or exit gas concentrations to be measured by the mass spectrometer (5). Compressed air and oxygen inputs are denoted by the two arrows *(far right)*.

Alternatively, the performance of the membrane lung can be determined by blood gas measurements on the blood entering and exiting from the membrane lungs. Sampling involves handling stopcocks attached to fragile luer-lock connectors at the top and bottom of the Sci-Med membrane lung. If one of these stopcocks is broken off, the membrane lung may have to be removed.

G. **Adjustment of membrane blood flow and gas flow.** That fraction of the patient's oxygen consumption and carbon dioxide production that needs to be transferred by the membrane lung depends on the inefficiency of gas exchange of the patient's injured lung and the level of ventilator support. In general, the lower the patient's FIO_2, PEEP, and respiratory rate and the greater his or her venous admixture and dead space, the greater the demands on the membrane lung's gas exchange.

1. **Choice of membrane lung blood flow.** In general, the higher the extracorporeal blood flow rate during V-V ECMO, the greater the

extracorporeal gas transfer. Thus, one should achieve the highest practical blood flow. The usual factor limiting the return flow from the extracorporeal circuit is the rate of blood inflow from the patient's veins into the reservoir bag through the drainage cannula. This flow through the extracorporeal drain cannula is determined by the position of the tip of the cannula, the radius of the drainage cannula, the CVP, and the height between the right atrium and the reservoir bag. Cannula position and size are almost impossible to change after the start of ECMO without heavy blood loss. However, the height between the right atrium and the reservoir bag can be changed rapidly by raising or lowering a motorized bed. The CVP increases mainly with intravenous volume infusion or decreases with hemorrhage. Care must be taken not to overtransfuse. Chronic elevation of the CVP above 25 mm Hg may cause hepatic venous congestion and peripheral edema. Pharmacologic alterations in venomotor capacitance can also change the CVP. Venodilation by endotoxin or nitroglycerin can enlarge the venous capacity, lower CVP, and decrease drainage. Venoconstrictors have the opposite effect. **There is little gain in raising the extracorporeal blood flow above the patient's cardiac output.**

However, more than the quantity of blood flow is involved. Even with ideal cannulae placement (Fig. 23-2), mass balance calculations predict that the pulmonary arterial SO_2 is unable to ever rise to 100%. This is true because the coronary venous return with its low SO_2 fails to drain into the extracorporeal circuit. Subsequently, the coronary sinus venous return mixes with the extracorporeal stream to form the mixed venous blood in the pulmonary artery. For example, let the outlet SO_2 of the membrane lung be equal to 1.0, the extracorporeal return flow be equal to 80% of the cardiac output, the coronary venous SO_2 be equal to 20%, and the coronary venous flow be equal to 20% of cardiac output. Then the maximum $S\bar{v}O_2$ will be 84%.

The SaO_2 attained after passage of the mixed venous blood through the pulmonary capillary bed depends on the $S\bar{v}O_2$ and the venous admixture of the injured lung. The venous admixture consists of regions of true shunt and low V_A/Q. The latter may improve their gas exchange with increased FIO_2. The maximum SaO_2 and PaO_2 attainable with V-V ECMO can be calculated assuming various venous admixtures (Table 23-4). Note that, with a 25% venous admixture while breathing room air, an SaO_2 of 94% and a PaO_2 of 74 mm Hg can be achieved when the extracorporeal blood flow equals the cardiac output! If the venous admixture is not all shunt, some improvement will occur by increasing the FIO_2. With a 100% venous admixture during a similar cardiac output and extracorporeal flow, the pulmonary and systemic arterial blood gas values become equal. That is, PaO_2 equals 49 mm Hg and SaO_2 equals 84%.

The expected gas transfer rates at any given blood and gas flows can be read from the operating performance curves (see Fig. 23-7A and B). For two membrane lungs mounted in parallel, the blood flow is assumed to be divided equally between them. The predicted oxygen and carbon dioxide transfer rates are read at half the total extracorporeal blood flow and then doubled.

2. **Choice of membrane lung gas flow.** Membrane lung carbon dioxide transfer is also strongly influenced by the inlet gas flow rate (Fig. 23-7C). Because there is some gain in extracorporeal carbon dioxide transfer with membrane lung hyperventilation, the gas flow rate is usually run at two to four times the blood flow rate. For two

Table 23-4. Calculated effect of venous admixture on arterial gas exchange during high efficiency V-V ECMO*

Venous admixture (%)	SaO_2 (%)	PaO_2 (mm Hg)
0	97	100
25	94	74
50	91	64
75	87	53
100	84	49

*Assumes:
1. FIO_2 equals 0.21
2. $PaCO_2$ equals 40 mm Hg
3. Cardiac output equals extracorporeal flow
4. Normal oxygen consumption and carbon dioxide production
5. Optimal cannula placement
6. Extracorporeal return at SO_2 of 100%

lungs in parallel, inlet gas flow rates of 10–20 liters/min are frequently used.

3. **Choice of membrane lung gas inlet oxygen concentration.** Prolonged exposure of the blood to high PO_2 within the membrane lung may cause oxidative damage to erythrocytes. This possibility can be avoided by reducing the gas inlet oxygen concentration until a PO_2 of 150 mm Hg or less is generated in the blood exiting from the membrane lung. Because reducing the PO_2 from 600 to 150 mm Hg produces only small changes in the SO_2 of the blood in the extracorporeal return, there is little effect on the mixed venous PO_2 in the pulmonary artery. This adjustment can be made without measurements on the blood samples exiting from the membrane lung. When measuring the membrane lung gas exchange while the inlet gas oxygen concentration is reduced, a point will be found at which the oxygen transfer of the membrane lung begins to drop precipitously. This is the minimal inlet oxygen concentration that should be used.

H. **Adjustment of mechanical ventilator.** The level of ventilator support required during ECMO depends on the efficiency of extracorporeal gas exchange and the resolution or worsening of lung injury. An optimal ventilation strategy during ECMO is undefined, but ventilator settings should be chosen to rest the injured lung and allow healing. Goals that are generally agreed on are lowering the FIO_2 to prevent further damage to the alveolar epithelium and endothelium from oxygen toxicity. During the first few hours of ECMO, the FIO_2 is slowly decreased to 0.2–0.3. What constitutes safe levels of inspired oxygen for the resolution of ARDS and the repair of acute lung injury remains unknown.

1. **Lowering ventilator rate.** Our second priority is to lower the ventilator rate to decrease mean airway pressure and lessen barotrauma. Simultaneously, while dropping the FIO_2, we slowly decrease the ventilator rate during the first few hours of ECMO to lower MAP. This usually requires hyperventilation of the membrane lung to prevent arterial hypercapnia. Despite the use of two 3.5-m^2 membrane lungs mounted in parallel, we have been unable to lower the ventricular rate to less than 10 breaths/min without elevating $PaCO_2$. This goal might be accomplished by mounting the same two mem-

brane lungs in series for further hyperventilation of the extracorporeal blood.

2. **Lowering tidal volume and PEEP.** The other two determinants of MAP are the tidal volume and the PEEP. The peak airway pressure depends largely on the tidal volume. For the first few hours of perfusion, we maintain the PEEP and tidal volume at their pre-ECMO levels. What level of PEEP and tidal volume should be used for lung inflation during ECMO remains unclear. Lower pressures may hasten the resolution of barotrauma but also cause total alveolar collapse. Such collapse occurred in three of our patients who went on to die in total pulmonary failure on ECMO. Consequently, we recommend that PEEP and tidal volume levels be decreased very slowly and that frequent chest radiographs be taken to assess lung aeration.

I. **Chest physiotherapy.** Rocker beds are an essential part of a patient's pulmonary management. The bed is rotated from side-to-side every 10 minutes. This enhances the mobilization of secretions into the central airways where they can be suctioned. Also, it provides a safe mechanism for rolling the patient for chest physiotherapy. With the ECMO cannulae fixed to the bed at the axis of rotation of the bed these movements are possible without dislodging the cannulae, which would likely be a fatal complication. Chest physiotherapy is vital in these patients to prevent infection and optimize pulmonary function. Periodically the rocker bed is locked at a 70-degree rotation to the right or left so that manual percussion and endotracheal suction can be performed. Mechanical vibration is applied to the chest wall every 2 hours.

J. **Infection control.** Infection control measures must be meticulous because uncontrolled sepsis makes extracorporeal circulation impossible. Major efforts must be made to avoid iatrogenic infection. Particularly susceptible are the cannulation sites in the groin and the neck. These sites need daily dressing changes with chemical debridement of the tissue using iodine-containing solutions and hydrogen peroxide. Daily wound cultures should be taken.

Equally important is the detection of bacteremia within the extracorporeal circuit. Any systemic venous bacteremia is likely to seed the extracorporeal circuit because almost the entire venous return is diverted into the drainage cannula. For this reason, anaerobic and aerobic blood cultures are taken from the reservoir bag of the extracorporeal circuit every 8 hours during perfusion.

Another possible source of sepsis is old blood left in stopcock hubs after blood sampling. All stopcocks attached to the extracorporeal circuit or patient must be rinsed after each use with an antibiotic solution containing 1 g of nafcillin and 80 mg of gentamicin in 500 ml of normal saline. After cleaning, every stopcock hub should be covered with a sterile locking cap between uses. Blood sampling and pressure monitoring from the extracorporeal circuit is kept at a minimum.

K. **Pharmacologic therapy.** Patients on ECMO **deserve adequate sedation and require profound muscle relaxation.** Occasional reversal of muscle relaxation and recovery from sedation is prudent to assess the possible onset of neurologic damage.

1. **Sedation.** The necessity for sedation is obvious and is best accomplished with continuous intravenous infusion of narcotics supplemented with benzodiazepines. Fentanyl doses as high as $10 \ \mu g \cdot kg^{-1} \cdot hr^{-1}$ and midazolam 2 mg/hr may be needed throughout the perfusion to achieve an amnestic, pain-free patient.

2. **Muscle relaxants.** Muscle relaxation is necessary for safety and to decrease shivering. An unparalyzed patient who is startled suddenly because of light sedation could occlude or dislodge the drainage and

reinfusion cannulae. By preventing shivering, muscle relaxants decrease carbon dioxide production and oxygen consumption, allowing mild hypothermia and reducing the ventilatory requirement. If bradycardia is present when the patient is disconnected for suctioning, pancuronium can minimize this effect. If renal or hepatic failure ensues, a switch to vecuronium or atracurium is wise. Infusion rates are titrated to reduce the train of 4 to 1 twitch. This goal frequently takes doses of 0.1 mg/kg/hr for vecuronium, or 0.1 or 1 mg/kg/hr for atracurium.

3. **Vasodilators.** Vasodilators have become popular in critical care medicine for treating low cardiac output states characterized by a high systemic vascular resistance (SVR). Intravenous infusions of sodium nitroprusside, nitroglycerin, and isoproterenol have been used for this purpose. Some have advocated their use in ARDS to treat the right ventricular dysfunction caused by pulmonary arterial hypertension. When used in patients with ARDS, these drugs also overwhelm the hypoxic vasoconstriction of the injured lung, which produces not only a drop in pulmonary vascular resistance (PVR) but also an increase in venous admixture and a fall in PaO_2. This may increase the need for a higher level of ventilator support. In theory, vasodilators may either worsen or ameliorate the pulmonary vascular damage in ARDS. Some argue that, because ARDS is an ischemic vascular injury of the lung, vasodilation of the injured regions will improve nutrient and oxygen flow. Others argue that removal of the arterial vasoconstriction exposes the injured capillary bed to the full elevated pulmonary arterial pressure and will cause further damage from overflow edema. Because the effects of vasodilators on the pulmonary circulation in ARDS are incompletely defined, we avoid their use unless they are absolutely needed for control of systemic arterial hypertension.

L. **Temperature control.** While the patient is paralyzed, body temperature is easily controlled by the built-in heat exchangers of the spiral coil lung. A temperature of 36–37°C is usually maintained, but it can be lowered rapidly to 30–32°C if one of the membrane lungs must be changed.

M. **Fluid balance.** Small doses of furosemide are usually needed to maintain diuresis. Excessive use of diuretics can be avoided by continuous removal of plasma water and electrolytes by hemultrafiltration. If renal function is normal, the ultrafiltration rate is set at 0.5 ml/kg/hr or less so that the urine output continues unabated. If renal function is impaired or renal failure is present, the ultrafiltration rate is chosen to be equal to the hyperalimentation and maintenance crystalloid input.

V-V hemultrafiltration may aid in clearing water from the injured lung. Because hemultrafiltration occurs within the extracorporeal V-V circuit, the plasma oncotic pressure of the blood returning in the extracorporeal line must be greater than that of blood being drained from the central veins. Thus, blood entering the pulmonary artery will have a higher oncotic pressure and may tend to pull water from the injured pulmonary capillary bed. The quantitative significance of this effect has not been established.

Fortunately, the circulating blood volume is generally easily augmented during ECMO. Care must be taken not to raise the central venous pressure above 25 mm Hg by fluid administration. This will avoid hepatic congestion and systemic edema. Sudden increases in venous return following the infusion of pressors can overfill the reservoir bag. Overfilling can be managed by quickly removing 200–300 ml of extracellular volume over a period of 30 minutes by rapid ultrafiltration. In edematous patients, large volumes of fluid may be ultrafiltered because excessive extracellular fluid is mobilized during recovery.

N. **Nutritional support.** Caloric intake during ECMO is provided by the intravenous infusion of 70% glucose with 4.25% amino acids through a central venous catheter. The accompanying fluid load is ultrafiltered. Fat emulsions are usually avoided during the acute injury phase for fear of further injury to the lung by the presence of hydroperoxides in the emulsion. Caloric input is given at a rate of 50–60 Kcal/kg/day and adjusted according to the patient's oxygen consumption, carbon dioxide production, and respiratory quotient. The oxygen consumption is taken as the sum of $\dot{V}o_2$ and $\dot{V}o_2$. Similarly, the carbon dioxide production is taken as the sum of $\dot{V}coO_2$ and $\dot{V}co_2$. Respiratory quotient is calculated as the ratio of carbon dioxide production to oxygen consumption.

VII. **Complications of ECMO and their emergency management**

A. **Hemorrhage.** Hemorrhage secondary to thrombocytopenia and disseminated intravascular coagulation can occur in any patient suffering from ARDS with or without ECMO. Systemic heparin infusions greatly increase this risk. Bleeding usually occurs at the sites of cannulation and is best controlled at the time of cannula insertion with careful surgical hemostasis. Often some bloody secretions will be obtained from the endotracheal tube during suctioning. Because insertion of nasogastric tubes may precipitate significant nasal hemorrhage, orogastric placement is preferable. Trauma patients are particularly subject to hemorrhage from open fractures and into contused tissue.

The onset of spontaneous bleeding requires investigation. An ACT should be done immediately, and coagulation studies including a prothrombin time, partial thromboplastin time, fibrinogen level, fibrin split products, and platelet count should be sent to the laboratory. Overheparinization and underheparinization with consumption of clotting factors need to be considered. The membrane lung manifolds should be checked for clot.

Packed red blood cells or whole blood are administered to maintain a hematocrit of 30. Fresh-frozen plasma is given to correct the prothrombin time. Fibrinogen levels less than 150 mg/dl are treated with cryoprecipitate. Platelet concentrates are given whenever the platelet count drops below 25,000/μl.

B. **Thrombus formation in the patient and extracorporeal circuit.** The reservoir bag, the transparent upper and lower surfaces of the hemultrafilter are illuminated frequently to check for in situ thrombosis formation or deposition of thromboemboli in the blood dispersal and collection manifolds. This is easily done with a flashlight to contrast the slightly translucent blood with the opaque clot. In the SciMed membrane lung the most frequent sites of thrombosis are along the four gas delivery tubes made of silicone rubber that pass through the blood phase of the dispersal and collection manifolds (items [15] and [18] in Fig. 23-6). In the reservoir bag the most frequent sites of thrombosis are the regions of stagnant flow at the corners of the bag or along the internal tubing. Small black or white thrombi start their growth at these sites.

Occasionally, clot may form unobserved on the internal blood surfaces of the membrane lung envelope. Its presence can be inferred by a decrease in membrane lung gas exchange and confirmed by disassembly of the membrane lung after its removal from the extracorporeal circuit. **Clot formation in the extracorporeal circuit has several implications:**

1. **If the patient is on V-A ECMO, the risk of systemic embolism.**

2. **If the patient is on V-V ECMO, the risk of pulmonary embolism.**
3. **Inadequate heparinization.**
4. **Impairment of membrane lung function.**
5. **Consumption of coagulation factors.**
Clot formation is usually accompanied by a rise in fibrin split products and may be treated by increasing the heparin infusion rate until the ACT is increased by approximately 100 seconds.

C. **Hemolysis.** Hemolysis may be induced by mechanically fragile erythrocytes passing through regions of high shear in the ECMO circuit or at the cannulae tips. The older the blood received from the blood bank for transfusion, the greater its mechanical fragility. Only the freshest blood should be used. Regions of high shear are seen at turbulent jets, where blood flows are accelerated to high velocities through expanded or contracted orifices. Turbulence can occur at the tip of the return cannula as well as at the entry to the reservoir bag. An overocclusive roller pump can also induce hemolysis.

The current rate of erythrocyte destruction is reflected by an increase in the plasma-free hemoglobin (normal values 0–10 mg/dl). Values seen during prolonged ECMO should not exceed 15 mg/dl. Cumulative erythrocyte destruction is reflected in the total bilirubin level. In the absence of hepatic and biliary dysfunction the conjugated bilirubin level should be less than 10 mg/dl during a prolonged ECMO perfusion.

D. **Sepsis.** Uncontrolled sepsis usually requires cessation of extracorporeal circulation. When bacteremia and sepsis ensue, one usually sees a drop in systemic arterial pressure with a very low systemic vascular resistance. These bouts of hypotension are initially corrected by dopamine or epinephrine but gradually become so extreme that vasopressors are ineffective even at high infusion rates. An ongoing lactic acidosis usually implies inadequate visceral perfusion or hepatocellular damage. This sign usually foretells death within the next few hours. To achieve adequate antibiotic levels within the perfusion circuit, antibiotics are infused into the reservoir bag.

E. **Neurologic damage.** A full neurologic examination is difficult during ECMO because most patients are chemically paralyzed. Periodically, the drug infusions are stopped, and paralysis is allowed to resolve by metabolism of the muscle relaxant so that neurologic function can be assessed. After decannulation, most patients remain on high-dose opiates for the remainder of the period of resolution of their ARDS. By 1 week after decannulation, most patients can respond verbally and follow three-step commands. All should have complete amnesia for their entire ICU experience. The most serious complications are permanent neurologic damage from ECMO. Cerebral hemorrhage, though common in neonates, is unusual during adult ECMO. During V-V pumping, the brain is usually protected from arterial thromboemboli from the membrane lung by the pulmonary circulation of the natural lung. However, during V-A pumping, cerebral emboli can occur. Hemorrhagic and embolic phenomena are usually diffuse with multiple neurologic signs. The prognosis for full recovery from either complication is poor. Survivors of ECMO, however, are often able to resume full neurologic functioning. One of our survivors went on to finish college and obtain a master's degree in business administration from an Ivy League school; he is currently employed as a stock broker.

F. **Equipment malfunction and operator error.** During use of the ECMO circuit, components can malfunction, fail, or be misused, with devastating results.

1. **Gas exchange failure of the membrane lung.** Clot may form on the membrane lung manifolds if the ACT is too low or if blood prod-

ucts are infused into the reservoir bag instead of into the patient's veins. Decreasing the pump flow rate also transiently decreases extracorporeal gas exchange and may cause the blood within the extracorporeal circuit to clot. Mounting two lungs in parallel allows one to be replaced while the other maintains some gas exchange (see [G1 and G2] in Fig. 23-3). Prior to replacing a malfunctioning membrane lung in the extracorporeal circuit, the new lung must be primed first in sterile fashion with carbon dioxide and then with saline.

2. **Roller pump failure.** When roller pump failure occurs, the cause is often a linear fracture of the PVC tubing under the pump rollers. Linear fracture occurs on both sides of the tubing at the edges of the tubing where it was flattening by the rollers. This problem will eventually occur regardless of the composition of the pump tubing. It will occur rarely if heavy duty PVC tubing is used as the pump tubing. For some time prior to failure, spallation (break-off of fragments of the inner tubing wall) occurs with subsequent embolization to the membrane lung and patient. Rupture is usually heralded by the appearance of a few drops of blood on the roller head track and may become manifest as a massive blood leak within minutes. The incidence and consequences of this problem can be minimized by always running two roller pumps mounted in parallel (see [G1 and G2] in Fig. 23-3). By alternating which pump runs at high speed, the wear can be distributed between the pump tubes. Both roller heads must always be rotating or clot will form at that site in the circuit. The pumps can be stopped one at a time for brief periods to move the tubing under the roller head. If the tubing under one of the pump roller heads fractures, the other pump can take over the entire extracorporeal blood flow without disrupting extracorporeal gas exchange. Meanwhile, the fractured tubing can be isolated by occlusive tubing clamps and replaced sterilely.

3. **Pump outflow occlusion.** Just as at the time of the initiation of ECMO, partial or total occlusion of the outflow of a roller pump at any time during the perfusion can be disastrous within seconds. If the reinfusion cannula is occluded even for a few seconds during ECMO with roller pumps, the connections between the connectors and the tubing on the high pressure side of the circuit distal to the roller pump may pop off, or the membrane lung may rupture. By securing all tubing connector junctions with nylon ties, pop-off tubing disconnections can be avoided during partial outflow occlusion.

4. **Pump inflow occlusion.** The volume of the reservoir bag is constant if the gravity drainage rate from the venous system equals the rate of removal by the roller pumps perfusing the membrane lungs. If the drainage line is occluded, the volume of the reservoir bag will rapidly diminish. An alert perfusionist will decrease the roller pump flow to avoid blood cavitation or degassing, which will occur if the bag empties completely. The time for the bag to empty following total inflow occlusion equals the quotient of the reservoir bag volume divided by the combined flow rates of the extracorporeal pumps perfusing the membrane lungs. Thus, a 2000-ml reservoir bag will empty in 30 seconds when the blood flow rate is 4000 ml/min.

5. **Stopcock fracture or displacement.** Care must be taken in handling stopcocks attached to tubing connectors and the membrane lung. A lateral, rotary force carelessly applied to a syringe that has been connected to the stopcock is transmitted to the junction of the Luer-lok with the surface of the membrane lung or with the body of the tubing connector. This force can shear off the Luer-lok or the stopcock and cause a large blood leak. This risk is reduced by minimizing the use of these stopcocks for sampling and infusion. When

manipulation is necessary, one hand must brace the body of the stopcock while the other hand attaches or detaches the syringe and turns the handle of the stopcock.

VIII. **When is ECMO discontinued at Penn State?**

A. **Success: weaning from ECMO.** Most patients show a transient improvement in natural lung gas exchange immediately after ECMO is started. This should not be confused with resolution of ARDS. During V-A ECMO, this improvement is partially due to a decreased pulmonary blood flow, which tends to perfuse only relatively uninjured regions of the lung. Because this transient improvement is also seen often during V-V ECMO, other mechanisms must be involved. Possibly the oncotic pressure of the extracorporeal prime at the beginning of perfusion is initially more than that of the patient's blood, thus drawing water transiently from the injured lung.

This early improvement is typically unsustained. During the next 6–12 hours the gas exchange deteriorates back to the preperfusion level or even becomes worse. The cause of this relapse is also unknown. The exposure of blood to the large surface of artificial membranes may activate complement through the indirect pathway, which then stimulates neutrophils to sequester in the pulmonary circulation. These activated phagocytes subsequently may attack the pulmonary endothelium. Other more likely possibilities include (1) too rapid a decrease in airway pressures, which leads to an increase in venous admixture, and (2) worsening of ARDS because of the natural progression of the pulmonary injury.

If sustained improvement is to occur due to resolution of ARDS, it usually begins within the first 2–7 days of perfusion. Occasionally improvement can occur as late as the third week of perfusion. Improvement is characterized by decreases in dead space, venous admixture, pulmonary hypertension, and PVR. Sometimes recovery is heralded by a thrombocytosis. This implies that, with the duration of perfusion permitted with current technology, ECMO acts to break the vicious cycle of oxygen toxicity or barotrauma as a cause or an aggravation of ARDS.

Whether or not a patient is ready to be weaned from ECMO can be decided without ever decreasing the extracorporeal blood flow rate. Maintaining high extracorporeal flows lessens the chance that thrombus will form in the circuit while ECMO weaning is attempted. The FIO_2 of the patient is increased to 0.6, the ventilator rate to about 20 breaths/min, and the PEEP to 10 cm H_2O. The contribution of membrane lung gas exchange is diminished by lowering the oxygen concentration and the flow rate of the gas ventilating the membrane lung. This maneuver results in a state in which up to 90% of the patient's carbon dioxide and oxygen consumption is transferred by the natural lung while as little as 10% is transferred in the membrane lung. Those patients who maintain a PaO_2 greater than 70 mm Hg for 6 hours under these conditions can be decannulated.

If successive positive blood cultures are drawn from the extracorporeal circuit, immediate attempts must be made to wean the patient from ECMO.

B. **Failure: terminating ECMO.** When ECMO continues for more than 1 week, the patient with ARDS usually dies. Death is preceded most often by a prolonged period of total pulmonary failure characterized by a dead space and venous admixture equal to 1.0. PaO_2 can fall as low as 35 mm Hg, and the SaO_2 can reach 80%. Extreme elevations of pulmonary arterial pressure and PVR are seen. Chest radiographs show complete opacification.

Three terminal scenarios are seen commonly. Most frequently, the chronic hypoxemia will progress to an agonal PaO_2. This is accompanied by presumptive sepsis with further progression of the hypermetabolic state and the development of a large colloid requirement to maintain the circulating blood volume. Bacteria or fungi may or may not be isolated from blood cultures. Occasionally, acute agonal hypoxemia will immediately follow the failure of components in the perfusion circuit. Rarely, hemorrhage will become increasingly severe, placing an unbearable strain on blood bank facilities.

Death is heralded by a progressive lactic acidemia and renal failure. The immediate cause of death is a hypoxic ventricular arrhythmia. Autopsy frequently reveals massive pulmonary fibrosis, but postmortem organ and blood cultures are usually negative.

IX. Medical Management after ECMO at Penn State

A. **Decannulation.** After being disconnected from the ECMO circuit, the patient is transported to the OR for decannulation. Usually the patient's gas exchange rate will be better than it was at the time of cannulation, and only a manual bag and PEEP valve are needed for ventilation. Surgery is performed under high-dose fentanyl and scopolamine anesthesia with vecuronium. After removal of the drainage cannula, the femoral vein is surgically repaired. After removal of the reinfusion cannula, the internal jugular vein is ligated. The neck and groin incisions are dressed and allowed to heal by secondary intent. Then the patient is returned to the ICU.

B. **Weaning from mechanical ventilation.** Ventilator support may be required for another 1–3 weeks. Opiate infusion rates are decreased to minimize respiratory depression. Muscle relaxants are stopped. A slow wean from the ventilator is attempted using intermittent mandatory ventilation. After 3 weeks of endotracheal intubation, a tracheostomy is performed to preserve laryngeal function. Vigorous chest physiotherapy is continued to mobilize alveolar debris.

C. **Rehabilitation.** Most of the posthospitalization care involves the patient's rehabilitation from other injuries. For example, the trauma patient with long bone fractures will require extensive physical therapy to regain active and passive range of motion.

D. **Slow recovery of pulmonary function.** After severe ARDS in adults requiring ECMO, the recovery of lung function is slow and incomplete. By 2 weeks after decannulation most patients have obtained a vital capacity in the range of 10 ml/kg and can be extubated or decannulated from their tracheostomy. Chest radiographs usually show complete clearing of infiltrates by the end of the second month. At this time pulmonary function tests show a decreased total lung capacity, a decreased vital capacity of about 50% normal, a FEV_1 of 70%, and a PaO_2 of 75–80 mm Hg and a saturation of 88–90% while breathing room air. Diffusion capacity for carbon monoxide is markedly decreased to 30% of normal. Follow-up testing at 6 and 12 months shows a gradual return of all parameters toward normal values. Vital capacity and FEV_1 usually reach control values. However, the diffusion capacity and arterial blood gas levels or saturation never completely return to normal levels. This condition probably represents an irreplaceable loss of pulmonary alveoli and capillaries that results in a slight but permanent V_A/Q mismatch.

E. **Resumption of activities of daily living.** Our three adult ECMO survivors returned to their normal activities of daily living within 6 months following the onset of ARDS. One year after their injury all have been able to maintain a moderate exercise tolerance without shortness of breath. With more severe exercise, some degree of arterial desaturation usually occurs. No problems with hypoxemia have been reported during flights on commercial aircraft or traveling to cities at a higher elevation.

X. Personnel requirements and roles. Camaraderie among all personnel is needed for the successful application of ECMO in ARDS. Knowledge of one another's primary responsibilities ensures that all tasks are performed and makes training team members straightforward.

 A. Anesthesiologist. Supervision of the transport of the patient to and from the ICU and the general anesthesia needed for cannulation and decannulation are provided by the anesthesiologists on the ECMO team.

 B. Surgeon. A thoracic surgeon performs the cannulation and decannulation of the internal jugular and common femoral veins in the operating room. On arrival in the ICU, he attaches the cannula to the extracorporeal circuit and assists at the start of ECMO. During the perfusion he changes the dressings on the cutdown sites and attempts to stop any surgical bleeding with electrocautery. At successful completion of ECMO, he decannulates the patient in the operating room and when possible repairs the veins.

 C. Physician management during ECMO. Our managing physician during ECMO is either a staff anesthesiologist or a surgeon who is in attendance for 8- to 12-hour shifts with the patient as his primary responsibility. He should be trained to fill the roles of all the other personnel in an emergency. He assumes primary responsibility for sedation, muscle relaxants, and all other primary orders. He must be ready to perform repeated bronchoscopies to supplement pulmonary toilet and to obtain sputum specimens for culture.

 A readily available physician who is intimately familiar with ECMO is essential because of the suddenness with which emergencies occur. Furthermore, because of the number of "routine" medical decisions that must be made during the conduct of ECMO, a physician's presence greatly decreases the nursing time spent in reporting to the physician. Also, an extra pair of hands and eyes make the care of ECMO patients easier and safer.

 D. Perfusionist. Qualified perfusionists are required to assemble the extracorporeal circuit, run the roller pumps, monitor extracorporeal gas exchange, and maintain bedside vigilance throughout the perfusion. They are most familiar with the ECMO circuit and best able to respond immediately to circuit emergencies.

 The actions of the perfusionist during the startup, maintenance, and termination of ECMO differ from the actions required during total CPB. Constant attention is needed to prevent, detect, and quickly correct pump inflow and outflow occlusion. A low circulating blood volume is usually detected as a drop in the volume of the reservoir bag. The managing physician and nurse must be notified quickly of the need to infuse blood products. Boredom must be fought actively during the long hours of uncomplicated perfusion. This is best avoided by short shifts and frequent breaks.

 There are many routine checks of circuit components, clerical duties and measurements to be performed. The reservoir bag and the manifolds of the membrane lung should be inspected frequently to detect the formation of thrombus. Tubing under the pump roller head must be checked frequently for signs of wear or fracture. Hourly records must be kept of extracorporeal blood and gas flow rates, heparin infusion rate, inlet oxygen concentration, inlet blood temperature, and hemultrafiltration rate. Extracorporeal gas exchange must be frequently measured. An ACT determination must be made from blood drawn from the arterial line every 1–3 hours and suitable alterations made in the heparin dosage. Perfusionists must draw any blood samples taken from the extracorporeal circuit.

Cleanliness is paramount if sepsis is to be evaded. Stopcocks in the circuit must be cleaned meticulously and sterilely to avoid sepsis. These stopcocks must be handled carefully to avoid breakage and displacement. Infusion of blood products into the circuit must be avoided to preserve membrane lung function. The tubing under the pump rollers must be advanced daily to reduce wear, spallation, and fracture. Because roller pump tubing or membrane lungs may have to be changed with little advance notice, 6–10 tubing clamps should be immediately available.

After the circuit is disconnected from the patient at the end of perfusion, it should be rinsed sterilely with saline until all blood is cleared. The sites of thrombus should be noted and specimens taken sterilely for culture.

E. Nurse. Critical care nursing staff familiar with ECMO and skilled in the care of critically ill patients is vital. Two nurses are usually needed for the startup of ECMO, termination of ECMO, and during emergencies. Most of the time during an uncomplicated perfusion, a single nurse can provide the needed care.

Routine critical care is complicated by the large cannulae that have been inserted in the neck and groin. The entire length of these tubes should be visible at all times. The nurse as well as the perfusionist must pay close attention to prevent and relieve their obstruction. Puncture of these tubes by needles or other sharp objects can bring a quick end to the perfusion. Aided by the respiratory therapist, the nurse should perform frequent percussion and vibration of the chest wall with endotracheal suctioning.

Meticulous infection control measures must be taken. All stagnant blood must be cleaned from stopcocks, which should be capped sterilely between sampling. Blood that has dripped from the cutdown sites and lies stagnant on the bed soon becomes infected and foul. The changing of bed linen and cleaning of the cushions of the rocker bed should be done at least once a shift and more often if bleeding becomes a problem. This requires many people if it is to be done quickly and safely while ECMO continues.

Chronic heparin therapy demands modification of routine care. Removal of oral and nasal secretions by vigorous suctioning and wiping can produce major blood loss. An intramuscular injection or a failed intravenous catheter placement can cause large hematomas.

There is a great need for psychological support for the patient and family. The patient is heavily sedated during ECMO. Survivors rarely have any recall of their clinical course, but there is no guarantee that this will be the case. On the other hand, the family is under intense stress. They must visit frequently an unresponsive, anesthetized loved one who is surrounded by a vast array of high technical life-support equipment in a relatively small room. Following the lead of the physician team, the nurses should encourage family members to have reasonable expectations.

F. Respiratory therapist. Mechanical ventilation for all patients with ARDS is provided by the respiratory therapist. Even higher demands are placed on the therapists during ECMO. They must provide mechanical ventilation for safe transport to and from the OR for cannulation. This requires the operation of a battery-powered, portable volume ventilator with its own mobile gas supply. It should be capable of generating PEEP as high as 45 cm water to minimize venous admixture and hypoxemia. It must also be capable of producing respiratory minute volumes in excess of 45 liters/min because of the large dead space characteristic of ARDS. Currently, we use the Servo 900C ventilator (Siemens, Solna, Sweden) for transport. Because intravenous anes-

Table 23-5. Additional cost of ECMO in adults (approximate costs—1989 dollars)

Equipment costs	
Durable	
Roller pump for main circuit	$3,800
Roller pump for hemultrafilter	695
Heater/cooler for heat exchange	3,600
ACT monitor	1,500
Disposable or rental	
3.5 m^2 membrane lung ($365/lung)	730
Hemultrafilter	70
Reservoir bag, tubing, connectors, cannulae	200
Rental rocker bed ($85/day)	85
Personnel	
Circuit setup by perfusionist (first day fee)	1,000
Perfusionist charge (subsequent daily fee)	950
Physician management fee (per day)	1,300
Anesthesia fee for cannulation and decannulation	1,000
Surgery fee for cannulation and decannulation	2,000
Biologic	
Blood ($150/500 ml unit)	150
Fresh-frozen plasma ($70/300 ml unit)	70
Platelets ($350/10 units)	350
Laboratory	
Blood cultures (every shift)	90
Daily plasma hemoglobin, coagulation profile	115
Blood gas determinations (approx. 20/day @ $33/sample)	660
Hospital charges	
OR fee for cannulation and decannulation	2,000
ICU charge (per day)	1,100
Perfusion fee (one time setup fee)	1,500

thesia is used for cannulation, the therapist remains in the operating room to aid the anesthesiologist in using the transport ventilator for life support. After cannulation, the therapist accompanies the patient and team back to the ICU for the startup of ECMO.

Immediately after ECMO begins, frequent decreases in the level of ventilator support must be made as extracorporeal gas exchange provided by V-V ECMO is maximized. Throughout ECMO the therapist aids the nurse in performing chest physiotherapy.

When ECMO ends successfully, the therapist aids in the transport of the patient back to the OR for decannulation. In the ensuing weeks, the therapist takes an active role in the weaning of the patient from mechanical ventilation.

XI. Costs

A. **Monetary costs.** The additional cost of treating an adult ARDS patient with ECMO (beyond the base cost of conventional ICU care with mechanical ventilation) depends on initial startup and ongoing daily expenditures (Table 23-5). If perfusion equipment cannot be spared from the operating room, the purchase of additional perfusion apparatus, heat exchange equipment, and anticoagulation monitor can cost approximately $10,000. This price is often amortized by life span or by the expected number of treated patients and is usually included in a hospital perfusion fee.

How do these individual items combine into the total cost to the patient? The total additional charge for the first day of perfusion usually amounts to $10,000. If there is no excessive hemorrhage, the cumulative cost for the first 5 days of perfusion including the first day amounts to $19,000. Most patients who survive will be able to be weaned from ECMO and can be decannulated by the fifth day. They will usually require two more weeks in the ICU if they survive on ECMO than if they had died while on conventional therapy. Counting only ICU bed costs and no other hospital costs or physician fees, this amounts to at least an additional $48,000 in the total cost of hospitalization when a patient survives ARDS on ECMO. This figure assumes that death would have occurred by the fifth day without ECMO. These costs do not include the expenses of rehabilitation.

Persisting on ECMO when the patient's outcome is hopeless costs the same or more. The cumulative cost of an uncomplicated 10-day perfusion with minimal blood loss in which the patient dies is approximately $43,000. If excessive hemorrhage occurs and laboratory testing is needed to attempt to treat multiple organ failure, the cost can double. An ultimately unsuccessful but uncomplicated ECMO treatment lasting 3 weeks may have a cumulative additional cost of $80,000. **In summary, whether or not a patient survives, the use of ECMO in adults as described here will result in an additional cost of at least $48,000 to the patient or his or her family. We believe that at present such expensive but potentially efficacious ECMO therapy should be applied only to those patients who are most likely to survive and should be withdrawn as soon as it is apparent that survival is hopeless.**

B. **Physiologic costs.** ECMO also has physiologic costs because it loads certain biochemical and physiologic systems within the body. Hemorrhage due to anticoagulation leads to problems of multiple blood transfusions. Blood loss in ARDS patients may be 10 times higher when ECMO is added to mechanical ventilation. Sublethal damage to erythrocytes due to extracorporeal pumping causes a shortened life span and hemolysis. This places an increased pigment load on the liver. Exposure of blood to large surface areas of artificial materials leads to complement activation and its sequelae. The extra number of sampling and infusion ports in the extracorporeal circuit makes bacterial contamination more likely.

XII. **Future developments.** Currently, attempts are being made at several centers to improve the survival rate of patients with ARDS who are treated with ECMO. These include the definition of better criteria for selecting more salvageable patients at an earlier time in the course of their acute lung injury; the testing of computer algorithms for making medical and ventilator management of patients with ARDS more uniform; the automation of pumping systems to make these safer and less labor intensive; and the development of percutaneously inserted cannulae. These advances, however, present only a refinement of existing technology.

Foremost among the new ideas that may come to fruition during the next 3–5 years is the **intravascular oxygenator.** This device was conceived, designed, and developed by J.D. Mortensen and will be commercially produced with the trade name IVOX (Cardiopulmonics Inc., Salt Lake City, UT). This device consists of a large number of membrane hollow fibers that are mounted in parallel on an intravenous catheter. (Fig. 23-10). This device will be inserted through a cutdown in the patient's femoral

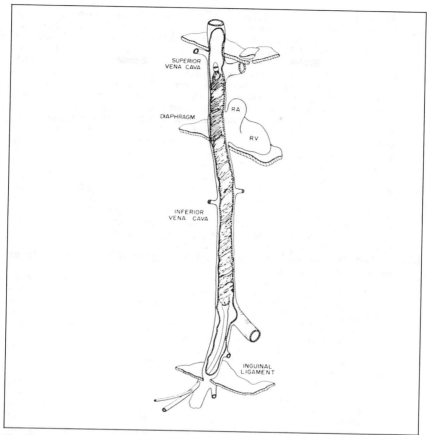

Fig. 23-10. Pictorial representation of Mortensen's intravascular oxygenator in the vena cava. The right ventricle is labeled RV and the right atrium RA. (From J. D. Mortensen. An intravenacaval blood gas exchange [IVCBGE] device. *Trans. Am. Soc. Artif. Intern. Organs* 33:570, 1987. With permission.)

vein and advanced so that its tip lies in the superior vena cava. The fibers are then unfurled so that the venous blood flow returning from the tissues flows around the fibers. Simultaneously, pure oxygen is sucked through the fibers at subatmospheric pressure. In vitro studies in circulatory models and in vivo studies in sheep indicate that one-half of man's basal oxygen consumption and carbon dioxide production may be transferred across this device. Phase one clinical studies for safety probably will begin by mid 1989. If efficacy of gas exchange can be demonstrated in man, the IVOX may revolutionize the treatment of ARDS.

XIII. Summary. Extracorporeal membrane oxygenation (ECMO) continues to be used successfully to treat patients with severe neonatal respiratory distress syndromes (NRDS) and severe adult respiratory failure (ARDS). At present, no classic randomized prospective study has shown a difference in survival of these patients when ECMO is added to mechanical ventilation. Nevertheless, in uncontrolled series, up to 80% of patients with

NRDS and 50% of patients with ARDS have survived following ECMO. Currently, adults with severe hypoxemia who have 9% or less probability of survival on mechanical ventilation should be considered candidates for veno-venous (V-V) ECMO. Of these patients, we use ECMO only in potentially salvageable patients who show signs of severe barotrauma with oxygen toxicity during maximal mechanical ventilation and whose primary disease process may resolve within 1–2 weeks of perfusion. Contraindications include prolonged irreversible lung injury, hemorrhage, sepsis, old age, multiple organ failure, and concomitant lethal disease.

We have presented our scenario for ventilator and medical treatment of ARDS that is designed to avoid ECMO. When we are unsuccessful with ventilator treatment alone, we have instituted V-V ECMO. But only a few patients are suitable. Our extracorporeal circuit and its use are outlined in detail. The special dangers that are present during ECMO are described along with advice on how to avoid and treat them. Finally, information is provided on how to wean the patient from ECMO without lowering the extracorporeal blood flow rate. Suggested roles and tasks for ECMO team members are described. Following our guidelines, we believe that as many as 50% of selected patients with ARDS and severe hypoxemia can be salvaged by life support with high-flow V-V ECMO, and these patients should be provided with this treatment.

XIV. **Appendix. Survival criteria based on degree of hypoxia and level of ventilator support**

Several criteria for predicting survival from ARDS have been proposed for identifying patients who might be candidates for ECMO. These criteria are based on the degree of hypoxemia shown at specified levels of ventilator support. The more severe the observed hypoxemia, the more severe the ARDS is assumed to be. Because the earliest forms of ARDS have not been identified and characterized, acute hypoxemia of noncardiac origin is assumed to be the earliest sign of ARDS. Not all patients with acute hypoxemia go on to develop ARDS. The following criteria have been recommended as indications of ECMO.

1. **Survival in acute hypoxemia of noncardiac origin.** Recently, collaborating investigators throughout Europe have defined simple criteria for estimating the survival rate of patients suffering from acute hypoxemia of noncardiac origin [1]. These investigators followed prospectively 591 patients who required endotracheal intubation and mechanical ventilation and were presumptive candidates for developing ARDS.

    The criteria for survival from acute hypoxemia of noncardiac origin consist of a single measurement of PaO_2 after the first 24 hours of mechanical ventilation. At the time of measurement the ventilator must be set at a FIO_2 of 0.50 or more and a PEEP of 5 cm H_2O.

    Patients attaining a PaO_2 of greater than 75 mm Hg had a 61% survival rate. Patients achieving a PaO_2 of less than 75 mm Hg had a 31% survival rate. Data combined from both groups implied a survival rate of 41% for any patient requiring mechanical ventilation for 24 hours. The number of these patients going on to develop ARDS was not reported.

2. **Survival of patients with severe ARDS.** During the NHLBI ECMO Study, severely hypoxic patients without left ventricular failure were selected randomly to be treated with either mechanical ventilation alone or with ECMO together with mechanical ventilation. Selection was made if one of two sets of criteria were met: fast entry criteria or slow entry criteria [7]. The survival rate of the 48 patients from the NHLBI ECMO Study who met these two sets of criteria and were

randomized to receive only mechanical ventilation can be used now to predict prospectively the outcome of patients currently suffering from ARDS. When applied prospectively, the slow entry criteria are more appropriately renamed the **criteria for survival from severe, slowly developing ARDS** and consist of:

a. A disease process of less than 21 days in duration.

b. Institution of maximum medical therapy for at least 48 hours.

c. A PaO_2 of 50 mm Hg or less observed on measurements made every 6 hours over a 12-hour interval. At the times of measurement the ventilator settings must have been maintained at a FIO_2 of 0.60 and a PEEP of 5 cm H_2O or more for at least 15 minutes. (Between criteria measurements any combination of FIO_2 and PEEP settings are permitted).

d. A venous admixture of more than 30% when the FIO_2 is 1.0 and the PEEP is at least 5 cm H_2O.

Patients meeting these criteria will have a predicted survival rate of only 9% if they receive only mechanical ventilation.

Similarly, when applied prospectively, the rapid entry criteria are more appropriately renamed the **criteria for survival from severe, rapidly developing ARDS** and consist of:

a. A disease process of less than 21 days in duration.

b. Institution of maximum medical therapy.

c. A PaO_2 of 50 mm Hg or less observed on measurements made every hour over a 2-hour interval. At the times of measurement the ventilator settings must have been maintained at a FIO_2 of 1.0 and a PEEP of 5 cm H_2O or more for at least 15 minutes. (Between criteria measurements any combination of FIO_2 and PEEP settings are permitted.)

Patients meeting these criteria will have a predicted survival rate of only 8% when they receive only mechanical ventilation.

3. Lethal ARDS. During the NHLBI ECMO study, patients who had been randomized to mechanical ventilation and went on to develop agonal hypoxia could be treated with ECMO as a heroic last resort. Applied prospectively, these agonal perfusion criteria are more appropriately renamed the **criteria for lethal ARDS** and consist of:

a. Fulfillment of either criteria for survival from ARDS of extreme severity.

b. Maximum medical management and ventilator support have been given.

c. A PaO_2 35 mm Hg or less observed on measurements made every 3 hours during a 6-hour interval. At the times of measurement the ventilator settings must have been maintained at a FIO_2 of 1.0 and a PEEP of at least 5 cm H_2O for at least 15 minutes.

Alternatively, a PaO_2 of 45 mm Hg or less observed on measurements made every 6 hours over a 12-hour interval. At the times of measurement the ventilator settings must have been maintained at a FIO_2 of 1.0 and a PEEP of at least 5 cm H_2O for at least 15 minutes. (Between criteria measurements any combination of FIO_2 and PEEP settings is permitted.)

Of the five patients meeting these criteria, none survived.

All existing criteria ignore defining the specific maximum medical therapy used, the ventilator I/E ratio employed, the severity of barotrauma, the prior duration and levels of oxygen exposure, and the cause of ARDS. As limited as the existing criteria are, physicians at many centers require that these be met or exceeded before patients with ARDS are considered candidates for ECMO. The number of patients in the severe and lethal ARDS groups is very small. Future studies may put a better bound on these rates. For example, the lethal ARDS group might eventually be found to have a survival rate with mechanical ventilation of 1% and be misnamed. The overall low survival rates are unlikely to change significantly as more patients are studied.

REFERENCES

1. Artigas, A. Adult Respiratory Distress Syndrome: Changing Concepts of Clinical Evolution and Recovery. In J. L. Vincent (ed.), *Update in Intensive Care and Emergency Medicine 5 Update, 1988*. Heidelberg: Springer-Verlag, 1988. Pp. 97–114.
2. Bartlett, R. H., Toomasian, J., Roloff, D., et al. Extracorporeal membrane oxygenation (ECMO) in neonatal respiratory failure—100 cases. *Ann. Surg.* 204:236–245, 1986.
3. Morris, A. H., Menlove, R. L., Rollins, R. J., et al. A controlled clinical trial of a new 3-step therapy that includes extracorporeal CO_2 removal for ARDS. *Trans. Am. Soc. Artif. Intern. Organs* 34:48–53, 1988.
4. Pesenti, A., Gattinoni, L., Kolobow, T., et al. Extracorporeal circulation in adult respiratory failure. *Trans. Am. Soc. Artif. Intern. Organs* 34:43–47, 1988.
5. Snider, M. T., Campbell, D. B., Kofke, W. A., et al. Venovenous perfusion of adults and children with severe acute respiratory distress syndrome—The Pennsylvania State University experience from 1982–1987. *Trans. Am. Soc. Artif. Intern. Organs* 34:1014–1020, 1988.
6. Snider, M. T., and Zapol, W. M. Assessment of Pulmonary Oxygenation during Veno-arterial Bypass with Aortic Root Return. In W. M. Zapol, and J. Qvist (eds.), *Artificial Lungs for Acute Respiratory Failure—Theory and Practice* New York: Academic Press, 1976. Pp. 263–273.
7. Zapol, W. M., Snider, M. T., Hill, J. D., et al. Extracorporeal membrane oxygenation in severe acute respiratory failure: A randomized prospective study. *J.A.M.A.* 242:2193–2196, 1979.
8. Zapol, W. M., Snider, M. T., and Schneider, R. C. Extracorporeal membrane oxygenation for acute respiratory failure. *Anesthesiology* 46:272–285, 1977.

SUGGESTED READING

Bartlett, R. H., Morris, A. H., Fairley, H. B., et al. A prospective study of acute hypoxic respiratory failure. *Chest* 89:684–689, 1986.

Borelli, M., Kolobow, T., Spatola, R., et al. Severe acute respiratory failure managed with continuous positive airway pressure and partial extracorporeal carbon dioxide removal by an artificial membrane lung. *Am. Rev. Respir. Dis.* 138:1480–1487, 1988.

Cleveland, K. J., Palanzo, D. A., Campbell, D. B., et al. Successful treatment of acute respiratory failure with veno-venous perfusion in a patient refractory to very high positive end-expiratory pressure. *Proc. Am. Acad. Cardiovasc. Perfusion* 4:159–163, 1983.

Friedman, L. I., Richardson, P. D., and Galletti, P. M. Blood oxygenator testing and evaluation. Part 2. Procedures and results. Medical Devices Application Program, National Heart and Lung Institute, Washington, D.C. 1973.

Hill, J. D., O'Brien, T. G., Murray, J. J., et al. Prolonged extracorporeal oxygenation for acute post-traumatic respiratory failure (shock-lung syndrome). *N. Engl. J. Med.* 286:629–634, 1972.

Hirschl, R. B., and Bartlett, R. H. Extracorporeal membrane oxygenation support in cardiorespiratory failure. *Adv. Surg.* 21:189–212, 1987.

Lakshminarayan S., Stanford, R. E., and Petty, T. L. Prognosis after recovery from adult respiratory distress syndrome. *Am. Rev. Respir. Dis.* 113:7–16, 1976.

Mortensen, J. D. An intravenacaval blood gas exchange (IVCBGE) device: A preliminary report. *Trans. Am. Soc. Artif. Intern. Organs* 33:570–572, 1987.

Rocker, G. M., Wiseman, M. S., Pearson, D., et al. Diagnostic criteria for adult respiratory distress syndrome: Time for reappraisal. *Lancet* 1:120–123, 1989.

Snider, M. T., Richardson, P. D., Friedman, L. I. et al. Carbon dioxide transfer rate in artificial lungs. *J. Appl. Physiol.* 36:233–239, 1974.

Zapol, W. M., and Falke, K. J. *Acute Respiratory Failure,* Vol. 24. New York: Marcel Dekker, 1985.

Brain Protection During Cardiac Surgery

G. Scott Wickey and Paul R. Hickey

I. **Incidence of neurologic dysfunction associated with cardiac surgery.** Particular vigilance must be directed to the brain during cardiac surgery because neurologic dysfunction remains a significant complication after cardiac surgery. An extensive review of studies concerning neuropsychiatric complications after cardiopulmonary bypass (CPB) reported a 7–44% incidence of transient and 1.6–23% incidence of permanent neuropsychiatric complications [9].

These broad ranges in incidence reflect progress in CPB during the past 20 years and differences between studies with reference to perspective of analysis, sensitivity of neurologic examinations performed (e.g., physical examination versus psychometric testing), type of CPB priming solution, and proportion of patients having intracardiac and extracardiac surgery. Neuropsychiatric abnormalities reported include motor and sensory deficits, discoordination, minimal brain dysfunction, disorientation, anorexia, depression, hostility, hallucinations, and delirium.

II. **Etiology of brain damage.** Causes of brain damage include hypoxia, ischemia, seizures, hypoglycemia, and possibly hyperglycemia. These disorders disrupt the normal integration of cerebral blood flow (CBF), metabolism, and neurotransmitter function to produce cerebral damage. Although hypoxia, seizures, hypoglycemia, and hyperglycemia can occur during anesthesia, **ischemia** is the most common cause of neurologic complications after surgery. Both focal and global ischemia can occur during cardiac surgery.

A. **Focal ischemia** is impaired perfusion of a region of the brain that produces localized sequelae and may be caused by
   1. **Embolism**
      a. **Most neurologic sequelae occurring after cardiac surgery are focal, and emboli have been implicated as the most common source of these focal events.**
      b. **Sources of emboli** during cardiac surgery include
         (1) Air
         (2) Atheromatous plaque
         (3) Microemboli
         (4) Left ventricular (LV) thrombus
         (5) Fat
         (6) Debris
   2. Hypoperfusion during systemic hypotension in the presence of localized cerebrovascular disease
   3. Hypoperfusion of "watershed" areas of the brain

B. **Global ischemia** is a generalized reduction in cerebral blood flow that may be complete or partial and results in diffuse brain dysfunction.
   1. **Complete global ischemia** may be due to
      a. Cardiac arrest
      b. Deep hypothermic circulatory arrest (DHCA)
   2. **Incomplete global ischemia** may be due to
      a. Hypotension
      b. Inadequate cardiopulmonary bypass flow

III. **Pathophysiology of brain damage.** A brief review of the pathophysiology of cerebral ischemia provides a theoretic basis for the current concepts in brain protection therapy (Fig. 24–1).

A. Ischemia produces a reduction in adenosine triphosphate (ATP) and phosphocreatine levels and increases in adenosine diphosphate and lactate levels because normal aerobic metabolism is disrupted.

B. The reduced energy state of the cell contributes to loss of cell membrane stability and dissipation of normal cellular ion gradients.

C. Accumulation of extracellular K^+ produces vasospasm, which exacerbates the ischemic process.

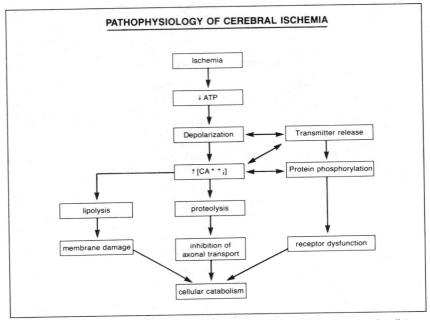

Fig. 24-1. The cascade of events triggered by cerebral ischemia (see text for details). (Modified from B. K. Siesjo and T. Wieloch. Cerebral metabolism in ischaemia: Neurochemical basis for therapy. *Br. J. Anaesth.* 57:59, 1985. With permission.)

D. Uptake of K^+ and CL^- by glial cells results in edema of astrocytic processes and compromise of neuronal substrate availability.

E. Dissipation of the Na^+ gradient allows Ca^{2+} to enter the cell so that intracellular calcium (Ca^{2+}_i) activity increases.

F. Normally, cellular processes including an ATP and Mg^{2+}-dependent Ca^{2+} pump and calcium-sodium exchange mechanism work to regulate Ca^{2+} levels; however, because these processes are saturable, Ca^{2+}_i increases.

G. Increased Ca^{2+}_i has several deleterious effects on the cell.
  1. Obligatory uptake of Ca^{2+} by mitochondria is energy consuming and diverts oxidation-derived energy from the production of ATP.
  2. Protein degradation results, leading to disruption of the cellular cytoskeleton.
  3. Lypolysis of membrane-bound phospholipids by Ca^{2+}-activated phospholipase A2 leads to accumulation of free fatty acids (FFA) and membrane damage.
  4. Disruption of synaptic activity by protein phosphorylation occurs.
  5. Enhanced neurotransmitter release is another effect.

H. Arachidonic acid (AA) is the predominant FFA that accumulates from lipolysis of membrane phospholipids.

I. Cyclooxygenase and lipooxygenase convert AA into prostaglandins, thromboxane, leukotrienes, and endoperoxides, which may contribute to neuronal damage during reperfusion.
  1. Thromboxane causes platelet activation and vasospasm.
  2. Endoperoxides may act as free radical oxidants.

J. Although metabolic pathways exist for conversion of FFA to superoxides or free radicals during reperfusion after ischemic injury, several studies have failed to document the presence of these cellular toxins. If present, superoxide could contribute to cell damage by attacking peroxide to produce very active oxidants like the hydroxyl radical, which can damage the structure of DNA.

K. Three aspects of the cellular derangement produced by cerebral ischemia warrant particular emphasis.

1. **Severity of the lactic acidosis** that develops during cerebral ischemia has a profound effect on the resulting cellular damage.
2. **Accumulation of intracellular Ca^{2+}** is an important factor mediating cell damage during cerebral ischemia.
3. Cell damage develops or matures during the **reperfusion and reoxygenation phase** after ischemia.

IV. Monitoring cerebral electrical activity. Detection of cerebral ischemia and administration of pharmacologic agents to provide cerebral protection depend on accurate, reliable monitoring of cerebral electrical activity.

A. Origin of electroencephalogram. The surface electroencephalogram (EEG) is a recording from the scalp of electrical activity in the underlying cerebral cortex. The EEG signal is generated by amplifying voltage differences between pairs of electrodes attached to the scalp. Each electrode pair constitutes a lead (channel). A single electrode reflects activity within a radius of approximately 2.5 cm, so the surface EEG provides no information concerning the function of structures deeper than the cortex.

B. Number of electrodes. As the number of electrodes in the EEG montage increases, the tissue area surveyed enlarges, and the capacity to detect regional differences in EEG activity is enhanced. The 21-electrode International 10–20 system is the EEG standard, but a two- or four-lead automated monitoring system utilizing fewer electrodes is more practical in the operating room. When a reduced number of electrodes is used, electrodes should be placed preferentially over the distribution of the middle cerebral artery.

C. Choice of electrodes

1. **Needle electrodes**
   a. Are easily and rapidly applied
   b. May be sterilized for use in a surgical field
   c. May cause bleeding in a heparinized patient
   d. Have a small surface area that decreases recording quality
   e. Are painful when inserted into awake patient, so awake baseline is precluded
   f. Can be satisfactorily placed in hair

2. **Silver/Silver chloride electrodes**
   a. Are easily applied after preparation of skin with abrasive electrolyte compound
   b. Are stable when applied to skin
   c. Are unsatisfactory for placement in hair

3. **Gold cup electrodes**
   a. Require tedious application with collodion or conductive paste after preparation of skin with abrasive compound
   b. Are very stable
   c. Have superior quality recording because of low impedance and tarnish resistance of gold
   d. Are satisfactorily placed in hair

4. **Electrode caps**
   a. Are rarely used
   b. Cause unstable electrode position

D. Impedance and interference

1. EEG signal information is generated from low voltages (50–100 μV) in an electrically hostile operating room environment.
2. Multiple sources of interference exist in the operating room.
   a. Electrical activity in skeletal and cardiac myofibrils
      (1) Shivering
      (2) Patient movement
   b. Electrical devices
      (1) ECG
      (2) Pacemaker
      (3) Electrosurgery units
   c. Electromechanical devices: CPB roller pumps
3. If electrode impedances are equal, interference is eliminated because the amplitude of interference is the same at each electrode and is canceled out when the EEG signal is processed. When electrode impedances are different, interference appears in the EEG signal as artifact. Interference artifact can be minimized by ensuring that electrode impedances are equal and as low as possible.
4. To ensure low electrode impedance (< 5 kohm) proper electrode contact with the scalp is imperative.

E. **Fundamental EEG rhythms.** Basic EEG rhythms are defined by their frequency (Table 24-1). Additional features of the EEG rhythm are amplitude of the activity, location on the scalp where the activity predominates, degree of organization and symmetry, reactivity to physiologic manipulations, and presence of abnormal patterns or rhythms. Special expertise is required to distinguish these aspects of the EEG.

F. **Data presentation.** The unprocessed EEG is the standard for monitoring cerebral electrical activity. Multiple channels are typically recorded simultaneously. Intraoperative analysis of the multichannel unprocessed EEG by anesthesiologists is not practical. The EEG tracing accumulates rapidly, and its analysis would be complex, distracting the anesthesiologist from patient care. Several methods have been developed to process the EEG signal into a format that is suitable for use in the operating room (Fig. 24-2).

1. **Power spectrum analysis.** Segments (time epochs) of the EEG are analyzed by Fourier transformation to quantitate the amplitude of component frequencies. Time, frequency, and amplitude (power) are then displayed in a two-dimensional format.
   a. **Compressed spectral array (CSA).** A graph of power versus frequency is plotted for each epoch of the analysis. High-power activity can obscure previously recorded low-power activity when the activities occur at similar frequencies.
   b. **Density modulation spectral array (DSA).** Power is represented by colors or shades of gray, which allows display of the spectral analysis without obscuring data; however, precision is lost in depicting amplitude data, particularly when a gray scale is used.
   c. With either form of spectral analysis the epoch analyzed should be short (2 seconds). When larger epochs are used, the averaging characteristics of the analysis may obscure features of the EEG rhythm such as burst suppression.
   d. CSA and DSA data are plotted for individual leads. Multiple displays can be combined into a single screen to evaluate several regions of cerebral cortex simultaneously.

2. **Aperiodic analysis.** Unlike Fourier transformation, which analyzes segments of the EEG, aperiodic analysis determines amplitude and frequency data by analyzing peaks and valleys in the unprocessed EEG on a wave-by-wave basis. Such analysis of the EEG may be more accurate than epoch analysis because the wave-by-wave anal-

Table 24-1. Characteristics of fundamental EEG rhythms

Rhythm	Frequency	Predominant amplitude	Predominant location	Associated physiologic state
Alpha	8–13 Hz	Medium	Occiput	Relaxed, awake
Beta	13–30 Hz	Low	Frontal	Alert, awake
Theta	4–8 Hz	High	Diffuse	Sleeping infant, child
Delta	0–4 Hz	High	Diffuse	Metabolic coma, cerebral ischemia, normal deep sleep, deep anesthesia

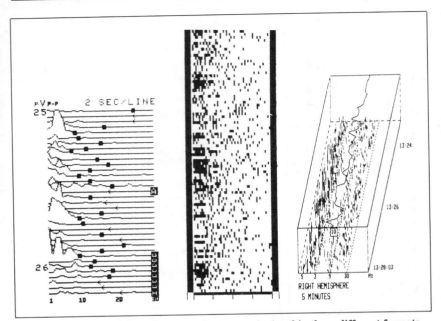

Fig. 24-2. EEG information from the same patient depicted in three different formats. Only one lead is presented for each format. In actual practice multiple leads (2–4) are usually displayed. *Left.* Compressed Spectral Array (CSA). Peaks on a line are used to represent amplitude of cerebral electrical activity across a frequency axis. Information is updated at a preselected interval by adding new lines, which progress down the recording. Large peaks may obscure previous data. A square is used to mark the spectral edge (frequency below which a preselected percentage of electrical activity occurs). The symbol A indicates recording artifact. *Center.* Density Modulation Spectral Array (DSA). A color gradient or gray scale is used to depict amplitude on a frequency axis so that data are not obscured. Precision is lost in amplitude interpretation. *Right.* Aperiodic Analysis. Spikes are recorded on a frequency axis to depict amplitude data. These spikes appear in a parallelogram so that new data can be added without obscuring previous data. A line on the top of the parallelogram plots the activity edge, which is the frequency below which a preselected percentage of the cerebral electrical activity occurs.

ysis eliminates the averaging of data inherent in Fourier transformation. Power, frequency, and time data are presented as parallelograms so that no data are obscured.

   3. Univariate descriptors of the EEG such as spectral edge (maximum frequency), mean frequency, peak power frequency, and activity edge (the frequency below which a preselected percentage of cerebral electrical activity occurs) can be derived from power spectrum analysis or aperiodic analysis of the EEG. These descriptors can then be used to signal changes in the EEG.

G. Interpretation of EEG data
   1. Despite the development of methods for processing the EEG into formats suitable for the operating room, interpretation of cerebral electrical activity still demands scrutiny and attention to detail.
   2. Univariate descriptors of the EEG are accurate for symmetric unimodal distributions of electrical activity. However, they may not

Table 24-2. EEG changes associated with drugs and altered physiology

Increased frequency
  Hyperoxia
  Hypercarbia: mild
  Hypoxia: initial
  Seizure
  Barbiturates: small dose
  Diazepam: ambulatory dose
  N_2O: 30–70%
  Inhalation agents: <1 MAC
  Ketamine

Decreased frequency, increased amplitude
  Hypoxia: mild
  Hypocarbia: moderate to extreme
  Hypothermia
  Barbiturates: moderate dose
  Etomidate
  Narcotics
  Inhalation agents: >1 MAC

Decreased frequency, decreased amplitude
  Hypoxia: marked
  Hypercarbia: severe
  Barbiturates: large dose

Electrical silence
  Brain death
  Hypoxia: severe
  Hypothermia: profound
  Barbiturates: coma dose
  Isoflurane: 2 MAC

Source: From J.H. Donegan. The Electroencephalogram. In C. D. Blitt (ed.), *Monitoring in Anesthesia and Critical Care Medicine.* New York: Churchill Livingstone, 1985. P. 334. With permission.

adequately describe the behavior of a complex EEG (which is frequently multimodal).

3. Accurate interpretation of the EEG requires familiarity with the general appearance of the unprocessed tracing, the processed graph (spectral analysis, aperiodic analysis), and any derived descriptors (spectral edge, mean frequency, peak power frequency). All of this data must be integrated into a unified impression of actual CNS electrical activity to prevent missed or misinterpreted data that can result from electrical interference or inherent deficiencies in the mathematical methods of EEG analysis.

H. EEG patterns associated with cardiac anesthesia
  1. Hypothermia, anesthesia, and changes in perfusion encountered during cardiac surgery produce dramatic changes in the EEG (Table 24-2).
  2. A variety of EEG patterns have been attributed to cerebral ischemia:
    a. Reduction of power at all frequencies.
    b. Reduction in maximum frequency with or without reduction of total power.
    c. Increase in power of low-frequency activity.
  3. Hypothermia produces EEG slowing followed by burst suppression and a flat EEG.
  4. Narcotics produce EEG slowing to delta sleep patterns.

Table 24-3. Brain protection during cardiopulmonary bypass

1. Monitor for cerebral ischemia
2. Use heart lung machine filters
3. Use glucose-free fluids. Avoid significant hyperglycemia
4. Maintain controlled temperature gradients
5. Use alpha stat management
6. Maintain appropriate perfusion pressure and flow during CPB
7. Consider pharmacologic brain protection
8. Utilize brain hypothermia during periods of reduced flow or perfusion pressure
9. Perform left ventricle de-airing maneuvers
10. Ensure high normal postoperative blood pressure

5. Barbiturates and isoflurane produce burst suppression at moderate doses and a flat EEG at high doses.
6. Enflurane produces dose-dependent seizure activity, which may be accompanied by motor activity.
7. It is evident that low-frequency, high-power activity and burst suppression may have several causes, so clinical correlation of the EEG is imperative.

V. **Prevention of cerebral insults during cardiac surgery.** Current methods utilized to prevent ischemic insults are designed to reduce the incidence of embolic phenomena, maintain appropriate CBF during CPB, and minimize metabolic derangements (Table 24-3). These goals require that the surgeon, perfusionist, and anesthesiologist act in concert to provide optimal conditions for brain protection.

A. **Embolic phenomena**
 1. **Manipulation of an atherosclerotic aorta**
  a. **Aortic cross-clamping and cannulation.** Careful assessment of the aorta for atherosclerotic lesions has been emphasized for patients requiring aortic cross-clamping or cannulation, so that these lesions can be avoided. Disruption and embolism of plaque could easily occlude the innominate, subclavian, or carotid arteries originating from the aortic arch. If severe atherosclerosis is palpated throughout the ascending aorta, cannulation of the femoral vessels may be preferred to prevent plaque embolism.
  b. **Unclamping the aorta.** In patients without carotid artery disease, gentle pressure may be applied to both carotid arteries when the aorta is unclamped so that any debris produced by cross-clamping will be directed away from the head vessels.
 2. **De-airing the left ventricle.** After procedures in which a cardiac chamber has been opened, the LV is aspirated with a needle and syringe before the aortic cross-clamp is removed. This procedure is combined with ventilation of the lungs, rocking the patient to dislodge air from the pulmonary arteries, and the Trendelenburg position to minimize air embolization into the systemic circulation. Next, the aorta is partially clamped to create a cupola, which is then vented to remove any air bubbles that could be ejected by the left ventricle into the systemic circulation (Fig. 24-3).
 3. **Filters**
  a. Several sources of embolic material are associated with use of a heart lung machine (HLM)
   (1) Small oxygen bubbles are formed by membrane and bubble oxygenators.
   (2) Microemboli are formed from platelet and leukocyte aggregates, and particulate debris from the surgical site and HLM components.

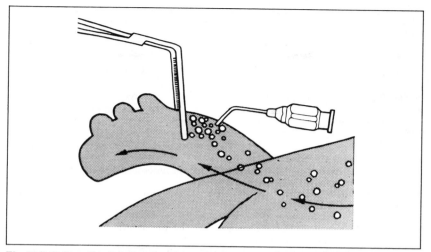

Fig. 24-3. Schematic view showing the cupola formed by partially cross-clamping the aorta to trap air bubbles. The air bubbles are aspirated through a needle vent in the aortic root during left ventricular deairing. (From G. M. Lemole and G. C. Pinder. A method of preventing air embolus in open-heart surgery. *J. Thorac. Cardiovasc. Surg.* 71:557, 1976. With permission.)

      b. Filters are used in the HLM circuit to remove embolic material before the blood is returned to the patient through the arteriotomy line. These filters can be used without impairing flow rates during CPB or significantly increasing destruction of blood components. Sites for these filters include
        (1) Arteriotomy line
        (2) Cardiotomy reservoir
  4. Control of the temperature gradient between venous return from the patient and the heat exchanger prevents dissolution of oxygen from supersaturated blood and resulting bubble formation.
  5. Meticulous de-airing of intravenous infusions avoids inadvertent infusion of air into the patient that could be shunted to the left heart by intracardiac defects such as a probe-patent foramen ovale, which is present in 30% of the general population.
B. Cerebral blood flow
  1. Acid-base management. Controversy about the optimal acid-base management during CPB continues. Two approaches have been advocated (Table 24-4).
      a. The **pH stat** method maintains a pH of 7.40 and a $PaCO_2$ of 40 mm Hg at the patient's actual body temperature (temperature-corrected values). Exogenous carbon dioxide must be added to the gases supplying the oxygenator during hypothermic CPB because as body temperature is reduced, carbon dioxide becomes more soluble in blood and carbon dioxide production decreases.
      b. The **alpha stat** method maintains a pH of 7.40 and a $PaCO_2$ of 40 mm Hg measured at 37°C, the temperature of the blood during blood gas analysis (uncorrected values). Since solubility of carbon dioxide increases under hypothermic conditions, the actual pH would be higher (7.5–7.6) and $PaCO_2$ lower (20–30 mm Hg) when corrected to actual body temperature. However, the carbon dioxide content of the blood remains constant.

Table 24-4. Comparison of acid-base management strategies

Alpha stat	pH stat
Rapid emergence since 1981	25 years of clinical use
Cerebral autoregulation preserved	Uncoupling of CBF and CMRO$_2$
Intracellular homeostasis preserved	Altered histidine charge state
Preserved myocardial performance	Myocardial depression

CBF = cerebral blood flow, CMRO$_2$ = cerebral oxygen consumption

    c. Advantages of the **alpha stat** management appear from current research to be preservation of
        (1) Coupling between cerebral metabolic rate and CBF, allowing maintenance of cerebral autoregulation. Conversely, pH stat management disrupts normal cerebral autoregulation and results in CBF that exceeds the metabolic demands of the hypothermic brain.
        (2) Buffering capacity of the alpha imidazole group of histidine, which preserves the electrochemical neutrality of the intracellular space. Electrochemical neutrality is required for optimal enzyme activity and retention of metabolic intermediates in the cell including high-energy phosphates. During pH stat management the charge state of histidine is altered, and cellular homeostasis is disrupted.
        (3) Myocardial performance as measured by LV peak pressure, lactate extraction, and coronary blood flow after short term (1 hour) ischemic cardiac arrest during systemic hypothermia. Similar measurements during pH stat management show prolonged myocardial depression.
    d. Ventilation and alpha stat management. The efficiency of ventilation during hypothermia has not been definitely established. Current literature indicates that ventilation of the hypothermic patient prior to initiating CPB should be maintained at normothermic or slightly reduced levels to preserve alpha stat management.
  2. Perfusion pressure and flow. The perfusion pressure and flow rate required to maintain adequate CBF and prevent postoperative neuropsychiatric dysfunction probably vary during the course of CPB because of changes in patient temperature, hematocrit, and acid-base status. Discrepancies in the literature concerning optimal CPB pressure and flow reflect advances in CPB technique during the past decade, differences in experimental design and patient populations, and varying sensitivity of methods for assessing neuropsychiatric dysfunction (Table 24-5).
    Clinical studies that involve normotensive patients without evidence of cerebrovascular disease may not be applicable to patients undergoing cardiac surgery, who are frequently hypertensive and have cerebrovascular disease.
    Despite these limitations, the present data suggest that flows of 2.0 liters $\cdot$ min^{-1} $\cdot$ m^{-2} and a perfusion pressure of 50 mm Hg are satisfactory during normothermic CPB in adults. Higher limits of perfusion pressure (70 mm Hg) may be prudent in older patients and in patients with symptomatic cerebrovascular disease. In children, especially infants and young children under 3 years of age, a lower

Table 24-5. Studies evaluating pressure and flow requirements during CPB

Reference	Date	Conclusion
Paneth et al. [8]	1957	A flow rate of 2.0 liters·min^{-1}·m^{-2} is adequate to supply cerebral metabolic needs of dogs during normothermic CPB.
Stockard et al. [10]	1973	Perfusion pressure (PP) during CPB should be at least 50 mm Hg, and 70 mm Hg if the patient has preexisting cerebrovascular disease.
Kolkka et al. [4]	1980	Perfusion pressure of 49 mm Hg and flow of 42 ml/kg/min during CPB do not increase the incidence of neurologic dysfunction.
Slogoff et al. [9]	1982	Perfusion pressures of less than 50 mm Hg for up to 18 minutes when hematocrit is maintained at less than 30% do not correlate with development of postoperative cerebral dysfunction.
Hickey et al. [3]	1983	After lowering body temperature to 25°C, flow can be reduced from 2.1 liters·min^{-1}·m^{-2} without changing whole body oxygen consumption, suggesting that tissue perfusion remains adequate.
Govier et al. [2]	1984	At 28°C there is no correlation between CBF and PP until PP is less than 30 mm Hg when flow is constant at 1.6 liters·min^{-1}·m^{-2}. This suggests that the limits of cerebral auto-regulation are extended by hypothermia.
Murkin et al. [6]	1987	Cerebral autoregulation is maintained during hypothermic CPB using alpha stat management when perfusion pressure is between 20 and 100 mm Hg.

limit of 30 mm Hg for arterial perfusion pressure is satisfactory in the absence of major anomalies or obstructions in either the venous or arterial tree. This assumes a reasonable rate of flow around 2.0 liters · min^{-1} · m^{-2} at normothermia.

3. High normal blood pressures should be maintained after CPB to prevent the "no reflow" phenomenon, in which microthrombi prevent restoration of blood flow to previously ischemic tissues. Aggressive treatment of hypertension is indicated after an ischemic insult to prevent hyperfusion syndromes associated with seizures and intra-cerebral hemorrhage.

4. Hemodilution will counteract the increased blood viscosity produced by hypothermia and improve oxygen delivery to body tissues. A hematocrit of 20–25% is generally accepted. However, lower hematocrits have been reported without apparent neurologic sequelae. Perfusion pressure is reduced by hemodilution during constant flow conditions.

C. Metabolic homeostasis

1. Glucose-free intravenous fluids will avoid exacerbating the lactic acidosis present during ischemia.

2. Blood pressure should be maintained within the patient's normal range during normothermic CPB.

3. Normocapnia should be maintained when the patient is normothermic.

4. Pharmacologic measures for brain protection should be considered (see sec. **VI** below).

VI. Pharmacologic brain protection

A. Metabolic suppression. Metabolic suppression is a mainstay of brain protection in clinical anesthesia and the only therapy for which a beneficial effect has been shown in humans. The purpose of metabolic suppression is to reduce cerebral oxygen consumption ($CMRO_2$) during periods of reduced oxygen delivery (ischemia, anoxia) so that oxygen debt is minimized.

1. **Cerebral metabolism.** The primary energy-consuming metabolic processes of the brain can be divided into **functional processes** subserving electrophysiologic function and **maintenance processes** that are responsible for cellular integrity. These two components of brain energy utilization distinguish the mechanisms by which hypothermia and anesthetic agents produce metabolic suppression.

2. **Hypothermic suppression.** Hypothermia causes a reduction in oxygen requirement by reducing both functional and maintenance requirements for oxygen. A reduction in body temperature by 10°C reduces oxygen requirements by about half, and further reductions in body temperature continue to lower $CMRO_2$. Hypothermia is routinely used during CPB to reduce cerebral oxygen consumption; however, during aortic cannulation and weaning from CPB the brain is normothermic and at most risk from ischemic insults. Anesthetic agents may be used for metabolic suppression during these high-risk periods.

3. **Pharmacologic suppression.** The anesthetics thiopental and isoflurane produce approximately a 50% reduction in $CMRO_2$ at doses that completely suppress EEG evidence of brain activity. Isoflurane is unique among the potent inhalation agents in that it produces a flat EEG at clinically relevant concentrations. Maintenance metabolic activity of the brain is **not** significantly affected, and increases in thiopental and isoflurane dose will not further reduce $CMRO_2$ once the EEG is flat. Isoflurane offers the advantage of rapid elimination postoperatively and a reduction in critical cerebral blood flow (cCBF) compared with other inhalation agents. However, isoflurane (unlike thiopental) does not produce uniform reductions in $CMRO_2$ throughout the brain and does produce cerebral vasodilation, which may result in substrate maldistribution and mismatching (steal).

4. **Significance of preexisting EEG activity.** These considerations suggest that both anesthetics and hypothermia will provide cerebral protection during incomplete ischemia as long as there is EEG activity. However, once the EEG is isoelectric, hypothermia but not anesthetic agents will produce further cerebral protection.

5. **Combined metabolic suppression.** Hypothermia and anesthetic agents may be used concurrently to produce metabolic suppression.

   a. When the risk of cerebral insult is not significant until after hypothermia is achieved (e.g., during an open ventricle cardiac procedure), hypothermia can be established, and thiopental can then be given to fully suppress the EEG if EEG activity is still present. Reduced doses of thiopental can be used because metabolic suppression is initiated with hypothermia.

   b. If the risk of cerebral insult is significant prior to hypothermia (e.g., during carotid endarterectomy followed by coronary artery revascularization), it may be prudent to initiate metabolic suppression with anesthetics before hypothermia begins. Larger doses of thiopental will be required under these circumstances, so increased side effects should be anticipated.

    c. If hypothermia alone has been sufficient to suppress the EEG, it may be prudent to give an empiric dose of thiopental (e.g., 8–10 mg/kg) because functional cerebral activity may be undetected by a limited-lead EEG. An empiric dose of thiopental may also be beneficial when circumstances preclude the use of an EEG monitor (e.g., emergency surgery).

B. Brain protection versus resuscitation. Therapy for major cerebral insults is usually limited to brain resuscitation after the insult has occurred (e.g., stroke victims). Anesthesiologists are in the unique position of being able to institute brain protective measures prior to a cerebral insult in patients whose medical history or operation place them at high risk for a cerebral insult. Although this therapy is largely empiric at the present time, an emphasis on early intervention in the ischemic process may have substantial impact on morbidity and mortality due to neuropsychiatric dysfunction after cardiac surgery. Two clinical studies have documented the importance of the level of preexisting cerebral metabolic activity in determining the efficacy of barbiturate brain protection.

    1. Abramson et al. [1] reported that high-dose thiopental loading (30 mg/kg) in patients resuscitated from severe **global** ischemic-anoxic cerebral insults (presumably with marked depression or obliteration of functional cerebral activity) did not significantly alter morbidity or mortality compared with patients not receiving thiopental.

    2. Nussmeier et al. [7] did show a protective effect from **focal** cerebral insults when thiopental was used to produce EEG suppression in patients undergoing open ventricle cardiac procedures during **normothermic** CPB.

    3. These two studies underscore the importance of administering barbiturates **prior to** the ischemic brain insult and in the setting of preexisting functional cerebral activity.

C. Adjunctive therapy. Medications used as part of brain protection protocols are selected for their theoretical benefit in reducing the derangement of normal cellular function that accompanies ischemia. Multiple medications are generally used; however, current brain protection protocols are empiric because there is very little evidence to support the clinical efficacy of these agents used alone or in combination. Current clinical practice supports the use of:

    1. Steroids for their membrane-stabilizing effects and reduction of postischemic cerebral edema (methylprednisolone 30 mg/kg IV).

    2. Mannitol for its free radical-scavenging properties and reduction of postischemic cerebral edema (mannitol 0.5 g/kg IV).

    3. Anticonvulsants for treatment of receptor dysfunction, modulation of synaptic function, and elevation of seizure threshold (diphenylhydantoin 1000 mg IV).

    4. Experimental therapies that may attain broader clinical use in the future are:

        a. Calcium channel blockers—nimodipine

        b. Calcium antagonists—magnesium

        c. Free radical scavengers—superoxide dismutase, catalase

        d. Cyclooxygenase inhibitors—(e.g., indomethacin) to decrease vasoactive prostaglandin formation

        e. Substrate augmentation—adenosine or inosine infusion (to restore depleted energy stores)

D. Side effects of pharmacologic therapy. Careful consideration must be given to the side effects of drug therapy. For example, cerebral protection with thiopental entails inotropic support, delayed awakening, and delayed extubation. The risk of these side effects must be compared with the possible benefit to each patient on an individual basis.

VII. Management of deep hypothermic circulatory arrest. DHCA is a clinical technique in which profound hypothermia (18–20°C) is achieved so that the patient can be exsanguinated into the HLM and CPB can be temporarily suspended to facilitate certain surgical procedures. In children DHCA appears to be safe for up to 1 hour. Tolerance of the adult nervous system to DHCA has not been established; however, it is probably less than 1 hour because of the presence of atherosclerosis and possibly a reduced tolerance for ischemia in the adult nervous system.

A. Features of DHCA
1. DHCA produces a stationary, bloodless surgical field so that CPB time is reduced and surgery is facilitated.
2. DHCA decreases blood trauma by reducing cardiotomy suctioning.
3. DHCA improves myocardial protection by reducing myocardial rewarming and preventing cardioplegia washout.

B. Clinical application of DHCA
1. **Frequently used in infants weighing less than 10 kg** for repair of complex congenital cardiac defects.
2. **Repair of aortic arch aneurysms**
   a. Primary considerations
   (1) Cerebral protection
   (2) Avoidance of emboli
   (3) Durable replacement of diseased aorta
   (4) Control of hemorrhage
   b. Cerebral perfusion techniques
   (1) Temporary or permanent bypass grafting of brachiocephalic vessels
   (2) CPB with separate brachiocephalic vessel perfusion
   (3) DHCA with cerebral protection
   c. DHCA has greatly simplified operative methods for aortic arch aneurysms and resulted in improved patient outcome.
   d. Hemorrhage with DHCA may be reduced by using moderate hypothermia (22–26°C), simplified operative procedures, and shorter circulatory arrest times to shorten the length of CPB. This approach, when combined with pretreatment of grafts to reduce graft hemorrhage, has been associated with improved patient outcome.
3. **Removal of intravascular tumor**
   a. Tumor thrombus must be added to the list of potential emboli that could injure the patient.
   b. Massive blood loss can be reduced by using DHCA to remove the intravascular portion of the tumor.
   c. Coronary artery bypass grafting (CABG) or carotid endarterectomy (CEA) may be indicated in conjunction with tumor excision to minimize ischemic injury during DHCA in patients with significant atherosclerotic vascular disease.
   d. Early institution of metabolic suppression should be considered because of the constant threat of tumor emboli; however, this action would preclude ischemia detection by EEG during a CEA and a large dose of anesthetic would be required, resulting in greater side effects.

C. Brain protection protocol for DHCA. Although there is insufficient clinical evidence to support a single method of managing circulatory arrest, theoretical considerations and current clinical practice support the following approach:
1. Prior to DHCA, adults should be evaluated for atherosclerotic vascular disease, and scans of the carotid arteries and coronary angiography should be performed if indicated.

2. Attenuate stress response to surgery (50–100 µg/kg fentanyl or equivalent).

3. Maintain brain hypothermia with both surface cooling and core cooling by means of CPB to promote even cooling and prevent premature rewarming of the brain (18°–20°C).

4. Use appropriate hemodilution (hematocrit mid 20s) during CPB.

5. Maintain optimal alpha stat acid-base status (pH 7.40 and $PaCO_2$ 40 mm Hg at 37°C).

6. Administer methylprednisolone 30 mg/kg and mannitol 0.5 g/kg prior to circulatory arrest.

7. Reduce total body oxygen consumption with muscle relaxants (pancuronium bromide 0.1 mg/kg) prior to circulatory arrest.

8. Monitor suppression of electrical (and metabolic) cerebral activity with hypothermia supplemented by thiopental prior to circulatory arrest.

9. Avoid hyperglycemia before and after DHCA by using glucose-free intravenous fluids and pump prime.

D. Complications of DHCA
   1. Transient seizures
   2. Neurologic deficits
   3. Structural central nervous system damage

VIII. Cardiac procedures associated with carotid artery disease
   A. Combined carotid endarterectomy and coronary revascularization
   1. Combined CEA and CABG is the most effective method of minimizing myocardial and cerebral ischemia in patients with coronary artery disease and carotid artery disease. Patients with symptomatic or bilateral carotid artery disease and concurrent unstable angina, left main, or left main equivalent coronary artery disease should have simultaneous procedures [5].

   2. When the two procedures are combined, most authors advocate performing CEA before CPB. Risks of performing CEA during CPB include excessive bleeding, prolongation of CPB, and reduced perfusion pressure and flow prior to hypothermia. However, the hypothermia, hemodilution, hemodynamic control, and heparinization that accompany CPB are advantageous for cerebral protection, and Minami et al. [5] reported a low incidence of neurologic sequelae in a small group of patients in which CEA and CABG were both performed during CPB.

   3. Management
      a. Patients with atherosclerotic carotid disease are frequently hypertensive and hypovolemic. They are therefore prone to hypotension on induction of anesthesia and to exaggerated hypertensive responses to stimulation. A gradual measured induction with judicious fluid loading and protection from the reflex responses to intubation are imperative.

      b. High-dose narcotic anesthesia produces EEG slowing, which may mask cerebral ischemia.

      c. Metabolic suppression with thiopental will interfere with EEG monitoring when given prior to CEA. Also, maintaining EEG suppression for the entire duration of CEA may require large doses of thiopental, with significant cardiovascular depression and delayed awakening.

      d. In patients with severe coronary artery disease, shunting during endarterectomy (with its associated risk of embolization) may be preferable to elevating blood pressure (with its associated risk of myocardial ischemia) to ensure adequate CBF.

B. Management of cardiac surgery in patients with inoperable carotid artery disease

1. Utilize CPB perfusion pressure (60–90 mm Hg) to maintain CBF. Increase blood pressure by raising pump flow to 2.5–3 liters • min^{-1} • m^{-2} before using vasopressors.
2. Maintain the patient's normal MAP and cardiac index before and after CPB with inotropic support and intraaortic balloon pump as needed.
3. Utilize moderate hypothermia during CPB (25°C)
4. Monitor the EEG for signs of cerebral ischemia.
5. Consider supplementing hypothermia-induced cerebral metabolic suppression with thiopental.

REFERENCES

1. Abramson, N. S., Safar, P., Detre, K., et al. Results of a randomized clinical trial of brain resuscitation with thiopental. *Anesthesiology* 59A:101, 1983.
2. Govier, A. V., Reves, J. G., McKay, R. D., et al. Factors and their influence on regional cerebral blood flow during nonpulsatile cardiopulmonary bypass. *Ann. Thorac. Surg.* 38:592–600, 1984.
3. Hickey, R. F., and Hoar, P. F. Whole-body oxygen consumption during low-flow hypothermic cardiopulmonary bypass. *J. Thorac. Cardiovasc. Surg.* 86:903–906, 1983.
4. Kolkka, R., and Hilberman, M. Neurologic dysfunction following cardiac operation with low-flow, low-pressure cardiopulmonary bypass. *J. Thorac. Cardiovasc. Surg.* 79:432–437, 1980.
5. Minami, K., Sagoo, K. S., Breymann, T., et al. Operative strategy in combined coronary and carotid artery disease. *J. Thorac. Cardiovasc. Surg.* 95:303–309, 1988.
6. Murkin, J. M., Farrar, J. K., Tweed, W. A., et al. Cerebral autoregulation and flow/metabolism coupling during cardiopulmonary bypass: The influence of $PaCO_2$. *Anesth. Analg.* 66:825–832, 1987.
7. Nussmeier, N. A., Arlund, C., and Slogoff, S. Neuropsychiatric complications after cardiopulmonary bypass: Cerebral protection by a barbiturate. *Anesthesiology* 64:165–170, 1986.
8. Paneth, M., Sellers, R., Gott, V. L., et al. Physiologic studies upon prolonged cardiopulmonary bypass with the pump-oxygenator with particular reference to (1) acid-base balance, (2) siphon caval drainage. *J. Thoracic. Surg.* 34:570–579, 1957.
9. Slogoff, S., Girgis, K. Z., and Keats, A. S. Etiologic factors in neuropsychiatric complications associated with cardiopulmonary bypass. *Anesth. Analg.* 61:903–911, 1982.
10. Stockard, J. J., Bickford, R. G., Schauble, J. F. Pressure-dependent cerebral ischemia during cardiopulmonary bypass. *Neurology* 23:521–529, 1973.

SUGGESTED READING

Frost, E. A. M. Therapy Following Major Brain Insult. In E. A. M. Frost (ed.), *Clinical Anesthesia in Neurosurgery*. Boston: Butterworth, 1984. Pp. 439–452.

Hickey, P. R., and Andersen, N. P. Deep hypothermic circulatory arrest: A review of pathophysiology and clinical experience as a basis for anesthetic management. *J. Cardiothoracic Anesth.* 1:137–155, 1987.

Marshall, L. Filtration in cardiopulmonary bypass: Past, present, and future. *Perfusion* 3:135–147, 1988.

Siesjo, B. K. Cell damage in the brain: A speculative synthesis. *J. Cereb. Blood Flow Metabl.* 1:155–185, 1981.

Steen, P. A., Newburg, L., Milde, J. H., et al. Hypothermia and barbiturates:

Individual and combined effects on canine cerebral oxygen consumption. *Anesthesiology* 58:527–532, 1983.

Utley, J. R., and Stephens, D. B. Prevention of major perioperative neurological dysfunction—A personal perspective. *Perfusion* 1:135–142, 1986.

Index

Index